HANDBOOK OF NEURODEVELOPMENTAL AND GENETIC DISORDERS IN CHILDREN

HANDBOOK OF NEURODEVELOPMENTAL AND GENETIC DISORDERS IN CHILDREN

Sam Goldstein
Cecil R. Reynolds

Editors

THE GUILFORD PRESS
New York   London

© 1999 The Guilford Press
A Division of Guilford Publications, Inc.
72 Spring Street, New York, NY 10012
http://www.guilford.com

Printed in the United States of America

This book is printed on acid-free paper.

Last digit is print number: 9 8 7 6 5 4 3 2 1

Library of Congress Cataloging-in-Publication Data

Handbook of neurodevelopmental and genetic disorders in children / Sam
  Goldstein, Cecil R. Reynolds, editors.
    p. cm.
   Includes bibliographical references and index.
   ISBN 1-57230-448-0 (hardcover : alk. paper)
   1. Developmental disabilities—Genetic aspects Handbooks, manuals,
etc. 2. Developmental neurobiology Handbooks, manuals, etc.
3. Genetic disorders in children Handbooks, manuals, etc.
4. Pediatric neuropsychology Handbooks, manuals, etc.
I. Goldstein, Sam, 1952–   . II. Reynolds, Cecil R., 1952–
III. Title: Neurodevelopmental and genetic disorders in children.
   [DNLM: 1. Abnormalities. 2. Child Development Disorders,
Pervasive. 3. Hereditary Diseases. 4. Mental Retardation. WS 107
H2365 1998]
RJ506.D47H36 1999
618.92'8588042—dc21
DNLM/DLC
for Library of Congress   99-21821
                                            CIP

For Janet, Allyson, and Ryan

To the strength, stamina, and perseverance of the children exemplified in this text, and to our ability to adjust expectations and meet their needs.

S. G.

To my wife and partner, Julia, for all of her good work in healing families.

C. R. R.

ABOUT THE EDITORS

Sam Goldstein, PhD, is a member of the faculty at the University of Utah. As a psychologist he specializes in child development, school psychology, and neuropsychology. He practices at the Neurology, Learning and Behavior Center in Salt Lake City. The Center provides evaluation, case management, and treatment services for individuals experiencing neurological and neuropsychological problems throughout the life span. Dr. Goldstein holds Fellow and Diplomate status in many disciplines and is a Fellow of the American Academy for Cerebral Palsy and Developmental Medicine. He is also Associate Editor of the *Journal of Attention Disorders* and serves on the editorial board of the *Archives of Clinical Neuropsychology*. A prolific author, Dr. Goldstein's previous ten texts have included works on classroom management, ADHD throughout the life span, controversial treatments, and depression.

Cecil R. Reynolds, PhD, ABPN, ABPP, is a professor of educational psychology and distinguished research scholar in the College of Education at Texas A&M University. He holds Diplomate status in Clinical Neuropsychology from the American Board of Professional Psychology; in School Psychology from the American Board of Professional Psychology; and from the American Board of Forensic Examiners. In addition, he is the author or editor of more than 300 scholarly publications, among them 24 books, including *Handbook of School Psychology, Encyclopedia of Special Education,* and *Handbook of Clinical Child Neuropsychology.* He is also Editor in Chief of the *Archives of Clinical Neuropsychology* and serves on the editorial boards of a number of journals. Dr. Reynolds has received multiple national awards for excellence in research, including the Lightner Witmer Award, and is a corecipient of the Society for the Psychological Study of Social Issues Robert Chin Award.

CONTRIBUTORS

Jenny Bartholomew, BS, Department of Psychology, Brigham Young University, Provo, Utah

Thomas L. Bennett, PhD, Brain Injury Recovery Program, Fort Collins, Colorado

Erin D. Bigler, PhD, Department of Psychology, Brigham Young University, Provo, Utah

Lynne W. Bradford, MS, Department of Educational Psychology, University of Utah, Salt Lake City, Utah

Michael Brooks, BS, Department of Psychology, Brigham Young University, Provo, Utah

Michael B. Brown, PhD, Department of Psychology, East Carolina University, Greenville, North Carolina

Robert T. Brown, PhD, Department of Psychology, University of North Carolina at Wilmington, Wilmington, North Carolina

Ronald T. Brown, PhD, Medical University of South Carolina, Children's Hospital, Charleston, South Carolina

John C. Carey, MD, MPH, Department of Pediatrics, University of Utah Health Sciences Center, Salt Lake City, Utah

Suzanne B. Cassidy, MD, Department of Genetics and Center for Human Genetics, Case Western Reserve University, and University Hospital of Cleveland, Cleveland, Ohio

Heather Cody, MEd, Department of Educational Psychology, University of Georgia, Athens, Georgia

Elisabeth M. Dykens, PhD, Division of Child and Adolescent Psychiatry, Neuropsychiatric Institute, University of California at Los Angeles, Los Angeles, California

Sam Goldstein, PhD, Neurology, Learning and Behavior Center, Salt Lake City, Utah

Randi J. Hagerman, MD, Department of Pediatrics, University of Colorado Health Sciences Center, and Fragile X Treatment and Research Center, Child Development Unit, The Children's Hospital, Denver, Colorado

Sarah L. Hoadley, BA, Department of Psychology, University of North Carolina at Wilmington, Wilmington, North Carolina

Maile Ho-Turner, PhD, Brain Injury Recovery Program, Fort Collins, Colorado

George Hynd, EdD, Center for Clinical and Developmental Neuropsychology, University of Georgia, Athens, Georgia

Sally Ingalls, PhD, Neurology, Learning and Behavior Center, Salt Lake City, Utah

Carolyn E. Ivers, PhD, Department of Pediatrics, Rainbow Babies and Children's Hospital, Cleveland, Ohio

Randy W. Kamphaus, PhD, Department of Educational Psychology, University of Georgia, Athens, Georgia

Ami Klin, PhD, Yale Child Study Center, Yale University, New Haven, Connecticut

Megan E. Lampe, BA, Fragile X Treatment and Research Center, Child Development Unit, The Children's Hospital, Denver, Colorado

Joan W. Mayfield, PhD, Baylor Pediatric Specialty Services, Dallas, Texas

William M. McMahon, MD, Department of Psychiatry and Pediatrics, University of Utah Health Sciences Center, Salt Lake City, Utah

Carolyn B. Mervis, PhD, Department of Psychology, University of Louisville, Louisville, Kentucky

Pamilla C. Morales, PhD, Department of Psychology, Bolton Institute, Bolton, Lancashire, United Kingdom

Colleen A. Morris, MD, Departments of Pediatrics (Genetics Division) and Pathology and Laboratory Medicine, University of Las Vegas School of Medicine, Las Vegas, Nevada

Dianne Nielsen, BS, Department of Psychology, Brigham Young University, Provo, Utah

David E. Nilsson, PhD, ABPP, Neurology, Learning and Behavior Center, Salt Lake City, Utah

Rene L. Olvera, MD, Department of Psychiatry, University of Texas Health Sciences Center at San Antonio, San Antonio, Texas

Steven R. Pliszka, MD, Department of Psychiatry, University of Texas Health Sciences Center at San Antonio, San Antonio, Texas

M. Paige Powell, PhD, Bluegrass Regional Mental Health Board, Lexington, Kentucky

Cecil R. Reynolds, PhD, ABPN, ABPP, Department of Educational Psychology, Texas A&M University, College Station, Texas

Timothy Schulte, EdS, Human Development Center/Shenandoah Valley Child Development Clinic, James Madison University, Harrisonburg, Virginia

Julien T. Smith, PhD, Neuropsychology Service, Department of Psychiatry, Primary Children's Medical Center, University of Utah, Salt Lake City, Utah

Phyllis Anne Teeter, EdD, Department of Educational Psychology, University of Wisconsin–Milwaukee, Milwaukee, Wisconsin

Fred R. Volkmar, MD, Yale Child Study Center, Yale University, New Haven, Connecticut

Susan E. Waisbren, PhD, Division of Genetics, Children's Hospital/Harvard Medical School, Boston, Massachusetts

Timothy B. Whelan, PhD, Department of Psychiatry, Baystate Medical Center, Springfield, Massachusetts

Elizabeth Wilde, BS, Department of Psychology, Brigham Young University, Provo, Utah

PREFACE

Our daily work as scientist–practitioners represents a blend of research, training, and clinical practice. As we participate in, read, and review current research, our clinical practice—what we do and how we do it—changes. As we train our students, our perceptions of ourselves, our ideas, and our clinical practice are sharpened. The pace at which these processes take place is increasing exponentially as we enter the new millennium. Though our society has been reluctant to acknowledge that there is a powerful biological basis for some children's problems (e.g., certain behavior and learning problems), it has at times almost too easily embraced biological determinism for other problems (e.g., Down syndrome, fragile X syndrome). But as the eminent neuropsychiatrist Dr. John Werry reminds us, biology is not destiny. As the longitudinal work of Emmy Werner and others has demonstrated, even significant biologically based problems can be and are affected significantly in their outcome by environmental consequences. Increasingly, we recognize as clinicians that biology very powerfully influences the neurodevelopment and behavior of many children with such problems as attention-deficit/hyperactivity disorder, learning disabilities, and anxiety disorders. However, we believe that the daily lives of all children are equally powerful in shaping the consequences of those symptoms. Thus, it is day-to-day life, particularly family life, that appears to determine whether an impulsive child will become a great pickpocket or a great shortstop.

The dramatic and rapid growth in medicine, psychology, and education at present is greatly improving our ability to prepare all children, even those with significant differences, for their adult lives. Clinicians in the next millennium will increasingly be expected to possess expertise not just in diagnosis and intervention, but in the medical and biological phenomena that have an impact on children's growth and development.

This text grew out of our mutual interest in educating our students and fellow clinicians in the powerful role genetics plays in shaping the development and lives of many children. It is our hope and intent that this text will serve as a ready and comprehensive reference, assisting clinicians to understand, evaluate, and ultimately help children with neurodevelopmental and genetic disorders.

SAM GOLDSTEIN, PhD
CECIL R. REYNOLDS, PhD

ACKNOWLEDGMENTS

We wish to thank our colleagues for their scholarly and thoughtful contributions to this text.

We also wish to thank Kathleen Gardner for her editorial organization, management, and secretarial skills, and Sharon Panulla, former senior editor at The Guilford Press, for her guidance and support.

CONTENTS

Human beings are individuals . . . just as genes are the only things that replicate, so individuals, not societies are the vehicles for genes . . . every individual is a specialist of some sort, whether he or she is a welder, a housewife, a playwright or a prostitute. In behaviour, as in appearance, every human individual is unique.

—MATT RIDLEY, *The Red Queen*

PART I

**Basic Principles
and Applications**

1

INTRODUCTION

SAM GOLDSTEIN
CECIL R. REYNOLDS

Neuropsychology is the study of brain–behavior relationships, and a clinical neuropsychologist is a clinician who applies the results of knowledge in this area to diagnosis and treatment of neurodevelopmental disorders, among other central nervous system (CNS) disturbances (e.g., CNS diseases, traumatic brain injury, cerebrovascular accidents, etc.). Clinical neuropsychology as practiced today traces its roots principally to the 1940s, although the contributions of earlier practitioners such as A. R. Luria were clearly important. As such, it is relatively young as a clinical discipline, but it is a burgeoning specialty within the broader discipline of psychology.

A MEDLINE search of articles published over a 5 year period from January 1993 through November 1998 yielded nearly 6,500 peer-reviewed research studies concerning chromosomal and genetic disorders in children. Over 4,000 studies published during the same period of time were identified as specifically dealing with the neuropsychological evaluation and treatment of children. Yet only 42 studies were found in this data base dealing with both issues. Even given the relative youth of the field, this seems too few papers. However, the nature of the studies and their appearance in mainstream medical and psychological journals indicate the need for even broader perspectives and interdisciplinary approaches to the diagnosis and treatment of children's neurodevelopmental disorders (ironically, at a time when the politics and costs of health care have given rise to the managed care model, which promotes singularity of treatment!).

A review of some of these 42 studies (which may not necessarily represent all published studies dealing with these two issues) reflects the increasing importance of a simultaneous view and understanding of these issues for neuropsychologists, physicians, and other medical and mental health professionals. For example, Mazzocco and Holden (1996) provided a neuropsychological profile of females with fragile X permutation. Devenny et al. (1996) described a longitudinal study of individuals with Down syndrome, and in doing so, defined the neurocognitive changes in this population over four decades. Lanoo, DePaepe, Leroy, and Thiery (1996) furnished data reflecting a profile characterized by difficulty with sustained visual attention and problems with visual construction, over and above the visual acuity problems and other phenomena associated with Marfan syndrome. Davalos et al. (1996) offered a neuropsychological profile reflecting a pattern of mild mental retardation, constructional apraxia, and expressive language impairment in a group of children presenting with proportionate short staure, delayed bone age, and peculiar faces. These children were subsequently identified as experiencing Floating–Harbor syndrome. Ross, Stefanatos, Roeltgen, Kushner, and Cutler (1995) described a longitudinal study providing a profile of neurocognitive changes in females with Turner syndrome. Finally, Watkins et al. (1998) evaluated and described the cognitive deficits in children with sickle cell disease suffering covert infarction and stroke.

When the known or likely contributions of genetics to more common childhood problems such as learning disabilities and attention-deficit/hyperactivity disorder are considered, together with the genetic contributions to many lower-incidence problems, the importance of beginning to develop a cohesive genetic–environmental model becomes immediately apparent. As Rutter (1997) has noted,

> Quantitative genetic research has been most informative in showing the importance of genetic influences on virtually all forms of human behavior. Behavior has to have a biological basis and it is necessary that we understand how the biology functions. Equally the same research has been crucial in its demonstration that environmental influences are also ubiquitous. (p. 396)

NATURE AND NURTURE

There are few topics as inflammatory, polemic, or controversial in psychology and related sciences as the so-called "nature–nurture controversy." Briefly stated, this controversy revolves around whether human development and human behavior (both overt and covert) are determined by human beings' genetic constitution (nature) or by the environment (nurture) in which people grow and develop. Few, if indeed any, contemporary scientists approach this question in such simplistic terms. The arguments now tend to center around the relative contributions of nature and nurture to human development and behavior, and the mechanisms of interaction and plausibility of transaction between them. It is also acknowledged that for specific human attributes, the answers will vary.

A "genotype" may be considered the raw material and blueprints (genes and chromosomes) provided through the melding of the parental genotypes. Except in the case of monozygotic twins and cloning, no two human genotypes are alike. The human organism then grows and develops in a unique environment to produce the visible, assessable, acting "phenotype"—the expression of the genotype in the unique environment. Attributes known to be "genetically determined" can often be altered in the course of development or even later in life. Height, known to have strong heritability in the human population, can be altered dramatically in an individual by manipulation of diet. As subsequent chapters of this volume indicate, many outcomes for some genetic disorders are entirely dependent on or at least strongly determined by changes in environment. Phenylketonuria (PKU) is a classic example. When phenylalanines are eliminated from the diet of youngsters with PKU, the outcomes for intellect, school adjustment, and other behavioral variables are all much improved. Even behaviors as complex as adult sexual behaviors and preference, which are strongly genetically influenced, can be altered by significant changes in the stress levels of the mother at particular times during pregnancy. There are certain critical periods during gestation when hormonal releases affect cell migration and organ development in a preprogrammed fashion. A mother under very high levels of stress may alter those hormonal release patterns in ways that affect adult sexual behavior in the offspring. It seems that few components of human behavior are too simple to be influenced by environment, or too complex to be related to the genotype. The complexity of the interaction and potential transaction is virtually incomprehensible when we recall that no two combinations of genotype and environment have been or ever will be identical.

To many scientists, ourselves included, it does appear that as our skills, insights, and techniques of investigation continue to grow in number and in sophistication, we learn that human biology has a more pronounced impact on behavior than we would prefer to believe. Even at the extremes of the hereditary influences argued by some scientists, there is much room for change, intervention, and environmental influence.

Take the controversial case of the heritability of human intelligence. The extremes of the various scientific arguments place the nature–nurture contributions to intelligence at 80% and 20% and at 20% and 80%, respectively (e.g., see Hernstein & Murray, 1994; Jensen, 1980; and Reynolds & Brown, 1984). One may argue urgently for relative contribution and interaction within these two extremes, but even in the most extreme genetic view (i.e., the view that 80% of the variance in human intelligence is genotype variation), two propositions remain inescapable:

1. Heritability statistics only apply to groups, and the genetic influence on intelligence for an individual may be more or less than the group heritability;
2. Even if 80% of an individual's intellectual level is genetically determined, changes in intellectual level as a function of environmental influences and transaction may be enormous.

The latter proposition requires some elaboration. Psychological variables such as intelligence and personality are measured with interval scales of measurement, which have no true zero point denoting the absence of the trait, such as zero reflects on a ratio scale of measurement. With a true zero point, the actual amount of a characteristic (e.g., height) can be determined, and such statements as "A height of 6 feet is twice a height of 3 feet" are accurate. However, interval scales, having no true zero point, begin measurement at the midpoint of a characteristic's distribution—the only point we can locate definitively. We then measure outward toward the two ends of a distribution, each of which is asymptotic to its axis. That is, we do not know where intelligence begins or ends, and an IQ of 100 does not reflect twice the intelligence of an IQ of 50. Herein lies the clinician's opportunity to intervene and potentially create meaningful results, even under the adversity of strong genetic determination. To increase an individual's intellectual level by a full 20% may mean an increase of 10, 20, 30, 40, or even more points on a psychometric scale. The same may hold true for other human characteristics that present as complex behavioral phenomena.

As later chapters of this book describe, many genetic disorders have high degrees of variable expressivity, often (but not always) for unknown reasons. We believe many of these reasons to be treatment-related, or at least associated with biological and environmental interplay. Early involvement of clinicians who understand brain–behavior relationships is necessary if children with neurodevelopmental disorders are to have the environmental and educational opportunities they need to achieve their highest possible level of functioning. All of this may be taken to mean that although genetics or biology may be destiny, it need not be.

Cortical development is genetically preprogrammed in many ways; however, not all genetic disorders have a full phenotypic impact at the same time. Environments may also alter the timing of development and change. As Bigler and Clement (1997) note so well, the process of maturation greatly complicates the evaluation of neurodevelopmental disorders in children and adolescents. The effects of the interaction between age and genetic expressivity in a disorder with CNS implications add to the complexity of all tasks with such children. A common change in CNS development may have radically different implications and outcomes, even in adulthood, if the age of occurrence is varied.

OBJECTIVES OF THIS VOLUME

Clinicians of the 21st century will need to possess a working knowledge of genetics as well as neuropsychology. Yet at this time, as the literature review described above reflects, the science of what we choose to term "behavioral genetics" remains in its infancy. The 21st-century clinician will need a sophisticated biopsychosocial model to rely upon. Clinicians will also continue to be called upon to assess the relationship between brain function and behavior. They will be asked to assess function by skills (e.g., the skills necessary to read efficiently). They will be asked to plan treatment, to monitor that treatment, and to assess progress. As ever more information is gathered concerning the influence of human genetics upon behavior, clinicians will be increasingly called upon to guide mental health, medical, and educational professionals in blazing new trails to improve the quality of life for children and adults with genetic disorders that affect their behavior and development. Clinicians who work with children must be knowledgeable about developmental psychology as well.

The primary objective of this text is to provide readers with a stand-alone compendium concerning the impact of genetics on neurodevelopment in children. In planning the volume, we realized quickly that this primary mission would entail creating a text similar in breadth and scope to those handbooks of neuropsychology that are familiar to each of us. The goal of those texts, as of this one, is to provide a comprehensive set of resource materials that will be available to readers as needed, organized in a framework that is understandable and immediately useful in clinical practice.

We have divided the text into three sections. Part I, "Basic Principles and Applications," offers our view of the role of neuropsychology in the assessment, treatment, and management of children with neurodevelopmental and genetic disorders. In Chapter 2, the role of neuropsychology in the assessment of these children is discussed. Chapter 3 is an overview providing readers with a basic model for understanding genetics, as well as up-to-date information concerning current trends and research in the field of human genetics. Chapter 4 examines current research concerning the use of neuroimaging to determine structural and biochemical differences in children with genetic disorders. Finally, psychosocial issues related to emotional, educational, familial, and behavioral problems are reviewed and discussed in Chapter 5. Together, these chapters provide a firm foundation for the discussions that follow concerning specific disorders in children. A working understanding of the information covered in Part I is essential for all practicing clinicians.

Part II of the volume contains chapters dealing with five disorders or groups of disorders that have accepted, though as yet not completely identified, genetic etiologies. Most of these disorders also occur relatively more frequently in the general population of children than do the disorders covered in Part III. Finally, these problems have a common theme, in that they primarily affect learning and behavior; thus topics that often do not find their way into genetics and neurobehavioral texts are included. The disorders covered here are learning disabilities, attention-deficit/hyperactivity disorder, Tourette syndrome, anxiety disorders, and autism and other pervasive developmental disorders. These five chapters, as well as those in Part III, provide readers with an overview of current genetic, behavioral, and developmental issues; guides to assessment; and discussions of treatment and management.

The third and by far lengthiest section, containing 14 chapters, offers overviews of disorders that (1) have a lower incidence in the general population than most of the disorders covered in Part II; (2) have specific genetic etiologies, for the most part (Noonan syndrome, Rett syndrome, and seizure disorders are exceptions); and (3) have overt physical/medical manifestations, as well as effects on learning and behavior. Despite the relative infrequency of these disorders, clinicians can expect to see children with these problems more and more often, especially within medical settings. Furthermore, the increasing recognition of the impact health impairments have upon children's functioning at school has now paved the way for many of these children to receive specialized services within school settings. Thus these problems are also likely to be faced more and more often by school psychologists, school nurses, and other educational staff members. The approach to education of children with these disorders can and usually does have a major impact on the quality of their lives. As an example, consider children with Down syndrome. In the not very distant past, Down syndrome children were rarely seen in public, and most were treated through residential placements in state facilities designed for children with severe developmental disorders. However, not all Down syndrome children also have mental retardation, and most of those who do are in the mild to moderate range. Decades of research have shown that Down syndrome children are best educated in a public school setting with maximum exposure to the normal school environment. Social and behavioral outcomes in particular are superior for these children when they are educated in public schools, according to a least-restrictive-environment model, as opposed to the isolation and restricted nature of an institutional setting. Increasingly, knowledge about the neuropsychological functioning of children with neurodevelopmental disorders and about ways to facilitate their development is intertwined with the public school systems of our nation—with good reason, for this is increasingly where the children are educated.

The path to success in life is neither simple nor easy for the majority of our youth as we enter the new millennium. This is all the more so for those with complex genetic and neurodevelopmental disorders. Given the medical community's increasing ability to provide for the health needs of these children, their subsequent increased survival rates, and the increased public recognition of and organized support for them, the path to success for these children has perhaps become slightly less convoluted and rocky. Yet the increasing educational, social, and family pressures placed upon children create an entirely new set of burdens for all youth. Neuropsychologists and other medical, mental health, and educational professionals will all play an increasing role in shaping the life path for children with genetic and neurodevelopmental disorders.

Although the liabilities of these children are of most interest to many professionals, their assets and tenacity in some cases must also be well defined and understood. Knowledgeable professionals can offer their patients, clients, and students a powerful sense of hope by providing accurate information, understanding, and support. Although much remains to be uncovered and understood about the impact of genetics and the interaction of genetics with the environment in shaping the lives of children, identification through careful assessment, as well as intervention and accommodation through thoughtful treatment, implementation, and support, will make a significant positive difference for children with genetic and neurodevelopmental disorders.

REFERENCES

Bigler, E. B., & Clement, P. F. (1997). *Diagnostic clinical neuropsychology.* Austin: University of Texas Press.

Davalos, I. P., Figuera, L. E., Bobadilla, L., Martinez-Martinez, R., Matute, E., Partida, M. D., Ganuelos, L. A., & Ramirez-Duenas, M. L. (1996). Floating–Harbor syndrome: A neuropsychological approach. *Genetic Counseling, 7,* 283–288.

Devenny, D. A., Silverman, W. P., Hill, A. L., Jenkins, E., Sersen, E. A., & Wisniewski, K. E. (1996). Normal aging in adults with Down's syndrome: A longitudinal study. *Journal of Intellectual Disability Research, 40,* 208–221.

Hernstein, R., & Murray, H. (1994). *The bell curve.* New York: Free Press.

Jensen, A. R. (1980). *Perspectives on bias in mental testing.* New York: Plenum Press.

Lanoo, E., DePaepe, A., Leroy, B., & Thiery, E. (1996). Neuropsychological aspects of Marfan syndrome. *Clinical Genetics, 49,* 65–69.

Mazzocco, M. M., & Holden, J. J. (1996). Neuropsychological profiles of three sisters homozygous for the fragile X premutation. *American Journal of Medical Genetics, 64*(2), 323–328.

Reynolds, C. R., & Brown, R. T. (1984). Bias in mental testing: An introduction to the issues. In R. T. Brown & C. R. Reynolds (Eds.), *Perspectives on bias in mental testing* (pp. 1–26). New York: Plenum.

Ross, J. L., Stefanatos, G., Roeltgen, D., Kushner, H., & Cutler, G. B. (1995). Ulrich–Turner syndrome: Neurodevelopmental changes from childhood through adolescence. *American Journal of Medical Genetics, 58,* 74–82.

Rutter, M. L. (1997). Nature–nurture integration: The example of anti-social behavior. *American Psychologist, 52,* 390–398.

Watkins, K. E., Hewes, D. K. M., Connelly, A., Kendall, B. I., Kingley, D. P. I., Evans, J. E. P., Gadian, D. G., Vargha-Khadem, F., & Kirkham, F. J. (1998). Cognitive deficits associated with frontal lobe infarction in children with sickle cell disease. *Developmental Medicine, 40,* 536–543.

2

NEUROPSYCHOLOGICAL ASSESSMENT IN GENETICALLY LINKED NEURODEVELOPMENTAL DISORDERS

CECIL R. REYNOLDS
JOAN W. MAYFIELD

Children in general have always posed special problems in clinical assessment and evaluation, and even more so from a psychometric standpoint. Infancy and childhood are the times of the greatest (and most rapid) breadth and depth of change in the human lifetime. This alone presents a significant challenge to those who would assess a child's status in order to make predictions about a child's future and about interventions that may be required to facilitate growth and development. Children who are developing normally or with only mild levels of disability can be difficult to assess accurately, for reasons related to the maturity of their language development, motor development, social skills, and attention, concentration, and memory skills. As the extent of disability increases, accurate assessment becomes ever more challenging.

Moreover, certain developmental periods pose special problems. During infancy in particular, a child's very limited language and motor skills prevent a thorough assessment of cognitive functions and higher cortical development. A pediatric neurologist can get a reasonable estimate, but only at a gross level, of neurodevelopmental status from a neurological examination that focuses on reflexes, muscle tone, and a review of cranial nerve functions. The neuropsychologist can add some additional details about higher cortical functions (i.e., thinking, reasoning, intellectual development, and language development), but our measures, even the most sophisticated (Bayley, 1969), remain crude. Except for very low levels of performance, scores on such instruments are relatively poor predictors of adult status. Little in the way of localization of function can be accomplished, and higher cortical systems of brain function are rarely assessed well. In these early years, we clinicians are often left with an unsatisfactory feeling about what we have accomplished with such assessments. However, an assessment at even these early stages by a neuropsychologist makes significant contributions to diagnosis and treatment.

   With infants changing so rapidly, it is imperative to have carefully constructed standards of normality if developmental problems are to be detected accurately. Minor variants of normal development need not be diagnosed as disorders, nor should significant problems be overlooked. It is in this context that psychometric testing has the most to offer. Psychologists are accustomed to using norm-referenced tests, such as the Bayley Scales of Infant Development (Bayley, 1969). Such tests have carefully constructed normative reference tables that define normal variations in development, typically considered as within two standard deviations of the mean of a normally functioning reference group. Tests constructed specifically for use with infants, despite involving much observation (as opposed to demand performances, as with older children and adults), compare relevant functions of infants to the distribution of the same functions for infants developing normally. Such quantitative approaches are a necessity for accurate diagnosis during times of rapid change. Informal or subjective observations and ratings place far too many cognitive demands on the clinician to produce consistent, reliable results.

   Neuropsychological testing is thus important to establish the presence of a cognitive disorder. Since neuropsychological testing is norm-referenced by chronological age, progress can be monitored via repeated or serial testing, and changing patterns of symptomatology can be detected. The effectiveness (or lack thereof) of interventions can be documented as well, and changes can be made as indicated.

   These same quantitative procedures are useful throughout childhood and adolescence, when cognitive development continues to be rapid and is often uneven. Quantitative tracking of change and the detection of change through psychometric methods providing age-corrected deviation scaled scores are necessities.

MONITORING AND MANAGING SYMPTOM EXPRESSION

All of the various disorders addressed in this volume are believed to have some degree of genetic linkage, and some are stronger and more obvious than others. However, they all show what is termed "variable expressivity" (i.e., the number and/or the severity of the symptoms defining the disorder vary across individuals). The variability of symptom expression must be monitored and will have clear treatment implications. The interaction between the genetic basis of a disorder on the one hand, and the individual's environmental circumstances and other biological predispositions (which may or may not be affected by the genetics of the primary disorder) on the other, will also alter the severity of symptoms. Phenylketonuria (PKU), for example, is an entirely genetic disorder. Yet the treatment compliance of both the family and the individual, along with the child's temperament, predisposition for intellectual development, and numerous other factors, will act to determine the cognitive symptoms displayed. This will have implications for whether special education programming for mental retardation, specific learning disabilities, or even serious emotional disturbance is required. Although dietary treatment is always indicated for PKU, one cannot assume what other treatments will be necessary. Rather, periodic formal neuropsychological testing should be conducted to detect cognitive changes that may require additional forms of intervention, and that may even provide some suggestive data about a patient's dietary compliance. Assessments of behavior and affect through norm-referenced, age-corrected methods (e.g., Reynolds & Kamphaus, 1992) are also necessary, as individuals with genetic disorders are commonly at increased risk of developing emotional and behavioral problems (see also Warzak, Mayfield, & McAlliston, 1996).

There is no cure or elimination of all symptoms for the disorders treated in this volume. Rather, most viable treatments center around symptom management. Neuropsychological and psychological assessment have two primary roles to play beyond assisting in diagnosis. The first, as noted above, is the evaluation of the severity of symptom expression; the second is the assessment of treatment effects through careful psychometric monitoring of changes in symptom expression.

Historically, neuropsychological evaluations were conducted with adults with known brain damage or injury, to determine lateralization or localization of lesion or injury. As Lezak (1995) points out, "[the] rapid evolution [of such evaluations] in recent years reflects a growing sensitivity among clinicians to the practical problems of identification, assessment, care, and treatment of brain damaged patients" (p. 7)—a comment that pertains as well to any patient with a compromised central nervous system (CNS), especially if higher cortical functions are involved. Neuropsychologists are often asked to provide information concerning prognosis for recovery, functional ability, and course of treatment. However, the practice of neuropsychology has broadened to include the need to clarify conditions where brain damage or CNS compromise has not been identified; in these cases, evaluations provide additional information for differential diagnoses, which result in more effective treatment planning.

As neuropsychologists gained more knowledge about brain–behavior relationships, they applied their knowledge to adults without known brain damage. After this, they turned their attention to problems of earlier development, which ultimately provided an understanding of brain–behavior functioning in children (Reitan & Wolfson, 1974). We agree that "child clinical neuropsychology has emerged as an important theoretical, empirical, and methodological perspective for understanding and treating developmental, psychiatric, psychosocial, and learning disabilities in children and adolescents" (Teeter & Semrud-Clikeman, 1997, p. 1).

The remaining purposes of this chapter are to give a functional definition of neuropsychology, to provide information concerning the necessary components of a neuropsychological evaluation, and to discuss their relationship to treatment. An overview of neuropsychological assessment processes is then presented, both historically and in the context of current practices, that incorporates the basic components of evaluation and encourages integrative, comprehensive assessment of CNS compromise. Furthermore, the chapter provides information concerning why children and adolescents are referred for neuropsychological evaluations, and how the results of such evaluations are relevant to their educational needs (in terms of effective remediation techniques, educational placement, and parental expectations).

WHAT IS NEUROPSYCHOLOGY?

Neuropsychology is the study of brain–behavior relationships. It requires acceptance of the idea that the brain, working as an interdependent, systemic network, controls and is all-inclusively responsible for behavior. Although this premise seems simple enough now, radical behavioral psychology in the 1960s and early 1970s ignored the brain, leading some to espouse the view that the brain was irrelevant to learning and behavior.

Neuropsychological assessment examines the relationship between brain functioning and behavior through tests that tap specific domains of functioning—typically much more specific domains than those that are represented on general tests of intelligence, such as attention, memory, forgetting, sensory functions, constructional praxis, and motor skills (Farmer & Peterson, 1995; Reitan & Wolfson, 1985). Neuropsychologists examine the functioning of the brain based on behavioral expression, and are able to determine whether a brain dysfunction exists or whether atypical patterns of neocortical development are present.

A neurologist looks at the anatomical construction of the brain. Working in conjunction with neurologists, neuropsychologists are able to determine the functioning sequelae of CNS dysfunction. Neurologists use advanced neuroimaging techniques, including magnetic resonance imaging (MRI), positron emission tomography (PET), and single-photon emission computed tomography (SPECT) of brain regions. Working in conjunction with neurologists, neuropsychologists focus on behavior and cognition in order to offer educational help and remediation strategies to teachers, counselors, and parents. Clinical neuropsychologists deal with a variety of issues as caregivers seek to understand the educational and psychological needs of children and youth who are coping with neurological deficits. Parents frequently want to know what they can do to provide the optimal learning environment to help their children reach their full potential. They seek to understand the specific deficits experienced by the children. On the basis of a child's medical, family, and developmental history, as well as the specific behavioral and educational concerns, a neuropsychological assessment is designed and conducted.

Although this chapter discusses specific neuropsychological tests and batteries of tests, neuropsychology is not a set of techniques. Rather, it is a way of thinking about behavior, often expressed as test scores; in essence, it is a paradigm for understanding behavior.

COMPONENTS OF A NEUROPSYCHOLOGICAL EVALUATION

A neuropsychological evaluation of a child will differ in design from that of an adult. Of necessity, it will include educational and behavioral measures that may not be necessary with adults. The most common neuropsychological batteries and approaches will thus need to be supplemented in specific ways, depending upon the referral questions posed. The following nine general guidelines should nevertheless prove useful and are derived from a variety of sources, including our own practices, the general teachings of Lawrence C. Hartlage, and other specific sources—in particular, Rourke, Bakker, Fisk, and Strang (1983).

1. *All (or at least a significant majority) of a child's educationally relevant cognitive skills or higher-order information-processing skills should be assessed.* This will often involve an assessment of general intellectual level (*g*) via a comprehensive IQ test, such as a Wechsler scale or the Kaufman Assessment Battery for Children (K-ABC; Kaufman & Kaufman, 1983a), although the latter also has specific applications in neuropsychology. Efficiency of mental processing as assessed by strong measures of *g* are essential to provide a baseline for interpreting all other aspects of the assessment process. Assessment of basic academic skills (including reading, writing, spelling, and math) will be necessary, along with tests such as the Test of Memory and Learning (TOMAL; Reynolds & Bigler, 1994), which also have the advantage of including performance-based measures of attention and concentration. Problems with memory, attention/concentration, and new learning are the most common of all complaints following CNS compromise and are frequently associated with more chronic neurodevelopmental disorders (e.g., learning disability, attention-deficit/hyperactivity disorder [ADHD]).

2. *Testing should sample the relative efficiency of the right and left hemispheres of the brain.* Asymmetries of performance are of interest on their own, but different brain

systems are involved in each hemisphere, and these have differing implications for treatment. Even in a diffuse injury such as anoxia, it is possible to find greater impairment in one portion of an individual's brain than in another. Specific neuropsychological tests like those of Halstead and Reitan or the Luria–Nebraska Neuropsychological Battery—Children's Revision (LNNB-CR; Golden, 1986) are useful here, along with measures of verbal and nonverbal memory processes. In neurodevelopmental disorders, uneven development often occurs.

3. *Testing should sample both anterior and posterior regions of cortical function.* The anterior portion of the brain is generative and regulatory, whereas the posterior region is principally receptive. Deficits and their nature in these systems will have a great impact on treatment choices. Many common tests, such as tests of receptive (posterior) and expressive (anterior) vocabulary, may be applied here, along with a systematic and thorough sensory perceptual examination and certain specific tests of motor function. In conjunction with point 2 above, this allows for evaluation of the integrity of the four major quadrants of the neocortex: right anterior, right posterior, left anterior, and left posterior.

4. *Testing should determine the presence of specific deficits.* Any specific functional problems a child is experiencing must be determined and assessed. In addition to such problems being of importance in the assessment of children with neurodevelopmental disorders, traumatic brain injury (TBI), stroke, and even some toxins can produce very specific changes in neocortical function that are addressed best by the neuropsychological assessment. Similarly, research with children with leukemia suggests the presence of subtle neuropsychological deficits following chemotherapy—deficits that may not be detected by more traditional psychological measures. Certain transplant patients will display specific patterns of deficits as well. Neuropsychological tests tend to be less g-loaded as a group and to have greater specificity of measurement than many common psychological tests. Noting areas of specific deficits is important in both diagnosis and treatment planning.

5. *Testing should determine the acuteness versus the chronicity of any problems or weaknesses found.* The "age" of a problem is important to diagnosis and to treatment planning. When a thorough history is combined with the pattern of test results obtained, it is possible, with reasonable accuracy, to distinguish chronic neurodevelopmental disorders such as dyslexia or ADHD from new, acute problems resulting from trauma, stroke, or disease. Particular care must be taken in developing a thorough, documented history when such a determination is made. Rehabilitation and habilitation approaches take differing routes in the design of intervention and treatment strategies, depending upon the age of the child involved and the acuteness or chronicity of the problems evidenced. As children with neurodevelopmental disorders age, symptoms will wax and wane as well, and distinguishing new from old symptoms is important when treatment recommendations are being made.

6. *Testing should locate intact complex functional systems.* The brain functions as a series of interdependent, systemic networks often referred to as "complex functional systems." Multiple systems are affected by CNS problems, but some systems are almost always spared except in the most extreme cases. It is imperative in the assessment process to locate strengths and intact systems that can be used to overcome the problems the child is experiencing. Treatment following CNS compromise involves habilitation and rehabilitation, with the understanding that some organic deficits will represent permanently impaired systems. As the brain consists of complex, interdependent networks of systems that produce behavior, the ability to ascertain intact systems is crucial to enhancing the probability of designing successful treatment. Identification of intact systems also suggests the

potential for a positive outcome to parents and teachers, as opposed to fostering low expectations and fatalistic tendencies on identification of brain damage or dysfunction.

7. *Testing should assess affect, personality, and behavior.* Neuropsychologists sometimes ignore their roots in psychology and focus on assessing the neural substrates of a problem. However, CNS compromise will results in changes in affect, personality, and behavior. Some of these changes will be transient, some will be permanent, and (because children are growing and developing beings) some will be dynamic. Some of these changes will be direct (i.e., the results of CNS compromise at the cellular and systemic levels), and others will be indirect (i.e., reactions to loss or changes in function, or to how others respond to and interact with the individual). A thorough history, including times of onset of problem behaviors, can assist in determination of direct versus indirect effects. As mentioned earlier, comprehensive approaches such as the Behavior Assessment System for Children (BASC; Reynolds & Kamphaus, 1992), which contain behavior rating scales, omnibus personality inventories, and direct observation scales, seem particularly useful. Such behavioral changes will also require intervention, and intervention will be not necessarily be the same if the changes noted are direct versus indirect or if premorbid behavior problems were evident.

8. *Test results should be presented in ways that are useful in school settings, not just to acute care or intensive rehabilitation facilities, or to physicians.* Schools are a major context in which children with chronic neurodevelopmental disorders must function. Children who have sustained insult to the CNS (e.g., TBI, stroke) will eventually return to a school or similar educational setting. This will be where the greatest long-term impact on a child's outcome after CNS compromise will be seen and felt. Results should speak to academic and behavioral concerns, reflecting what a child needs to be taught next in school, how to teach to the child's strengths through the engagement of intact complex functional systems, how to motivate the child, and how to manage positive behavioral outcomes. For a child with TBI, additional information regarding the potential for recovery and the tenuousness of evaluation results immediately postinjury need to be communicated, as does the need for reassessment of both the child and the intervention program at regular intervals. The changing nature of symptoms in a neurodevelopmental disorder must be followed and explained to those who believe that symptom expressivity is within an affected individual's control; such beliefs are all-too-common problems, especially in cases of ADHD, Tourette syndrome, XXY syndrome, and temporal lobe seizure disorder, and even in more common psychopathological disorders (e.g., depression).

9. *If consulting directly with a school system, an evaluator must be certain that the testing and examination procedures are efficient.* School systems, which is where one finds children, do not often have the resources for funding the types of diagnostic workups neuropsychologists prefer. Therefore, when one is consulting with a school system, it is necessary to be succinct and efficient in planning a neuropsychological evaluation. If the school can provide the results of a very recent intellectual and academic assessment, as well as of a behavioral assessment, this can be then integrated into the neuropsychological assessment. If a recent intellectual and academic assessment has not been completed, it may be cost-efficient for qualified school district personnel to complete this portion of the assessment for later integration with other data obtained and interpreted by the neuropsychologist. For children in intensive rehabilitation facilities or medical settings, it may be appropriate for school personnel to participate in the evaluation prior to discharge. This collaborative involvement can facilitate program planning with the receiving school district and is preferable to eliminating needed components of the neuropsychological evaluation.

ASSESSMENT APPROACHES AND INSTRUMENTS

There are two major conceptual approaches to neuropsychological assessment. In the first approach, a standard battery of tasks designed to identify brain impairment is used. The Halstead–Reitan Neuropsychological Test Battery for Children (for ages 9–14) and the Reitan–Indiana Neuropsychological Test Battery for Children (for ages 5–8) are the most commonly used batteries. "The second approach to neuropsychological assessment of children favors the use of a flexible combination of traditional psychological and educational tests. The composition of this battery varies depending upon a number of child variables, including the age, history, functioning level, and presenting problem of the particular child" (Telzrow, 1989, p. 227). The major theoretical premise of both the Halstead–Reitan and the Reitan–Indiana batteries is the proposition that behavior has an organic basis (i.e., the brain controls behavior), and thus that performance on behavioral measures can be used to assess brain functioning (Bigler, 1996; Dean, 1985; Grant & Adams, 1986). In order to infer brain functioning based on behavioral measures, it was necessary to validate these measures on children with known brain damage (Nussbaum & Bigler, 1989).

The Halstead–Reitan Neuropsychological Test Battery for Older Children (for ages 9–14; see Table 2.1) was adapted from the original Halstead–Reitan Neuropsychological Test Battery, which was designed for adults. The two batteries share much of the same equip-

TABLE 2.1. Halstead–Reitan Neuropsychological Test Battery for Older Children (Ages 9–14)

Test administered	Function or skills assessed	Hypothesized localization
Lateral Dominance Aphasia Screening Test	Language	Language items relate to left hemisphere; constructional items related to right hemisphere
Finger Tapping Test	Motor	Frontal lobe
Grip Strength	Motor	Frontal lobe
Sensory–Perceptual Examination	Sensory–perceptual	
Tactile Perception Test		Contralateral parietal lobe
Auditory Perception Test		Temporal lobe
Visual Perception Test		Visual pathway; visual fields
Tactile Form Recognition		Parietal lobe
Fingertip Writing Perception Test		Peripheral nervous system; parietal lobe
Finger Localization Test		Unilateral errors implicate contralateral parietal lobe—can also occur with bilateral errors
Rhythm Test	Alertness and concentration	Global
Speech Sounds Perception Test	Alertness and concentration	Global; anterior left hemisphere
Trail Making Test		
Part A	Visual–spatial	Global
Part B	Reasoning	Global
Tactual Performance Test		
Total Time	Motor	Frontal lobe
Memory	Immediate memory	Global
Localization	Immediate memory	Global
Category Test	Reasoning	Global; sensitive to right frontal lobe dysfunction in older children

Note. Data from Reitan and Wolfson (1985).

ment and many of the same tests; however, there are some changes in the children's battery. The Tactual Performance Test uses a 6-hole board instead of the 10-hole board. On the Speech Sounds Perception Test, the child underlines the correct sound from three alternatives instead of four. The Category Test has been reduced from 208 slides to 168 slides. Likewise, Parts A and B of the Trail Making Test (Trails A and B) have been reduced in length.

Further modifications have been made with the Reitan–Indiana Neuropsychological Test Battery (for ages 5–8; see Table 2.2). Trails A and B, Speech Sounds Perception Test, and Rhythms have been omitted. Numerous tests have been added: Matching Pictures, Matching V's and Figures, Star Drawing, Concentric Square, Target Test, Marching Test, Color Form Test, and Progressive Figures. On the Category Test, the number of items has been further reduced to 80, and the number caps have been replaced with color caps. The same 6-hole board is used for the Tactual Performance Test as that used for the Halstead–Reitan version; however, the board is placed horizontally rather than vertically. The Aphasia Screening Test uses the same booklet, but some of the items have been omitted and replaced with more age-appropriate items. Because young children have difficulty manipulating the manual finger tapper, an electric tapper was developed for the Finger Tapping Test.

TABLE 2.2. Reitan–Indiana Neuropsychological Test Battery for Children (Ages 5–8)

Test administered	Function or skills assessed	Hypothesized localization
Lateral Dominance Aphasia Screening Test	Language	Language items relate to left hemisphere; constructional items related to right hemisphere
Finger Tapping Test	Motor	Frontal lobe
Grip Strength	Motor	Frontal lobe
Matching Pictures	Visual–spatial	Global right hemisphere
Matching V's and Figures	Visual–spatial	Association areas
Concentric Square and Star Drawing	Visual–spatial	Global right hemisphere
Target Test	Visual–spatial	Association areas
Marching Test	Motor	Global
Color Form Test		
Reasoning	Global	Global
Progressive Figures	Alertness and concentration	Global
Sensory–Perceptual Examination	Sensory–perceptual	
Tactile Perception Test		Contralateral parietal lobe
Auditory Perception Test		Temporal lobe
Visual Perception Test		Visual pathway; visual fields
Tactile Form Recognition		Parietal lobe
Fingertip Writing Perception Test		Peripheral nervous system; parietal lobe
Finger Localization Test		Unilateral errors implicate contralateral parietal lobe—can also occur with bilateral errors
Tactual Performance Test		
Total Time	Motor	Frontal lobe
Memory	Immediate memory	Global
Localization	Immediate memory	Global
Category Test	Reasoning	Global; sensitive to right frontal lobe dysfunction in older children

Note. Data from Reitan and Wolfson (1985).

Right–left differences, dysphasia and related deficits, and cutoff scores that differentiate normal from brain-damaged children for each battery are used to determine the score on the Neuropsychological Deficit Scale, which is the child's level of performance. Based on normative comparisons, raw scores are weighted as "perfectly normal" (score = 0), "normal" (score = 1), "mildly impaired" (score = 2), or "significantly impaired" (score = 3). Separate tables are available for the test results of older children and younger children.

In contrast to the use of standard batteries, the process approach uses a flexible battery of developmental and psychological tests, which permits the clinician to select tasks appropriate to the specific referral question, functioning levels, and response limitations of the child. Client variables such as "age, gender, handedness, familial handedness, educational and occupational background, premorbid talents, patient's and family's medical, neurological, and psychiatric history, drug or alcohol abuse, use of medications (past and present), etiology of the central nervous system (CNS) dysfunction, and laterality and focus of the lesion" (Kaplan, 1990, p. 72) all provide valuable information in developing the assessment. Furthermore, this process provides an analysis of the child's neuropsychological assets, rather than focusing on a diagnosis or a specific localization of brain impairment, for which the standardized batteries have been noted. The flexible-battery approach purportedly translates more directly into educational and vocational interventions, and a major goal of conducting a neuropsychological assessment is to aid in the planning of such interventions. Finally, since this method uses more traditional educational and psychological tests that are more familiar to school personnel, this assessment is more directly applicable to school settings. Schools provide the most affordable and available habilitation and rehabilitation opportunities for children with neuropsychological impairment; therefore, it is imperative that the assessment data be transferred into these settings (Telzrow, 1989). A major concern about the process approach is the difficulty in establishing validity for the innumerable versions of batteries used, as interpretations may not be uniform or reliable. This issue has been addressed inadequately thus far.

REASON FOR REFERRAL

Children are initially referred to neuropsychologists for a variety of reasons. If a child has a congenital brain defect, the child is frequently brought to a neuropsychologist early in his or her development, particularly if developmental delays, language deficits, or behavioral problems are observed. Depending on the results of the neuropsychological evaluation, the child may qualify for early intervention programs or other special programs through the public school system.

In other cases, as a child grows, parents may seek a diagnosis of ADHD as they cope with the child's problems at home and at school because of "hyper-ness" or "inability to sit still." At this time the neuropsychologist seeks to discover the cause of the inattentiveness—whether it is truly ADHD or a learning disability, developmental delay, or psychiatric problem that is causing the behavior problems exhibited by the child.

Children who have experienced a TBI are frequently referred for a neuropsychological evaluation to determine the extent of the brain injury in terms of the child's cognitive strengths, weaknesses, and reentry into the school environment. On the basis of this evaluation, the neuropsychologist makes appropriate recommendations to the parents and school.

Even when the parents are unable to define specific referral questions, the driving forces behind the majority of neuropsychological referrals are problems in the educational setting. Teachers are often unprepared to address these difficulties and do not understand the specific learning problems of children with brain dysfunction. No two brain dysfunctions or injuries are the same. Two children can experience the same type of injury and still require different modifications in the classroom. Parents as well as teachers are looking for answers—ways to teach their children and to provide appropriate educational opportunities. A neuropsychological evaluation helps to furnish that information; it provides data for answering the question "So what do we do now?" after a diagnosis has been made. The information gained from a neuropsychological evaluation enables the neuropsychologist to make recommendations concerning attention, learning and memory, intellectual functioning, cognitive strengths and weaknesses, problem-solving abilities, and so forth to the parents and the educators.

TEACHING TO THE CHILD'S STRENGTHS

One of the primary reasons for conducting a neuropsychological evaluation is not to determine "what has been impaired," but rather to determine "what has been spared." Educators and parents supply numerous examples of what a child is unable to do: "He cannot follow instructions," "She can't remember anything," "He cannot read." Very seldom does a referral source approach an evaluation with a list of the activities or skills that the child is able to accomplish with ease and proficiency. But whether or not the source realizes it at the time of the referral, such a list contains the very information that is urgently needed for the child to move forward in the educational process. It is essential that we teach to the child's strengths instead of his or her weaknesses. As pointed out by Reynolds (1981a), teaching to a child's weaknesses focuses on brain areas that are damaged or dysfunctional. When teaching methods focus on cortical areas that are not intact, the child's potential for failure is increased, and this is harmful to the child. Reynolds (1981a) also points out that research on these remedial practices (referred to as "deficit-centered models" of remediation) has found them to be ineffective.

In contrast, teaching to a child's strengths has a number of advantages. This method may be especially helpful for children who are resistant to focused remediation of weaknesses (Rourke et al., 1983). When self-confidence is low or when a failure syndrome emerges as a result of frustration, a strength-centered approach should be adopted. Second, teaching to the child's strengths may reduce the possibility of the child's falling farther and farther below peers in academic areas. Finally, Luria (1966) suggested that recovery of function following cortical damage can be achieved "by the replacement of the lost cerebral link by another which is still intact" (p. 55). "For example, a child with an impaired auditory system could be taught to differentiate simple sounds using visual or nonverbal images" (Teeter & Semrud-Clikeman, 1997, p. 364). More details on strength-centered models of remediation may be found in Reynolds and Hickman (1987).

OTHER INFORMATION NEEDED FOR ASSESSMENT

When a child is initially referred to a neuropsychologist, the child's history is the first critical piece of information. This history should include prenatal, perinatal, developmental, and medical history. It is also important to include familial information about educational or learning problems, discipline, and family structure. If the child has had a TBI or illness, age of onset, duration of illness of injury, and time since illness or trauma all provide important information.

A child's school history provides invaluable information as well. The child's grades and other school records allow the neuropsychologist to look at trends in the student's educational process, and they provide a means of comparing the student's abilities with those of peers. School transcripts may also be helpful in evaluating individual motivational factors, study habits, and daily classroom performance. IQ tests or other standardized academic tests (e.g., the Woodcock–Johnson Psycho-Educational Battery, the Wide Range Achievement Test, Wechsler Individualized Achievement Tests) provide standardized scores, which give further information about a child's cognitive and academic strengths and weaknesses. If a student has been receiving special services, one cannot assume that the existing services will meet the child's present needs; these services may need to be expanded or modified to meet the actual needs of the child.

On the basis of the historical information obtained, the trained neuropsychologist conducts a structured interview, which culminates in a list of referral questions and specific concerns about the child.

HABILITATION AND REHABILITATION CONSIDERATIONS

When one is making recommendations for rehabilitation of the child with a focal injury or TBI, several additional considerations are evident. It is important to determine what type of functional system is impaired. Impaired systems may, for example, be modality-specific or process-specific. The nature or characteristics of the impairments must be elucidated before an intelligent remedial plan can be devised.

The number of systems impaired should be determined. In addition, because children may not be able to work on everything at once, a system of priorities should be devised so that the impairments with the most important impact on overall recovery are the first and most intensely addressed. The degree of impairment, a normative question, will be important to consider in this regard as well. At times, this will require the neuropsychologist to reflect on the indirect effects of a child's disorder or injury, as an impaired or dysfunctional system may adversely affect other systems that are without true direct organic compromise.

As noted earlier, the quality of the neuropsychological strengths that exist will also be important; this tends to be more of an ipsative than a normative determination. Certain strengths are more useful than others as well. Preserved language and speech are of great importance, for example, whereas an intact sense of smell (an ability often impaired in TBI) is of less importance in designing treatment plans and outcome research. Even more important to long-term recovery are intact planning and concept formation skills. The executive functioning skills of the frontal lobes takes on greater and greater importance with age, and strengths in these areas are crucial to long-term planning (as are weaknesses). These will change with age, however, as the frontal lobes become increasingly prominent in behavioral control after age 9 years, again through puberty, and continuing into the 20s.

BASES FOR EDUCATIONAL MODIFICATIONS

After the neuropsychologist makes his or her assessment and recommendations, the school personnel and the parents hold a multidisciplinary team meeting. The purposes of this meeting are to make appropriate modifications in the classroom that will enable the child to reach his or her academic potential, and to develop an individualized education plan

(IEP) for the child. In many cases, educational modifications that teachers are currently using in their regular classrooms (e.g., small groups, modified assignments, individualized instruction) are the only modifications needed. Cohen (1991) suggests developing active learning situations, slowing down, assuring that lesson tasks address the appropriate deficits, teaching the process of the activity, teaching students to become more independent, and developing strategies that can be used in various situations. In other cases, the needed modifications include scheduling or placement issues that involve much more than the regular classroom setting. Placement options include the regular classroom, with no provision or support in the classroom; modified regular education, which could include a lighter course load or special tutorial sessions; a collapsed or half-day schedule; or special education services ranging from part-time to full-time. Class size may also be a consideration. Homebound or residential education programming may be yet another option. Fatigue is common during recovery from a head injury or stroke, and a schedule that allows for a structured rest time may also be a needed option (Cohen, 1991).

Educational support materials, such as computers, calculators, tape records, writing aids, positioning equipment, or augmentative communication devices, may be essential equipment in providing an appropriate educational environment. The use of such classroom aids should be implemented in consultation with the occupational therapist, physical therapist, and neuropsychologist, and should be included on the IEP.

Throughout this process, school personnel must collaborate with the child's parents. Open communication and cooperation between the parents and the school will assure the parents that their requests, apprehensions, and concerns will be addressed, and that their child will be provided with the most appropriate education. The neuropsychologist and school personnel can also make appropriate recommendations for the parents. With this information, the parents are able to formulate appropriate guidelines for behaviors and expectations for their child's educational potential.

MEMORY AND LEARNING

In cases of TBI, including closed head injury, problems with memory and attention are the most common, frequent complaints at all age levels. However, memory and learning problems seem to characterize nearly any CNS disorders in which higher cortical systems are involved (e.g., see Gillberg, 1995; Knight, 1992; and Reynolds & Bigler, 1997). Table 2.3 provides a listing of the primary neurodevelopmental disorders in which the clinician can anticipate memory and learning deficits.

The approach to assessment proffered herein would seem to require an assessment of children's memory and immediate learning skills. The neuropsychological batteries primarily in use with children, even when accompanied by a thorough assessment of intellect (as they should be), provide only a brief screening of memory and learning skills. Comprehensive assessment of children's memory and learning skills is a relatively recent phenomenon: The first comprehensive batteries for evaluating memory in children were not published until the 1990s (Reynolds & Bigler, 1994; Sheslow & Adams, 1990). By contrast, adult batteries, notably the Wechsler Memory Scale, have been available since the 1930s. Nevertheless, memory assessment in children was seen as important in evaluating children's skills at least as early as the work of Binet in the 1890s, and at least one measure of short-term memory appears in every Wechsler scale and most other major intelligence tests (e.g., the various Kaufman batteries, the McCarthy scales, and the various versions of the Detroit

TABLE 2.3. Primary Neurodevelopmental Disorders in Which Memory and Learning Are Likely to Be Compromised

Attention-deficit/hyperactivity disorder (ADHD)	*In utero* toxic exposure (e.g., neonatal cocaine addiction, fetal alcohol syndrome)	Neurofibromatosis
Autism		Prader–Willi syndrome
Cerebral palsy	Juvenile Huntington disease	Rett syndrome
Down syndrome	Juvenile parkinsonism	Schizophrenia
Endocrine disorders	Learning disability	Seizure disorders
Extremely low birth weight	Lesch–Nyhan syndrome	Tourette syndrome
Fragile X syndrome	Mental retardation	Turner syndrome
Hydrocephalus	Myotonic dystrophy	Williams syndrome
Hypoxic–ischemic injury	Neurodevelopmental abnormalities affecting brain development (e.g., anencephaly, microcephaly, callosal dysgenesis)	XXY syndrome
Inborn errors of metabolism (e.g., phenylketonuria [PKU], galactosemia)		XYY syndrome

Note. After Reynolds and Bigler (1997).

Tests of Learning Aptitude). A brief review of the neurobiology of memory shows why it is so crucial to assess memory when organic deficiencies are suspected.

Basic Neurobiology of Memory

"Attention" leaves tracks or traces within the brain that become memory. "Memory," as commonly conceived of, is the ability to recall some event or information of various types and forms. Biologically, memory functions at two broad levels: the level of the individual cell, and a systemic level. With the creation of memories, changes occur in individual cells (e.g., see Cohen, 1993; Diamond, 1990; Scheibel, 1990), including alterations in cell membranes and synaptic physiology.

At the systems level, there exists a division of sorts in the formation of memory and memory storage. There is considerable evidence for distributed storage of associative memory throughout the cortex, which may even occur in a statistical function (Cohen, 1993). At the same time, evidence indicates more localized storage of certain memories and localized centers for memory formation and for classical and operant conditioning. The medial aspect of the temporal lobe—particularly the hippocampus and its connecting fibers within the other limbic and paralimbic structures—is particularly important in the development of associative memory. The limbic system (with emphasis on the posterior hippocampal regions) also mediates the development of conditioned responses, and some patients with posterior hippocampal lesions may not respond to operant paradigms in the absence of one-to-one reinforcement schedules. Damage to or anomalous development of either the medial temporal lobe and its connecting fibers, or the midline structures of the diencephalon, typically results in the difficulties in formation of new memories (anterograde amnesia); however, it may also disrupt recently formed memories preceding the time of injury (retrograde amnesia). Various regions within the limbic and paralimbic structures have stronger roles in formation of certain types of memory, and simple conditioned memories may occur at a subcortical level. Through all the interactions of these systems, related mechanisms of attention, particularly in the brain stem and the frontal lobes, are brought to bear and will influence memory formation directly and indirectly. Memory is a complex function of the interaction of brain systems (with unequal contributions), and damage to one or more of many structures may impair the ability to form new memories.

In right-handed individuals, there is a tendency for damage to or abnormal developmental patterns within the left temporal lobe and adjacent structures to affect verbal and sequential memory more strongly. Damage to the cognate areas of the right hemisphere affects visual and spatial memory more adversely.

Through distributive storage of memory, the entire brain participates in memory functioning. The recall of well-established memories tends to be one of the most robust of neural functions, whereas the formation of new memories, sustained attention, and concentration tend to be the most fragile of neural functions. Neurological dysfunction of most types is associated with a nonspecific lessening of memory performance, along with disruptions of attention and concentration; this is of greater consequence when temporolimbic, brain stem, or frontal lobe involvement occurs. However, a variety of psychiatric disturbances, especially depression, may also suppress fragile anterograde memory systems. A careful analysis of memory, forgetting, affective states, history, and comprehensive neuropsychological test results may be necessary before one can conclude that memory disturbances are organic in origin, especially in the complex case of neurodevelopmental disorders.

Assessing Memory

The two most widely regarded and recommended memory batteries for children are the Wide Range Assessment of Memory and Learning (WRAML; Sheslow & Adams, 1990) and the Test of Memory and Learning (TOMAL; Reynolds & Bigler, 1994). The WRAML consists of nine subtests divided equally into three scales, Verbal Memory, Visual Memory, and Learning, followed by brief delayed-recall tasks to assess rapidity of the decay of memory. The WRAML represented a substantial improvement over existing measures of memory in children when it appeared in 1990, but it still provided a somewhat limited scope of assessment. To increase the breadth and depth of assessment of memory and learning functions in children with a coordinated battery of diverse tasks, Reynolds and Bigler (1994) developed the TOMAL. The TOMAL is featured here as "the most comprehensive of its kind . . . and will undoubtedly be a useful tool for assessing memory functioning in children and adolescents in many clinical, research, and educational settings" (Ferris & Kamphaus, 1996, p. 256). The many well-normed, reliable subtests of the TOMAL provide examiners with the maximum flexibility in evaluating various referral questions and with the choice of the most comprehensive assessments available. The individual subtests also have good reliability and specificity of measurement.

The Test of Memory and Learning

The TOMAL is a comprehensive battery of 14 memory and learning tasks (10 core subtests and 4 supplementary subtests) normed for use with children and youth from ages 5 years, 0 months, 0 days through 19 years, 11 months, 30 days. The 10 core subtests are divided into the content domains of Verbal Memory and Nonverbal Memory, which can be combined to derive a Composite Memory Index. A Delayed Recall Index is also available; this requires a repeat recall of the first four subtests' stimuli 30 minutes after their first administration.

As noted above, memory may behave in unusual ways in an impaired brain, and traditional content approaches to memory may not be useful. The TOMAL thus provides alternative groupings of the subtests into five supplementary indexes: Sequential Recall, Free Recall, Associative Recall, Learning, and Attention and Concentration. These supplementary indexes were derived by having a group of "expert" neuropsychologists sort the 14 TOMAL subtests into logical categories (Reynolds & Bigler, 1994). To provide greater flexibility to the clinician, a set of four purely empirically derived factor indexes—Complex Memory, Sequential Recall, Backward Recall, and Spatial Memory—has been made available as well (Reynolds & Bigler, 1996).

Table 2.4 gives the names of the subtests and summary scores, along with their metrics. The TOMAL subtests are scaled to the familiar metric of a mean of 10 and a standard

TABLE 2.4. Core and Supplementary Subtests and Indexes Available for the Test of Memory and Learning (TOMAL)

	M	SD
Core subtests		
Verbal		
Memory for Stories	10	3
Word Selective Reminding	10	3
Object Recall	10	3
Digits Forward	10	3
Paired Recall	10	3
Nonverbal		
Facial Memory	10	3
Visual Selective Reminding	10	3
Abstract Visual Memory	10	3
Visual Sequential Memory	10	3
Memory for Location	10	3
Supplementary subtests		
Verbal		
Letters Forward	10	3
Digits Backward	10	3
Letters Backward	10	3
Nonverbal		
Manual Imitation	10	3
Summary scores		
Core indexes		
Verbal Memory Index	100	15
Nonverbal Memory Index	100	15
Composite Memory Index	100	15
Delayed Recall Index	100	15
Supplementary indexes (expert-derived)		
Sequential Recall Index	100	15
Free Recall Index	100	15
Associative Recall Index	100	15
Learning Index	100	15
Attention and Concentration Index	100	15
Factor indexes (empirically derived)		
Complex Memory Index	100	15
Sequential Recall Index	100	15
Backward Recall Index	100	15
Spatial Memory Index	100	15

deviation of 3 (range = 1 to 20). Composite or summary scores are scaled to a mean of 100 and a standard deviation of 15. All scaling was done using the method of rolling weighted averages and is described in detail in Reynolds and Bigler (1994).

The 10 core and 4 supplementary TOMAL subtests require about 60 minutes for a skilled examiner if the subtests for the Delayed Recall Index are also administered. The subtests were chosen to provide a comprehensive view of memory functions and, when used *in toto*, provide the most thorough assessment of memory available (Ferris & Kamphaus, 1996). The subtests are briefly described in Table 2.5.

The TOMAL subtests systematically vary the format of both presentation and response, so as to sample verbal, visual, and motoric modalities and combinations of these. Multiple trials to a criterion are provided on several subtests, including the Selective Reminding subtests, so that learning or acquisition curves may be derived. Multiple trials (at least five are necessary, according to Kaplan [1996], and the TOMAL provides up to eight) are provided on the Selective Reminding subtests to allow an analysis of the depth of processing. In the Selective Reminding format (wherein examinees are reminded only of stimuli "forgotten" or unrecalled), when items once recalled are unrecalled by an examinee on later trials, problems are revealed in the transference of stimuli from working memory and immediate memory to more long-term storage. Cueing is also provided at the end of certain subtests, to add to the examiner's ability to probe depth of processing.

Subtests are included that sample sequential recall (which tends strongly to be mediated by the left hemisphere, especially temporal regions; e.g., see Lezak, 1995) and free recall in both verbal and visual formats to allow localization. To assess more purely right-hemisphere functions, tests of pure spatial memory are included; these are very difficult to confound via verbal mediation.

Well-established memory tasks (e.g., recalling stories) that correlate well with school learning are also included, along with tasks more common to experimental neuropsychology that have high (e.g., Facial Memory) and low (e.g., Visual Selective Reminding) ecological salience. Some subtests employ highly meaningful material (e.g., Memory for Stories), whereas others use highly abstract stimuli (e.g., Abstract Visual Memory).

Aside from allowing a comprehensive review of memory function, the purpose of such a factorial array of tasks across multiple dimensions is to allow a thorough, detailed analysis of memory function and of the sources of any memory deficits that may be discovered. The task of the neuropsychologist demands subtests that have great specificity and variability of presentation and response, and that sample all relevant brain functions, in order to solve the complex puzzle of dysfunctional brain–behavior relationships. Kaufman (1979) first presented a detailed model for analyzing test data in a comprehensive format (later elaborated; Kaufman, 1994), which likens the task of the clinician to that of a detective. The thoroughness, breadth, and variability of the TOMAL subtests, coupled with their excellent psychometric properties, make the TOMAL ideal for use in a model of "intelligent testing" and particularly in the analysis of brain–behavior relationships associated with memory function.

ASSESSMENT OF BRAIN–BEHAVIOR RELATIONSHIPS
THROUGH LURIAN PROCESSING MODELS

The previously reviewed approaches to assessing brain–behavior relationships focus on specificity of aptitudes or mental skills (i.e., their relative distinctiveness from one another) as a model for their assessment. Processing models of brain function focus more heavily

TABLE 2.5. Description of TOMAL Subtests

Core subtests

Memory for Stories
  A verbal subtest requiring recall of a short story read to the examinee. Provides a measure of meaningful and semantic recall, and is also related to sequential recall in some instances.

Facial Memory
  A nonverbal subtest requiring recognition and identification from a set of distractors: black-and-white photos of people of various ages, both genders, and various ethnic backgrounds. Assesses nonverbal meaningful memory in a practical fashion and has been extensively researched. Sequencing of responses is unimportant.

Word Selective Reminding
  A verbal free-recall task in which the examinee learns a word list and repeats it; the examinee is only reminded of words left out in each case. Tests learning and immediate recall functions in verbal memory. Trials continue until mastery is achieved or until eight trials have been attempted; sequence of recall is unimportant.

Visual Selective Reminding
  A nonverbal analogue to Word Selective Reminding. Examinees point to specified dots on a card, following a demonstration by the examiner, and are reminded only of items recalled incorrectly. As with Word Selective Reminding, trials continue until mastery is achieved or until eight trials have been attempted.

Object Recall
  The examiner presents a series of pictures, names them, has the examinee recall them, and repeats this process across four trials. Verbal and nonverbal stimuli are thus paired and recall is entirely verbal, creating a situation found to interfere with recall for many children with learning disabilities, but to be neutral or facilitative for children without disabilities.

Abstract Visual Memory
  A nonverbal task. Assesses immediate recall for meaningful figures when order is unimportant. The examinee is presented with a standard stimulus and required to recognize the standard from any of six distractors.

Digits Forward
  A standard verbal number recall task. Measures low-level rote recall of a sequence of numbers.

Visual Sequential Memory
  A nonverbal task requiring recall of the sequence of a series of meaningless geometric designs. The ordered designs are shown, followed by a presentation of a standard order of the stimuli, and the examinee indicates the order in which they originally appeared.

Paired Recall
  A verbal paired-associates learning task, in which easy and hard pairs are provided by the examiner. Measures immediate associative recall and learning.

Memory for Location
  A nonverbal task that assesses spatial memory. The examinee is presented with a set of large dots distributed on a page and asked to recall the locations of the dots in any order.

Supplementary subtests

Manual Imitation
  A psychomotor, visually based assessment of sequential memory. The examinee is required to reproduce a set of ordered hand movements in the same sequence as presented by the examiner.

Letters Forward
  A language-related analogue to common digit span tasks, using letters as the stimuli in place of numbers.

Digits Backward
  This is the same basic task as Digits Forward, except that the examinee recalls the numbers in reverse order.

Letters Backward
  A language-related analogue to the Digits Backward task, using letters as the stimuli instead of numbers.

on the manipulative demands of a mental task than on the content demands. Cognitive tasks can thus be grouped according to these processing demands for more reliable and detailed assessment, leading to conclusions about brain function with direct implications for intervention (e.g., see Kamphaus & Reynolds, 1987; Reynolds, 1981a, 1981b; and Hartlage & Reynolds, 1981).

Lurian Theories

From a clinical perspective, the neuropsychological models of information processing espoused by Luria are of the greatest utility. "Alexander R. Luria's theory of higher cortical function has received international acclaim. His conceptual schemes of the functional organization of the brain are probably the most comprehensive currently available" (Adams, 1985, p. 878). Much of Luria's work elaborated and extended the earlier work of Sechenov (1863/1965) and Vygotsky (1978).

Luria defined mental processes in terms of two sharply delineated groups, "simultaneous" and "successive," following Sechenov's suggestions. The first process involves the integration of elements into simultaneous groups. Luria further qualified Sechenov's original meaning, indicating that simultaneous processing means the synthesis of successive elements (arriving one after the other) into simultaneous spatial schemes, whereas successive processing means the synthesis of separate elements into successive series.

Luria (1966) divided the brain into three blocks. Block One consists of the brain stem and reticular system and is responsible principally for regulating level of consciousness, arousal, and the overall tone of the cortex. Block Two consists of the parietal, occipital, and temporal lobes of the brain (the lobes posterior to the central sulcus) and is responsible for receiving and encoding sensory input. Block Three consists of those regions of the brain anterior to the central sulcus (the frontal lobes and the prefrontal regions) and is responsible for the self-regulation of behavior, including such variables as attention, planning and execution of behavior, and other tasks generally referred to as "executive functions." In Luria's model, various zones and regions of the brain interact in a transactional manner to produce complex behavior; thus the functional localization of complex mental tasks is seen as dynamic, defying efforts at highly specific anatomical localization. Luria's approach lends itself to strength-centered intervention models, wherein the clinician actively seeks intact complex functional systems within the brain that can be used to habilitate and facilitate learning, rather than to models focusing on remediating dysfunctional or damaged brain systems (e.g., see Reynolds, 1981a, 1997; Riccio & Reynolds, 1998).

Two neuropsychological batteries for children are based primarily on Luria's theory of brain function. The first to be published was the Kaufman Assessment Battery for Children (K-ABC; Kaufman & Kaufman, 1983a), followed soon thereafter by the Luria–Nebraska Neuropsychological Battery—Children's Revision (LNNB-CR; Golden, 1986). Each of these batteries has a stronger focus on process than the typical neuropsychological test per se, with the possible exception of the TOMAL, but the TOMAL focuses on memory processes more specifically.

The Kaufman Assessment Battery for Children

The K-ABC was designed and is standardized for use with children ages 2½ years through 12½ years. It is divided into three scales: the Sequential Processing Scale, the Simultaneous

Processing Scale (these two are summed to provide a global score, the Mental Processing Composite), and the Achievement Scale (a measure of previously acquired information). Table 2.6 describes the subtests that constitute these three scales.

The K-ABC is a useful scale for applications in the neuropsychological evaluation of children. Detailed discussions of its use in neuropsychology are provided in Kamphaus and Reynolds (1987), Reynolds and Kamphaus (1997), and Reynolds, Kamphaus, Rosenthal, and Hiemenz (1997); the following summary draws directly from these sources.

In the K-ABC, the Kaufmans define mental processes in a manner similar to Luria's and provide a standardized assessment of these functions. "Simultaneous processing" here refers to the child's mental ability to integrate input simultaneously in order to solve a problem correctly. Simultaneous processing frequently involves spatial, analogical, or organizational abilities (Kaufman & Kaufman, 1983b), as well as problems solved through the application of visual imagery. The Triangles subtest of the K-ABC (an analogue of Wechsler's Block Design task) is a prototypical measure of simultaneous processing. To solve these items correctly, one must mentally integrate the components of the design to

---

TABLE 2.6. Subtests and Scales of the Kaufman Assessment Battery for Children (K-ABC)

Sequential Processing Scale

Hand Movements (ages 2½–12½ years): Imitating a series of hand movements in the same sequence as the examiner performed them.

Number Recall (ages 2½–12½ years): Repeating a series of digits in the same sequence as the examiner said them.

Word Order (ages 4–12½): Touching a series of pictures in the same sequence as they were named by the examiner, with more difficult items employing a color interference task.

Simultaneous Processing Scale

Magic Windows (ages 2½–4): Identifying a picture that the examiner exposes by moving it past a narrow slit or "window," making the picture only partially visible at any one time.

Face Recognition (ages 2½-4): Selecting from a group photograph the one or two faces that were exposed briefly in the preceding photograph.

Gestalt Closure (ages 2½–12½): Naming the object or scene pictured in a partially completed "inkblot" drawing.

Triangles (ages 4–12½): Assembling several identical triangles into an abstract pattern that matches a model.

Matrix Analogies (ages 5–12½): Selecting the picture or abstract design that best completes a visual analogy.

Spatial Memory (ages 5–12½): Recalling the placement of pictures on a page that was exposed briefly.

Photo Series (ages 6–12½): Placing photographs of an event in chronological order.

Achievement Scale

Expressive Vocabulary (ages 2½–4): Naming the object pictured in a photograph.

Faces and Places (ages 2½–12½): Naming the well-known person, fictional character, or place pictured in a photograph or illustration.

Arithmetic (ages 3–12½): Answering a question that requires knowledge of math concepts or the manipulation of numbers.

Riddles (ages 3–12½): Naming the object or concept described by a list of three characteristics.

Reading/Decoding (ages 5–12½): Naming letters and reading words.

Reading/Understanding (ages 7–12½): Acting out commands given in written sentences.

"see" the whole. Such a task seems to match up nicely with Luria's qualifying statement about the synthesis of separate elements (each triangle) into spatial schemes (the larger pattern of triangles, which may form squares, rectangles, or larger triangles). Whether the tasks are spatial or analogical in nature, the unifying characteristic of simultaneous processing is the mental synthesis of the stimuli to solve the problem, independent of the sensory modality of the input or the output.

"Sequential processing," on the other hand, emphasizes the arrangement of stimuli in sequential or serial order for successful problem solving. In every instance, each stimulus is linearly or temporally related to the previous one (Kaufman & Kaufman, 1983b), creating a form of serial interdependence within the stimulus. The K-ABC includes subtests that tap various modalities of sequential processing. Hand Movements involves visual input and a motor response; Number Recall involves auditory input with a response involving the auditory output channel only; and Word Order involves the visual channel for input and an auditory response. Therefore, the mode of presentation or mode of response is not what determines the scale placement of a task; rather, it is the mental processing demands of the task that are important (Kaufman & Kaufman, 1983b). By providing systematic variation of modality of input and modality of response, the K-ABC provides a clinical vehicle for locating intact complex functional systems, as well as for specifying where any potential breakdown may have occurred in a faulty functional system. Qualitative evaluation of a child's performance on the K-ABC can be most useful in such instances and can lead to more effective rehabilitation plans. Table 2.7 reviews definitions of the primary processes assessed by the K-ABC.

No one with an intact brain uses only a single type of information processing to solve problems. These two methods of information processing are constantly interacting (even in the so-called "split brain" following commissurotomy), although one approach will often take a lead role in processing. Which method of processing takes the lead role can change according to the demands of the problem or (as is the case with some individuals) can persist across problem type, forming habitual modes of processing. In fact, any problem can be solved through either method of processing, but in most cases one method is clearly superior to another. What makes the K-ABC a valuable tool is that the two mental processing scales are primarily, not exclusively, measures of sequential or simultaneous processing. "Pure" scales (i.e., scales measuring only one process) do not exist. Careful observation of a child's performance, which should be the order of the day during any evaluation, will be particularly important to any neuropsychological assessment or neuropsychological interpretation of K-ABC test results; observation in many cases will be a primary source of information regarding which mental processes a child has invoked on any given task, regardless of its scale.

An equally important component of the K-ABC is the Achievement Scale. This scale measures abilities that serve to complement the mental processing scales. Performance on the Achievement Scale is viewed as an estimate of children's success in the application of their mental processing skills to the acquisition of knowledge from the environment (Kaufman, Kamphaus, & Kaufman, 1985). This scale contains measures of what have been identified traditionally as verbal intelligence, general information, and acquired school skills. Keeping in mind that it is not possible to separate entirely what individuals know (achievement) from how well they think (intelligence), the Kaufmans attempted to differentiate the two variables more clearly than traditional measures of intelligence generally do. From a clinical-neuropsychological standpoint, the K-ABC allows one to assess information-processing skills without as much contamination from prior learning. Measurement of children's academic skills, however, is a traditional component of the comprehensive neuro-

TABLE 2.7. Definitions of the Two Types of Mental Processing That Underlie the K-ABC Intelligence Scales, from the K-ABC Manual and from Several Theoretical Perspectives

Source	Label for process	Definition
K-ABC manual: Kaufman & Kaufman (1983a)	Sequential	Places a premium on the serial or temporal order of stimuli when solving problems.
	Simultaneous	Demands a gestalt-like, frequently spatial integration of stimuli to solve problems with maximum efficiency.
Cerebral specialization: Nebes (1974) (summarizing model of Bogen, Levy-Agresti, and Sperry)	Analytic/propositional/ left-hemisphere	Sequentially analyzes input, abstracting out the relevant details, with which it associates verbal symbols in order to manipulate and store the data more efficiently.
	Synthetic/appositional/ right-hemisphere	Organizes and treats data in terms of complex wholes, being in effect a synthesizer with a predisposition for viewing the total rather than the parts.
Luria/Das: Das, Kirby, & Jarman (1979)	Successive	Processes information in a serial order. The important distinction between this type of information processing and simultaneous processing is that in successive processing the system is not totally surveyable at any point in time. Rather, a system of cues consecutively activates the components.
	Simultaneous	Synthesizes separate elements into groups, with these groups often taking on spatial overtones. The essential nature of this sort of processing is that any portion of the result is at once surveyable without dependence on its position in the whole.
Cognitive psychology: Neisser (1967)	Sequential/serial	Viewed as a constructive process; constructs only one thing at a time. The very definitions of "rational" and "logical" also suggest that each idea, image, or action is sensibly related to the preceding one, making an appearance only as it becomes necessary for the aim in view.
		A spatially "serial" activity is one that analyzes only a part of the input field at any given moment. On the other hand, "sequential" refers to the manner in which a process is organized; it is appropriate when the analysis consists of successive, interrelated steps simultaneously, or at least independently.
	Simultaneous	Carries out many activities simultaneously, or at least independently.

psychological assessment. The inclusion of the Achievement Scale in the K-ABC affords the opportunity to observe the application of processing skills to complex learning tasks, to assess functional academic levels, and to estimate long-term memory ability. For a thorough review of interpretation of the K-ABC Achievement Scale, see Kamphaus and Reynolds (1987).

Majovski (1984) noted the high degree of fit between Luria's theory and the K-ABC and recommended that the test be used as an integral part of a neuropsychological battery for children (see also Spreen & Strauss, 1991). It is a good complement to nearly any choice of neuropsychological instruments. Majovski found the K-ABC particularly useful in contrasting problem-solving skills with acquisition of facts and in evaluating how a child solves a particular problem.

When young children (below age 6) are being assessed, the K-ABC should be the neuropsychologist's test of choice for measuring intellectual skill. The K-ABC mental processing subtests are child-oriented and much briefer than (. . . but with comparable reliability to) those of its major competitor, the Wechsler Preschool and Primary Scale of Intelligence—Revised (Wechsler, 1989). For assessing mental processes, the K-ABC seems far superior to other measures of intelligence, since it is far less dependent on prior learning and exposure to the mainstream Anglo culture (e.g., see Kamphaus & Reynolds, 1987). When one is assessing the intellectual processes of non-native English speakers, the independence of the K-ABC mental processing scales is particularly important, so as not to confound cultural experiences and cultural dependence of test items with neuropsychological processing (e.g., see Ardila, Roselli, & Puente, 1994). A growing body of literature shows the appropriateness of the K-ABC across a broad range of U.S. ethnic minorities.

Support for use of the K-ABC in the context of neuropsychological assessment also comes from a variety of sources in cerebral specialization research. In a comprehensive review of research concerning the lateralization of human brain functions, Dean (1984) concluded that the K-ABC is well suited to clinical use and in research with children.

It has been proposed that sequential processing and simultaneous processing are lateralized to the left and right hemispheres, respectively (e.g., Reynolds, 1981a). Many other dichotomies have been suggested. Some find the research on cerebral specialization difficult to coalesce. Indeed, the many seeming contradictions in the results of cerebral specialization studies have prompted at least one pair of leading researchers to remark: "[To] say that the field of hemispheric specialization is in a state of disarray and that the results are difficult to interpret is an understatement. The field can best be characterized as chaotic" (Tomlinson-Keasey & Clarkson-Smith, 1980, p. 1). On the other hand, reviews by Dean (1984) and Reynolds (1981b) have noted some consistencies, especially when one focuses on process specificity and not the content of the task stimulus.

For the vast majority of individuals, the left cerebral hemisphere appears to be specialized for linguistic, propositional, serial, and analytic tasks, and the right hemisphere for more nonverbal, oppositional, synthetic, and holistic tasks. The literature includes a large number of studies of hemispheric specialization that have attempted to provide anatomical localization of performance on specific, yet higher-order, complex tasks. Much of the confusion in the literature stems from the apparently conflicting data of many of these studies. However, Luria's principle of dynamic functional localization, and the knowledge that any specific task can potentially be performed through any of the brain's processing modes, should give some insight into the conflicting results that appear in the literature. In this regard, it is most important to remember that cerebral hemispheric asymmetries of function are process-specific and not stimulus-specific. Shure and Halstead (1959) noted early in this line of research that manipulation of stimuli is at the root of hemispheric differences—a notion that is well supported by current empirical research (e.g., Ornstein, Johnstone, Herron, & Swencionis, 1980) and thought (e.g., Reynolds, 1981a, 1981b). The confusion of the content and sensory modality through which stimuli are presented with the process by which they are manipulated, particularly in the secondary and tertiary regions of each lobe of the neocortex, seems to be at the root of the chaos. How information is manipulated while in the brain is not dependent on its modality of presentation and not necessarily dependent on its content, though the latter may certainly be influential. The variations in content and in method of presentation of the tasks that make up the three scales of the K-ABC allow one to tease out any modality or content effects that may nevertheless occur for a specific child, though clearly the emphasis of the K-ABC is on process, not content.

We think that a process-oriented explanation provides a better organizing principle than does a focus on content. The "content-driven" attempts at explaining hemispheric differences fail to recognize the possibilities for processing any given set of stimuli or particular content in a variety of processing modes. Bever (1975) emphasized this point and elaborated on two modes of information processing that are of interest here because of their similarity to simultaneous and sequential cognitive processes.

The K-ABC also taps most of the functions identified by Dean (1984) in his review of the literature on cerebral specialization, with the exceptions of depth, haptic, and melodic perceptions. These skills are assessed by other traditional neuropsychological batteries, although such tasks are virtually nonexistent for the very young child. Careful observation may still provide insight into neuropsychological processing deficits, especially if one pays particular attention to the manner in which errors are made. Qualitative and quantitative data are complementary, not interchangeable; Kaufman's (1994) philosophy of "intelligent testing" is just as crucial to neuropsychological assessment as to any other area of clinical evaluation.

The Luria–Nebraska Neuropsychological Battery– Children's Revision

The LNNB-CR (Golden, 1986) is a downward extension of the Luria–Nebraska Neuropsychological Battery for adults. Originally, in its research form, it was administered down to age 5, but reliable performance could only be obtained beginning at age 8 (Golden, 1997). After age 12, the adult battery is used.

There are 11 scales on the LNNB-CR, and each is listed and described in Table 2.8. As Golden (1997) describes, the LNNB-CR lends itself to three levels of interpretation: scale, item, and qualitative. Each of the 11 scales yields a T-score, and the resulting profile has been the subject of significant empirical work. However, the items within these scales vary in modality and other demand characteristics, and an analysis of item scores is also used. Finally, Luria was a renowned clinician and approached patients individually; Golden (1986) thus designed the LNNB-CR to allow qualitative analysis as a supplement to the typical Western psychological approach of quantitative analysis of performance on the various scales. As Table 2.8 indicates, the LNNB-CR has some scales and items where process is the dominant feature, but others where content and learned behavior predominate. Careful review of LNNB-CR performance at all three levels (scale, item, and qualitative) is not just possible but necessary. In a qualitative analysis, an examiner is more concerned with wrong answers than with correct ones and analyzes the nature of the errors committed by the examinee. For example, was the inability to write to dictation caused by

TABLE 2.8. Scales of Luria–Nebraska Neuropsychological Battery—Children's Revision (Ages 8–12)

Scales	Description of abilities assessed
Motor Skills	Motor speed, complex coordination, imitation of motor movements, constructional praxis
Rhythm	Attention, perceiving and repeating rhythmic patterns, analyzing groups of tones
Tactile	Finger localization, arm localization, two-point discrimination, movement discrimination, shape discrimination, stereognosis, verbal–tactile integration
Visual	Visual recognition, visual discrimination, spatial perception
Receptive Speech	Following simple commands, comprehending verbal directions, decoding phonemes, naming
Expressive Language	Reading and repeating words and simple sentences, naming object from description, using automated speech, discerning missing words
Writing	Analyzing letter sequences, spelling, writing from dictation, copying
Reading	Letter and word calling, sentence and paragraph reading, nonsense syllable reading
Arithmetic	Simple calculation, number writing, number recognition (Arabic and Roman)
Memory	Verbal and visual memory, some interference tasks
Intelligence	Vocabulary, verbal reasoning, picture interpretation, social reasoning, deduction, scanning

a visual–motor problem, a visual–perceptive deficit, a failure of comprehension, or a planning, attention, or execution problem? Only through careful observation and a review of successful tasks can these questions be answered. Examiners must have extensive experience with normal individuals, however, to avoid overinterpretation. This process of interpretation at multiple levels continues to be consistent with Kaufman's (1979, 1994) philosophy of "intelligent testing" and is advisable for use with all assessment devices discussed herein. However, the LNNB-CR was devised with these approaches in mind, making it more amenable to multilevel analysis. A revision of the LNNB-CR is underway that is intended to expand the scale from its currently very limited age range, extending it downward to age 5 years. This will certainly make the battery more useful for children with various neurodevelopmental disorders.

The Boston Process Approach

Another, newer effort at evaluating process in neuropsychological assessment is known as the Boston Process Approach (BPA) and is described in detail in Kaplan (1988, 1990). This model also tries to integrate quantitative and qualitative approaches to interpretation and analysis of performance on various cognitive tasks. The BPA alters the format of items on traditional tests such as the various Wechsler scales, and BPA versions of the Wechsler Intelligence Scale for Children—III and the Wechsler Adult Intelligence Scale—III are available. Additional, supplementary tests have been devised specifically for the BPA over many years, including the Boston Naming Test, the Boston Diagnostic Aphasia Examination, and the California Verbal Learning Test, along with others. As with other methods of assessment, examiners are advised to use BPA assessments in conjunction with history and interview data and observations of the patient.

The strength of the BPA lies in its flexibility, which enables a neuropsychologist to tailor the assessment to the referred problem. There is quite a bit of research on individual aspects of the BPA (e.g., see White & Rose, 1997), but research on the BPA as a whole is lacking. The modifications made to well-designed, carefully standardized tests such as the Wechsler scales also have unpredictable and at times counterintuitive outcomes in patient examination (e.g., Slick et al., 1996). Slick et al. (1996) found that changes made to the BPA version of the Wechsler Adult Intelligence Scale—Revised caused a substantial number of individuals to earn lower scores on the modified items than on the corresponding standardized versions of the items, even though the intent of the modification was in part to make the items easier. This could easily draw a clinician into overinterpretation and overdiagnosis of pathology. Slick et al. (1996) correctly conclude that whenever changes are made to standardized instruments, comprehensive norms are required under the new testing conditions. They also conclude that clinical interpretation of such modified procedures prior to the development and purveyance of the norms is questionable from an ethical standpoint.

The lack of good normative or reference data has been a long-term problem for neuropsychological assessment (e.g., see Reynolds, 1997). This causes a variety of problems related to test interpretation, not the least of which is understanding the relationship of status variables such as gender, ethnicity, and socioeconomic status to test performance. The BPA, because of its principal strengths, also makes inordinate cognitive demands on the examiner. Until the normative and data integration problems of BPA are solved, it is recommended here primarily only as a research approach (albeit a most promising one). It may be useful now, but only to a small group of clinicians with extensive, supervised training in its use from one of its progenitors.

CONCLUDING REMARKS

There are many methods and models of neuropsychological assessment. The field of pediatric neuropsychology is young as clinical disciplines go. Controversies continue over the training and credentialing of neuropsychologists as well. However, the field has proven itself to be of value in contributing to patient care, and thereby it will continue to grow and even thrive. Clinicians must recognize that patient care is the ultimate goal and must provide carefully integrated, treatment-relevant data. A clinician writing a report on a child's neuropsychological examination should pay particular attention to the following suggestions:

1. *Write reports that go beyond a simple descriptive presentation of test data and findings.* A clinician should integrate data across the history and across data sources. Data should be interpreted for the reader.

2. *Write professionally.* A clinician should use proper grammar and formal language structures in presenting reports.

3. *Use language that is easily understood.* Reports on children will be used in many arenas, and writing a child's neuropsychological report in such a way as to be interpretable only by a physician or another neuropsychologist does not facilitate treatment. The report of the neuropsychologist is of no value if it cannot be understood. Reports should be cognitively accessible to school personnel (including teachers, counselors, and school psychologists), rehabilitation staff (e.g., occupational therapists, speech therapists, physical therapists), and parents, in addition to referring physicians.

4. *Write reports about children, not about tests.* Too often the neuropsychological evaluation of a child reads like a test recital (i.e., test after test is presented, and the child's performance is noted). No data integration is attempted, and it is common to find contradictory statements in such rote reports. Parents often interpret such impersonal reports as lacking in concern or interest for their child.

5. *Draw diagnostic conclusions.* Whenever possible, the examining clinician should proffer a diagnostic summary for consideration of other sources. Diagnosis is treatment-relevant and should be noted.

6. *Describe treatment implications of neuropsychological findings.* Although no one clinician can reasonably be expected to know all treatment implications of a set of findings, clinicians should note, to the extent of their knowledge, treatment implications of the findings of their own examinations. Neuropsychological results may indicate a need for specific interventions (e.g., neurocognitive therapy, speech therapy) or for specific methods of intervention within a known class (e.g., reading instruction via phonics vs. whole language, inefficacy of certain behavior therapies in the face of particular neuropsychological findings).

Neuropsychologists have much of value to offer in the care of children with neuro-developmental disorders. Data and recommendations related to symptom expressivity, new problems, effectiveness of treatment, and possible behavioral interventions are some of their most valuable offerings. In this age of cost containment, it is crucial to provide useful, scientifically supported conclusions that contribute to treatment and other facets of patient care, and to maximize the benefit of the neuropsychological examination for the child.

REFERENCES

Adams, K. (1985). Review of the Luria–Nebraska Neuropsychological Battery. In J. V. Mitchell (Ed.), *Ninth mental measurements yearbook*. Lincoln, NE: Buros Institute of Mental Measurement.

Ardila, A., Roselli, M., & Puente, A. (1994). *Neuropsychological evaluation of the Spanish-speaker*. New York: Plenum Press.

Bayley, N. (1969). *Bayley Scales of Infant Development*. New York: Psychological Corporation.

Bever, T. G. (1975). Cerebral asymmetries in humans are due to the differentiation of two incompatible processes: Holistic and analytic. In D. Aronson & R. Reiber (Eds.), *Developmental psycholinguistics and communication disorders*. New York: New York Academy of Sciences.

Bigler, E. D. (1996). Bridging the gap between psychology and neurology: Future trends in pediatric neuropsychology. In E. S. Batchelor, Jr., & R. S. Dean (Eds.), *Pediatric neuropsychology* (pp. 27–54). Needham Heights, MA: Allyn & Bacon.

Cohen, R. A. (1993). *The neuropsychology of attention*. New York: Plenum Press.

Cohen, S. B. (1991). Adapting educational programs for students with head injuries. *Journal of Head Trauma Rehabilitation*, 6(1), 47–55.

Das, J. P., Kirby, J. R., & Jarman, R. F. (1979). *Simultaneous and successive cognitive processes*. New York: Academic Press.

Dean, R. S. (1984). Functional lateralization of the brain. *Journal of Special Education*, 8, 239–256.

Dean, R. S. (1985). Foundation and rationale for neuropsychological bases of individual differences. In L. Hartlage & K. Telzrow (Eds.), *Neuropsychology of individual differences* (pp. 7–39). New York: Plenum Press.

Diamond, M. C. (1990). Morphological cortical changes as a consequence of learning and experience. In A. B. Scheibel & A. F. Wechsler (Eds.), *Neurobiology of higher cognitive function* (pp. 1–12). New York: Guilford Press.

Farmer, J. E., & Peterson, L. (1995). Pediatric traumatic brain injury: Promoting successful school reentry. *School Psychology Review, 24*(2), 230–243.

Ferris, L. M., & Kamphaus, R. W. (1996). Review of the Test of Memory and Learning. *Archives of Clinical Neuropsychology, 11,* 251–256.

Gillberg, C. (1995). *Clinical child neuropsychiatry.* Cambridge, England: Cambridge University Press.

Golden, C. J. (1986). *Manual for the Luria–Nebraska Neuropsychological Battery—Children's Revision.* Los Angeles: Western Psychological Services.

Golden, C. J. (1997). The Nebraska–Neuropsychological Children's Battery. In C. R. Reynolds & E. Fletcher-Janzen (Eds.), *Handbook of clinical child neuropsychology* (2nd ed., pp. 237–251. New York: Plenum Press.

Grant, I., & Adams, K. M. (Eds.). (1986). *Neuropsychological assessment of neuropsychiatric disorders* (2nd ed.). New York: Oxford University Press.

Hartlage, L. C., & Reynolds, C. R. (1981). Neuropsychological assessment and the individualization of instruction. *Neuropsychological assessment and the school-aged child* (pp. 355–378). New York: Grune & Stratton.

Kamphaus, R. W., & Reynolds, C. R. (1987). *Clinical and research applications of the K-ABC.* Circle Pines, MN: American Guidance Service.

Kaplan, E. (1988). A process approach to neuropsychological assessment. In T. Boll & B. K. Bryant (Eds.), *Clinical neuropsychology and brain function: Research, measurement, and practice.* Washington, DC: American Psychological Association.

Kaplan, E. (1990). The process approach to neuropsychological assessment of psychiatric patients. *Journal of Neuropsychiatry, 2*(1), 72–87.

Kaplan, E. (1996). *Discussant.* Symposium on assessment of children's memory at the annual meeting of the National Association of School Psychologists, Atlanta, GA.

Kaufman, A. S. (1979). *Intelligent testing with the WISC-R.* New York: Wiley-Interscience.

Kaufman, A. S. (1994). *Intelligent testing with the WISC-III.* New York: Wiley-Interscience.

Kaufman, A. S., Kamphaus, R. W., & Kaufman, N. L. (1985). The Kaufman Assessment Battery for Children: K-ABC. In C. S. Newark (Ed.), *Major psychological assessment instruments.* Boston: Allyn & Bacon.

Kaufman, A. S., & Kaufman, N. L. (1983a). *Kaufman Assessment Battery for Children.* Circle Pines, MN: American Guidance Service.

Kaufman, A. S., & Kaufman, N. L. (1983b). *K-ABC interpretation manual.* Circle Pines, MN: American Guidance Service.

Knight, R. G. (1992). *The neuropsychology of degenerative brain diseases.* Hillsdale, NJ: Erlbaum.

Lezak, M. D. (1995). *Neuropsychological assessment* (3rd ed.). New York: Oxford University Press.

Luria, A. R. (1966). *Human brain and psychological processes.* New York: Harper & Row.

Majovski, L. (1984). The K-ABC: Theory and applications for child neuropsychological assessment and research. *Journal of Special Education, 18,* 266–268.

Nebes, R. D. (1974). Hemispheric specialization in commisurotomized man. *Psychological Bulletin, 81,* 1–14.

Neisser, V. (1967). *Cognitive psychology.* New York: Appleton-Century-Crofts.

Nussbaum, N. L., & Bigler, E. D. (1989). Halstead–Reitan Neuropsychological Test Batteries for Children. In C. R. Reynolds & E. Fletcher-Janzen (Eds.), *Handbook of clinical child neuropsychology* (pp. 181–192). New York: Plenum Press.

Ornstein, R., Johnstone, J., Herron, J., & Swiencionis, C. (1980). Differential right hemisphere engagement in visuospatial tasks. *Neuropsychologia, 18,* 49–64.

Reitan, R. M., & Wolfson, D. (1974). *Clinical neuropsychology: Current status and applications.* Washington, DC: Winston.

Reitan, R. M., & Wolfson, D. (1985). *The Halstead–Reitan Neuropsychological Battery: Theory and clinical interpretation.* Tucson, AZ: Neuropsychological Press.

Reynolds, C. R. (1981a). The neuropsychological basis of intelligence. In G. Hynd & J. Obrzut (Eds.), *Neuropsychological assessment and the school-aged child* (pp. 87–124). New York: Grune & Stratton.

Reynolds, C. R. (1981b). Neuropsychological assessment and the habilitation of learning: Considerations in the search for the aptitude × treatment interaction. *School Psychology Review, 10,* 343–349.

Reynolds, C. R. (1997). Measurement and statistical problems in neuropsychological assessment of children. In C. R. Reynolds & E. Fletcher-Janzen (Eds.), *Handbook of clinical child neuropsychology* (2nd ed., pp. 180–203). New York: Plenum Press.

Reynolds, C. R., & Bigler, E. D. (1994). *Manual for the Test of Memory and Learning.* Austin, TX: PRO-ED.

Reynolds, C. R., & Bigler, E. D. (1996). Factor structure, factor indexes, and other useful statistics for interpretation of the Test of Memory and Learning. *Archives of Clinical Neuropsychology, 11,* 29–43.

Reynolds, C. R., & Bigler, E. D. (1997). Clinical neuropsychological assessment of child and adolescent memory with the Test of Memory and Learning. In C. R. Reynolds & E. Fletcher-Janzen (Eds.), *Handbook of clinical child neuropsychology* (2nd ed., pp. 296–319). New York: Plenum Press.

Reynolds, C. R., & Hickman, J. A. (1987). Remediation, deficit-centered models of. In C. R. Reynolds & L. Mann (Eds.), *Encyclopedia of special education* (pp. 1339–1342). New York: Wiley-Interscience.

Reynolds, C. R., & Kamphaus, R. W. (1992). *Behavior Assessment System for Children.* Circle Pines, MN: American Guidance Service.

Reynolds, C. R., & Kamphaus, R. W. (1997). The Kaufman Assessment Battery for Children: Development, structure, and applications in neuropsychology. In A. Horton, D. Wedding, & J. Webster (Eds.), *The neuropsychology handbook* (2nd ed., Vol. 1, pp. 291–330). New York: Springer.

Reynolds, C. R., Kamphaus, R. W., Rosenthal, B., & Hiemenz, J. (1997). Applications of the Kaufman Assessment Battery for Children (K-ABC) in neuropsychological assessment. In C. R. Reynolds & E. Fletcher-Janzen (Eds.), *Handbook of clinical child neuropsychology* (2nd ed., pp. 252–269). New York: Plenum Press.

Riccio, C. A., & Reynolds, C. R. (1998). Neuropsychological assessment of children. In M. Hersen & A. Bellack (Series Eds.) & C. R. Reynolds (Vol. Ed.), *Comprehensive clinical psychology: Vol. 4. Assessment* (pp. 267–302). New York: Elsevier Science.

Rourke, B. P., Bakker, D. J., Fisk, J. L., & Strang, J. D. (1983). *Child neuropsychology.* New York: Guilford Press.

Scheibel, A. B. (1990). Dendritic correlates of higher cortical function. In A. Scheibel & A. Wechsler (Eds.), *Neurobiology of higher cognitive function* (pp. 239–270). New York: Guilford Press.

Sechenov, I. (1965). *Reflexes of the brain.* Cambridge, MA: MIT Press. (Original work published 1863)

Sheslow, W., & Adams, W. (1990). *Wide Range Assessment of Memory and Learning.* Wilmington, DE: Jastak Associates.

Shure, G. H., & Halstead, W. (1959). Cerebral lateralization of individual processes. *Psychological Monographs: General and Applied, 72*(12).

Slick, D., Hopp, G., Strauss, E., Fox, D., Pinch, D., & Stickgold, K. (1996). Effects of prior testing with the WAIS-R NI on subsequent retest with the WAIS-R. *Archives of Clinical Neuropsychology, 11*(2), 123–130.

Spreen, O., & Strauss, E. (1991). *A compendium of neuropsychological tests.* London: Oxford University Press.

Teeter, P. A., & Semrud-Clikeman, M. (1997). *Child neuropsychology: Assessment and intervention for neurodevelopmental disorders.* Needham Heights, MA: Allyn & Bacon.

Telzrow, C. F. (1989). Neuropsychological applications of common educational and psychological tests. In C. R. Reynolds & E. Fletcher-Janzen (Eds.), *Handbook of clinical child neuropsychology* (pp. 227–246). New York: Plenum Press.

Tomlinson-Keasey, C., & Clarkson-Smith, L. (1980). *What develops in hemispheric specialization?* Paper presented at the annual meeting of the International Neuropsychological Society, San Francisco.

Vygotsky, L. S. (1978). *Mind in society.* Cambridge, MA: Harvard University Press.

Warzak, W. J., Mayfield, J. W., & McAllister, C. (1996, November). *Integrating neuropsychological and behavioral data to develop comprehensive assessment strategies in brain injured individuals.* Paper presented at the 30th Annual Convention of the Association for Advancement of Behavior Therapy, New York.

Wechsler, D. (1989). *Wechsler Preschool and Primary Scale of Intelligence—Revised.* San Antonio, TX: Psychological Corporation.

White, R. F., & Rose, F. E. (1997). The Boston Process Approach: A brief history and current practice. In G. Goldstein & T. Incagnoli (Eds.), *Contemporary approaches to neuropsychological assessment* (pp. 171–212). New York: Plenum Press.

3

NEUROBEHAVIORAL DISORDERS AND MEDICAL GENETICS

An Overview

JOHN C. CAREY
WILLIAM M. McMAHON

The entrance of the discipline of medical genetics into the care of children with neuro-developmental disorders is a relatively recent but highly significant event. The application of the principles of genetics to medicine in general is crucial, because of the important role of genes in the causation of human developmental disorders: About one-third of children with developmental disabilities have a congenital malformation or other genetic condition as the primary etiology of the problem. Moreover, at least 50% of sensory disabilities are caused by genetic mechanisms (Carey, 1997). In addition, a precise diagnosis of a genetic condition or syndrome is of importance to a child, a family, and the practitioner caring for the child. Parents of children with disabilities and differences of any sort frequently ask questions about the risk of a disorder's occurring again in future pregnancies.

Medical genetics has only recently emerged as a bona fide specialty in medicine. In the 1960s, the fields of biochemical genetics, clinical cytogenetics, and dysmorphology developed and paved the way for the delineation of this discipline. Now, with the recently publicized advances in the mapping and cloning of human disease genes, interest about genetics and its roles in human disorders is commonplace; indeed, these have become topics of everyday conversations. The purpose of this chapter is to summarize the body of knowledge and principles of medical genetics needed for the discussion of the neurobehavioral disorders presented in this book. This review will ideally provide a foundation in genetic science for all readers, regardless of their professional or personal background. The first section of the chapter provides an overview of basic concepts in medical genetics. The second section is a primer of the principles of medical genetics. The chapter closes with a brief discussion of the concept of behavioral phenotypes in dysmorphic syndromes.

BASIC CONCEPTS IN MEDICAL GENETICS

Genomic Structure

The influence of genetics as we know it today is primarily the result of research accomplished during this past century. The basic foundation of the field of genetics is the understanding of genomic structure. The "genome" is the term applied to the total complement of deoxyribonucleic acid (DNA). DNA molecules are organized into 50,000–100,000 functional units, which are called "genes." Alterations in these genes, either alone or in combination with alterations in other genes, can produce the diseases that we call "genetic disorders." From a molecular point of view, genes are simply defined functional strips of DNA. They are clumped together in orderly arrangements in the cell, in a microscopically visible set of structures called "chromosomes." The basic biology of DNA and chromosomes was established in the 1950s and 1960s. Thus most of our knowledge of the molecular, chromosomal, and even biochemical basis of human disease has been acquired in just the latter half of the 20th century.

Each human cell, with the exception of the "gametes" (i.e., sperm or egg cells), contains 23 pairs of different chromosomes for a total of 46. One member of each pair is derived from an individual's father, while the other is derived from the mother. One pair of chromosomes is designated as sex chromosomes and consists of what is called "XX" in a female and "XY" in a male. The remaining 22 pairs of chromosomes are called "autosomes" and are numbered from 1 to 22. A gamete or germ cell is different from a somatic cell, in that it contains only one chromosome from each pair. The reader is referred to basic texts of biology and genetics that discuss cell division and meiosis in more detail (e.g., Jorde, Carey, & White, 1995).

Types of Genetic Disorders

Genetic disorders in humans are classified into several major groups:

1. *Chromosome disorders.* In these conditions, the entire chromosome (or segments of a chromosome) is missing or duplicated. They are divided into conditions of abnormal number and conditions of abnormal structure. Human chromosome disorders are defined simply by performing a "karyotype" (chromosome study) of a body tissue—usually blood, but almost any tissue in which cells can grow can be utilized. A number of disorders discussed in this text, including Down and Turner syndromes, have their biological basis as a disorder of human chromosomes. Some of the important concepts that relate to chromosome syndromes are discussed below.

2. *Monogenic (mendelian) conditions.* These are disorders in which a single gene or pair of genes contains a mutation (alteration of DNA structure) that is the primary cause of the disease. They are divided into "autosomal dominant," "autosomal recessive," and "X-linked" conditions. The term "mendelian" refers to Gregor Mendel, the 19th century scientist who established the basic laws of heredity in his study of pea plants.

3. *Multifactorial or polygenic disorders.* These are conditions caused by a combination of multiple effects, either multiple genes (hence the term "polygenic") or gene–environment interactions. Epidemiological and family studies indicate that there is a genetic basis for these conditions, but the conditions do not follow the simple, regular rules of inheritance established for single-gene disorders (Mendel's laws). Many human diseases fall into this less well-defined category. These include nonsyndromal congenital malformations, such

as cleft lip and neural tube defects, as well as several psychiatric disorders (e.g., schizophrenia and bipolar disorders). In this context, the genetic basis of human behavior has recently been reviewed (Sherman et al., 1997; Smalley, 1997).

4. *Mitochondrial disorders.* This nontraditional group of disorders includes a relatively small number of recently defined diseases caused by alterations of the small cytoplasmic mitochondrial chromosome.

For the purposes of this text, the chromosome and monogenic disorders as well as their principles are reviewed in some detail in this chapter. Although discussions of multifactorial and mitochondrial disorders are highly important in any review of genetic diseases, these groups are not covered in detail here. The reader is referred to recent texts of medical genetics for more detail on multifactorial and mitochondrial disorders (Jorde et al., 1995; Gehlerter & Collins, 1998; Thompson, McInnes, & Willard, 1991).

Table 3.1 summarizes the various types of human genetic disorders defined above, with examples in each category. This table also lists three other nontraditional forms of inheritance—"mosaicism," "genomic imprinting," and "anticipation," which are defined and discussed later in this chapter. All of the concepts in the table are discussed as well in the chapters on individual conditions.

Population Prevalence of Human Genetic Disorders

Although genetic disorders are often thought of as rare and exotic, these conditions constitute an important cause of human mortality and morbidity, especially in children. The most common causes of infant mortality as of the mid-1980s were congenital malformations, most of which have some genetic basis. By the 1970s, 50% of all deaths in childhood were found to be attributable to genetic causes (Jorde et al., 1995).

The calculation of incidence and prevalence figures for genetic disorders is very complex. Difficulties in establishing disease registries and standardization in diagnosis and recording practices make estimates difficult at best. Various investigations that have attempted to estimate the frequency of monogenic disorders, chromosome disorders, and congenital malformations derive figures of about 3–7% for the likelihood of an individual's developing one of these well-established genetic disorders during his or her lifetime. These figures, however, do not include cases of common adult diseases such as coronary artery disease, diabetes mellitus, and cancer, all of which have some genetic basis (Jorde et al., 1995). Moreover, most epidemiologists presently would not classify human disease as purely

TABLE 3.1. Types of Human Genetic Disorders

Inheritance	Exemplary disorders
Traditional	
Chromosome	Down syndrome, Turner syndrome
Monogenic/mendelian	Neurofibromatosis type 1, Lesch–Nyhan syndrome
Multifactorial/polygenic	Neural tube defects, schizophrenia
Nontraditional	
Mitochondrial	Kearns–Sayre syndrome
Mosaicism	Osteogenesis imperfecta, chromosome mosaicism
Genomic imprinting	Prader–Willi and Angelman syndromes
Anticipation	Fragile X syndrome, myotonic dystrophy

environmental/acquired or purely genetic. Rather, causation of human disease represents a continuum: At one end of the spectrum are those disorders that are strongly determined by genes, especially monogenic and chromosome disorders, while at the other end are those that are strongly determined by environment. However, there is now increasing evidence that many infectious diseases or even types of resistance to infectious diseases (e.g., resistance to HIV) have a genetic basis, and thus most diseases are multifactorial in the strict sense of the word.

Types of Genetic Services

With the development of medical genetics as a specialty in mainstream medicine, clinical genetic services have become an integral part of the health care delivery system in North America and Europe. Most university medical centers in the Western Hemisphere have a program or clinic in genetics. The major objective of clinical genetic programs is to provide genetic diagnosis and counseling services for the referred patient population.

The cornerstone of medical genetics is the art and science of genetic counseling. Although the term "counseling" implies that this service is in the domain of mental health or psychotherapy, genetic counseling in fact is a marriage of human genetics and behavioral science. In 1975, the American Society of Human Genetics adopted a definition that was proposed by an assigned working group. This definition, which has basically stood the test of time, is as follows:

> Genetic counseling is a communication process which deals with the human problems associated with the occurrence, or the risk of occurrence, of a genetic disorder in a family. This process involves an attempt by one or more appropriately trained persons to help the individual or family to: (1) comprehend the medical facts including the diagnosis, probable cause of the disorder, and available management; (2) appreciate the way heredity contributes to the disorder and the risk of occurrence in specified relatives; (3) understand alternatives for dealing with the risk of reoccurrence; (4) choose a course of action which seems to them appropriate in the view of their risk, their family goals, and the standards and act in accordance with that decision, and (5) make the best possible adjustments to the disorder in the affected family member and/or to the risk of the occurrence of that disorder. (Ad Hoc Committee on Genetic Counseling, 1975, p. 241)

This well-established definition illustrates the complex tasks presented to the practitioner of medical genetics. The first task involves establishing the diagnosis and discussing the natural history and management of the disorder in question. The second task requires an understanding of the basic tenets of medical genetics. The third and fourth objectives of the genetic counseling process underlie the primary differentiation between the genetic model suggested here and the traditional biomedical approach. Here the tasks involve a discussion of reproductive options and a facilitation of decision making, respectively. Implicit in the definition is the notion of respect for the family members' autonomy and for their perception of the risk. This approach is often different from the traditional medical approach, which often has recommendations as its basic theme. The final task of the genetic counseling process involves helping the family cope with the condition, its impact, and its potential heritability.

The practice of clinical genetics actually involves a diverse array of services. As mentioned above, a genetic program or clinic provides diagnosis, management, genetic counseling, and consultation. These occur in a variety of settings, including university outpatient clinics, community clinics, hospital wards, and specialty clinics, often with a multidisciplinary team approach. For example, medical geneticists are often involved in organizing or coordinating team clinics for such disorders as craniofacial malformations, neurofibromatosis, and spina bifida. Genetic services also include prenatal screening, which is presently done in conjunction with obstetricians and perinatologists. Moreover, genetic practitioners are closely involved with the development, orchestration, and delivery of genetic screening programs, which serve prenatal, neonatal, and general populations. The various types of clinical genetic services are discussed in detail elsewhere (Rimoin, Connor, & Pyeritz, 1996)

One of the hallmarks of evaluation in a clinical genetic setting is the documentation of the family history. It is now considered standard for practitioners evaluating a child with a potential genetic disorder to construct an accurate family history and place it in the patient's chart. This is usually done as a drawing called a "pedigree." The reader is referred to any standard medical text for reference on symbols used in the construction of a pedigree and the actual mechanics of documenting this important data set. (See also Figures 3.4 and 3.5, below.)

PRINCIPLES OF MEDICAL GENETICS: A PRIMER

In this section, the basic principles of medical genetics required to understand the biological basis of the syndromes described in this book are summarized. Our goal here is not to provide a comprehensive summary of the science, but rather to highlight the important points. The key terms important in clinical discussion of these genetic disorders are emphasized throughout the discussion (see also Jorde et al., 1995, and Rimoin et al., 1996).

Chromosome Disorders

Figure 3.1 is a standard karyotype, showing the chromosome arrangement of a normal female. Note that the chromosomes are paired and numbered from 1 to 22. There are stripes on each chromosome, which are called "bands." A system for the numbering of bands on the various chromosomes has been established in the field of cytogenetics. Each chromosome is lined up in a standard way, with the central constriction (called a "centromere") representing a landmark. The shorter of the two longitudinal chromosome "arms" is called the "p arm," and the longer one is called the "q arm." In a chromosome such as 1, 2, or 3, where the centromere is just about in the middle of the chromosome, the standards committee has decided which of the two arms should be called the p and the q. Different groupings of the chromosomes vary according to the size and location of the centromere. Thus, chromosomes 1 through 3 have a centrally placed centromere (called "metacentric"), while chromosomes 4 and 5 have a submetacentric construction. Details of the banding/numbering system are not discussed here and are available in all genetic texts. Figure 3.2 shows two chromosome diagrams and their designated bands.

Most chromosomal studies done in a clinical setting utilize a "Giemsa-banding" or "G-banding" technique. The average number of bands on all 23 pairs of chromosomes in a standard chromosome study will be about 450. In a more recently developed technique called "high-resolution banding," the process stops the cell in an early part of the cell cycle and allows for more stretched-out chromosomes, and thus for more bands. This particular technique is more time-intensive, and decisions about size and missing or extra pieces require more study. Suffice it to say, however, that high-resolution banding techniques do

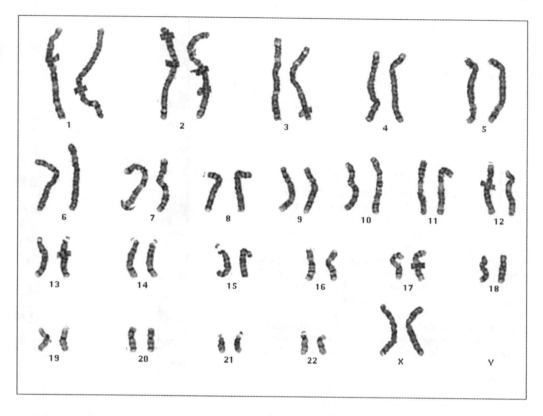

FIGURE 3.1. A standard G-banded karyotype of a normal (XX) female. Note that there are 23 pairs of chromosomes arranged in a specific, orderly array. The autosomes are numbered from 1 through 22, and the sex chromosomes are conventionally placed at the bottom right-hand portion of the karyotype. The individual pattern of G-bands determines the chromosome. (Courtesy of Dr. Art Brothman, University of Utah Health Science Center.)

allow for the recognition of more subtle chromosome disorders. This is the technique that allowed a cytogeneticist in the early 1980s to recognize that some patients with Prader–Willi syndrome had a subtle but definite missing piece (deletion) of the upper most band on the long arm of chromosome 15 (15q, the band called q11–13). However, high-resolution banding was not sensitive enough to pick up the recently recognized deletion seen in individuals with Williams syndrome. In this situation, the diagnosis of the characteristic deletion of Williams syndrome requires a newer technique using DNA fluorescent probes, called "fluorescent *in situ* hybridization" (FISH). This technique is of significance because it is now the technique of choice for detecting the subtle deletions of Prader–Willi, Angelman, Williams, and velocardiofacial/DiGeorge syndromes. Also, it is sometimes utilized to pick up more subtle submicroscopic deletions in relatively well-known deletion syndromes, such as 5p or 4p deletion. Figure 3.3 is a black-and-white photograph of FISH in a patient with the 4p deletion (also known as Wolf–Hirschhorn syndrome). This important condition is a common autosomal disorder in humans.

As mentioned above, chromosome disorders can be divided into disorders of chromosome number and structure. Disorders of chromosome number (also called "aneuploidy") are those conditions in which there is either an entirely extra chromosome or a missing

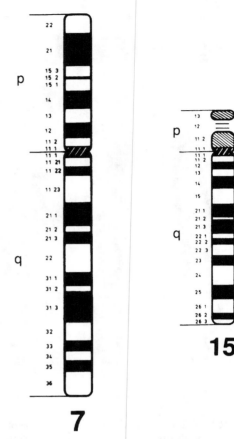

FIGURE 3.2. A standard diagram of banding patterns in chromosomes 7 and 14, two important chromosomes for neurobehavioral disorders. Chromosome 7 is a typical "metacentric" chromosome (i.e., the centromere is located right in the middle). The banding pattern above this is called the "short arm" or "p arm"; the pattern below this is called the "long arm" or "q arm." This is determined by convention. Chromosome 15 is called an "acrocentric" chromosome, because the centromere is near the designated top and the short arm contains what is called the "satellite material." Note on both chromosomes that the band numbers move consecutively away from the centromere. Note also that the chromosome arms are divided broadly into segments and then into the individual bands. They are numbered by segment and then by band; the band that is deleted in the Prader–Willi syndrome is the 15q11–13. (Courtesy of Dr. Art Brothman, University of Utah Health Science Center.)

chromosome. Down syndrome, or trisomy 21, involves the presence of an extra chromosome 21 (usually the entire chromosome) and represents the prototypical chromosome condition of abnormal number (see Cody & Kamphaus, Chapter 17, this volume). Turner syndrome, which is monosomy X, and Klinefelter syndrome, or 47,XXY, represent other disorders of abnormal chromosomal number (see Powell & Schulte, Chapter 11, and Cody & Hynd, Chapter 18, this volume).

Disorders of abnormal structure involve conditions where a segment of a chromosome is either missing (deletion) or extra (duplication). The terms "partial monosomy" and "partial trisomy," respectively, are also utilized. The most common deletion syndromes include 5p deletion (also known as *cri du chat* syndrome), 4p deletion (Wolf–Hirschhorn syndrome), and 18q deletion. Note here that the letter p or q refers to the fact that the deletion is of that particular chromosomal arm. Using that designation, however, does not tell one where the actual deletion is; the banding number is also needed. A more comprehensive discussion of chromosome biology is available in most textbooks of human and medical genetics.

In the 1980s, as noted above, a number of chromosome deletion syndromes involving very subtle deletions were described. These have come to be known as the "microdeletion" syndromes. Prader–Willi, Angelman, and Williams syndromes all fall into this category. Because the deletions are subtle and are thought to affect a potentially definable cluster of neighboring genes, the microdeletion syndromes are sometimes referred to as "contiguous-

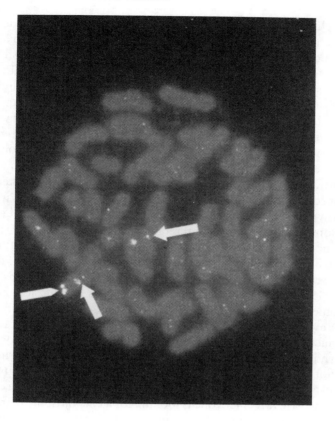

FIGURE 3.3. An abnormal FISH study of a girl who has the 4p deletion. The two 4 chromosomes are lined up next to each other. The normal one shows two signals, while the other chromosome is missing a DNA signal. Thus there is a missing piece of DNA in the critical region consistent with this syndrome. From Jorde, Carey, and White (1995). Copyright 1995 by C. V. Mosby and Year Book Medical Publishers. Reprinted by permission.

gene syndromes." (Prader–Willi and Angelman syndromes are discussed further in the section below on nontraditional inheritance.)

From a clinical point of view, chromosome disorders are associated with characteristic syndromes. In each of these conditions, there is a recognizable and relatively reproducible pattern of physical manifestations, minor anomalies, and sometimes major congenital malformations, often consistent enough to be recognized by the experienced clinician. The syndrome thus represents the "phenotype," or the manifestations that we actually observe physically or clinically. The concept of phenotype is contrasted with the term "genotype," which refers to the individual's genetic constitution. For example, the phenotype in the Down syndrome is the constellation of physical findings first described recognized by Dr. J. Langdon Down; the genotype is the chromosomal constitution of 47,XY +21. (About 90–95% of persons with Down syndrome have the chromosomal finding of trisomy 21, while the remaining 5–10% have other structural changes; see Cody & Kamphaus, Chapter 17.) The concept of the syndrome and the usefulness of minor anomalies of structure in the diagnosis of syndromes, especially in the neurobehavioral setting, are discussed in more detail later.

One of the clinical decisions that often confronts the practitioner is the question of when to order a chromosome study. The most common reason for such a study is to confirm the presence of a well-established chromosome syndrome, such as Down or Turner syndrome. Since autosomal chromosome disorders produce syndromal patterns of multiple anomalies, usually with psychomotor retardation, a karyotype is indicated in a person who has this type of clinical picture. Thus, in the evaluation of an individual with developmental delay or mental retardation, a chromosome study is obviously indicated when a child has multiple major and minor anomalies or features different from those of his or her family background. The question of doing a karyotype in a person who has mental retardation or developmental delay without dysmorphic signs or minor anomalies is somewhat more controversial. However, since the dysmorphic features can often be quite subtle even in established syndromes (e.g., 5p deletion/*cri du chat* syndrome and 17p deletion/Smith–Magenis syndrome), most geneticists seriously consider doing a karyotype for any child with developmental delay or mental retardation (Curry et al., 1997). In more recent years, many clinicians in the field have also considered doing a karyotype for any child with autism who has no associated medical diagnosis. This is because of the recent recognition of the inverted duplication 15 syndrome, where the clinical signs are quite subtle (Battaglia et al., 1997). The yield of chromosome studies looking for this finding or for other chromosome disorders in large populations of children with autism with no medical diagnosis is not available. Certainly this testing can be pursued on a case-by-case basis. Also of importance in ordering a karyotype, when one is considering one of the specific microdeletion syndromes (i.e., Prader–Willi, Angelman, Williams, or Shprintzen syndrome), is the fact that not only high-resolution banding but also FISH is warranted.

Another reason for a chromosome study is to study a parent when a child has a disorder of chromosome structure. Here one is looking for a chromosome rearrangement (e.g., translocation). There are a number of other indications for performing chromosome studies that are not as relevant to the neurodevelopmental arena and are not discussed in detail here; these include recurrent miscarriages, an undiagnosed stillborn infant, concern about one of the chromosomal instability syndromes, and diagnosis of certain malignancies. Again, comprehensive discussions of these indications are available in the texts cited earlier in the chapter.

Monogenic Disorders

Monogenic disorders are those conditions resulting from a mutation, either as a single copy or as a double copy of a gene. Prior to the 1980s, the notion of a monogenic disorder was really one that involved simply an assumption. Now that the genes for over 1,000 human disorders have been mapped to a chromosomal location, or in many cases identified (cloned), the notion of the gene is no longer a theoretical construct. Some elements of this relatively new DNA technology are discussed later.

Monogenic disorders, also known as mendelian conditions, can be divided into autosomal dominant, autosomal recessive, and X-linked conditions. The determination of the inheritance pattern was known long before the new DNA technology became available; it was based simply on interpretation of pedigree structure. Thus, when a condition was recognized to occur through generations in a vertical fashion, the assumption that the condition was an autosomal dominant disorder was usually made. This was the logic that permitted the recognition of neurofibromatosis type 1 (NF1) as an autosomal dominant condition long before the gene was identified in 1990. (NF1 is utilized in this section to illustrate principles.)

The concept of a dominant gene means that one gene in the homologous gene pair possesses a mutation, while the other is the normal or "wild-type" gene (often called the "wild allele"). "Alleles" are different variations of a gene, and in recent years these have been determined at a molecular level for many conditions. Thus, in an autosomal dominant disorder, when a person has such a mutation, the chance of transmitting the mutation to offspring is one in two (or 50%) with each pregnancy. This is why the pedigree structure of a dominant trait will often be multigenerational. Figure 3.4 shows a typical autosomal dominant pedigree in a family with NF1. Note that there is transmission in this particular family tree from a father to a son (i.e., male-to-male transmission), confirming that this is an autosomal trait and not an X-linked trait (in an X-linked trait, a male cannot transmit the trait to a male offspring, because the father transmits his Y to a son and his X to a daughter). In many autosomal dominant traits, a condition starts off with a person who is often called the "progenitor." In that situation it is assumed that there is a *de novo* (new) mutation for the gene. Thus, in many autosomal dominant conditions there will be no family history, because the particular person in question is the progenitor for the disorder. This is often the case in NF1, where in the clinical setting about 50% of all patients who present to a medical genetic clinic have their disorder as a *de novo* mutation. (The other 50%, of course, inherit the gene from one of their parents.) This illustrates the point that the absence of any family history of a condition by no means excludes genetic causation. In fact, in X-linked and autosomal recessive conditions (where there is often no family history) as well, the impression that the lack of family history mitigates against a genetic disorder is inaccurate.

An autosomal recessive disorder is one in which both genes in a gene pair have a mutation of the gene in question. In an autosomal recessive pedigree, each parent is assumed to carry a mutant copy of the gene, and thus the parents are called "carriers" or "heterozygotes." The term "homozygote" is used when a person has two mutant genes or two copies. Because of the segregation pattern that occurs in recessive situations, the chance

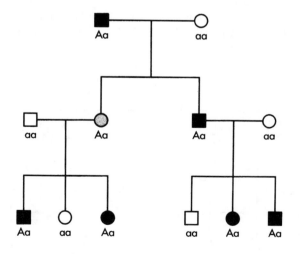

FIGURE 3.4. This family pedigree illustrates the typical inheritance pattern of an autosomal dominant trait, NF1. Note the transmission from a father to son in the first to second generation. The letters refer to the heterozygous state. Individuals with NF1 are designated as "Aa," with the normal being "aa." From Jorde, Carey, and White (1995). Copyright 1995 by C. V. Mosby and Year Book Medical Publishers. Reprinted by permission.

that a family that has one child with an autosomal recessive condition will have another is one in four (or 25%) with each pregnancy. Most inborn errors of metabolism, such as phenylketonuria (see Waisbren, Chapter 19, this volume), are inherited in an autosomal recessive fashion. These biochemical conditions represent disorders of intermediary metabolism, and a homozygous deficiency of an enzyme accounts for each such disorder. Moreover, the hemoglobinopathies, including sickle cell anemia (see Smith, Chapter 16, this volume), are also inherited in an autosomal recessive fashion. A comprehensive discussion of the principles of population genetics that are important in any discussion of autosomal recessive diseases can be found in the textbooks cited earlier.

The third type of disorder transmitted in a mendelian fashion is an X-linked disorder. The X-linked disorders are conditions that from pedigree structures (and now DNA technology) are known to be mutations on the X chromosome. In this situation, a female (who typically has two X chromosomes) will "carry" the gene for the condition and may or may not express it, while the male (who only has a single X) will almost invariably express the condition. Again, just as in autosomal dominant disorders, some individuals who have an X-linked disorder may have it because of a new mutation of the gene on the X chromosome. Figure 3.5 shows a typical X-linked pedigree of a family with color blindness seen in a clinical setting. Conditions of significance in the neurobehavioral arena with X-linked inheritance include fragile X, Hunter syndrome, Lesch–Nyhan syndrome (see Morales, Chapter 21, this volume), and X-linked aqueductal stenosis/hydrocephalus.

Decisions about patterns of inheritance are complex and often controversial in the field of medical genetics. Knowledge of the genetic basis for many conditions is now being acquired through recent developments in DNA technology. Detailed discussions of the evidence for inheritance pattern of human diseases and phenotypes are available in the classic multivolume text *Mendelian Inheritance in Man*. V. A. McKusick, the author, is often considered the father of medical genetics, and has produced 12 editions of this seminal work. One is now able to look up conditions or phenotypes and discover key and recent citations on clinical and genetic aspects as well as molecular biology (McKusick, 1998). This work is currently available on-line through the World Wide Web (http:\\www3.ncbi. nlm.nih.gov/omim/). This is an incomparable and invaluable resource for current knowledge about the genetic and molecular basis of almost any condition. The 11th edition

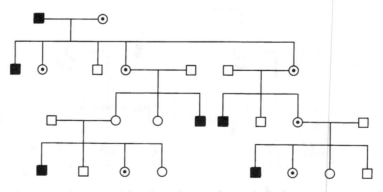

FIGURE 3.5. This is a rather typical family pedigree of an X-linked recessive trait, color blindness. Solid symbols represent affected individuals and dotted symbols represent heterozygous carriers. Note in the first generation the female carrier mated with a male with the condition. From Jorde, Carey, and White (1995). Copyright 1995 by C. V. Mosby and Year Book Medical Publishers. Reprinted by permission.

(McKusick, 1994) described 6,678 different conditions, while the 12th edition (McKusick, 1998) includes 8,587 entries. The reader is referred to this work whenever this type of information is needed.

Genotype–Phenotype Relationships: Basic Tenets

Although the discussion thus far seems to be relatively straightforward, the actual evaluation of a patient with a potential genetic condition is not so clear-cut. As mentioned above, an abnormality of chromosome structure or a gene mutation produces a phenotype that is recognizable and often discrete. However, the relationship between the gene alteration and the disease state is complex, as there is marked variability in the clinical picture, regardless of the genotype. Various conditions seem to have their own intrinsic degree of variability. For these reasons, geneticists over the century have developed concepts that explain the often fuzzy relationship between the genotype and the phenotype. These tenets include the following concepts: "expressivity," "penetrance," "heterogeneity," "pleiotropy," and "mutation." These are discussed individually in the ensuing paragraphs.

"Expressivity" is a term utilized in genetics to refer to the variability in clinical severity seen in a given condition. Various members of the same family with a certain genetic trait have exactly the same mutation, yet the degree of involvement can range from minimal to severe. The study of the clinical aspects of NF1 illustrates this point (see Nilsson & Bradford, Chapter 15, this volume). About 50–70% of patients with NF1 simply have *café au lait* spots or dermal neurofibromas, and their disorder is of mild significance. Approximately 30–50% of patients have one of the many listed serious manifestations of NF1, including optic pathway tumors, neurofibrosarcomas, or scholeosis. Even within the same multigenerational kindred, there will be marked variability. This discussion also applies to Noonan syndrome (see Teeter, Chapter 14, this volume). Again, even within the same pedigree, there will be marked variability in the clinical signs (short stature, pulmonic stenosis, etc.), even though all patients will have at least the facial features.

"Penetrance" is the frequency of expression of a genotype. Some individuals who carry a gene in a mendelian disorder will have no observed clinical signs of the condition. There are other monogenic disorders in which penetrance (usually expressed as a percentage of those who express the conditions to some extent) is 100%. Thus the absence of any signs of such a disorder will give the impression that the gene in question has skipped a generation. The concept of incomplete penetrance or lack of penetrance is an attempt to explain the clinical picture where the genotype and phenotype do not match, as one would expect. All of the monogenic conditions described in this book essentially have 100% penetrance. For example, in NF1, individuals who have the trait have some cutaneous or eye signs of NF1—usually by the age of 5, but certainly by the age of 20 years. Sometimes it may be difficult to exclude the presence of the gene in a young child, but usually by adulthood, the *café au lait* spots, dermal neurofibromas, and Lisch nodules of the iris have made their appearance. In examination of NF1 pedigrees, one does not see examples of three-generation pedigrees where the gene has skipped. On the other hand, in tuberous sclerosis, there have been cases reported in which there are two affected children of normal, unaffected parents. This particular pedigree structure could be described as incomplete penetrance; however, one does not see three generations of people with tuberous sclerosis where the person in the middle generation lacks any signs. Most geneticists currently think that families with tuberous sclerosis represent "germ-line mosaicism" (i.e., mutation occurring in multiple gametes and not in somatic cells, putting the parents at increased risk for recurrence).

Mosaicism is now thought to occur more often than previously recognized in the field. In Table 3.1 it is listed as one of the nontraditional modes of inheritance, and it is discussed a bit further below.

The concept of "heterogeneity" presently has a number of usages in medical genetics. The traditional concept is "genetic heterogeneity," in which a certain phenotype (e.g., retinitis pigmentosa or cataracts) is known to be caused by different genetic alterations (i.e., autosomal dominant, autosomal recessive, or X-linked). With the recent advances in DNA technology, the existence of genetic heterogeneity has been proven. For example, in tuberous sclerosis, some families with this autosomal dominant gene map to the chromosome 16 and have a mutation of a certain tumorous suppressor gene, whereas other families map to chromosome 9 and have the disorder because of mutations of a different gene. This can be referred to as either "locus heterogeneity" or "genetic heterogeneity." The term is also used to refer to a mixture of phenotypes as well. For example, when it was recognized in the 1980s that bilateral acoustic neuromas were really a condition not seen in classical neurofibromatosis, the notion of phenotypic heterogeneity of the neurofibromatoses was proposed. Even before the two separate genes were mapped and cloned, clinicians and scientists were referring to multiple forms of NF. Now the terms NF1 and NF2 are used for the classic condition (NF1) and for bilateral acoustic neuromas (NF2).

The concept of "pleiotropy" refers to the idea that diverse manifestations in different organs and systems can have a single-gene cause. Again, NF1 illustrates this concept nicely. In this syndrome one sees manifestations that do not seem on first glance to be tied together pathogenically (i.e., *café au lait* spots, neurofibromas, optic pathway tumors, learning disabilities, skeletal findings, etc.). The notion here is that a single gene has multiple roles in development and cell biology, and thus that a mutation in this gene has multiple effects. In the case of NF1, the common denominator is presumably in the control of cells derived from the developing neural crest of the embryo. To give another example, the pleiotropic manifestations of Noonan syndrome include the characteristic face, short stature, pectus excavatum, and pulmonic stenosis. Again, this diverse array of effects appears to be due to the single mutation. The concept of pleiotropy moves to the essence of how a gene produces the phenotype (i.e., its pathogenesis), and it relates to the idea of the syndrome.

As mentioned in various places in the chapter, "mutation" refers to the specific alteration of the DNA molecule in a particular condition. In recent years, with the advances in DNA technology, the defined and specific mutations that cause many disorders have been detected. For example, after the gene for NF1 was identified in 1990, about 10% of individuals with NF1 had a detectable mutation. In the other 90%, the scientists were just not technically able to find the gene alteration, presumably because of the size of the NF1 gene. Since 1990, because of the new techniques, laboratory scientists have become able to detect the disease-causing mutations in 70% of NF1 patients (Gutmann et al., 1997). Of note is the fact that about 80% of the mutations are ones in which the gene is basically inactivated (i.e. there is simply one operating gene, while the other is not operating). In some cases the entire gene is deleted, while in others a small deletion of only a few nucleotides is present. Most cases are caused by a single nucleotide change that either results in a shortened protein or affects function of the protein. In other conditions, the specific type and location of gene mutations affect the phenotype. For example, Apert syndrome is due to relatively specific mutations of a gene that encodes a protein called fibroblast growth factor receptor 2 (Webster & Donoghue, 1997). This is a cell receptor protein that sits on the outside of a cell and, when signaled by a growth factor, sends a message to the nucleus of the cell. It is now known that Apert syndrome is due to mutations of the gene that alter the extracellular portion of this growth factor receptor. Mutations of other parts of this same gene produce different phenotypes and recognized syndromes that have manifestations overlapping with those of Apert syndrome, but that represent different patterns. These other syndromes, which include Crouzon and Pfeiffer syndromes, are not discussed here in detail.

In summary, the area of genotype–phenotype correlation is a timely topic. Ideally, better understanding of how mutations in specific genes produce specific phenotypes will clarify the pathogenesis of human diseases of this nature.

Recently Delineated Concepts: Nontraditional Inheritance

As mentioned above, the concepts of variability, pleiotropy, and heterogeneity were basically created to explain observed discrepancies between genotypes and phenotypes. In the 1980s and 1990s, a number of newer, nontraditional categories of inheritance have been recognized. One of these, "mosaicism," has been mentioned above. Here there are essentially two cell lines—usually one that is normal and one that contains gene mutation or chromosomal alteration. Other concepts that have been proposed in the last decade include "genomic imprinting" and "anticipation." These concepts have altered thinking about the clinical and genetic aspects of a number of important conditions. These concepts are discussed below as they relate to two of the conditions described in this text (i.e., the Prader–Willi and fragile X syndromes), as well as to Angelman syndrome.

The principle of "genomic imprinting" challenged the central dogma of genetics that arose from Mendel's experiments with peas. Originally it was thought that a trait was inherited from a mother or a father, and that the parent of origin made no difference. Recently, however, it has become increasingly apparent that in some genes the parent of origin does make a difference and has an effect on phenotype and disease manifestation. Here the idea is that the expression of a gene is influenced by the parental origin of the gene, and that the activity level depends on this origin. The concept of genomic imprinting in humans is best illustrated by the Prader–Willi and Angelman syndromes. As mentioned earlier, it has been known since the early 1980s that a microdeletion on chromosome 15 in the upper portion of the long arm could produce Prader–Willi syndrome (see Dykens & Cassidy, Chapter 23, this volume). A similar deletion was recognized in some patients with Angelman syndrome. (Angelman syndrome is a condition of profound developmental disability, seizure disorder, muscle tone abnormalities, small head size, and a characteristic face.) Now it is known that if a deletion arises on the paternal chromosome 15, the offspring will develop Prader–Willi syndrome; if the deletion arrives on the maternal chromosome 15, the child will develop Angelman syndrome. Thus there is a definite parent-of-origin effect. It is now clear that a gene (or genes) within the crucial segment of chromosome 15 is normally only active on the paternal chromosome and not the maternal one (the maternal copy is said to be "imprinted"). In a case when the critical gene (or genes) is deleted on the paternal chromosome and thus inactivated, this deletion results in Prader–Willi syndrome. Conversely, the gene for Angelman syndrome has also been identified, and the logic is the reverse. Although most cases of Prader–Willi syndrome and Angelman syndrome are sporadic, without a family history, this parent-of-origin effect results in some unusual pedigrees that would not at first glance fit any of the simple rules of single-gene disorders discussed above (see Jorde et al, 1995).

The other recently proposed concept that is classified as nontraditional is that of "anticipation." Since the early part of the 20th century, it has been observed that some genetic

diseases display an earlier age of onset and have more severe expression in later generations of the family tree. Such disorders are said to exhibit anticipation. Until recently, most
investigators felt that this was probably a bias of ascertainment and not a real biological
phenomenon. In the early 1990s, the genes for a number of dysplasias or novel mutational
mechanisms were identified through the positional cloning approach. These included fragile
X syndrome (see Hagerman & Lampe, Chapter 12, this volume), myotonic dystrophy, and
Huntington chorea. These three conditions share a unique mutation mechanism, that of
the expanded DNA repeat; they have thus been labeled the "trinucleotide repeat-expansion
disorders." There are repeat sequences of DNA nucleotides that are normally present in
all individuals; persons with repeat-expansion disorders have an increased number of these
nucleotide repeat sequences. Somehow such an expansion affects the way the DNA works
or the way the protein functions, and therefore it produces the disease. Thus of these conditions actually explain the phenomenon of anticipation and give it a biological basis. Like
genomic imprinting, this phenomenon provides the biological and molecular basis for several unusual pedigrees.

DNA Technology and Linkage

The tools and strategies to localize a particular gene for a mendelian disorder to its particular chromosome (or chromosomes) only arose in the late 1970s and early 1980s. The
combination of the development of DNA probes, complicated computer programs, and
restriction endonucleases laid the groundwork for the application of this technology. The
basic point here is that for the overwhelming majority of genetic disorders (except the biochemical disorders), the biological bases were almost entirely unknown. One could speculate that a condition like NF1 was due to some disorder of neural crest biology, or that
Apert syndrome was due to a developmental disorder of the skeleton, but the real basis of
the pleiotropy in each case was essentially unclear. For this reason, the concept that one
can map a gene by utilizing the incredible and well-known variation in DNA structure arose.
The idea is that an individual's variations of DNA should "run" with the disease genes in
question. By using these complicated computer programs and already linked DNA probes,
one can (with luck and hard work) map a gene. Once a disease gene is mapped, the first
step toward being able to isolate the actual causative gene is accomplished. The isolation
of the gene for a condition is referred to as "gene identification" or "cloning." If the basic
structure of the DNA is known, one can then derive the amino acid sequence and the pep-
tide structure. The strategy, once called "reverse genetics" and now referred to as "positional cloning," has been highly successful in the 1980s and 1990s in identifying important
disease genes. The first gene mapped by this approach was Huntington chorea. In the late
1980s, the genes for cystic fibrosis, Duchenne muscular dystrophy, and NF1 were mapped
and then cloned. Correlation of the detected mutations in these conditions with specific
genotypes is now ongoing for these and all other conditions in which there has been gene
identification.

Figure 3.6 illustrates this paradigm. First, families with a particular dominant or recessive condition are collected. If, by chance, some patients have an associated chromosomal rearrangement that suggests a gene location, the success rate in mapping the gene is
improved. Once a gene is mapped, linkage testing in the clinical arena is available. For
example, in familial cases of NF1, the families that are interested in prenatal diagnosis or
early-infancy diagnosis (often before any *café au lait* spots have developed) now have this

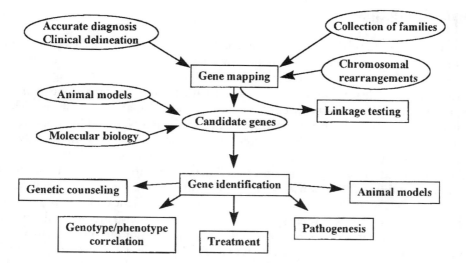

FIGURE 3.6. The gene-cloning paradigm: The chronology of the mapping and identifying of a disease gene, with its resulting consequences. Note that after a gene is mapped, the possibility that linkage testing can be used in the clinical arena occurs. Cloning a gene creates the potential for understanding pathogenesis and perhaps orchestrating strategies for treatment and prevention.

option. Once a gene has been mapped or localized, perusal of the existing gene map may show "candidate genes" in the same region that may be the basis for the disorder in question. This approach was used to clone the gene responsible for Apert syndrome. Once the gene for a related but different condition called Crouzon syndrome (referred to above) was mapped to chromosome 10, and it was discovered that there was a candidate gene on chromosome 10 that encodes fibroblast growth factor receptor 2, mutations were detected in patients with Crouzon syndrome. The logical hypothesis was that perhaps different mutations of the same gene cause related disorders, including Apert syndrome. This turned out to be the case, and it is now known that the gene for fibroblast growth factor receptor 2 is the causative gene in Apert syndrome (Webster & Donoghue, 1997). As mentioned above, this paradigm was also successful in mapping and cloning the important gene in fragile X syndrome. At present if a person is recognized to have fragile X syndrome and this is confirmed on a molecular basis, DNA testing can be offered to other members of the family who are at risk. Direct mutation testing for the expanded repeat of fragile X syndrome is currently available in most clinical molecular laboratories in North America (see Hagerman & Lampe, Chapter 12, this volume).

The ultimate aim of this strategy is to understand the molecular pathogenesis of these single-gene conditions. If the protein is detected and in its role in cell biology is sorted out, then one has the beginnings of the tools to propose treatments that can alter or modify the sequence of events in the cell pathway in question. For example, the gene for NF1 is a tumor suppressor gene that is involved in signal transduction within the cell. The encoded protein neurofibromin is known to slow down growth within the cell. Thus, if a mutation occurs, the expected brakes on cell growth will not be present and will predispose a person to develop benign or malignant tumors. If one could figure out how to alter some of the elements of the pathway, then one could perhaps prevent the occurrence of benign or malignant tumors in NF1.

Diagnostic Principles

For many of the genetic disorders described in this chapter and in this text, clinicians and investigators have set forth criteria that allow a practitioner to arrive at a secure diagnosis. The idea of developing these criteria arose in the 1980s as gene linkage studies progressed. It became clear to both clinicians and scientists that in order for one to attempt to map a gene, there had to be a consensus on who was affected and who was not. The diagnostic criteria for NF1 illustrate this principle. In 1987, at a National Institutes of Health (NIH) conference on NF1 and NF2, criteria were proposed for making the diagnosis of this condition. Table 3.2 presents these criteria. A basic premise here is that if a patient's manifestations fulfill the required items, the clinician can settle upon a highly secure diagnosis of the condition (NIH Consensus Development Conference, 1988). Diagnostic criteria are not widely available or established for many other genetic conditions. However, in certain circumstances (e.g., Apert syndrome), diagnostic criteria are not really necessary, since the distinctiveness of the pattern is clear-cut. In addition, for conditions where the diagnosis can be made on a molecular basis (e.g., Prader–Willi syndrome), diagnostic checklists or criteria are not needed as much (except sometimes to help a clinician decide who needs to be evaluated). The concept of diagnostic criteria is emphasized here simply to underscore the subjective nature and occasional difficulty of arriving at the diagnosis of a genetic disorder or syndrome. This concept is further discussed below in regard to syndromes (and, later, to behavioral phenotypes).

Syndrome Diagnosis

The term "syndrome" is utilized in a specific way in the field of medical genetics. It refers to a recognizable and consistent pattern of multiple manifestations known to have a specific etiology. The cause is usually a mutation of a single gene, a chromosome alteration, or an environmental agent. In other words, a syndrome is a specific phenotype that usually has a known cause. The notion of syndrome is related closely to the concept of pleiotropy, described earlier. The diagnosis of malformation or developmental syndromes in general is a challenge, as over 1,000 syndromes involving multiple congenital anomalies are listed in catalogs and diagnostic computer programs (see Jones, 1997; Gorlin, Cohen, & Levin, 1990).

TABLE 3.2. NIH Consensus Statement: Diagnostic Criteria for NF1

The diagnostic criteria for NF1 are met in an individual if two or more of the following are found:

- Six or more *café au lait* macules of over 5 mm in greatest diameter in prepubertal individuals and over 15 mm in greatest diameter in postpubertal individuals.
- Two or more neurofibromas of any type or one plexiform neurofibroma.
- Freckling in the axillary or inguinal regions.
- Optic glioma.
- Two or more Lisch nodules (iris hamartomas).
- A distinctive osseous lesion such as sphenoid dysplasia or thinning of the long bone cortex with or without pseudoarthrosis.
- A first-degree relative (parent, sibling or offspring) with NF1 by the above criteria.

Note. From NIH Consensus Development Conference (1988).

In addition to knowledge of the more common disorders, the clinician who approaches the area of syndromology needs knowledge and skill in the recognition of minor anomalies of structure, which often provide phenotypic clues for a diagnosis. Thus, for example, diagnosing Williams syndrome can be difficult in early childhood or infancy unless one is familiar with the physical characteristics of the face in the context of the developmental condition. Even such signs as curly hair and characteristic voice are part of the component manifestations that are helpful in diagnosis. Since no individual feature or manifestation is obligatory in almost any syndrome, one has to be familiar with the clinical variability in order to secure the diagnosis. The diagnosis of chromosome syndromes can often be straightforward if the clinician has the appropriate index of suspicion; ordering the chromosome study confirms the diagnosis. As mentioned earlier, if one is considering a microdeletion syndrome, the appropriate chromosome study (including FISH) needs to be performed. By constrast, if the condition in question possesses relatively consistent features (e.g., as the multiple *café au lait* spots of NF1), and diagnostic criteria are available to establish the diagnosis, the diagnostic reasoning process can be fairly simple.

One of the important points in this discussion is that the concept of a syndrome encompasses a multiplicity of manifestations, all of which are variable within the constellation. In chromosome syndromes in general and in the syndromes discussed in this book, some disorder of development is invariably present. In that sense, mental retardation is accepted widely as a component manifestation of many of these syndromes. In the same sense, alterations in cognition, personality, and behavior can be variable manifestations in many of these syndromes, just like the more clearly defined manifestation of mental retardation. This point is the essence of the concept of "behavioral phenotype," which is discussed later.

Environmental Syndromes

In addition to syndromes of single-gene or chromosome etiology, there exist several syndromes caused by teratogenic agents. A "teratogen" is an agent external to the fetus that induces structural malformations, growth deficiency, or functional alterations during prenatal development. Although teratogens cause only a small percentage of developmental disabilities and birth defects, they are an important group because of the potential for prevention. In the neurobehavioral arena, the most important and common condition is fetal alcohol syndrome (FAS). This condition has a recognizable pattern of malformation consisting of prenatal growth deficiency (low birth weight, low stature), postnatal growth deficiency (short stature, failure to thrive), microcephaly (small head), and a characteristic pattern of minor facial anomalies (Streissguth, Clarren, & Jones, 1985). Although on first glance the facial anomalies may seem nonspecific, taken together they are diagnostic of FAS. These facial alterations include short palpebral fissures (small eyelids on horizontal measurement), short upturned nose, long philtrum (distance from nasal septum to upper lip), and relatively thin upper lip. The facial gestalt of older children with FAS is quite characteristic, and a clinician who has experience with the disorder can make a secure clinical diagnosis in the context of maternal alcohol abuse. The full syndrome occurs in 10–40% (depending on the study) in mothers who drink excessively and abuse alcohol (Stratton, Howe, & Battaglia, 1996). While the issue of whether moderate or less frequently used amounts of alcohol cause adverse effects is controversial and not clear-cut, there is no question that maternal alcoholism is a significant risk factor for this recognizable syndrome.

One of the component manifestations of FAS is neurodevelopmental difficulty. A majority of children with FAS have learning disabilities, but some actually have enough developmental disability to be diagnosed as having mental retardation. In addition to this, a behavioral phenotype has been suggested but not well documented in the literature (Stratton et al., 1996). This particular behavioral profile includes attention deficits, hyperactivity, an unusual degree of memory loss, and conduct problems. The last component indicates a deficiency in the person's awareness of the consequences of his or her actions. Although none of these components of the behavioral profile are specific, taken together in the context of full FAS, they appear to represent a consistent manifestation of the overall pattern. A clinical dilemma frequently arises when a child who has a vague or undocumented history of maternal alcohol abuse, often in an adoptive or foster care situation, has one or more components of this stated behavioral profile. We would suggest that it is inappropriate to draw a causal inference based simply on the nonspecific behavioral disorder, *without* the physical manifestations and phenotype of FAS. However, this issue is somewhat controversial within the field. The National Academy of Sciences' Institute of Medicine has produced a scholarly document that identifies the complex issues surrounding the diagnosis and developmental aspects of FAS (Stratton, et al., 1996). This group, like others (Aase, Jones, & Clarren, 1995), suggests the abandonment of the term "fetal alcohol effects," which has sometimes been used in the diagnostic arena. We would agree, and we recommend not utilizing the term "fetal alcohol effects" because of our uneasiness about drawing diagnostic conclusions from a child with a behavioral disorder without the physical signs.

Some of the other teratogenic syndromes are known to involve developmental difficulties, but all require additional investigation before any firm conclusions can be drawn. For instance, some children with the fetal valproate syndrome have been said to have autism (Christianson, Chesler, & Kromberg, 1994); this requires further investigation. Children with fetal hydantoin and isotretinoin syndromes have also been recognized to have developmental disabilities, but, again, further study on the learning profile is needed.

Benefits of Diagnosis

Often the diagnosis of a neurobehavioral disorder or dysmorphic syndrome is relegated to the area of the exotic. However, as has been emphasized throughout this chapter, diagnosis is important for the child, the family, and the practitioners who are caring for the child. Table 3.3 summarizes the benefits of making the diagnosis of a genetic condition or syndrome. These can be illustrated in the diagnosis of a child with Williams syndrome. Once a diagnosis has been established, and the deletion of the elastin gene has been confirmed with FISH, recurrence risk counseling can occur; if a parent does not have Williams syndrome (which is usually the case), the deletion is certainly *de novo*, and the recurrence risk approaches that of the background. Prenatal diagnosis with the FISH technique is possible in future pregnancies but is probably not necessary, given the low recurrence risk in sporadic cases. The diagnosis helps the clinician in stating some predictions about prognosis—especially the neurodevelopmental outcome, but also the natural history of the condition. Children with Williams syndrome will need a cardiac evaluation due to a 60% occurrence of heart defects (especially supravalvular aortic stenosis), and this is important for follow-up care. In addition, a higher index of suspicion for hearing loss, visual difficulties, urinary tract infections, and hypertension should occur, and this should further modify the primary care practitioner's health supervision plan. A diagnosis makes it possible to avoid unnecessary laboratory testing. A child with Williams syndrome who has developmental delay should not require any metabolic testing or neuroimaging—tests that are frequently done in the diagnostic evaluation of a child with this presentation. Moreover, knowledge

TABLE 3.3. Benefits of Diagnosis in a Genetic Condition or Syndrome

- *Recurrence risk in genetic counseling.* The recognition of an established disorder of known etiology provides information on cause and genetic aspects of the condition, including risk of recurrence.
- *Prediction of prognosis.* Each disorder has its own particular natural history and outcome. Knowledge of the degree of disability that occurs on average is often helpful to parents.
- *Appropriate laboratory testing and screening.* Precise diagnosis can eliminate the need for many tests frequently considered in the evaluation of a child with a developmental disorder; appropriate screening can be planned according to natural history.
- *Guidelines for management.* Knowledge of the natural history of a syndrome allows for the establishment of guidelines for routine care, including suggestions for educational interventions.
- *Family support.* In some families, the knowledge of a condition helps in dealing with the uncertainty of the situation. A diagnosis provides a biological basis for a condition.

of the natural history of the developmental profile in Williams syndrome at least allows for some initial steps in planning educational intervention in the preschool and elementary school settings. Although it is certainly true that a "cookbook"-type plan cannot be laid out, there is a profile of strengths and weaknesses in children with Williams syndrome that can help the educator. (See Chapter 24, this volume). Finally, making a diagnosis of a specific condition often helps a family with the experience of uncertainty, as often a general diagnosis of a developmental disability conveys a sense of meaninglessness and confusion. A diagnosis of a particular syndrome, even an uncommon one, gives a biological basis and often credibility to the child's difficulties.

BEHAVIORAL PHENOTYPES IN DYSMORPHIC SYNDROMES

The term "behavioral phenotype" has been used for the last few decades in the fields of child psychiatry and medical genetics. There is no consensus on its definition, and it is used by different people to mean different things. Turk and Hill (1995) provide an excellent summary of the issues in their review. They assert that "a number of conditions, recognizable by a common physical phenotype, single gene defect or chromosomal abnormality, seem also to have a constellation of behaviors or cognitive anomalies which are characteristic" (p. 105). Flint and Yule (1994) take a stricter view of this concept and require that before the term is used, there must be a distinctive behavior that occurs in almost every case and rarely in other conditions. However, we would agree with Turk and Hill that this more restrictive view is not applied in the inclusion of particular nonbehavioral manifestations in the definition of syndromes. For example, the atrioventicular canal defect seen in 20–30% of children with Down syndrome is relatively characteristic, as almost two-thirds of children with this defect have Down syndrome. However, there are clearly other causes of this defect other than trisomy 21, and not all patients with Down syndrome have it. Similarly, only about 20% of individuals with Turner syndrome have a left-sided obstructive lesion of the heart, and the overwhelming majority of cases who have this heart lesion do not have Turner syndrome. Thus, as illustrated here, most clinicians would not require the physical defects of the heart to occur completely consistently and specifically before including them as part of the syndrome. The same concept then, we believe, should hold true for behavioral components.

In the literature, the term "behavioral phenotype" is used without its users' necessarily clarifying whether it refers to a psychological/cognitive profile, a behavioral disorder, or a personality trait (Turk & Hill, 1995). In this context, we would propose a modification of the definition of the term suggested by Turk and Hill. As we see it, a behavioral phenotype is a profile of behavior, cognition, or personality that represents a component of the overall pattern seen in many or most individuals with a particular condition or syndrome. Although the profile may not be specific, it is consistent in the syndromal pattern. The challenge for the next decade (as stated in many of the chapters in this book) is continued documentation of these parameters with state-of-the-art tools. The diagnosis of a dysmorphic syndrome needs to be rigorous and clear-cut, and the documentation of the neurodevelopmental and neuropsychological profile demands the best current strategies. At present, a glance through review papers, like those of Turk and Hill (1995) and Flint and Yule (1994), gives one the impression that there is not much specificity to the behavioral patterns described in the literature reviewed. However, this perusal is not very different from one's first glance through a catalog of listed facial features and minor anomalies in chromosome syndromes. Yet the consistency in the facial features of children of the same age with chromosome disorders illustrates the reproducibility of these syndromes. Recognition of facial features and documentation of their pattern are often difficult without tools for quantification. These same kinds of issues apply to documentation in the neurobehavioral realm, especially in the profiles of behavioral disorders and personality traits. The principles should be the same: Just as the facial features differ from those of the family background in such conditions as Williams syndrome and Down syndrome, there is an alteration of the biological basis of behavior and personality beyond the family background in these conditions.

Table 3.4 lists the dysmorphic syndromes that have been found to have a relatively specific or characteristic behavioral profile. The chromosomal location or identified gene is listed as well, when this is known. The reader is referred to the above-mentioned review papers. Moreover, the chapters in this text summarize the behavioral profiles of several of these syndromes.

A behavioral phenotype is generally defined by beginning with a sample of subjects with a specific dysmorphic syndrome and then studying specific cognitive, affective, or behavioral characteristics, as compared to a relevant control group. Some syndromes, such as Williams and Prader–Willi syndromes, have been associated with chromosomal regions as well as with behavioral patterns. A complementary approach has recently made use of several large affected families, extensive cognitive testing, and DNA markers to find linkages for components of a complex cognitive phenotype—developmental dyslexia. In six large families containing 94 adults affected with reading disability (documented in childhood), defective phonological awareness was linked to markers on chromosome 6, and defective single-word reading was linked to chromosome 15 (Grigorenko et al., 1997). Success in using genetics to dissect this complex phenotype first required careful study of the reading disability phenotype through state-of-the-art cognitive science (Pennington, 1997). Future progress in understanding genotype–phenotype relationships in neurobehavioral disorders, such as autism or Tourette disorder, is likely to rely on an interplay of approaches from psychology, genetics, neuroimaging, and other disciplines.

CONCLUSION

The field of medical and molecular genetics has blossomed in the last decade. The basic paradigm provides the potential for a newer understanding of human disease pathogenesis, similar to the advances in infectious diseases and immunology earlier in the 20th cen-

TABLE 3.4. Dysmorphic Syndromes Thought to Have a Characteristic Behavioral Phenotype

Syndrome	Cause
Chromosome	
Williams syndrome	7q microdeletion
Velocardiofacial/DiGeorge syndrome	22q11 deletion
Prader–Willi syndrome	15q11–13 microdeletion[a]
Angelman syndrome	15q11–13 microdeletion[a]
Smith–Magenis syndrome	17p11 microdeletion
Down syndrome	Trisomy 21
Klinefelter syndrome	XXY
Monogenic	
Neurofibromatosis type 1 (NF1)	Mutation on 17
Noonan syndrome	Autosomal dominant gene on 12
Fragile X syndrome	Mutation of X
Rett syndrome	Mutation of X
Multifactorial/undefined	
de Lange syndrome	Unknown, presumed mutation
Environmental	
Fetal alcohol syndrome	Maternal alcohol abuse
Fetal valproate syndrome	Maternal use of valproate

[a]Imprintable genes; see text. See also Dykens and Cassidy (Chapter 23, this volume).

tury. The principles necessary to apply this approach in the clinical setting can be mastered with some effort and are valuable in the care of patients with neurodevelopmental disorders. The diagnosis of genetic disorders and syndromes is of vital importance to patients, their families, and care providers. The relatively recently proposed concept of behavioral phenotype fits quite well into the paradigm of medical genetics. Ongoing work utilizing current techniques in phenotype analysis, medical genetics, and neuropsychology will be necessary to delineate the behavioral profiles, specific or nonspecific, of various syndromes. An understanding of the biological basis of the neurodevelopmental aspects in these genetic conditions can provide fresh insight into well-known and common symptomatic disorders, such as learning disabilities and autism.

REFERENCES

Aase, J. M., Jones, L. K., & Claren, S. K. (1995). Do we need the term "FAE"? *Pediatrics, 95*, 428–430.

Ad Hoc Committee on Genetic Counseling. (1975). Report to the American Society of Human Genetics. *American Journal of Human Genetics, 27*, 240–242.

Battaglia, A., Gurrieri, F., Bertini, E., Bellacosa, A., Pomponi, M. G., Paravatou-Petsotas, M., Mazza, S., & Neri, G. (1997). The inv dup(15) syndrome: A clinically recognizable syndrome with altered behavior, mental retardation, and epilepsy. *Neurology, 48*, 1081–1086.

Carey, J. C. (1997). Genetic services in the care of children with disabilities. In H. M. Wallace, R. F. Biehl, J. C. MacQueen, & J. A. Blackman (Eds.), *Mosby's resource guide to children with disabilities and chronic illness*. St. Louis, MO: Mosby–Year Book.

Christianson, A. L., Chesler, N., & Kromberg, J. G. R. (1994). Fetal valproate syndrome: Clinical and neuro-developmental features in two sibling pairs. *Developmental Medicine and Child Neurology, 36*, 361–369.

Curry, C. J., Stevenson, R. E., Cunniff, C., Aughton, D., Byrne, J., Carey, J. C., Cassidy, S., Graham, J. M., Jr., Jones, M. C., Kaback, M. M., Moeschler, J., Schaefer, G. B., Schwartz, S., Tarleton, J., & Opitz, J. (1997). Evaluation of mental retardation: Recommendations of a consensus conference. *American Journal of Human Genetics, 72*, 468–477.

Flint, J., & Yule, W. (1994). Behavioural phenotypes. In M. Rutter, E. Taylor, & L. A. Hersov (Eds), *Child and adolescent psychiatry: Modern approaches*. Oxford: Blackwell Scientific.

Gelehrter, T. D., & Collins, F. S. (1998). *Principles of genetics* (2nd ed). Baltimore: Williams & Wilkins.

Gorlin, R. J. K., Cohen, M. M., Jr., & Levin, L. S. (1990). *Syndromes of the head and neck* (3rd ed.). New York: Oxford University Press.

Grigorenko, E. L., Wood, F. B., Meyer, M. S., Hart, L. A., Speed, W. C., Shuster A., & Pauls, D. L. (1997). Susceptibility loci for distinct components of developmental dyslexia on chromosomes 6 and 15. *American Journal of Human Genetics, 60*, 27–39.

Gutmann, D. H., Aylsworth, A., Carey, J. C., Korf, B., Marks, J., Pyeritz, R. E., Rubenstein, A., & Viskochil, D. (1997). The diagnostic evaluation and multidisciplinary management of neurofibromatosis 1 and neurofibromatosis 2. *Journal of the American Medical Association, 278*, 51–57.

Jones, K. L. (1997). *Smith's recognizable patterns of human malformation* (5th ed.). Philadelphia Saunders.

Jorde, L. B., Carey, J. C., & White, R. L. (1995). *Medical genetics*. St. Louis, MO: Mosby–Year Book.

McKusick, V. A. (1994). *Mendelian inheritance in man* (11th ed.). Baltimore: Johns Hopkins University Press.

McKusick, V. A. (1998). *Mendelian inheritance in man* (12th ed.). Baltimore: Johns Hopkins University Press.

National Institutes of Health (NIH) Consensus Development Conference. (1988). Neurofibromatosis. *Archives of Neurology, 45*, 575–578.

Pennington, B. F. (1997). Using genetics to dissect cognition. *American Journal of Human Genetics, 60*, 13–16.

Rimoin, D. L., Connor, J. M., & Pyeritz, R. E. (Eds.). (1996). *Emery and Rimoin's principles and practice of medical genetics* (3rd ed.). New York: Churchill Livingstone.

Sherman, S. L., DeFries, J. C., Gottesman, I. I., Loehlin, J. C., Meyer, J. M., Pelias, M. Z., Rice. J., & Waldman, I. (1997). Behavioral genetics '97: ASHG statement recent developments in human behavioral genetics: Past accomplishments and future directions. *American Journal of Human Genetics, 60*, 1265–1275.

Smalley, S. L. (1997). Behavioral genetics '97: Genetic influences in childhood-onset psychiatric disorders: Autism and attention-deficit/hyperactivity disorder. *American Journal of Human Genetics, 60*, 1276–1282.

Stratton, K., Howe, C., & Battaglia, F. (1996). *Fetal alcohol syndrome: Diagnosis, epidemiology and treatment*. Washington, DC: National Academy Press.

Streissguth, A. P., Clarren, S. K., & Jones, K. L. (1985). National history of the fetal alcohol syndrome: A 10-year follow-up of eleven patients. *Lancet, ii*, 85–91.

Thompson, M. W., McInnes, R. R., & Willard, H. F. (1991). *Thompson and Thompson's genetics in medicine* (5th ed.). Philadelphia: Saunders.

Turk, J., & Hill, P. (1995). Behavioural phenotypes in dysmorphic syndromes. *Clinical Dysmorphology, 4*, 105–115.

Webster, M., & Donoghue, D. J. (1997). FGFR activation in skeletal disorders: Too much of a good thing. *Trends in Genetics, 13*, 178–182.

4

NEUROIMAGING AND GENETIC DISORDERS

ERIN D. BIGLER
DIANNE NIELSEN
ELIZABETH WILDE
JENNY BARTHOLOMEW
MICHAEL BROOKS
LYNNE W. BRADFORD

Contemporary imaging methods provide exquisite visualization of gross brain anatomy and pathology. For example, the images provided in Figure 4.1, based on magnetic resonance (MR) scanning, permit detailed examination of surface, cortical, and subcortical brain structures. The interpretation of such images is based on two simple principles that characterize the brains of normal individuals: "symmetry" and "similarity." Symmetry is readily apparent in Figure 4.1, taken from a normal subject. In the normal brain, what is present in one hemisphere is duplicated in the other. Similarity is the consistent reproducibility of basic brain structures across individuals. For example, Figure 4.2 compares MR images of five normal subjects, all at the thalamus–basal ganglia level. An image at a given level in one normal subject parallels that seen in all other subjects at similar levels. These two principles provide the basis for clinical interpretation of brain imaging findings when one is examining any clinical case (see also Bigler, Nilsson, Burr, & Boyer, 1997). A further example is provided in Figure 4.3. This is a case of congenital agenesis of the corpus callosum. When the midsagittal section of the MR scan is compared to that of a normal subject, it is obvious that the corpus callosum is missing. Although the absence of the corpus callosum is the most obvious abnormality, it is not the only abnormality present. The cingulate gyrus has not developed properly, and the temporal horns of the lateral ventricle are dilated, probably representing malformation of the temporal lobe. Applying the rules of symmetry and similarity in this manner to the interpretation of scans from individuals being assessed for genetic disorders provides important clinical information about the structural and functional integrity of the brain.

(a)

(b)

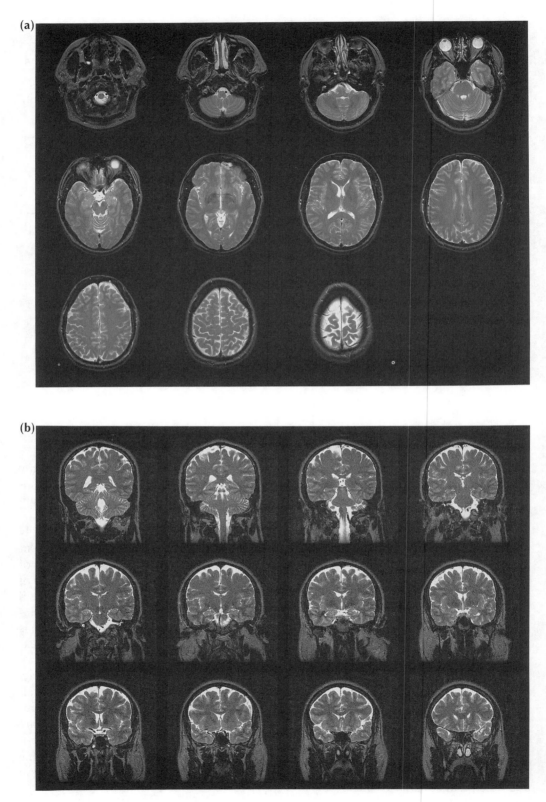

(c)

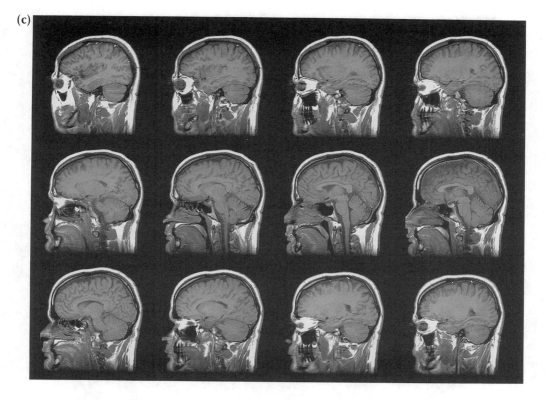

FIGURE 4.1. MR imaging in the three standard planes: (a) axial, (b) coronal, and (c) sagittal. Note, regardless of the plane, the general symmetry of the brain when one side is compared to its counterpart in the opposite hemisphere. Because of the closeness with which one hemisphere mirrors the other, features that show up in one hemisphere and not in the other can be signs of underlying pathology.

Based on the interpretive principles reviewed above, this chapter provides an overview of neuroimaging findings in some of the common genetic disorders. Further details on clinical interpretation of scan findings and contemporary research can be found in Bigler (1996a, 1996b), Osborn (1995), and Wolpert and Barnes (1992). In addition, Peterson (1995) provides an excellent review of neuroimaging in child and adolescent neuropsychiatric disorders, many of which have a genetic basis. This chapter focuses primarily on MR imaging, because it is the most widely used imaging method and provides excellent anatomical detail. The reference books cited above review other imaging techniques, such as computerized tomography (CT), single-photon emission computed tomography (SPECT), positron emission tomography (PET), functional magnetic resonance imaging (FMRI), and MR spectroscopy. Although these other imaging methods are sometimes used to assess children with genetic disorders, the primary imaging tool for this purpose is MR, and thus it is the one addressed in this chapter.

Often in genetic disorders, associated morphological brain abnormalities coexist with skeletal, skin, or other organ abnormalities. Brain embryogenesis often relates to other organ abnormalities, in that some early parent cells or cellular mechanisms share a common origin that may simultaneously influence brain, skin, muscles, bone, or other organs. An example of this can be found in the congenital muscular dystrophies (CMDs), which have an autosomal recessive mode of inheritance. The focus in CMDs has been on the clinicopatho-

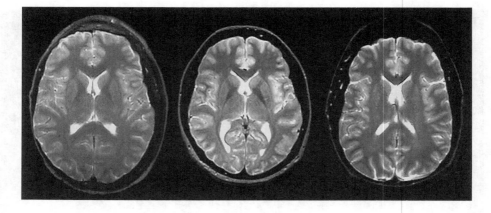

FIGURE 4.2. This figure demonstrates the principle of similarity across the brains of three patients all scanned at approximately the same level (thalamus–caudate nucleus). Note the almost identical appearance of the anterior horns when the three patients are compared. Because of this similarity of one scan to another in normal individuals, when the general anatomy of the brain is known, comparisons can be made to the more pathological changes seen with various disorders.

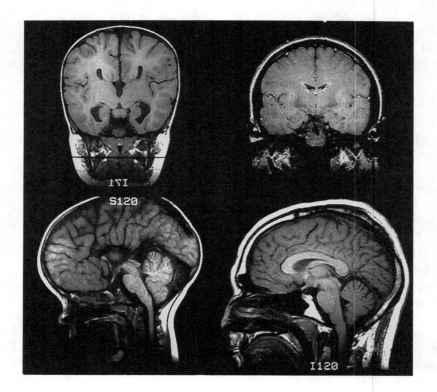

FIGURE 4.3. The MR scans on the left (top, coronal; bottom, sagittal) are from a child with agenesis of the corpus callosum. This is readily apparent when these scans are compared to normal coronal (top right) and sagittal (bottom right) sections. Also, compare this case to the scans depicted in Figure 4.1. Although absence of the corpus callosum is the most striking abnormality, others are present as well. For example, the cingulate gyrus cannot be visualized, and the temporal lobe appears malformed (large, dilated temporal horns and an exceptionally large posterior fossa).

logical features of generalized hypotonia and muscular weakness, their confirmation by muscle biopsy, and their inexorable course of muscle wasting. Because of the devastating outward appearance of CMDs, in the past such disorders have been characterized as peripheral nerve–muscle disorders. Although some CMDs are restricted to purely peripheral involvement, a number of CMD variants have been described in which significant cerebral abnormalities exist. For example, van der Knaap et al. (1997) have demonstrated a variety of brain abnormalities identified by MR imaging in children with CMDs. An example of such abnormalities in a CMD child is given in Figure 4.4.

Neuroimaging is a relatively new development in radiology. Clinical application of CT was introduced circa 1974, followed by the introduction of MR imaging about a de-

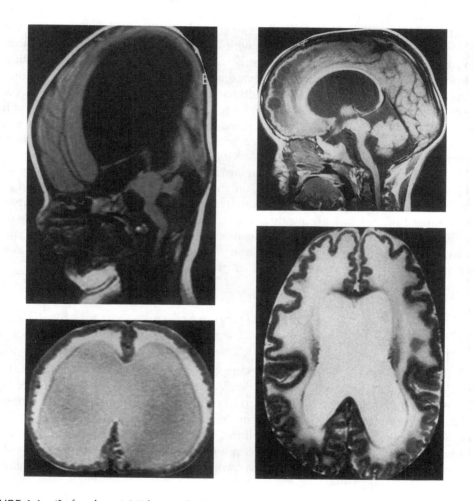

FIGURE 4.4. (Left column) Midsagittal MR view (top) and coronal section of a child with a congenital muscular dystrophy (CMD) who had marked cerebral abnormalities, including hydrocephalus, hypoplasia of the pons, fused superior and inferior colliculi, cerebellar vermis hypoplasia, and agyric polymicrogyria. (Right column) A different child, also with a CMD and abnormal brain development. Sagittal MR view (top) depicts thin corpus callosum, dilated ventricular system, fused colliculi, and pons and vermis hypoplasia. Also, diffuse white matter abnormalities are present (bottom). From van der Knaap et al. (1997). Copyright 1997 by Lippincott Williams & Wilkins. Reprinted by permission.

cade later (see Bigler, Yeo, & Turkheimer, 1989). With the fast-moving changes in computer technology, both CT and MR imaging rapidly improved from the mid-1980s to the present. Because the early technology was relatively crude, few systematic studies involving genetic disorders were performed in the early days of imaging. Furthermore, because of the rapid changes in technology, some of the early studies (i.e., those performed before 1985) may not represent contemporary findings. Thus the field has seen a dramatic change in the last decade. Review of the clinical and research literature in this area indicates that only the most common genetic disorders have received any systematic research attention; most reports that deal with less common genetic disorders tend to be single-case, anecdotal finds. In an example of the more systematic research, Jernigan, Bellugi, Sowell, Doherty, and Hesselink (1993), by applying new techniques for image analysis and quantification in their seminal work on Down syndrome (DS), have demonstrated the expected—namely, that DS subjects have smaller brain volume than normal, age-matched controls. Moreover, Jernigan et al. (1993) have demonstrated that adolescents with Williams syndrome (WS)—a genetic disorder producing characteristic faces and cognitive deficits, but some sparing of linguistic ability—also have smaller brain volume, but that quantitative differences between DS and WS subjects are present. For example, DS subjects have significantly less gray matter. This work represents one of the earliest efforts to attempt to quantify differences in the brains of individuals with DS and WS. Within 10 years, standardized quantitative normative data bases will be available so that any child, of any age, with any type of disorder can be compared to a normative sample (Steen, Ogg, Reddick & Kingsley, 1997).

Undoubtedly, the number of neuroimaging studies in genetic disorders is rapidly growing. Nonetheless, for the current chapter, only recent neuroimaging findings for a select few of the most common genetic disorders are reviewed. The chapter also briefly discusses neuroimaging findings in learning disabilities, attention-deficit/hyperactivity disorder (ADHD), and pervasive developmental disorders (PDDs), which may all have some genetic underpinnings. Some of the neuroimaging findings in various disorders have already been summarized by Peterson (1995) and are presented in Table 4.1.

ANGELMAN SYNDROME

Both CT and MR studies have indicated generalized cerebral atrophy in Angelman syndrome (Boyd & Patton, 1988; Dorries, Spohr, & Kunze, 1988; Ganji & Duncan, 1989; Robb, Pohl, Baraitser, Wilson, & Brett, 1989; Volpe & Yamada, 1990; Williams & Frias, 1982). Angelman syndrome is considered to be related to a deletion error on chromosome 15, the same region of deletion apparent in Prader–Willi syndrome and WS. As already stated, WS subjects have reduced brain volume. In Prader–Willi syndrome, because of the characteristics of insatiable appetite and corresponding obesity, MR imaging studies have focused on the hypothalamic–pituitary axis, where not all but some subjects display abnormalities (Swaiman, 1994).

APERT SYNDROME

No large imaging studies have been done on children with Apert syndrome. However, since the syndrome is associated with skull abnormalities (in particular, craniosynostosis), these malformations can be associated in turn with a variety of structural abnormalities in the brain (Kragskov, Sindet-Pedersen, Gyldensted, & Jensen, 1996). For example, Wider, Schwartz, Carmel, and Wood-Smith (1995) reported on a case of Apert syndrome in which the child developed hydrocephalus and the frontal lobe had herniated through a bony cavity created in the frontal bone created by the synostosis.

DOWN SYNDROME

The most commonly reported abnormalities in DS have been related to reduced volume of various cortical and subcortical structures when DS subjects are compared to age-matched normal controls (Jernigan & Bellugi, 1990; Jernigan et al., 1993; Peterson, 1995; Raz et al., 1995; P. P. Wang, Doherty, Hesselink, & Bellugi, 1992; Weis, 1991). Premature aging is also detectable in persons with DS who routinely receive MR scans (Emerson et al., 1994; Emerson, Kesslak, Chen, & Lott, 1995; Prasher, Barber, West, & Glenholmes, 1996; Roth, Sun, Greensite, Lott, & Dietrich, 1996). MR imaging can therefore be useful in detecting a dementing process in the DS child (Kesslak, Nagata, Lott, & Nalcioglu, 1994). Recently, Aylward et al. (1997) have shown that while cerebellar volumes are smaller in DS, they do not diminish significantly with age. It may be that comparison to changing status of cerebral structures to the more age resistant cerebellar structures will aid in detecting deterioration.

FRAGILE X SYNDROME

The quantitative analyses of MR scans from subjects with fragile X syndrome by Reiss, Freund, Tsang, and Joshi (1991) probably represent the most comprehensive studies of brain abnormalities in this syndrome to date. Reiss et al.'s results indicated morphological differences in the temporal lobes (particularly the hippocampus) and reduced size of the cerebellum.

FRIEDREICH ATAXIA

Although individuals with various ataxic disorders may have cerebellar and brain stem atrophy, the study by Ormerod et al. (1994) found no specific central nervous system (CNS) abnormalities on MR scans of subjects with Friedreich ataxia. These authors compared cortical/subcortical, cerebellum, brain stem, and cervical cord findings in patients with early and late Friedreich ataxia, normal controls, and patients with ataxic disorders other than Friedreich ataxia.

INBORN ERRORS OF METABOLISM

Infants and children with inborn errors of metabolism have numerous structural and metabolic abnormalities of the brain. One of the most common of these disorders is adrenoleukodystrophy, in which extensive white matter degeneration occurs (see Figure 4.5 and Patel et al., 1995; Vanhanen, Raininko, Autti, & Santavuori, 1995a; Vanhanen, Raininko,

TABLE 4.1. Summary of Major Neuroimaging Findings in Various Developmental Disorders

Condition	Ventricles	Cortex	Subcortex	Other
Autism	Possibly increased cortical and ventricular CSF	High frequency of regional structural abnormalities that included localized parietal and frontal volume loss, localized pachygyria, and micro- and macrogyria, suggestive of neuronal migration abnormalities Diffuse regional abnormalities in rCBF and metabolism may correspond to the presence of regional structural abnormalities MRS studies suggest hypermetabolism and abnormal cell membrane metabolism in prefrontal cortex Possibly increased cortical CSF	None described	Possibly altered size of vermian lobules VI and VII; hypo- and hyperplastic subtypes may exist No alterations in cerebellar blood flow have been seen Possibly reduced size of midbrain and medulla
Fragile X syndrome	Increased fourth ventricle size	Bilaterally increased hippocampal volumes Bilaterally decreased size of the superior temporal gyrus Hippocampal and superior temporal gyrus volume changes may be correlated with increasing age	None described	Size reductions of vermian lobules VI and VII that may correlate with sex-specific differences in the degree of genetic loading
Down syndrome	None described	Decreased whole brain and gray matter volumes, with a disproportionately large reduction in frontal gray matter volume Abnormal regional intercorrelations of frontal and parietal cortices	Relative sparing of lenticular nucleus and diencephalon	Reduced size of the anterior regions of the corpus callosum Reduced cerebellar volumes and reduced size of all vermian lobules

Schizophrenia	Increased VBR Increased size of temporal horn of left lateral ventricle Ventricular size in at-risk individuals appears to be determined by the interaction of genetic and environmental risk factor exposure	Decreased metabolism and rCBF in frontal cortex Probably reduced frontal cortex volumes Reduced volumes of anterior superior temporal gyrus (auditory association cortex), and possibly increased rCBF during auditory hallucinations Possibly reduced amygdala and hippocampus (esp. gray matter) volumes Possibly reduced asymmetries of temporal lobe and cortical surface Increased cortical CSF	Variable volumetric changes in basal ganglia, possibly increased Decreased metabolism and rCBF in basal ganglia that may normalize with treatment Reduced basal ganglia volumetric and metabolic asymmetries Increased right-sided basal ganglia metabolism with neuroleptics Inconsistent findings of increased striatal dopamine receptor density Thalamic lesions, esp. on the right	Inconsistent reports of increased size of all cerebellar vermian lobules
TS	Possibly enlarged ventricles with abnormal asymmetries	Possibly reduced metabolism in frontal, cingulate, and insular cortices Abnormal T2 asymmetries in frontal white matter	Left-sided lenticular nucleus volume reductions and absence of asymmetry in children and adults Reduced basal ganglia metabolism, possibly more pronounced in ventral portions Abnormal T2 asymmetries in basal ganglia Possibly increased level of presynaptic dopamine transporter sites	Reduced midsagittal cross-sectional area of the corpus callosum in adults Possibly abnormal T2 times in red nucleus and amygdala

(cont.)

TABLE 4.1. (cont.)

Condition	Ventricles	Cortex	Subcortex	Other
ADHD	No obvious ventricular size abnormalities	Possibly sulcal widening Variable functional findings, including reduced metabolic rates in sensory–motor, auditory, and occipital regions in adolescents; reductions in global rates and regional normalized rates in premotor and sensory–motor regions in adults	Possibly reduced left lenticular nucleus volumes in ADHD subjects with comorbid TS Possibly reduced striatal metabolism in adolescents Possibly absence of normal caudate nucleus asymmetry	Reduced cross-sectional area of corpus callosum subregions, variably seen in anterior (genu, rostrum) and posterior (rostral body, isthmus, splenium) portions
Dyslexia	None described	Varying reports of abnormal asymmetries in the planum temporale Tissue may be distributed differently between the temporal and parietal banks of the planum in dyslexic subjects Multiple Heschl gyri often seen on either side in the planum temporale Metabolic activation of the left posterior planum may be reduced, and activation of medial portions may be increased bilaterally during phonological processing tasks	None described	None

Note. See the corresponding portions of the text for a more complete discussion of these summary findings and citations of the studies reporting them. CSF, cerebrospinal fluid; rCBF, regional cerebral blood flow; MRS, magnetic resonance spectroscopy; VBR, ventricle–brain ratio; ADHD, attention-deficit/hyperactivity disorder; TS, Tourette syndrome. Adapted from Peterson (1995). Copyright 1995 by the American Academy of Child and Adolescent Psychiatry. Adapted by permission from Lippincott Williams & Wilkins.

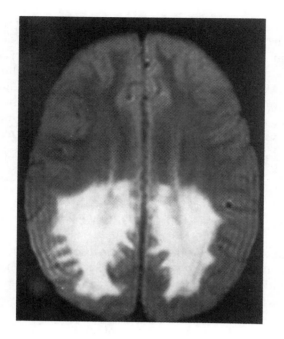

FIGURE 4.5. MR image obtained from a 6-year-old boy with adrenoleukodystrophy. The "white" regions clearly depicted bilaterally signify white matter degeneration, which is extensive and bilateral. The white matter (darker gray) seen in the frontal region is the normal signal seen with white matter. This type of extensive degenerative change is associated with significant cognitive decline in these children. From Wolpert and Barnes (1992). Copyright 1992 by C. V. Mosby and Year Book Medical Publishers. Reprinted by permission.

Santavuori, Autti, & Haltia, 1995b). These disorders tend to have devastating neurological effects, often resulting in early death. One inborn error of metabolism, phenylketonuria (PKU), is discussed separately below.

KLINEFELTER SYNDROME

Most MR reports dealing with Klinefelter syndrome are single-case or anecdotal reports (Heausler et al., 1992; Miyamoto, Kitawaki, Koida, & Nagao, 1993). No consistent abnormality has been reported, but various abnormalities have been seen in subjects with this syndrome, including ventricular dilation, hypoplasia of subcortical structures, and focal lesions.

NEUROFIBROMATOSIS

Neurofibromatosis (NF) is one of the genetic disorders most frequently studied with CT and MR imaging, because of the characteristic abnormalities that represent the CNS extensions of the classic cutaneous lesions associated with NF. Most studies have demonstrated lesions to be most likely in the basal ganglia and while matter of the brain

(Boardman, Anslow, & Renowden, 1996; Castillo et al., 1995; DiMario, Ramsby, Breenstein, Langshur, & Dunham, 1993; Es, North, McHugh, & de Silva, 1996; Ferner, Chaudhuri, Bingham, Cox, & Hughes, 1993; Hofman, Harris, Bryan, & Denckla, 1994; Itoh et al., 1994; Menor, & Marti-Bonmati, 1992; Menor, Marti-Bonmati, Mulas, Cortina, & Olague, 1991; Moore, Ater, Needle, Slopis, & Copeland, 1994; North et al., 1994; Terada, Barkovich, Edwards, & Ciricillo, 1996). A number of studies have attempted to relate the number of central NF lesions to cognitive and/or behavioral deficits, but no clearly systematic relationships have been characterized (see Denckla et al., 1996; DiMario et al., 1993; Ferner et al., 1993; Hofman et al., 1994; Moore, Slopis, Schomer, Jackson, & Levy, 1996).

RETT SYNDROME

Rett syndrome is a progressive neurodevelopmental disorder that occurs in young females. These children display autistic-like behavior, gait ataxia and generalized apraxia, and microcephaly. Cognitively, significant intellectual compromise is present where the child deteriorates after meeting "normal" perinatal developmental milestones. Subramaniam, Naidu, and Reiss (1997) have examined the neuroanatomy of Rett syndrome demonstrating global reductions in white and gray matter volumes along with preferential reduction in caudate nucleus volume.

NEUROPSYCHIATRIC DISORDERS

Considerable genetic loading is present in many of the major neuropsychiatric disorders (Peterson, 1995). Table 4.1 summarizes the imaging findings in several of these disorders, including autism, schizophrenia, ADHD, and dyslexia. From a neuroimaging perspective, schizophrenia and ADHD are probably the most widely studied of the neuropsychiatric disorders. The consensus of this work, as summarized in Table 4.1, is that these disorders are associated with underlying structural aberrations, none of which are diagnostic.

Attention-Deficit/Hyperactivity Disorder and Learning Disabilities

With regard to ADHD, one of the most comprehensive studies performed recently is that by Filipek et al. (1997). These authors found that ADHD subjects had smaller volumes in the following structures: left total caudate and caudate head, right anterior superior (frontal) region and white matter, bilateral anterior inferior region, and bilateral retrocallosal (parietal–occipital) region white matter. These localized structural anomalies appear to be concordant with theoretical models of abnormal frontal–striatal and parietal function. Castellanos et al. (1996) have provided supporting evidence for the hypothesized dysfunction of right-sided prefrontal–striatal systems in ADHD. They found that ADHD subjects had a 4.7% smaller total cerebral volume, a significant loss of normal right-greater-than-left asymmetry in the caudate, smaller right globus pallidus, smaller right anterior frontal region, smaller cerebellum, and reversal of normal lateral ventricular asymmetry. Giedd et al. (1994) found that the rostrum and rostral body of the corpus callosum were significantly smaller in the ADHD group than in controls.

Neuroimaging studies in learning disabilities up to the early 1990s were summarized by Bigler (1992). More recently, Schultz, Cho, Staib, and Kier (1994) completed a comprehensive study of dyslexic children and the planum temporale (a temporal lobe structure thought to be related to learning ability), but no consistent abnormalities were identified. However, Hynd et al. (1995) did find smaller corpus callosum size in children with dyslexia than in controls (see also Hynd & Semrud-Clikeman, 1989).

Pervasive Developmental Disorders

Over the last decade, a number of larger studies have been conducted on children with various PDDs. For example, a study by Delacato, Szegda, and Parisi (1994) included CT and MR clinical evaluations performed on 474 children diagnosed with autism. They found that 81% of these subjects had some degree of ventricular enlargement, a nonspecific indication of possible injury or maldevelopment (see also Piven, Arndt, Bailey, & Andreasen, 1996; Piven et al., 1995). Various structural abnormalities have been reported by other researchers, including cerebellar vermal hypoplasia and hyperplasia (Courchesne et al., 1994a; Courchesne, Townsend, & Saitoh, 1994b; Hashimoto et al., 1995), decreased volume in midbrain and brain stem structures (Hashimoto, Murakawa, Miyazaki, Tayama, & Kuroda, 1991a; Hashimoto et al., 1991b; Hashimoto, Tayama, Miyazaki, Murukawa, & Kuroda, 1993; Hashimoto et al., 1992, 1995), decrease in the parietal lobe cortex volume and white matter (Courchesne, Press, & Yeung-Courchesne, 1993), and larger hemisphere or lobe size (Bailey et al., 1993; Filipek et al., 1992; Piven et al., 1992, 1995, 1996). Other studies have begun to investigate structures such as the hippocampus in autistic patients (Filipek et al., 1992; Saitoh, Courchesne, Egaas, Lincoln, & Schreibman, 1995).

Recent studies involving CT and MR in Rett syndrome have indicated other findings, including frontal atrophy, global brain hypoplasia, progressive cerebellar atrophy with increasing age, reduced hemisphere and caudate nuclei sizes, and reduced gray and white matter. However, some of these findings may be complicated by superimposed factors, such as seizure activity, use of anticonvulsants, or poor nutrition (Atlas, 1996). Studies involving small numbers of individuals with Asperger syndrome include findings of cortical dysplasias in the frontal and temporal lobes (Berthier, Starkstein, & Leiguarda, 1990), and of decreased gyri and increased sulci widths in anterior perisylvian and posterior parietal areas (Berthier, 1994). However, to date, studies of patients with PDDs suggest no specific structural abnormality that appears to encompass the spectrum of PDDs (Atlas, 1996; Filipek, 1996a, 1996b). In fact, there seems to be considerable heterogeneity in the type and degree of abnormalities associated with PDDs (Courchesne et al., 1993, 1994a, 1994b; Holttum, Minshew, Sanders, & Phillips, 1992; Jambaque, Cusami, Curatolo, & Cortesi, 1991).

PHENYLKETONURIA

Various imaging abnormalities have been reported with PKU—in particular, diffuse signal irregularities throughout the brain (especially the white matter) and calcifications of the basal ganglia (Cleary et al., 1994; Hasselbach et al., 1996; Ishimaru, Tamasawa, Baba,

Matsunga, & Takebe, 1993; Leuzzi, Trasmeni, Gualdi, & Antonozzi, 1995). The study by Cleary et al. (1994) also looked for a relationship between the number of MR abnormalities and IQ, but no specific relationship was identified. PET imaging studies as well as MR spectroscopy have demonstrated regions of greatest phenylalanine concentrations; these are especially prominent in the basal ganglia and cerebellum (Kreis, Pietz, Penzien, Herschkowitz, & Boesch, 1995; Paans, et al., 1996).

SICKLE CELL DISEASE

Neuroimaging abnormalities associated with sickle cell disease (SCD) are related to the greater likelihood of SCD children to have vascular lesions and strokes. Kugler et al. (1993) compared SCD children with age-matched normal children and found that over 90% of the SCD children followed over time had vascular lesions and white matter hyperintensities. The most common lesion associated with SCD is a small infarct in the periventricular region of the brain, with small-vessel disease the neuropathological substrate (Hajnal et al., 1992; Z. Wang et al., 1992).

TOURETTE SYNDROME

Several MR imaging studies of Tourette syndrome (TS) have been done (Hyde et al., 1995; Peterson, Gore, Riddle, Cohen, & Leckman, 1994; Peterson et al., 1993; Singer et al., 1993). Mild ventricular enlargement, white matter hyperintensities, basal ganglia abnormalities, and reduced corpus callosum area have all been reported. TS subjects also have been evaluated with metabolic imaging methods including SPECT and PET; these studies have demonstrated abnormalities in basal ganglia, as well as in some limbic structures (Braun, Stoetter, & Randolph, 1993; Chase, Geoffrey, Gillespe, & Burrows, 1986). A comparison of TS patients with and without Asperger syndrome found all but one TS patient without this PDD to have normal MR scans, whereas five of the seven patients with both syndromes had developmental brain anomalies (Berthier, Bayes, & Tolosa, 1993). Thus structural cortical and subcortical abnormalities are more common in individual with concurrent TS and Asperger syndrome than in those with TS alone. Dysfunction of frontal–subcortical systems is implicated in the pathophysiology of concurrent TS and Asperger syndrome. In addition, Peterson (1995) found reduced midsagittal cross-sectional area of the corpus callosum in nearly 20% of TS subjects.

A case study (Leckman et al., 1993) described a 40-year-old man with severe TS, characterized by self-injurious motor tics, coprolalia, and obsessive–compulsive disorder. He had bilateral anterior cigulotomies and bilateral infrathalamic lesions placed stereotactically during two neurosurgical procedures, after which he developed a marked dysarthia and severe gait disturbance with postural instability, bradykinesia, axial rigidity, micrographia, and a profound swallowing disorder. His MR showed asymmetrical (left > right) low-density areas in an infrathalamic region, as well as low-density areas bilaterally in the anterior cingulate gyri. The tics and obsessive–compulsive symptoms improved, though the self-injurious motor tics and other motor and phonic tics recurred. In addition, the patient's speech remained largely unintelligible for 8 months following the last surgery, and other neurological deficits remained unchanged. In another case study (Patoni, Poggesi, Repice, & Inzitari, 1997), a 48-year-old man with TS experienced relief from his motor tics after the onset of a midbrain syndrome related to thiamine deficiency (Wernicke encephalopathy). His MR scan showed a lesion in the dorsal area of the midbrain, suggesting that loops in the midbrain tegmentum may influence the presence of motor tics.

TURNER SYNDROME

Turner syndrome stems from a partial or complete absence of the X chromosome. Physical characteristics include short stature, webbing of the neck, lack of pubertal maturation, and various degrees of cognitive limitations. MR imaging has demonstrated reduced brain volume in subjects with Turner syndrome. Three studies have used MR methods to evaluate children with Turner syndrome in more detail, and these studies demonstrated various morphological differences (Reiss et al., 1993). As with other syndromes, no pathognomonic MR features are diagnostic of Turner syndrome, but these studies tend to indicate smaller brain structures than normal.

INFANTILE NEURONAL CEROID LIPOFUSCINOSIS

Infantile neuronal ceroid lipofuscinosis is transmitted as an autosomal recessive trait, with the gene located on chromosome 1. Early development may be normal, but by 6 to 18 months of age, deterioration begins; this includes muscular hypotonia, truncal ataxia, mental retardation, visual impairment, epilepsy, and eventually death. Figure 4.6 demonstrates the extensive pathological changes associated with infantile neuronal ceroid lipofuscinosis as visualized on MR imaging (Vanhanen et al., 1995b).

THE CENTRAL THEME: BRAIN MALFORMATION

The central theme of most of the discussion above is that brain malformation is often associated with some established genetic aberration. As an extreme example, Figure 4.7 is an MR image of a child with hydranencephaly, a condition where the cerebrum essentially does not develop. A common consequence of many other brain malformations is some degree of hydrocephalus. A severe form of hydrocephalus is illustrated in Figure 4.8. In both Figures 4.7 and 4.8, excess cerebrospinal fluid is present to fill the void created by the absence of brain tissue. Often some of the most significant changes in brain structure may be manifested in ventricular abnormality. Also, there are a variety of disorders that affect primarily hindbrain development. Ramaekers, Heimann, Reul, Thron, and Jaeken (1997) have shown that the majority of children with cerebellar structural abnormalities had some form of an autosomal recessively inherited disease. The importance of identifying any abnormalities, including deviations from normal size, is that such abnormalities often have a significant effect on cognitive and neurobehavioral development (Reiss, Abrams, Singer, Ross, & Denckla, 1996).

CONCLUSIONS

Most genetic disorders that influence the brain are associated with structural abnormalities that can be detected by standard neuroimaging techniques. The nature and degree of

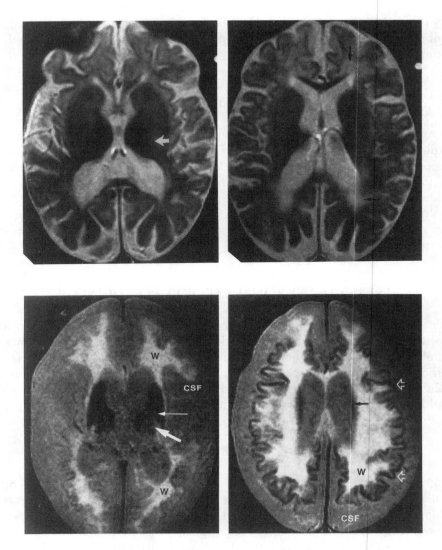

FIGURE 4.6. MR abnormalities in infantile neuronal ceroid lipofuscinosis. (Top) MR scan from a 17-month-old girl with moderately enlarged sulci and third ventricle. The corpus callosum is thin. Signal abnormalities are also present: The white arrow indicates striking hypointensity in the thalamus, whereas the dark arrows indicate hyperintense regions in the periventricular regions. (Bottom) Axial MR section from an 8-year-old boy (left); axial MR section from an 11-year-old girl (right). W, white matter; CSF, cerebrospinal fluid. Note the extensive loss of brain substance, with the void filled with cerebrospinal fluid. In the scan on the left, the arrows denote signal abnormalities in the basal ganglia (thin white arrow) and thalamus (thick white arrow). In the scan on the right, the cortex can be barely discerned between the white matter and the outer cortical mantle (open white arrows). Signal abnormality is also observed in the caudate (thin black arrow). From Vanhanen, Raininko, Santavuori, Autti, and Haltia (1995b). Copyright 1995 by B. C. Decker Inc. Publisher. Reprinted by permission.

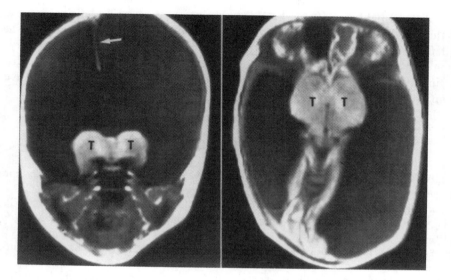

FIGURE 4.7. A case of hydranencephaly. Note that the cerebral hemispheres are essentially replaced by cerebrospinal fluid. (Left) Coronal view. Arrow points to the falx, but note the absence of any cerebral tissue. (Right) Axial view showing prominent thalami (T) and a thin remnant of the posterior medial temporal lobe and inferior occipital lobe. Note again the absence of cerebral tissue. From Wolpert and Barnes (1992). Copyright 1992 by C. V. Mosby and Year Book Medical Publishers. Reprinted by permission.

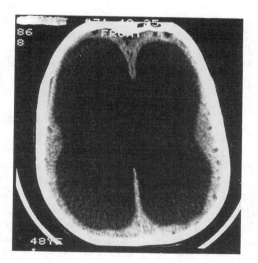

FIGURE 4.8. Axial CT scan from an individual with hydrocephalus. Note that just a thin mantle of tissue is left around the cortical rim. In such cases of hydrocephalus, massive structural abnormality is present in the brain. However, unlike the case presented in Figure 4.7 (where the brain did not develop, resulting in ventricular expansion to fill the void), for the individual in this figure, the expanding pressure of cerebrospinal fluid in the ventricle produced brain damage by compressing tissue. This patient had achondoplasia dwarfism.

structural abnormality are often related to behavioral and cognitive deficits associated with a genetic disorder. Although this is not a linear relationship, generally the greater the structural defect, the greater the neurobehavioral and cognitive deficits. Contemporary neuroimaging techniques are a vital part of any workup in individuals with genetic disorders. These findings should be reviewed by the neuropsychologist as part of comprehensive evaluation and treatment planning.

REFERENCES

Atlas, S. W. (1996). *Magnetic resonance imaging of the brain and spine*. Philadelphia: Lippincott–Raven.

Aylward, E. H., Habbak, R., Warren, A. C., Pulsifer, M. B., Barta, P. E., Jerram, M., & Pearlson, G. D. (1997). Cerebellar volume in adults with Down syndrome. *Archives of Neurology, 54*, 209–212.

Bailey, A., Luthert, P., Bolton, P., Le Couteur, A., Rutter, M., & Harding, B. (1993). Autism and megalencephaly. *Lancet, 341*, 1225–1226.

Berthier, M. L. (1994). Corticocallosal anomalies in Asperger's sydnrome [Letter]. *Journal of Roentgenology, 162*, 236–237.

Berthier, M. L., Bayes, A., & Tolosa, E. S. (1993). Magnetic resonance imaging in patients with concurrent Tourette's disorder and Asperger's syndrome. *Journal of the American Academy of Child and Adolescent Psychiatry, 32*, 633–639.

Berthier, M. L., Starkstein, S. E., & Leiguarda, R. (1990). Developmental cortical anomalies in Asperger's syndrome: Neuroradiological findings in two patients. *Journal of Neuropsychiatry and Clinical Neurosciences, 2*, 197–201.

Bigler, E. D. (1992). The neurobiology and neuropsychology of adult learning disorders. *Journal of Learning Disabilities, 25*, 488–506.

Bigler, E. D. (1996a). *Neuroimaging: Vol. 1. Basic science*. New York: Plenum Press.

Bigler, E. D. (1996b). *Neuroimaging: Vol. 2. Clinical applications*. New York: Plenum Press.

Bigler, E. D., Nilsson, D. E., Burr, R. B., & Boyer, R. S. (1997). Neuroimaging in pediatric neuropsychology. In C. R. Reynolds & E. Fletcher-Janzen (Eds.), *Handbook of clinical child neuropsychology* (2nd ed., pp. 342–355). New York: Plenum Press.

Bigler, E. D., Yeo, R. A., & Turkheimer, E. (1989). *Neuropsychological function and brain imaging*. New York: Plenum Press.

Boardman, P., Anslow, P., & Renowden, S. (1996). Pictoral review: MR imaging of neuronal migration anomalies. *Clinical Radiology, 51*, 11–17.

Boyd, S. G., Homer, A. H., & Patton, M. A. (1988). EEG in early diagnosis of Angelman's (happy puppet) syndrome. *European Journal of Pediatrics, 147*, 508–513.

Braun, A. R., Stoetter, B., & Randolph, C. (1993). The functional neuroanatomy of Tourette's syndrome: An FDG-PET study, I. Regional changes in cerebral glucose metabolism differentiating patients and controls. *Neuropsychopharmacology, 9*, 277–291.

Castellanos, F. X., Giedd, J. N., Marsh, W. L., Hamburger, S. D., Vaiturzis, A. D., Dickstein, D. P., Sarfatti, S. E., Vauss, Y. C., Snell, J. W., Lange, N., Kaysen, D., Krain, A. L., Ritchie, G. F., Rajapakse, J. C., & Rapoport, J. L. (1996). Quantitative brain magnetic resonance imaging in attention-deficit hyperactivity disorder. *Archives of General Psychiatry, 53*, 607–616.

Castillo, M., Green, C., Kwock, L., Smith, K., Wilson, D., Schiro, S., & Greenwood, R. (1995). Proton MR spectroscopy in patients with neurofibromatosis type 1: Evaluation of hamartomas and clinical correlation. *American Journal of Neuroradiology, 16*, 141–147.

Chase, T. N., Geoffrey, V., Gillespe, M., & Burrows, G. H. (1986). Structural and functional studies of Gilles de la Tourette syndrome. *Review of Neurology* (Paris), *142*, 851–855.

Cleary, M. A., Walter, J. H., Wraith, J. E., Jenkins, J. P., Alani, S. M., Tyler, K., & Whittle, D. (1994). Magnetic resonance imaging of the brain in phenylketonuria. *Lancet, 344*, 87–90.

Courchesne, E., Press, G. A., & Yeung-Courchesne, R. (1993). Parietal lobe abnormalities detected with MR inpatient with infantile autism. *American Journal of Roentgenology, 160,* 387–393.

Courchesne, E., Townsend, J., Akshoomoff, N. A., Saitoh, O., Yeung-Courchesne, R., Lincoln, A. J., James, H., Haas, R. H., Schreibman, L., & Lau, L. (1994a). Impairment in shifting attention in autistic and cerebellar patients. *Behavioral Neuroscience, 108,* 848–865.

Courchesne, E., Townsend, J., & Saitoh, O. (1994b). The brain in infantile autism: Posterior fossa structures are abnormal. *Neurology, 44,* 214–223.

Delacato, D. F., Szegda, D. T., & Parisi, A. (1994). Neurophysiological view of autism: Review of recent research as it applies to the Delacato theory of autism. *Developmental Brain Dysfunction, 7,* 129–131.

Denckla, M., Hofman, K., Mazzocco, M., Melhem, E., Reiss, A., Bryan, R., Harris, E., J, L., Cox, C., & Schuerlolz, L. (1996). Relationship between T2-weighted hyperintensities (unidentified bright objects) and lower IQs in children with neurofibromatosis-1. *American Journal of Medical Genetics (Neuropsychiatric Genetics), 67,* 98–102.

DiMario, F., Ramsby, G., Breenstein, R., Langshur, S., & Dunham, B. (1993). Neurofibromatosis type 1: Magnetic resonance imaging findings. *Journal of Child Neurology, 3,* 32–39.

Dorries, A., Spohr, H. L., & Kunze, J. (1988). Angelman ("happy puppet") syndrome—seven new cases documented by cerebral computed tomography: Review of the literature. *European Journal of Paediatrics, 148,* 270–273.

Emerson, J. F., Chen, P. C., Shankle, W. R., Greesite, F. S., Foltz, E. L., Lott, I. T., & Nalcioglu, O. (1994). Cortical CSF volume fluctuations by MRI in brain aging, dementia and hydrocephalus. *Neuroreport, 5,* 27–30.

Emerson, J. F., Kesslak, J. P., Chen, P. C., & Lott, I. T. (1995). Magnetic resonance imaging of the aging brain in Down syndrome. *Progress in Clinical and Biological Research, 393,* 123–138.

Es, S., North, K., McHugh, K., & de Silva, M. (1996). MRI findings in children with neurofibromatosis type 1: A prospective study. *Pediatric Radiology, 26,* 478–487.

Ferner, R., Chaudhuri, R., Bingham, J., Cox, T., & Hughes, R. (1993). MRI in neurofibromatosis 1: The nature and evolution of increased intensity T2 weighted lesions and their relationship to intellectual impairment. *Journal of Neurology Neurosurgery, and Psychiatry, 56,* 492–495.

Filipek, P. A. (1996a). Structural variations in measures in the developmental disorders. In R. W. Thatcher, G. R. Lyon, J. Rumsey, & N. Krasnegor (Eds.), *Developmental neuroimaging: Mapping the development of brain and behavior* (pp. 169–186). San Diego, CA: Academic Press.

Filipek, P. A. (1996b). Brief report: Neuroimaging in autism—the state of the science 1995. *Journal of Autism and Developmental Disorders, 26,* 211–215.

Filipek, P. A., Richelme, C., Kennedy, D. N., Rademacher, J., Pitcher, D. A., Zidel, S. Y., & Caviness, V. S. (1992). Morphometric analysis of the brain in developmental language disorders and autism. *Annals of Neurology, 32,* 475. (Abstract)

Filipek, P. A., Semrud-Clikeman, M., Steingard, R. J., Renshaw, P. F., Kennedy, D. N., & Biederman, J. (1997). Volumetric MRI analysis comparing subjects having attention-deficit hyperactivity disorder with normal controls. *Neurology, 48,* 589–601.

Ganji, S., & Duncan, M. C. (1989). Angelman's (happy puppet) syndrome: Clinical, CT scan and serial electroencephalographic study. *Clinical Electroencephalography, 20,* 128–140.

Giedd, J. N., Castellanos, F. X., Casey, B. J., Kozuch, P., King, A. C., Hamburger, S. D., & Rapoport, J. L. (1994). Quantitiative morphology of the corpus callosum in attention deficit hyperactivity disorder. *American Journal of Psychiatry, 151,* 665–669.

Hajnal, J. V., Bryant, D. J., Kasuboski, L., Pattany, P. M., De Coene, B., Lewis, P. D., Pennock, J. M., Oatridge, A., Young, I. R., & Bydder, G. M. (1992). Use of fluid attenuated inversion recovery (FLAIR) sequences in MRI of the brain. *Journal of Computed Assisted Tomography, 16,* 841–844.

Hashimoto, T., Murakawa, K., Miyazaki, M., Tayama, M., & Kuroda, Y. (1991a). Magnetic resonance imaging of the brain structures in the posterior fossa in retarded autistic children. *Acta Paediatrica, 81,* 149–153.

Hashimoto, T., Tayama, M., Miyazaki, M., Murukawa, K., & Kuroda, Y. (1993). Brainstem and cerebellar vermis involvement in autistic children. *Journal of Child Neurology, 8,* 149–153.

Hashimoto, T., Tayama, M., Miyazaki, M., Murakawa, K., Sakurama, N., Yoshimoto, T., & Kuroda, Y. (1991b). Reduced midbrain and pons size in children with autism. *Tokushima Journal of Experimental Medicine, 38,* 15–18.

Hashimoto, T., Tayama, M., Miyazaki, M., Sakurama, N., Yoshimiti, T., Murakawa, K., & Kuroda, Y. (1992). Reduced brainstem size in children with autism. *Brain and Development, 14,* 94–97.

Hashimoto, T., Tayama, M., Murakawa, K., Yoshimoto, T., Miyazaki, M., Harada, M., & Kuroda, Y. (1995). Development of the brainstem and cerebellum in autistic patients. *Journal of Autism and Developmental Disorders, 25,* 1–18.

Hasselbach, S., Knudsen, G. M., Toft, P. B., Hogh, P., Tedeschi, E., Holm, S., Videbaek, C., Henriksen, O., Lou, H. C., & Paulson, O. B. (1996). Cerebral glucose metabolism is decreased in white matter changes in patients with phenylketonuria. *Pediatric Research, 40,* 21–24.

Heausler, G., Frisch, H., Guchev, F., Hadziselimovic, A., Neuhold, A., & Vormittag, W. (1992). Hypoplasia of the corpus callosum and growth hormone deficiency in the XXXXY syndrome. *American Journal of Medical Genetics, 44,* 230–232.

Hofman, K., Harris, E., Bryan, R., & Denckla, M. (1994). Neurofibromatosis type 1: The cognitive phenotype. *Journal of Pediatrics, 124,* S1–S8.

Holttum, J. R., Minshew, N. J., Sanders, R. S., & Phillips, N. E. (1992). Magnetic resonance imaging of the posterior fossa in autism. *Biological Psychiatry, 32,* 1091–1101.

Hyde, T. M., Stacey, M. E., Coppola, R., Handel, S. F., Rickler, K. C., & Weinberger, D. R. (1995). Cerebral morphometric abnormalities in Tourette's syndrome: The influence of comorbid attention-deficit/hyperactivity disorder. *Neurology, 47,* 1176–1182.

Hynd, G. W., & Semrud-Clikeman, M. (1989). Dyslexia and brain morphology. *Psychological Bulletin, 106,* 447–469.

Hynd, G. W., Hall, J., Novey, E. S., Eliopulos, D., Black, K., Gonzalez, J. J., Edmonds, J. E., Riccio, C., & Cohen, M. (1995). Dyslexia and corpus callosum morphology. *Archives of Neurology, 52,* 32–38.

Ishimaru, K., Tamasawa, N., Baba, M., Matsunga, M., & Takebe, K. (1993). Phenylketonuria with adult-onset neurological manifestation. *Rinsho-Shinkeigaku, 33,* 961–965.

Itoh, T., Magnaldi, S., White, R., Denckla, M., Hofman, K., Naidu, S., & Bryan, R. (1994). Neurofibromatosis type 1: The evolution of deep gray and white matter MR abnormalities. *American Journal of Neuroradiology, 15,* 1513–1519.

Jambaque, I., Cusami, R., Curatolo, P., & Cortesi, F. (1991). Neuropsychological aspects of tuberous sclerosis in relation to epilepsy and MRI findings. *Developmental Medicine and Child Neurology, 33,* 698–705.

Jernigan, T. L., & Bellugi, U. (1990). Anomalous brain morphology on magnetic resonance images in Williams syndrome and Down syndrome. *Archives of Neurology, 47,* 529–533.

Jernigan, T. L., Bellugi, U., Sowell, E., Doherty, S., & Hesselink, J. R. (1993). Cerebral morphologic distinctions between Williams and Down syndromes. *Archives of Neurology, 50,* 186–191.

Kesslak, J. P., Nagata, S. F., Lott, I., & Nalcioglu, O. (1994). Magnetic resonance imaging analysis of age-related changes in the brains of individuals with Down's syndrome. *Neurology, 44,* 1039–1045.

Kragskov, J., Sindet-Pedersen, S., Gyldensted, C., & Jensen, K. L. (1996). A comparison of three-dimensional computed tomography scans and stereolithographic models of evaluation of craniofacial anomalies. *Journal of Oral and Maxillofacial Surgery, 54,* 402–411.

Kreis, R., Pietz, J., Penzien, J., Herschkowitz, N., & Boesch, C. (1995). Identification and quantitation of phenylalanine in the brain of patients with phenylketonuria by means of localized *in vivo* 1H magnetic resonance spectroscopy. *Journal of Magnetic Resonance-B, 107,* 242–251.

Kugler, S., Anderson, B., Cross, D., Sharif, Z., Sano, M., Haggety, R., Prohovnick, I., Hurlet-Jensen, A., Hilal, S., Mohr, J., & DeVivo, D. C. (1993). Abnormal cranial magnetic resonance imaging scans in sickle-cell disease. *Archives of Neurology, 50,* 629–635.

Leckman, J. F., de Lotbiniere, A. J., Marek, K., Cracco, C., Scahill, L., & Cohen, D. J. (1993).

Severe disturbances in speech, swallowing and gait following stereotactic infrathalamic lesions in Gilles de la Tourette's syndrome. *Movement Disorders, 11,* 563–566.

Leuzzi, V., Trasimeni, G., Gualdi, G. F., & Antonozzi, I. (1995). Biochemical, clinical and neuroradiological (MRI) correlations in late-detected PKU patients. *Journal of Inherited Metabolic Disorders, 18,* 624–634.

Menor, F., & Marti-Bonmati, L. (1992). CT detection of basal ganglion lesions in neurofibromatosis type 1: Correlation with MRI. *Pediatric Radiology, 21,* 227–235.

Menor, F., Marti-Bonmati, L., Mulas, F., Cortina, H., & Olague, R. (1991). Imaging considerations of central nervous system manifestations in pediatric patients with neurofibromatosis type 1. *Pediatric Radiology, 21,* 389–394.

Miyamoto, A., Kitawaki, K., Koida, H., & Nagao, K. (1993). MRI and SPECT of Klinefelter's syndrome with various neuropsychiatric symptoms: A case report. *Japanese Journal of Psychiatry and Neurology, 47,* 863–867.

Moore, B., Ater, J., Needle, M., Slopis, J., & Copeland, D. (1994). Neuropsychological profile of children with neurofibromatosis, brain, tumor, or both. *Journal of Child Neurology, 9,* 363–377.

Moore, B., Slopis, J., Schomer, D., Jackson, E., & Levy, B. (1996). Neuropsychological significance of areas of high signal intensity on brain MRIs of children with neurofibromatosis. *Neurology, 46,* 1660–1668.

North, K., Joy, P., Yuille, D., Cocks, N., Mobbs, E., Hutchings, P., McHugh, K., & de Silva, M. (1994). Specific learning disability in children with neurofibromatosis type 1: Significance of MRI abnormalities. *Neurology, 44,* 878–883.

Ormerod, I. E. C., Harding, A. E., Miller, D. H., Johnson, G., MacManus, D., du Boulay, E. P. G. H., Kendall, B. E., Moseley, I. F., & McDonald, W. I. (1994). Magnetic resonance imaging in degenerative ataxic disorders. *Journal of Neurology, Neurosurgery and Psychiatry, 57,* 51–57.

Osborn, A. G. (1995). *Diagnostic neuroradiology.* St. Louis, MO: Mosby.

Paans, A. M., Pruim, J., Smit, G. P., Visser, G., Willemsen, A. T., & Ullrich, K. (1996). Neurotransmitter positron emission tomographic studies in adults with phenylketonuria: A pilot study. *European Journal of Pediatrics, 155,* 78–81.

Patel, P. J., Kolawole, T. M., Malabarey, T. M., Al-Herbish, A. S., Al-Jurrayan, N. A. M., & Saleh, M. (1995). Adrenoleukodystrophy: CT and MRI findings. *Pediatric Radiology, 25,* 256–258.

Patoni, L., Poggesi, L., Repice, A., & Inzitari, D. (1997). Disappearance of motor tics after Wernicke's encephalopathy in a patient with Tourette's syndrome. *Neurology, 48,* 381–383.

Peterson, B. S. (1995). Neuroimaging in child and adolescent neuropsychiatric disorders. *Journal of the American Academy of Child and Adolescent Psychiatry, 34,* 1560–1567.

Peterson, B. S., Gore, J. C., Riddle, M. A., Cohen, D. J., & Leckman, J. F. (1994). Abnormal magnetic resonance imaging T2 relaxation time asymmetries in Tourette's syndrome. *Psychiatry Research, 55,* 205–221.

Peterson, B. S., Riddle, M. A., Cohen, D. J., Katz, L. D., Smith, J. C., Hartin, M. T., & Leckman, J. F. (1993). Reduced basal ganglia volumes in Tourette's syndrome using three-dimensional reconstruction techniques from magnetic resonance images. *Neurology, 43,* 941–949.

Piven, J., Arndt, S., Bailey, J., & Andreasen, N. (1996). Regional brain enlargement in autism: A magnetic resonance imaging study. *Journal of the American Academy of Child and Adolescent Psychiatry, 35,* 530–536.

Piven, J., Arndt, S., Bailey, J., Havercamp, S., Andreasen, N. C., & Palmer, P. (1995). An MRI study of brain size in autism. *American Journal of Psychiatry, 152,* 1145–1149.

Piven, J., Nehme, E., Simon, J., Barta, P. E., Pearlson, G., & Folstein, S. E. (1992). Magnetic resonance imaging in autism: Measurement of the cerebellum, pons, and fourth ventricle. *Biological Psychiatry, 31,* 491–504.

Prasher, V. P., Barber, P. C., West, R., & Glenholmes, P. (1996). The role of magnetic resonance imaging in the dignosis of Alzheimer disease in adults with Down syndrome. *Archives of Neurology, 53,* 1310–1313.

Ramaekers, V.Th., Heimann, G., Reul, J., Thron, A., & Jaeken, J. (1997). Genetic disorders and cerebellar structural abnormalities in childhood. *Brain, 120,* 1739–1751.

Raz, N., Torres, I. J., Briggs, S. D., Spencer, W. D., Thornton, A. E., Loken, W. J., Gunning, F. M., McQuain, J. D., Driesen, N. R., & Acker, J. D. (1995). Selective neuroanatomic abnormalities in Down's syndrome and their cognitive correlates: Evidence from MRI morphometry. *Neurology*, *45*, 356–366.

Reiss, A., Freund, L., Tsang, J., & Joshi, P. (1991). Neuroanatomy in fragile X females: The posterior fossa. *American Journal of Human Genetics*, *49*, 279–288.

Reiss, A. L., Abrams, M. T., Singer, H. S., Ross, J. L., & Denckla, M. (1996). Brain development, gender and IQ in children: A volumetric imaging study. *Brain*, *119*, 1763–1774.

Reiss, A. L., Freund, L., Plotnick, L., Baumgardner, T., Green, K., Sozer, A. C., Reader, M., Boehm, C., & Denckla, M. B. (1993). The effects of X monosomy on brain development: Monozygotic twins discordant for Turner's syndrome. *Annals of Neurology*, *34*, 95–107.

Robb, S. A., Pohl, K. R. E., Baraitser, M., Wilson, J., & Brett, E. M. (1989). The "happy puppet" syndrome of Angelman: Review of the clinical features. *Archives of Disease in Childhood*, *64*, 83–86.

Roth, G. M., Sun, B., Greensite, F. S., Lott, I. T., & Dietrich, R. B. (1996). Premature aging in persons with Down syndrome: MR findings. *American Journal of Neuroradiology*, *17*, 1283–1289.

Saitoh, O., Courchesne, E., Egaas, B., Lincoln, A. J., & Schreibman, L. (1995). Cross-sectional area of the posterior hippocampus in autistic patients with cerebellar and corpus callosum abnormalities. *Neurology*, *45*, 317–324.

Schultz, R. T., Cho, N. K., Staib, L. H., & Kier, L. E. (1994). Brain morphology in dyslexic children: The influence of sex and age. *Annals of Neurology*, *35*, 732–742.

Singer, H. S., Reiss, A. L., Brown, J. E., Aylward, E. H., Shih, B., Chee, E., Harris, E. L., Reader, M. J., Chase, G. A., & Bryan, R. N. (1993). Volumetric MRI changes in basal ganglia of children with Tourette's syndrome. *Neurology*, *43*, 950–956.

Steen, R. G., Ogg, R. J., Reddick, W. E., & Kingsley, P. B. (1997). Age-related changes in the pediatric brain: Quantitative MR evidence of maturational changes during adolescence. *American Journal of Neuroradiology*, *18*, 819–828.

Subramaniam, B., Naidu, S., & Reiss, A. L. (1997). Neuroanatomy in Rett syndrome: Cerebral cortex and posterior fossa. *Neurology*, *48*, 399–407.

Swaiman, K. F. (1994). *Pediatric neurology: Principles and practice*. St. Louis, MO: Mosby.

Terada, H., Barkovich, A., Edwards, M., & Ciricillo, S. (1996). Evolution of high-intensity basal ganglia lesions on T1-weighted MR in neurofibromatosis type 1. *American Journal of Neuroradiology*, *17*, 755–760.

van der Knaap, M. S., Smit, L. M. E., Barth, P. G., Catsman-Berrevoets, C. E., Brouwer, O. F., Begeer, J. H., de Coo, I. F. M., & Valk, J. (1997). Magnetic resonance imaging in classification of congenital muscular dystrophies with brain abnormalities. *Annals of Neurology*, *42*, 50–59.

Vanhanen, S. L., Raininko, R., Autti, T., & Santavuori, P. (1995a). MRI evaluation of the brain in infantile neuronal ceroid-lipofuscinosis: Part 2. MRI findings in 21 patients. *Journal of Child Neurology*, *10*, 444–450.

Vanhanen, S. L., Raininko, R., Santavuori, P., Autti, T., & Haltia, M. (1995b). MRI evaluation of the brain in infantile neuronal ceroid-lipofuscinosis: Part 1. Postmortem MRI with histopathologic correlation. *Journal of Child Neurology*, *10*, 438–443.

Volpe, K. A., & Yamada, J. J. (1990). Angelman's syndrome in infancy. *Developmental Medicine and Child Neurology*, *32*, 1005–1011.

Wang, P. P., Doherty, S., Hesselink, J. R., & Bellugi, U. (1992). Callosal morphology concurs with neurobehavioral and neuropathological findings in two neurodevelopmental disorders. *Archives of Neurology*, *49*, 407–411.

Wang, Z., Bogdan, A. R., Zimmerman, R. A., Gusnard, D. A., Leigh, J. S., & Ohene-Frempong, K. (1992). Investigation of stroke in sickle cell disease by H nuclear magnetic resonance spectroscopy. *Neuroradiology*, *35*, 57–65.

Weis, S. (1991). Morphometry and magnetic resonance imaging of the human brain in normal controls and Down's syndrome. *Anatomical Record*, *23*, 593–598.

Wider, T. M., Schwartz, T. H., Carmel, P. W., & Wood-Smith, D. (1995). Internal brain herniation in a patient with Apert's syndrome. *Annals of Plastic Surgery, 34,* 420–423.

Williams, C. A., & Frias, J. I. (1982). The Angelman ("happy puppet") syndrome. *American Journal of Medical Genetics, 11,* 453–460.

Wolpert, S. M., & Barnes, P. D. (1992). *MRI in pediatric neuroradiology.* St. Louis, MO: Mosby–Year Book.

5

INTEGRATIVE DEVELOPMENTAL NEUROPSYCHOLOGY

A General Systems and Social-Ecological Approach to the Neuropsychology of Children with Neurogenetic Disorders

TIMOTHY B. WHELAN

The development of children with neurological and genetic disorders occurs, as it does for all children, in a dynamic web of exchange. As neuropsychologists, our focus has traditionally been on the pathophysiology of the nervous system and its consequences expressed cognitively, academically, motorically, affectively, and so forth. Our expertise is thus unique in attempting to grasp the meaning of relationships between the brain and behavior, and yet we are at risk of painting clinical portraits of children that are too narrow or monochromatic unless we constantly consider influences at other levels of functioning. In this chapter, selected aspects of the literature on children, illness, and psychosocial functioning are discussed and illustrated with case material.

To set the stage, it is important to emphasize that the incidence of adjustment difficulties among children with disabling medical conditions is high: It is generally accepted that they are at 1½ to 3 times greater risk for behavioral, social, and psychological maladjustment than their healthy peers (Perrin, 1986; Pless, 1984). Results of epidemiological studies indicate that children with chronic illness experience lower academic achievement, greater absenteeism, and increased behavioral difficulties such as nervousness and aggression (Pless & Roghmann, 1971; Rutter, Tizard, & Whitmore, 1970). Furthermore, when the affected organ—the brain—is itself the organ most intimately related to the capacity to adjust, the prognosis for successful coping drops still further. Rutter, Graham, and Yule (1970) reported from the classic Isle of Wight study that the occurrence of psychiatric disorders among children with non-neurological chronic disease was 11.6%; among those with epilepsy and no other pathology, the incidence was 37.5%; and among children and adolescents with epilepsy associated with organic brain disease, it was 58.3%. Breslau (1985) also noted a higher incidence of psychological adjustment difficulties among children with brain-based disease than among either healthy children or those with other systemic diseases. More recently, Howe, Feinstein, Reiss, Molock, and Berger (1993) found, not surprisingly, that adolescents with brain-related illnesses had more academic difficulties than peers with non-brain-related illnesses. In their extensive review of the literature, Thompson and Gustafson (1996, p. 130) concluded that "children with chronic physical illness are at risk for difficulties in social adjustment and peer relationships as well as school adjustment and performance. These difficulties may vary as a function of illness type, with children with illnesses that affect the [central nervous system] being at particular risk."

A word of caution is nevertheless in order, though: Some seemingly pathological behaviors may actually be adaptive in those with chronic illness (Drotar & Bush, 1985; Van Dongen-Melman & Sanders-Woudstra, 1986). For example, a child incessantly retelling traumatic events leading to hospitalization may be coping appropriately despite creating discomfort within caregivers who must repeatedly listen to those events (Broufman, Campis, & Koocher, 1998). Moreover, not all children are negatively affected, and resilience may be equally impressive (Stabler, 1988).

OVERARCHING CONCEPTS

It is not unusual in the fields of psychology and medicine to organize a conceptual framework for understanding disease and health within general systems theory—a general science of "wholeness," examining sets of elements standing in interrelationship (Bertalanffy, 1968). Within this theory, the human organism exists as a hierarchy of systems ranging from the molecular level of the biological realm, to larger organ systems, to cognitive and intrapsychic levels, and on to family and social spheres. It is assumed that these systems are interrelated, that events at one level of the hierarchy have effects up and down the system, and that the system maintains a state of homeostasis during periods of stress or stability. Therefore, because changes at one level have ramifications at many other levels, one may elect to treat the experience of dysphoria by selectively inhibiting serotonin reuptake, or to utilize behavioral techniques with patients who have painful spinal degeneration.

This conceptualization was the basis for seminal writings by George Engel (1977, 1980), which led health care practitioners to the reconceptualization of disease as a biopsychosocial phenomenon, and one can see this influence in the earlier literature on families with illness (Gochman, 1985; Kerns & Curley, 1985; Kerns & Turk, 1985; Leventhal, Leventhal, & Van Nguyen, 1985) and clinical health psychology (Millon, Green, & Meagher, 1982). Moreover, this conceptual framework is undoubtedly becoming increasingly central in the era of capitated medical care.

In addition to consideration of a general systems organization of the individual, it is important to link our understanding to the developmental psychology of families and children. Bronfenbrenner (1979) has written about "social ecology," defined as "the study of the relation between the developing human being and the settings and contexts in which that person is actually involved" (Kazak, 1989, p. 26). According to Kazak, who has applied these theories in families of chronically ill children—including children with physical handicaps (Kazak, 1986), phenylketonuria (Kazak, Reber, & Smitzer, 1988), and AIDS (Kazak, 1989)—the presumption in social ecology is that the child is at the center of concentric spheres of influence, with nearby rings representing family, school, and neighborhood, and with more distant impact coming from social values and culture. Again, the impact of events is bidirectional: The child is influenced by the family, for instance, and the family is influenced by the child. Thus, if the father of an adolescent boy with Duchenne muscular dystrophy whose muscles have wasted to the point of personal immobility throws himself into his office work, this may immediately affect the son and his mother, who become occupied with more intimate personal care.

As a colleague and I have previously pointed out (Whelan & Walker, 1997), any model of child clinical neuropsychology requires additional complexity, because processes of development must be taken into account. The child is conceptualized on multiple levels standing in interrelationship, with the hierarchy of systems set in temporal motion. Bernstein and Waber (1990) have also written in this vein on their goal in developmental neuropsychological assessment "not to diagnose deficits in a child, but rather to construct a *Child–World System* that characterizes the reciprocal relationship of the developing children and the world in which that child functions" (p. 312). Their approach was derived from the systemic traditions of Luria and Vygotsky, as well as the Wernerian approach most thoroughly elaborated in neuropsychology by Edith Kaplan. Bernstein and Waber's model considers manifestations of neurological and cognitive structures, neurological and psychological timetables of development, alternative mechanisms (pathways and strategies), and context (including the role of experience and environmental interactions). Any attributions of difficulty are thus shifted from the child to the system, and temporal/developmental processes are considered central.

This shift in thinking—from an individual child with a neurological or genetic disorder to the dysfunction of systems within and surrounding the child—is difficult to maintain. After all, professional training and individual academic interests tend to draw us toward specific domains of expertise in our practices. Moreover, there are powerful societal influences on our own thinking and on the thinking of others in the child's social ecology. As described by Resnick (1984a) well over a decade ago, to understand the sociological destiny of those with disability, it is necessary to understand the genesis of attitudes and expectations surrounding them. Resnick reviewed an extensive literature indicating a number of significant, though unfortunate, trends with implications for psychological health, school success, and vocational life. First, children in general may prefer interactions with able-bodied peers rather than with disabled children, and this bias may increase as they get older (Ryan, 1981; Voeltz, 1980; Weinberg, 1976; Weinberg & Santana, 1978). Second, teachers may hold negative attitudes toward disabled students (Good & Brophy, 1978; Martinek & Karper, 1981); and, third, there are persistent biases against employment of the disabled (Bender, 1981; Conley, 1973). Such findings contribute to the concept of "handicapism," a social experience involving prejudice, stereotype, and discrimination. In essence, says Resnick, there is a social construction of the reality of the disabled individual, in which people and events are "instantaneously assessed in their compatibility or discordance with the mainstream values" (1984a, p. 33). Moreover, we ourselves may inadvertently occupy an important place in this social construction, as our well-intentioned professional assistance sometimes places an identified patient in a position of continual dependence and gratitude within a larger culture that values self-reliance and independence.

As we have previously discussed (Whelan & Walker, 1997), a dilemma exists in regard to the societal doctrine of normality, where certain behaviors and physical characteristics are acceptable and where occurrences outside these bounds are regarded as deviant. This point of view may not be necessary or helpful for children who are born with genetic or neurological disorders, since such children may have always viewed their so-called "deficits" as part of their identity. "Handicap" is thus defined from an "outsider's perspective" (Shontz, 1982), and "insiders" may not perceive that there is anything about their condition to overcome (Massie, 1985). The critical question within such an individual's system shifts to this: How does the individual achieve a complete sense of fulfillment, given his or her uniqueness?

CRITICAL VARIABLES

Throughout the 1970s and 1980s, researchers were accumulating data indicating that a conceptual grasp of the nature of coping and adjustment of children with chronic illness encompasses a broad array of factors. (For a complete account of the progress of research and the many directions of study, see Thompson & Gustafson, 1996—a book that guided the development of this section.) In the mid-1970s, Monat and Lazarus (1977, p. 3) developed the notion that "stress" is a situation "in which environmental demands, internal demands, or both tax or exceed the adaptive resources of an individual, social system, or tissue system." Researchers began to consider the ways in which children may adjust to these stresses when they involve illness. For example, Pless and Pinkerton (1975) described "coping style" and "self-concept" as central to psychological adjustment to illness. They placed these concepts against a backdrop including family characteristics, the social environment, the type of illness, and so forth. Thus not only were they considering biological factors in illness; they were implying that other sections of the child's hierarchy of systems and the social environment in which they exist are important in adaptation. These domains, in turn, are available as potential targets of intervention.

Adjustment to stress also came under scrutiny, and what clinical psychologists had typically considered defense mechanisms began to be seen in a different, more positive light. Even earlier (Kroeber, 1964), parallels were drawn between more pathological "ego defense mechanisms" (isolation, projection, repression) and "coping mechanisms" (objectivity, empathy, suppression), the latter implying more active and effective attempts to deal with conflict. Lazarus (1983) struggled especially with the conditions under which people may deceive themselves; he tried to distinguish "classical denial" (the negation of impulse, feeling, thought, or external reality) from "partial denial" (a temporary suspension of belief during periods of health crisis). Moreover, he considered it possible that denial may reduce distress when there is no direct action one can take to improve the situation at one point in a disease process, whereas at another point it may be critical to perceive dysfunction accurately in order to take available steps to remedy or rehabilitate the situation.

Apart from traditional models of psychological adjustment, cognitive and developmental psychologists were contributing to the field. For instance, as ideas of self-worth and self-concept were explored, some studies reported that children with chronic illness were negatively affected (e.g., Lineberger, Hernandez, & Brantley, 1984). In contrast, others (e.g., Kellerman, Zeltzer, Ellenberg, Dash, & Rigler, 1980; Simmons et al., 1985) reported no significant group differences between ill and healthy children. In general, though, ill children with neurological involvement seemed at risk for poorer self-concept and lower self-esteem (Lindemann & Stranger, 1981).

In 1977, Moos and Tsu developed a "life crisis" model of adjustment to childhood illness, in which the outcome of crisis precipitated by illness involves cognitive appraisals of the meaning of the illness, adaptive tasks (i.e., dealing with symptoms of the illness and its treatments, maintaining emotional balance and interpersonal relationships), and various aspects of coping skills involving defenses and problem solving. They considered all levels of a systems hierarchy, including physical and illness-related factors, personal background, and social and environmental factors. These elements contribute to a set of adaptive tasks, such as dealing with stress associated with the condition itself and its treatment, maintaining relationships with caregivers, managing distressing emotions, preserving family and social relationships, and anticipating the future.

Moos and Tsu (1977) described coping skills as involving multiple factors, including minimizing the seriousness of the situation, seeking information and support, emphasizing problem-solving skills, and finding meaning in illness. Perhaps the most statistically sophisticated studies of the nature of coping are those reported by Tobin, Holroyd, Reynolds, and Wigal (1989), who developed a rigorous hierarchical model of coping by means of factor analysis of the Coping Strategies Inventory administered to young adults. This model included eight identified primary factors (problem solving, cognitive restructuring, emotional expression, social support, problem avoidance, wishful thinking, self-criticism, and social withdrawal), organized into two types of activities, problem-focused and emotion-focused. These in turn fell into broad factors of engagement and disengagement. The degree to which such a model is applicable to children is uncertain.

MODELS

As the literature focusing on particular influences such as those described above expanded, some researchers began to assemble more general models incorporating these various specific trains of thought. The disability–stress–coping model (Wallander & Varni, 1992; Wallander, Varni, Babani, Banis, & Wilcox, 1989) identifies both risk and resistance factors. Among the former are qualities specific to the disease, such as diagnosis, visibility, and brain involvement. Resistance factors are both within the individual (e.g., competence and effectance motivation) and within the social ecology (e.g., family environment, social support).

In addition to perspectives from social learning and attribution theories, concepts of intrinsic motivation are important. It is generally assumed that humans naturally strive for effective interaction with their environment, and that successful mastery produces feelings of efficacy and competence. These feelings in turn lead to further efforts to master additional tasks (Stipek & Weisz, 1981). Elsewhere (Whelan, 1986), however, I have suggested that the situation is not always straightforward. When I examined perceptions of competence among children with genetically based neuromuscular disease, perceptions of physical competence were more closely related to general self-worth than to actual neuropsychological measures of motor output, suggesting that children may have distorted appraisals of components of their functioning in the service of maintaining positive global self-perceptions. The implication is that children with specific neurodevelopmental disorders may not follow patterns of intrinsic motivation established in groups of healthy children.

Perhaps the most encompassing of the efforts to organize specific functional components of study is the transactional stress and coping model of adjustment to childhood illness developed by Thompson, Gil, Burbach, Keith, and Kinney (1993a, 1993b) and Thompson, Gustafson, Hamlett, and Spock (1992a, 1992b), which is derived from Bronfenbrenner's (1977) ecological–systems theory. As shown in Figure 5.1 and as explained in detail by Thompson, Gustafson, George, and Spock (1994), typical demographic variables are noted, as are unique disease factors. Cognitive processes and coping methods are emphasized, as is family functioning. What is especially significant is the interface between child and maternal adjustment as determining the outcome of the entire system. In other words, their model assumes that the adjustment of the child is affected by the experiences

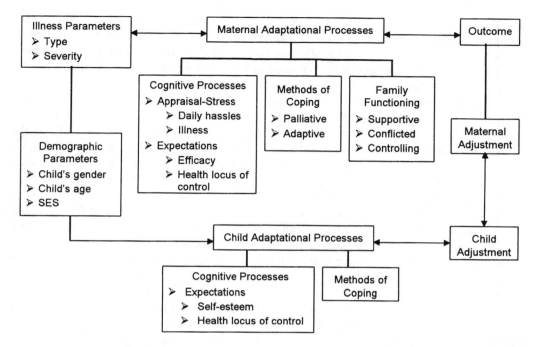

FIGURE 5.1. Transactional stress and coping model of adjustment to chronic illness. From Thompson, Gustafson, George, and Spock (1994). Copyright 1994 by Plenum Publishing Corp. Reprinted by permission.

of stress and symptoms by the mother and other family members—a notion directly derived from social-ecological theory. Thompson and colleagues have utilized this model to understand the functioning of children with cystic fibrosis, sickle cell disease, and spina bifida. In the end, after considering the host of models that have now been proposed, Thompson and Gustafson (1996, p. 156) suggested that "stress processes, social support, and parenting are currently the most prominent intervention targets."

DIAGNOSIS IN SYSTEMS AND SEQUENCES

Adam, the only child of an intact marriage, was born following a full-term pregnancy complicated by maternal dehydration in the first 4 months, which required several hospitalizations. There was no maternal medication or substance abuse. He was delivered following a 37-hour labor, and although there was some meconium staining, there was no need for intensive care. However, at 1 week of age he developed a fever of 105°F with gastrointestinal distress, and this persisted. At age 6 months, he was diagnosed with transient hypogammaglobulinemia and clostridium-difficile, but treatment did not relieve chronic diarrhea, pain, and sleep disturbance. He was fed by nasogastric tube and was intermittently hospitalized for 4 years. Additional problems developed, including apnea, very occasional partial and generalized seizures, stroke-like episodes, irregular heart rate, stomach and leg pain, labile emotions, and unpredictable and sometimes markedly dysregulated behaviors. Apart from primary nighttime enuresis, developmental motor and language milestones were met in a timely way. Adam was diagnosed at an early age with an intestinal pseudo-obstruction, and he had a bowel resection. Only shortly before neuropsychological assessment at age 13, muscle biopsies were found to be consistent with mitochondrial myopathy in both mother and child. A gastrostomy tube had recently been placed, and a psychotherapist was consulted in regard to Adam's behavior problems and in order to assist him with relaxation in the face of pain.

It might seem that a child with such a lengthy history of intense medical difficulties, even though an encompassing diagnosis was exceptionally elusive, would receive supportive services without debate or hesitation, but this was not initially the case. Prior to the diagnosis of mitochondrial myopathy, the combination of vague somatic complaints such as belly or diffuse limb pain, disruptive behavior, and efforts to retreat from the demands of the classroom because of fatigue were suspected to represent a psychiatric condition. More malignant was the suggestion by some health care professionals that this was a case of Munchausen syndrome by proxy. That accusation polarized the situation dramatically: The school system became suspicious and withholding, and the parents became horrified that they were accused of causing their son's symptoms. Suits and charges were considered; the family system reached a point at which instructional efforts (many of which were entirely appropriate) were rejected as unhelpful; and Adam was increasingly drawn away from school.

With the formal diagnosis of mitochondrial myopathy in both Adam and his mother, the parents were no longer accused. They embraced the disorder publicly, with Adam becoming a regional poster child, and with his mother becoming the subject of local newspaper articles on the disorder. Though this was medically unlikely, the mother continued to believe that her own life was precarious. Neuropsychological evaluation was able to define the direction of academic modifications acceptable to both the school system and the family, and Adam's functioning in school improved. Interestingly, the family soon withdrew from psychotherapy, which could have helped them negotiate ongoing threats to the adjustment of each individual.

In this case, when all the many influences on Adam within family and social systems recognized his illness, he got better. The improvements did not result from more closely targeted medical treatments at a biological level; rather, the framework of expectations changed, promoting alterations in system relationships and a shift in affect. In a curious way, impotence, guilt, and rage were diminished when the etiology of Adam's compromises changed from a psychological to a genetic realm, and the psychological health of the family system improved when the family members organized around this rare illness. In the sense of social ecology, the family had reached a new state of homeostasis—one seeming more functional to the outsider, though still constrained within what Resnick (1984a, p. 41) has described as the "public relations representative" role, in which the individual or family members have placed upon them(selves) a constant burden of explaining and interpreting.

It should be pointed out that diagnosis is not a one-time event. Kupst et al. (1984) have studied different temporal reactions to the diagnosis of a child with cancer, as initial anxiety over the meaning of the diagnosis evolves during the course of actual treatment. Also, familiarity with a diagnosis may result in a more advanced conceptual understanding; for example, a preschooler may apply more sophisticated causal reasoning to a cold than to a newly diagnosed neurological disorder (Siegel, 1988). Similarly, there are developmental considerations in children's understanding of the nature of a genetic or neurological disorder, and an extensive literature within pediatric psychology advises health care professionals to take the nature of cognitive functioning in a Piagetian sense into account when they are conveying medical diagnostic and treatment information to children of different ages (Brodie. 1974; Campbell, 1975; Mechanic, 1964; Neuhauser, Amsterdam, Hines, & Steward, 1978; Palmer & Lewis, 1976).

Specific information concerning stages of child cognitive functioning in a pediatric context may be found in Perrin and Gerrity (1981), Whitt, Dykstra, and Taylor (1979), and Bibace and Walsh (1979). In some ways, one can trace children's movement toward more systemic thinking when it comes to their own health. Thus a child functioning at a preoperational level (between ages 2 and 7) may consider illness prevention and recovery to be associated with a rigid set of rules surrounding immediate and concrete perceptions of experience—avoiding the touch of friends, or staying in bed. Later, with the emergence of formal operations, illness may be conceptualized not only in terms of internal organs whose malfunctions are manifested in external symptoms, but also in terms of psychological events as disease symptoms and causes of internal dysfunction—the etiology of headache, for example, may included too much worry. The concepts of neurological and genetic disorders may be especially difficult to communicate when they affect academic adjustment, and many parents and professionals have found the books by Mel Levine (1990, 1993) especially helpful.

PATTERNS OF FAMILY INTERACTION

Susan was a 10-year-old girl with a rare variant of a rare disorder, leukodystrophy, which had resulted in a broad set of impairments. She became progressively ataxic, often using a wheelchair, but still able to walk slowly and to participate in swimming. Purposeful movements could precipitate striking titubation. There were concerns about early optic atrophy and the development of horizontal nystagmus. Her seizures were under control, but she was struggling to manage abrupt moments of bowel urgency, especially given her motoric difficulties with self-toileting. Her cognitive functioning dropped to the range of mild mental retardation, and she was placed in a substantially separate special educational setting. The prognosis for this leukodystrophy was grave—gradually progressive and devastating neurological compromises, and a greatly restricted lifespan.

Such disturbances in the growth and development of a child are terrible in and of themselves, as the expressions of a still-forming nervous system in increasing disarray because of progressive white matter disease. At issue in the context of this chapter are the various other influences in the ecology of Susan's life. Susan developed symptoms of anxiety and marked dependence upon her mother, and she made increasing demands upon her. The mother was the only one she permitted to assist her in toileting, and if she was unavailable (at school, for instance), Susan would not eat beforehand. Separation became difficult. Indeed, she was demanding ever more complex nighttime rituals: She wouldn't go to sleep unless certain lights were on; her mother not only had to be holding Susan's hand, but also had to be facing her daughter with her eyes open until Susan fell asleep; and she was expected to be in the same position when Susan woke. They had discontinued attending a support group for parents of children with academic special needs, because their situation was so profoundly different from that of the other parents.

In considering this system from a traditional neuropsychological point of view, one might focus on Susan herself and on the nature of her cognitive and motor impairments. And, in fact, she did participate with motoric benefit in experimental drug trials coordinated at a national level for the treatment of leukodystrophy. At another level in the system hierarchy, however, she had developed symptoms of an anxiety disorder with an obsessive–compulsive quality, as well as a measure of almost omnipotent control over parental behaviors. There were minimal efforts to target these symptoms with psychotropic medication, because of the potential for negative side effects in a child with great medical complexity. Efforts thus became psychotherapeutic, assisting Susan in decreasing her fears and apprehensions—some of which were primitive, vague, and nameless, but probably connected with fears of death. For the mother, there were efforts to reframe "caring" as taking on the frightening task of letting her daughter "suffer" limit setting, in the service of ultimately acquiring greater autonomy in some things as she became more dependent in others. Nevertheless, it was not the parents' goal to establish a typical set of boundaries and roles in parent–child or marital relationships, simply because they felt they had precious little time with Susan and did not wish to spend it in active conflict. Thus in many ways the family had reached a point of homeostasis. As Kazak (1989, p. 26) points out, the construct of "homeostasis" may be used to appraise patterns of family interaction that serve to maintain a sense of stability. In other words, "reactions that tend to be viewed as maladaptive (i.e. overprotectiveness, enmeshed family relationships, denial) may actually function to maintain a protective homeostasis for the family."

On the other hand, as Kazak adds, a family system may become too harmful to its members; abuse must be dealt with as an indicator of a family system gone astray, rather than simply as a homeostatic variant. Interventions leading to a new steady state must be implemented, as in the following case.

Gail was a child adopted in infancy by enormously caring parents with gentle temperaments; the adoptive father was a minister and academic at an exclusive liberal arts college. It wasn't long, however, before it was clear that the child's tempo and style of interpersonal interaction were markedly different from the parents'. Gail ultimately developed severe attention-deficit/hyperactivity disorder with highly impulsive features, as well as comorbid symptoms of oppositional defiant disorder. The contrast between parents and child was sharp, and before these diagnoses were made and interventions were implemented, the situation had deteriorated into regular and routine outbursts of harsh, abusive physical punishment of Gail by the father. His image of himself as a progressive-minded humanitarian was shattered as he was pressed beyond the heretofore unsuspected limits of his capacity to manage the situation. The presumption was that this child with a genetically based disorder was being raised by parents who did not share her biology and whose style was so different as to be nearly irreconcilable. Even though a combination of medications, behavioral and psychotherapeutic interventions, and respite greatly diminished the misfit between parents and child, the father still needed to take daily refuge in books and music within his library, which was specially constructed for soundproofing and inaccessibility. In this way, a new homeostasis was created.

Every disease has a natural history, and the capacity of a family system surrounding a child to adjust may be a function of the interplay between normal developmental challenges and the nature of the disease impact. One of the most poignant accounts of this interaction may be found in Resnick (1984b, p. 302):

> While his age cohorts were arguing with parents over the length of their hair, he needed help washing his; while they were resisting doing assigned chores, he was unable to perform any; while they were battling curfews, he needed not only permission, but physical assistance in order to be out. Instead of sharing his peers' increased independence from parents and others, symbolized by mild acting out behaviors, this patient could merely fantasize his acting out, with his illness providing a constant reminder of his chronic dependent status.

Some researchers have proposed stages of parental adjustment, which, at some points and in some families, may include the experiences of fear, shock, numbness or detachment, relief, helplessness, denial, sadness or depression, anxiety, and guilt (Drotar, Baskiewicz, Irvin, Kennell, & Klaus, 1975; Hobbs, Perrin, & Ireys, 1985; McCollum, 1981). Readers are referred to Whelan and Walker (1997) for further discussion of these issues within families.

Whereas the field of clinical psychology has often focused on such painful human conditions, it is also possible to consider alternatives, and hope is one. This is a construct with a complex religious and philosophical history: Hope was one of the evils in Pandora's box in Greek tradition, and it is a virtue and central theme of the Judeo-Christian message (Menninger, 1963). In more contemporary times, researchers have attempted to operationalize the meaning of hope (Petiet, 1983). It can be classified as a coping mechanism incorporating a realistic appraisal of current circumstances, a future orientation, expectant cognition, optimistic affect, and resultant motivation. As such, hope is seen as a desirable state during medical procedures and rehabilitation (Brackney & Westman, 1992; Brody, 1981; Lillis & Prophit, 1991; Rabkin, Williams, Neugebauer, Reimien, & Goetz, 1990; Ruvelson, 1990), though developmental correlates in children have yet to be defined.

SOCIAL CULTURE

Little has been written concerning contemporary cultural issues influencing the functioning of children with neurodevelopmental or genetic disorders, and this level of analysis will not occupy a prominent position in this chapter. Still, there is reason on several counts to consider these broad-system issues. For example, some genetic disorders may express themselves according to the culture in which they arise. As a particular instance, in many U.S. cities, a family with Duchenne muscular dystrophy—a relentlessly progressive and ultimately fatal neuromuscular disorder that has an X-linked pattern of inheritance—may be looked upon as pathologically irresponsible if the mother continues to have children, despite genetic counseling concerning the probability of having another affected son. Most families with this disorder in mainstream U.S. culture are therefore relatively small, with few affected individuals. By contrast, in San Antonio, which has a high density of families with ties to the traditions of the Catholic Church and of Mexico, large families with many affected individuals across the generations may be more common and more likely to be viewed with a charitable eye.

One of the best examples of writing concerning cultural and sociological issues, and political/economic correlates in the care of children with chronic illness, is the edited volume by Hobbs and Perrin (1985). In it they organize representative chapters on specific conditions, including some with clear neurodevelopmental consequences (e.g., neuromuscular disease, sickle cell disease, and spina bifida). The direction of that text, as well as of another by Hobbs et al. (1985) and of work by Nelson (1984), Resnick (1984a), Silber (1984), and Strax and Wolfson (1984), extends to public policy. These writings probe such topics as health care expenditure, integrating federal programs at the state level, defining parental opportunity costs and other economic costs of disabling conditions, the role of ethics and values in shaping public policy, and preparing professionals for new roles.

The last issue—preparing professionals for new roles—deserves a personal comment. Perhaps a decade ago, I began to lament to colleagues who were also supervising doctoral psychology trainees in my teaching hospital that there was a creeping trend away from a "pure" opportunity for teaching neuropsychological theory and clinical technique, and toward inclusion of more emphasis on the politics of health care delivery. As we in the community of health care providers continue to find our way in the shifting culture of professional politics and managed care, our relationships to our field and to our patients fluctuate, and we remain challenged in our practice and teaching to advocate for excellent patient care within redefined roles and product lines. At this level, we ourselves are in our patients' hierarchy of systems, and they are in ours.

SUMMARY

In this chapter, the professional literature has been reviewed in a highly selective fashion, with the intent of providing the reader with some of the "industry standard" reference points for understanding psychosocial contributions to the development of emotional, educational, and behavioral problems in children with neurobehavioral and genetic disorders. As well, some specific topics and clinical examples have been included that represent unique personal interests. The field appears robust, not only given its state at the moment, but also in historical context; clearly, the empirical research being derived from existing descriptive models of the ways in which children adjust to illness is much more integrated and detailed than it was a decade ago. Clinically, too, there has been a movement toward improved integration of information from traditional clinical psychology and neuropsychology with practices derived from developmental pediatric psychology and (because of the typical ecology of children) from school psychology. This type of cross-fertilization suggests a productive future and holds promise for continued efforts at excellence in professional practice.

ACKNOWLEDGMENT

I wish to acknowledge the creative and intellectually challenging input of Muireann McNulty in the development of this chapter.

REFERENCES

Bender, L. F. (1981). 1980 presidential address to the American Academy for Cerebral Palsy and Developmental Medicine. *Developmental Medicine and Child Neurology, 23,* 103–108.

Bernstein, J. H., & Waber, D. P. (1990). Developmental neuropsychological assessment. In A. A. Boulton, G. B. Baker, & M. Hiscock (Eds.), *Neuropsychology: Vol. 17. Neuromethods* (pp. 311–371). Clifton, NJ: Humana Press.

Bertalanffy, L. von. (1968). *General systems theory.* New York: Braziller.

Bibace, R., & Walsh, M. E. (1979). Developmental stages in children's conceptions of illness. In G. C. Stone, F. Cohen, & N. E. Adler (Eds.), *Health psychology* (pp. 285–301). San Francisco: Jossey-Bass.

Brackney, B. E., & Westman, A. S. (1992). Relationships among hope, psychosocial development, and locus of control. *Psychological Reports, 70,* 864–867.

Breslau, N. (1985). Psychiatric disorder in children with physical disabilities. *Journal of the American Academy of Child Psychiatry, 24,* 87–94.

Brodie, B. (1974). View of healthy children toward illness. *American Journal of Public Health, 64,* 1156–1159.

Brody, H. (1981). Hope. *Journal of the American Medical Association, 246,* 1411–1412.

Bronfenbrenner, U. (1977). Toward an experimental ecology of human development. *American Psychologist, 32,* 513–531.

Bronfenbrenner, U. (1979). *The ecology of human development*. Cambridge, MA: Harvard University Press.

Broufman, E. T., Campis, L. B., & Koocher, G. P. (1998). Helping children to cope: Clinical issues for acutely injured and medically traumatized children. *Professional Psychology: Research and Practice, 29*, 574–581.

Campbell, J. D. (1975). Illness is a point of view: The development of children's concepts of illness. *Child Development, 46*, 92–100.

Conley, R. W. (1973). *The economics of mental retardation*. Baltimore: Johns Hopkins University Press.

Drotar, D., Baskiewicz, A., Irvin, N., Kennell, J., & Klaus, M. (1975). The adaptation of parents to the birth of an infant with a congenital malformation: A hypothetical model. *Pediatrics, 56*, 710–717.

Drotar, D., & Bush, M. (1985). Mental health issues and services. In N. Hobbs & J. M. Perrin (Eds.), *Issues in the care of children with chronic illness* (pp. 514–550). San Francisco: Jossey-Bass.

Engel, G. (1977). The clinical application of the biopsychosocial model. *American Journal of Psychiatry, 137*, 535–544.

Engel, G. (1980). The need for a new medical model: The challenge for biomedicine. *Science, 196*, 129–136.

Gochman, D. S. (1985). Family determinants of children's concepts of health and illness. In D. Turk & R. Kerns (Eds.), *Health, illness, and families* (pp. 23–50). New York: Wiley.

Good, T., & Brophy, J. (1978). *Looking in classrooms*. New York: Holt, Rinehart & Winston.

Hobbs, N., & Perrin, J. M. (Eds.). (1985). *Issues in the care of children with chronic illness*. San Francisco: Jossey-Bass.

Hobbs, N., Perrin, J. M., & Ireys, H. T. (1985). *Chronically ill children and their families*. San Francisco: Jossey-Bass.

Howe, G. W., Feinstein, C., Reiss, D., Molock, S., & Berger, K. (1993). Adolescent adjustment to chronic physical disorders: I. Comparing neurological and non-neurological conditions. *Journal of Child Psychology and Psychiatry, 14*, 1153–1171.

Kazak, A. E. (1986). Families with physically handicapped children: Social ecology and family systems. *Family Process, 25*, 265–281.

Kazak, A. E. (1989). Families of chronically ill children: A systems and social-ecological model of adaptation and challenge. *Journal of Consulting and Clinical Psychology, 57*, 25–30.

Kazak, A. E., Reber, M., & Snitzer, A. (1988). Childhood chronic disease and family functioning: A study of phenylketonuria. *Pediatrics, 81*, 224–230.

Kellerman, J., Zeltzer, L., Ellenberg, L., Dash, J., & Rigler, D. (1980). Psychological effects of illness in adolescence. *Journal of Pediatrics, 97*, 126–131.

Kerns, R., & Curley, A. (1985). A biopsychosocial approach to illness and the family: Neurological diseases across the life span. In D. Turk & R. Kerns (Eds.), *Health, illness, and families* (pp. 146–182). New York: Wiley.

Kerns, R., & Turk, D. (1985). Behavioral medicine and the family: Historical perspectives and future directions. In D. Turk & R. Kerns (Eds.), *Health, illness, and families* (pp. 338–353). New York: Wiley.

Kroeber, T. C. (1964). The coping functions of ego mechanisms. In R. W. White (Ed.). *The study of lives* (pp. 178–198). New York: Atherton.

Kupst, M. J., Schulman, J. L., Maurer, H., Honig, G., Morgan, E., & Fochman, D. (1984). Coping with pediatric leukemia: A two-year follow-up. *Journal of Pediatric Psychology, 9*, 149–163.

Lazarus, R. S. (1983). The costs and benefits of denial. In S. Breznetz (Ed.), *Denial of stress*. New York: International Universities Press.

Leventhal, H., Leventhal, E., & Van Nguyen, T. (1985). Reactions of families to illness: Therapeutic models and perspectives. In D. Turk & R. Kerns (Eds.), *Health, illness, and families* (pp. 108–145). New York: Wiley.

Levine, M. (1990). *Keeping a head in school*. Cambridge, MA: Educators.

Levine, M. (1993). *All kinds of minds*. Cambridge, MA: Educators.

Lillis, P. P., & Prophit, P. (1991). Keeping hope alive. *Nursing, 21,* 65–67.

Lindemann, J. E., & Stranger, M. E. (1981). Progressive muscle disorders. In J. E. Lindemann (Ed.), *Psychological and behavioral aspects of physical disability* (pp. 273–300). New York: Plenum Press.

Lineberger, H. P., Hernandez, J. T., & Brantley, H. T. (1984). Self-concept and locus of control in hemophiliacs. *International Journal of Psychiatry in Medicine, 14,* 243–251.

Martinek, T. J., & Karper, W. B. (1981). Teachers' expectations for handicapped and non-handicapped children in mainstreamed physical education classes. *Perceptual and Motor Skills, 53,* 327–330.

Massie, R. K. (1985). The constant shadow: Reflections on the life of a chronically ill child. In N. Hobbs & J. Perrin (Eds.), *Issues in the care of children with chronic illness.* San Francisco: Jossey-Bass.

McCollum, A. T. (1981). *The chronically ill child: A guide for parents and professionals.* New Haven, CT: Yale University Press.

Mechanic, D. (1964). The influence of mothers on their children's health attitudes and behaviors. *Pediatrics, 33,* 444–453.

Menninger, K. (1963). *The vital balance.* New York: Viking Press.

Millon, T., Green, C., & Meagher, R. (Eds.). (1982). *Handbook of clinical health psychology.* New York: Plenum Press.

Monat, A., & Lazarus, R. S. (Eds.). (1977). *Stress and coping: An anthology.* New York: Columbia University Press.

Moos, R. H., & Tsu, U. D. (1977). The crisis of physical illness: An overview. In R. H. Moos (Ed.), *Coping with physical illness* (pp. 3–21). New York: Plenum Press.

Nelson, R. P. (1984). Political and financial issues that affect the chronically ill adolescent. In R. W. Blum (Ed.), *Chronic illness and disabilities in childhood and adolescence* (pp. 1–15). Orlando, FL: Grune & Stratton.

Neuhauser, C., Amsterdam, B., Hines, P., & Steward, M. (1978). Children's concepts of healing: Cognitive development and locus of control factors. *American Journal of Orthopsychiatry, 48,* 335–341.

Palmer, B., & Lewis, C. (1976). Development of health attitudes and behaviors. *Journal of School Health, 46,* 401–402.

Perrin, J. M. (1986). Chronically ill children: An overview. *Topics in Early Childhood Education, 5,* 1–11.

Perrin, J. M., & Gerrity, P. S. (1981). There's a demon in your belly: Children's understanding of illness. *Pediatrics, 67,* 841–849.

Petiet, C. A. (1983). *Hope: The major predictor of positive resolution after marital loss.* Paper presented at the 91st Annual Conference of the American Psychological Association, Anaheim, CA.

Pless, I. B. (1984). Clinical assessment: Physical and psychological functioning. *Pediatric Clinics of North America, 31,* 33–45.

Pless, I. B., & Pinkerton, P. (1975). *Chronic childhood disorders: Promoting patterns of adjustment.* Chicago: Year Book Medical.

Pless, I. B., & Roghmann, K. J. (1971). Chronic illness and its consequences: Observations based on three epidemiologic surveys. *Journal of Pediatrics, 79,* 351–359.

Rabkin, J. G., Williams, J. B. W., Neugebauer, R., Remien, R. H., & Goetz, R. (1990). Maintenance of hope in HIV-spectrum homosexual men. *American Journal of Psychiatry, 147,* 1322–1327.

Resnick, M. (1984a). The social construction of disability and handicap in America. In R. W. Blum (Ed.), *Chronic illness and disabilities in childhood and adolescence* (pp. 29–46). Orlando, FL: Grune & Stratton.

Resnick, M. (1984b). The teenager with cerebral palsy. In R. W. Blum (Ed.), *Chronic illness and disabilities in childhood and adolescence* (pp. 299–326). Orlando, FL: Grune & Stratton.

Rutter, M., Graham, P., & Yule, W. (1970). *A neuropsychiatric study in childhood* (Clinics in Developmental Medicine Nos. 35 and 36). London: Spastics International Heinemann Medical.

Rutter, M., Tizard, J., & Whitmore, K. (1970). *Education, health, and behavior: Psychological and medical study of childhood development.* London: Longman.

Ruvelson, L. (1990). The tense tightrope: How patients and their therapists balance hope and hope-lessness. *Clinical Social Work Journal, 18,* 145–155.

Ryan, K. M. (1981). Developmental differences in reactions to the physically disabled. *Human Development, 24,* 240–256.

Shontz, F. C. (1982). Adaptation to chronic illness. In T. Millon, C. Green, & R. Meagher (Eds.), *Handbook of clinical health psychology* (pp. 153–172). New York: Plenum Press.

Siegel, M. (1988). Children's knowledge of contagion and contamination as causes of illness. *Child Development, 59,* 1353–1359.

Silber, T. (1984). Ethical considerations in the care of the chronically ill adolescent. In R. W. Blum (Ed.), *Chronic illness and disabilities in childhood and adolescence* (pp. 17–27). Orlando, FL: Grune & Stratton.

Simmons, R. J., Corey, M., Cowen, L., Keenan, N., Robertson, J., & Levison, H. (1985). Emo-tional adjustment of adolescents with cystic fibrosis. *Psychosomatic Medicine, 47,* 111–122.

Stabler, B. (1988). Perspectives on chronic childhood illness. In B. H. Melamed, K. A. Matthews, D. K. Rauth, B. Stabler, & N. Schneiderman (Eds.), *Child health psychology.* Hillsdale, NJ: Erlbaum.

Stipek, D., & Weisz, J. R. (1981). Perceived personal control and academic achievement. *Review of Educational Research, 51,* 101–137.

Strax, T., & Wolfson, S. (1984). Life-cycle crisis of the disabled adolescent and young adult: Impli-cations for public policy. In R. W. Blum (Ed.), *Chronic illness and disabilities in childhood and adolescence* (pp. 47–57). Orlando, FL: Grune & Stratton.

Thompson, R. J., Gil, K. M., Burbach, D. J., Keith, B. R., & Kinney, T. R. (1993a). Psychological adjustment of mothers of children and adolescents with sickle cell disease: The role of stress, coping methods, and family functioning. *Journal of Pediatric Psychology, 18,* 549–559.

Thompson, R. J., Gil, K. M., Burbach, D. J., Keith, B. R., & Kinney, T. R. (1993b). Role of child and maternal processes in the psychological adjustment of children with sickle cell disease. *Journal of Consulting and Clinical Psychology, 61,* 468–474.

Thompson, R. J. & Gustafson, K. E. (1996). *Adaptation to chronic childhood illness.* Washington, DC: American Psychological Association.

Thompson, R. J., Gustafson, K. E., George, L. K., & Spock, A. (1994). Change over a 12-month period in the psychological adjustment of children and adolescents with cystic fibrosis. *Jour-nal of Pediatric Psychology, 19,* 189–203.

Thompson, R. J., Gustafson, K. E., Hamlett, K. W., & Spock, A. (1992a). Psychological adjust-ment of children with cystic fibrosis: The role of child cognitive processes and maternal adjust-ment. *Journal of Pediatric Psychology, 17,* 741–755.

Thompson, R. J., Gustafson, K. E., Hamlett, K. W., & Spock, A. (1992b). Stress, coping, and fam-ily functioning in the psychological adjustment of mothers of children with cystic fibrosis. *Journal of Pediatric Psychology, 17,* 573–585.

Tobin, D. L., Holroyd, K. A., Reynolds, R. V., & Wigal, J. K. (1989). The hierarchical factor struc-ture of the Coping Strategies Inventory. *Cognitive Therapy and Research, 13,* 343–361.

Van Dongen-Melman, J. E., & Sanders-Woudstra, J. A. (1986). Psychological aspects of childhood cancer: A review of the literature. *Journal of Child Psychology and Psychiatry, 27,* 145–180.

Voeltz, L. M. (1980). Children's attitudes toward handicapped peers. *American Journal of Mental Deficiency, 84,* 455–464.

Wallander, J. L., & Varni, J. W. (1992). Adjustment in children with chronic physical disorders: Programmatic research on a disability–stress–coping model. In A. M. La Greca, L. Siegel, J. L. Wallander, & C. E. Walker (Eds.), *Stress and coping in child health* (pp. 279–298). New York: Guilford Press.

Wallander, J. L., Varni, J. W., Babani, L., Banis, H. T., & Wilcox, K. T. (1989). Family resources as resistance factors for psychological maladjustment in chronically ill and handicapped children. *Journal of Pediatric Psychology, 14,* 157–173.

Weinberg, N. (1976). Social stereotyping of the physically handicapped. *Rehabilitation Psychology, 23,* 115–124.

Weinberg, N., & Santana, R. (1978). Comic books: Champions of the disabled stereotype. *Rehabilitation Literature, 15,* 25–33.

Whitt, J. K., Dykstra, W., & Taylor, C. (1979). Children's conceptions of illness and cognitive development. *Clinical Pediatrics, 18,* 327–339.

Whelan, T. (1986). *Neuropsychological performance, reading achievement, and perceptions of competence in boys with Duchenne muscular dystrophy.* Paper presented at the 14th Annual Meeting of the International Neuropsychological Society, Denver, CO.

Whelan, T., & Walker, M. (1997). Coping and adjustment of children with neurological disorder. In C. Reynolds & E. Fletcher-Janzen (Eds.), *Handbook of clinical child neuropsychology* (2nd ed., pp. 688–711). New York: Plenum Press.

PART II

Disorders Primarily Affecting
Learning and Behavior

6

LEARNING DISABILITIES

SALLY INGALLS
SAM GOLDSTEIN

Learning disabilities (LDs),* including reading disabilities, are the most prevalent group of neurobehavioral disorders affecting children and adults. As research has demonstrated and is continuing to confirm, there is frequently a strong genetic component to these disabilities; therefore, a chapter that addresses the neurobehavioral and genetic aspects of LDs is appropriate for inclusion in this text. However, unlike most other disorders described in this text, LDs are not a single, relatively well-defined entity or syndrome. Rather, LDs are an extremely heterogeneous group of learning problems with diverse characteristics that can result from a variety of biological influences, including genetic factors, environmental insults to the brain, and possibly (as recent research on brain development suggests) extreme lack of early environmental stimulation. As a result, the multifaceted field of LD is complex and often contentious, with many competing theories, definitions, diagnostic procedures, and suggested avenues of intervention.

Within the framework of this chapter, it is not possible to adequately describe or attempt to integrate the many competing viewpoints and claims surrounding the construct of LD. This task has been undertaken admirably by other writers in the field, who have approached LDs from a broad historical perspective as well as from the viewpoint of best current practices (Lerner, 1993; Mercer, 1991; Torgesen, 1998). In line with the focus of this text on genetics and the neurology of behavior, this chapter approaches LDs from biomedical, neuropsychological, and information-processing perspectives. Alternative formulations of the construct of LD are mentioned but are not given equal emphasis. The broad scope of the field of LD is condensed sufficiently to enable us to do the following:

- Trace the historical development of the concept and the field of LD.
- Consider the complex issues surrounding the prevalence of LD.

---

*In this chapter, the abbreviation "LD" is used to refer to both the noun "learning disability" and the adjective "learning-disabled." "LDs" is used to refer to "learning disabilities" in the plural.

- Discuss the etiology of LDs, by reviewing the accumulating information concerning both environmental and genetic factors.
- Summarize the search for subtypes of LD.
- Suggest a simple interim model to assist practitioners to organize the disparate characteristics associated with different subtypes of LD.
- Outline an approach to the assessment and diagnosis of LDs.
- Present a perspective for developing intervention plans and selecting instructional materials for LDs.
- Discuss important issues concerning LDs across the lifespan, sociocultural issues pertaining to LDs, and comorbid conditions associated with LDs.
- Summarize ongoing issues in the field of LD.

HISTORICAL DEVELOPMENT OF THE CONCEPT AND THE FIELD

The concept of LD as a category of human exceptionality evolved from the observations of physicians and educators as they studied and attempted to assist brain-injured children. Alfred Strauss and Laura Lehtinen published their classic work, *Psychopathology and Education of the Brain-Injured Child*, in 1947. In 1966, Clements, as head of a task force sponsored by the Department of Health, Education and Welfare, strongly supported use of the term "minimal brain dysfunction," which became popularized as "MBD" (Mercer, 1991).

The terms "minimal brain injury" or "MBD" were used to describe children of normal intelligence who appeared similar to some individuals with known brain injury, in that they exhibited a combination of hard or soft signs of neurological deficiency concomitantly with educational and sometimes with behavioral disorders. MBD was believed to be responsible for observed deficits in processes such as auditory and visual perception, symbol learning, short- and long-term memory, concept formation and reasoning, fine and gross motor functions, and integrative functions—deficits resulting in disorders of receptive and expressive language, reading, writing, mathematics, physical skill development, and interpersonal adjustment. In addition, behavioral traits such as distractibility, impulsivity, perseveration, and disinhibition were often found in children with MBD (Cruickshank, Bentzen, Ratzeburg, & Tannhauser, 1961; Gardner, 1973; Johnson & Myklebust, 1967). Thus, from the first, the field of LD centered around a medical model, with the label of MBD being applied to an extremely heterogeneous group of individuals.

Johnson and Myklebust (1967) discussed the limitations of terminologies extant at that time. They suggested that "minimal" was an inappropriate term to describe individuals whose resulting disabilities had a much greater than minimal impact on their learning functions, and that the words "brain injury" or "brain dysfunction" were viewed as too stigmatizing by many affected individuals and their parents.

In 1963, at a national conference of concerned parents and professionals held in Chicago, Samuel Kirk proposed use of the term "LD" (Lerner, 1993). This term was quickly accepted by parents, and it gained ascendance when federal and state governments adopted it at the time special education services were expanded to include students of average or better intelligence with otherwise unexplained academic learning problems (Mercer, 1991). Kirk viewed LDs from a psycholinguistic perspective: He proposed that underlying deficiencies in specific central nervous system (CNS) functions result in deficits in psychoneurological learning processes, which in turn explain observed LDs. Drawing on the psycholinguistic-process model of Charles Osgood, Kirk described LDs according to learning channels (auditory–verbal or visual–motor), learning levels (rote or conceptual), and specific processes (perception, reception, memory, integration, expression, etc.) (Kirk & Kirk, 1971).

Kirk's influence on the developing field of LD was reflected in the definition of LD adopted by the U.S. government in 1975 as part of Public Law (P.L.) 94-142, the Education for All Handicapped Children Act. This definition was reiterated in P.L. 101-476, the Individuals with Disabilities Education Act (IDEA) of 1990, and in P.L. 105-17, the IDEA Amendments of 1997. The federal definition, though one of many and unacceptable to some, remains the most widely referenced:

> The term "children with specific learning disabilities" means those children who have a disorder in one or more of the basic psychological processes involved in understanding or in using language, spoken or written, which disorder may manifest itself in imperfect ability to listen, think, speak, read, write, spell, or to do mathematical calculations. Such disorders include such conditions as perceptual handicaps, brain injury, minimal brain dysfunction, dyslexia, and developmental aphasia. Such term does not include children who have learning problems which are primarily the result of visual, hearing, or motor handicaps, of mental retardation, of emotional disturbance, or of environmental, cultural or economic disadvantage. (Quoted in Lerner, 1993, p. 9)

In an attempt to provide operational guidelines that would assist in the process of implementing P.L. 94-142, the U.S. Office of Education issued and reissued additional regulations further delineating criteria for identifying LD students. Primary operational components of the regulations, as outlined in the *Federal Register* of December 29, 1977, stipulate that a child has a specific LD if, when provided with appropriate learning experiences, the child exhibits a severe discrepancy between intellectual ability and achievement in one or more of seven specified achievement areas: listening comprehension, oral expression, basic reading skill, reading comprehension, written expression, mathematical calculation, and mathematical reasoning (U.S. Office of Education, 1977, cited in Mercer, 1991).

Other governmental, professional, and parental groups, dissatisfied with the federal definition of LD, have set forth their own definitions to remedy perceived deficiencies or oversights. At issue have been such questions as whether to include or exclude the concept of LD as a processing deficit, whether to include or exclude the concept of a CNS dysfunction, and whether or not such things as social deficits or attention-deficit/hyperactivity disorder (ADHD) should be included as primary forms of LD or viewed as comorbid disorders. Since the field of LD has always been an interdisciplinary one, it is not surprising that a multiplicity of conflicting viewpoints and definitions should arise.

Although the view of LDs as neurologically based process deficits remained widespread, during the 1970s a more behavioral approach to the topic was promulgated. Process deficits were roundly criticized as hypothetical constructs that could not be diagnosed validly or reliably, and that had little or no demonstrable relationship to effective interventions (Hammill & Larsen, 1974; Larsen, Parker, & Hammill, 1982). Proponents of this view advocated criterion-referenced or curriculum-based assessment of a multitude of specific skills, and interventions based on a detailed analysis of the component parts of each skill to be taught/learned, along with ecological analysis and modification of the learning environment. Well-designed and group-validated approaches to curriculum instruction were held to be appropriate and effective for all students, including slow learners, without reference to supposed internal processing deficits or disabilities.

While this debate raged, a third approach to understanding and assisting those with LD added a new dimension. Based on research centered at the University of Virginia

(Hallahan, 1980) and the University of Kansas (Schumaker, Deshler, Alley, & Warner, 1983), cognitive learning models were applied to the understanding and treatment of LDs. Within a cognitive framework, learners are viewed as directing their own learning by focusing on topics and skills that are personally meaningful and by developing active strategies for information acquisition. One outgrowth of cognitive theory has been the holistic or constructivist approach to teaching and learning, including whole-language methods of reading instruction. Although the tenets of cognitive theory have been applied to the LD population in a number of ways, a major emphasis has been on helping students to develop more reflective, accurate, and efficient approaches to learning tasks (i.e., on helping them learn how to learn). Students are taught to consciously employ self-monitoring strategies and effective learning/study strategies.

During the 1980s, concern mounted regarding the urgent need for a nationally coordinated program of neurobiological research to address the persistent and perplexing issues surrounding diagnosis and treatment of LDs. In 1985 the U.S. Congress passed P.L. 99-158, the Health Research Extension Act, which initially set up the Interagency Committee on Learning Disabilities—a consortium of representatives from numerous federal agencies dealing with education and public health, whose mission was to study the issues and recommend a research agenda. The work of the committee culminated in a report to Congress on the status of research needs in LD (Wyngaarden, 1987). With funding from Congress, and under the direction of the National Institute of Child Health and Human Development (NICHD), the Learning Disabilities Research Network was inaugurated in 1987 and charged with the following research goals: to identify the etiology and map the developmental course of different types of LD; to develop early predictors and prevention strategies for each type of LD; to identify co-occurring disorders and secondary social and behavioral characteristics associated with LD; and to identify effective treatments and teaching methods for different types of LD (Cannon, 1997). The first appropriation of $7.25 million in 1989 expanded, during the "Decade of the Brain" (declared by President George Bush and Congress) to an annual expenditure of $21 million as of 1996 (McElgunn, 1996). This money helps fund the research activities of a number of university-based research centers, which to date have pursued the stated research goals primarily in the areas of linguistic, reading, and spelling disabilities. Dr. G. R. Lyon, director of LD research programs for NICHD, noted that as of 1996 the combined efforts of the Research Network had yielded over 2,000 journal articles and a large number of books (McElgunn, 1996). Major findings from LD research programs supported by NICHD have been summarized by Lyon (1995, 1996b). Research in the neurosciences is beginning to provide some understanding of the neurobiological basis of LDs; longitudinal research in the area of reading is beginning to yield empirically validated interventions in that critical area of instruction. We are at the frontier of a new era in LD, in which research may lead to a functional integration of the neurological, behavioral, and cognitive approaches in the process of establishing a scientific foundation for this multifaceted and important field.

PREVALENCE

Determining prevalence rates, or the frequency of occurrence, of LD in the population might at first glance appear to be a relatively straightforward process. However, since the determination of a prevalence rate for any disease or disability is dependent on having a clear-cut definition of the disorder under consideration, and since there is no consensually accepted or experimentally validated definition of LD, the process of determining the prevalence of

LD is a quagmire. At the present time, prevalence figures for this nondefinitive disorder or group of disorders cannot be determined precisely and are essentially broad estimates. Keeping in mind the indeterminate status of the field, in this section we discuss some of the issues surrounding the prevalence of LD and present what is known, as far as current definitional and diagnostic practices permit.

Important considerations regarding the determination of LD prevalence have been presented by MacMillan (1993) and Lyon (1996b). In a discussion of operationalizing disability definitions, MacMillan described "prevalence rate" as referring to the total percentage of the population that is affected by a disorder, whereas "detection rate" refers to the number of known or identified cases. For LD, prevalence and detection rates may, and indeed probably do, differ. Depending on the stringency of identification criteria, prevalence estimates for LD have varied from as low as 1% to as high as 30% of the school-age population (Lerner, 1993). Mercer (1991) suggested that approximately 1.5% of students may have severe specific LD, while the inclusion of students with mild LD could raise that figure to about 4% or 5%.

Prior to the record-keeping and child-counting requirements of P.L. 94-142, which was first implemented during the 1976–1977 school year, there was no national data base for estimating the prevalence of LD. Johnson and Myklebust's (1967) comprehensive text on LD (a standard reference during the late 1960s and early 1970s) made no mention of the prevalence of LD, suggesting only that it affects a substantial number of children. Since the implementation of P.L. 94-142, the U.S. Department of Education (USDE) issues annual reports to Congress that include a count of the number of children in the United States enrolled in special education under each disability category. Depending on the method used for determining percentages, in the year 1976–1977 approximately 1.2% of all students were classified as LD (Lerner, 1993). This figure rose steadily until in 1993, 5% of school children aged 6 to 21 were so identified (Lyon, 1996b). In 1976–1977, the number of LD students served was just under 800,000; by 1990 this figure had increased to over 2,000,000 (U.S. Department of Education [USDE], 1991, cited in Lerner, 1993). The sharp rate of increase in the identification of LD subsequent to the implementation of P.L. 94-142 has begun to level off in recent years. As of 1994, the category of LD accounted for just over 50% of all students served in special education (Office of Special Education Programs [OSEP], 1994, cited in Reschly, 1996).

There are many factors associated with what some view as the burgeoning or even epidemic identification rate for LD. These factors can be divided into four groups: those related to definition/classification, available diagnostic instrumentation, systems operation, and sociopolitical realities. The four groups are discussed in detail here, because they are central to some of the most important and persistently ineluctable issues in the field of LD.

As was mentioned, the primary factors underlying widely varying prevalence estimates for LD are lack of a clear-cut definition and lack of classification procedures derived from coherent theory. As Lyon (1996b) has put it, "Valid prevalence estimates depend upon a set of criteria for identification that are clear, observable, measurable, and agreed upon" (p. 58). Although research-based theory building in terms of definition and classification is proceeding apace in the areas of phonological reading disorders and nonverbal learning disabilities (NLD; Torgesen, 1993), for the broad field of LD this remains a distant goal. As noted earlier, the concept of LD is multifaceted. Diverse views are engendered by a wide array of associated medical and pedagogical disciplines, including neurology, psychology, neuropsychology, speech and language pathology, optometry, occupational and physical therapy, and education, as manifested through university research, regular education, special education, and private clinical assessment/tutoring. Each profession brings its own set of theoretical considerations, methodologies, and predilections. In addition, there is much variability within professional orientations. For example, among public school special education programs, the criteria for designating students as LD vary widely. Mercer, Forgnone, and Wolking (1976) and Mercer, King-Sears, and Mercer (1990) documented the range of definitions of LD and the lack of agreement in the diagnostic criteria adopted by state boards of education across the United States. The concept of IQ–achievement discrepancy (which is presently the central feature of LD diagnosis in public schools) is operationalized differently by different states, with arbitrary cutoff points for both intellectual level and achievement level. One result of highly flexible decision making is that the percentage of children labeled as LD differs from state to state, varying from 2.2% to 7.8% (Lerner, 1993).

Another set of factors affecting the detection rate for LD involves the availability of an appropriate range of reliable and valid assessment measures. Although there is currently much criticism of IQ–achievement discrepancy as the basis for determining the presence or absence of LD (Lyon, 1996b; MacMillan, 1993; Mather & Roberts, 1994; Stanovich, 1993; Toth & Siegel, 1994; Zigmond, 1993), intelligence and achievement will probably always be essential constructs for understanding individuals with LD, and therefore they must be measured as accurately as possible. In addition, to the extent that LDs are viewed as reflecting specific process deficits or information-processing deficiencies, there must be a variety of well-standardized instruments for quantifying processing strengths and weaknesses. For a given individual, it may be important to assess any of the following: phonemic awareness, phonological segmentation, grammatical and semantic comprehension, rapid automatic naming (quick label retrieval), digit/sentence repetition, oral expression, tactile perception, directional perception, spatial organization, social perception, verbal and nonverbal concept formation, concrete and abstract problem solving, processing speed, and motor coordination in its many forms. Although there are measures available to assess these constructs, their specificity, adequacy, quality of standardization, and breadth of dissemination are highly variable. The development of psychometrically sound diagnostic instruments remains a primary goal; it will reduce misidentification and eventually have a positive impact on our understanding of the prevalence of LD, as well as of specific subtypes of LD.

A third important (though somewhat overlooked) group of factors affecting LD prevalence rates consists of what MacMillan (1993) has termed "system identification variables." This group of factors overlaps to some degree with the fourth set of factors, the effects of sociopolitical realities. Broadly, "system identification" encompasses the ecological processes within families, schools, and clinics that increase or decrease the likelihood that a given individual will be referred for evaluation and classified as LD. Family system variables affecting whether parents seek LD assessment for a child, or whether an individual seeks assessment for himself or herself, may include socioeconomic status (SES), family values regarding educational attainment for males and for females, the presence or absence of comorbid conditions that create additional functional difficulties, the presence or absence of medical insurance coverage, and so forth. Variables within educational systems that influence the prevalence of LD include the educational philosophy of the school system, financial incentives for identification, the nature and quality of basic education provided for all students, class size, training of regular class teachers to accept and deal with diversity, availability of other types of supportive services for students and teachers, training/competence of special education diagnosticians, and the like. LD prevalence rates are also affected by sociopolitical factors, such as increased attention to LDs as a result of public awareness and political advocacy; ambiguity in the definitions and overlap of disability categories; and the social desirability of an LD classification rather than a classification of intellectual disability or mental retardation. (Keogh, 1993; Macmillan, 1993). In addition, MacMillan (1993, citing Zigler & Hodapp, 1986) has suggested that for LD, "the ratio of detected to undetected cases may (and probably does) vary by age, IQ level, racial group, gender, and socioeconomic status" (p. 143).

Within school populations, data have been gathered on the prevalence of LD by age, race, and gender. A report from OSEP (1994, cited by Reschly, 1996) presented data showing that LD students aged 6 to 11 constitute 41% of the total special education population for that age range, while LD students aged 12 to 17 make up 63% of all special education students in that age group. Lerner (1993, citing USDE, 1991) reported that the number of LD children served in special education at each age level increases rapidly from 6 years to 9 years, peaks and levels off for children aged 10 to 12, and then gradually declines to age 18. Thus it appears that the majority of LD children are first identified during their primary and intermediate years of elementary school, and that far fewer students are first identified during secondary school. Lerner (1993) has also suggested that the decrease in the number of LD students served during their teen years partially may be accounted for by the number of teenagers with LD who drop out of school.

The U.S. Office of Civil Rights has been concerned about the number of students from racial and ethnic minority groups who are identified as disabled and enrolled in special education. A survey by that office (OSEP, 1994, cited by Reschly, 1996) reported that a total of 8% of African American students, 6.5% of European Americans students, and 5.6% of Hispanic students were enrolled in special education under the categories of mild mental retardation, severe emotional disability, and LD. Although African American students may be overrepresented and Hispanic students underrepresented overall, according to this survey the percentage of students from each group categorized as LD was relatively constant: 5.0% of African Americans, 5.0% of European Americans, and 4.7% of Hispanics.

The prevalence of LD by gender has long been a topic of discussion and concern. Lerner (1993, citing U.S. General Accounting Office, 1981) reported that of the special education students classified as LD at that time, approximately 72% were boys and 28% were girls. Research studies of individuals with reading disability have typically estimated that the gender ratio of males to females ranges from 2:1 to 5:1 (Huston, 1992). Various explanations have been suggested to account for the preponderance of males with reading disability—for example, genetic factors, factors associated with differences in prenatal brain development, sex-linked differences in hemispheric specialization, postnatal maturational differences, and system identification variables (Kelley, 1993; Pennington, 1991; Thomson, 1990). Although some of the variation in male–female prevalence or severity of reading disability can probably be attributed to biological differences, findings from three of the universities in the Learning Disabilities Research Network indicate that nearly equal numbers of males and females manifest dyslexia (Lyon, 1996b; Kolata, 1990; Shaywitz, Shaywitz, Fletcher, & Escobar, 1990). When prevalence estimates are determined through research-based epidemiological studies in which every child in a given cohort of children is assessed for reading disability, the ratio of males to females is close to 1:1; when estimates are determined through prevalence figures for school-identified or clinic-identified populations based on teacher or parent referral, the ratio of males to females is much higher. System identification variables resulting in gender-based ascertainment bias appear to account for the majority of this difference. As is true for boys in general, boys with reading difficulty display more behavioral problems, including regulation of activity level, than do girls. Since their functional difficulties are more readily perceived as problematic, more boys than girls are referred for assessment, and consequently more are classified to receive special education services (Shaywitz et al., 1990).

Studies of several samples of adopted children have shown that LDs are diagnosed four to five times more frequently in these groups than in equivalent groups of nonadoptees (Kenny, Baldwin, & Mackie, 1967; Silver, 1970, 1989). Because information about the biological parents of adoptees is often limited or confidential, it is difficult to determine the reasons for the high rate of LD among adopted children.

ETIOLOGY

Background: Neurobiological Findings

From the time of the earliest medical reports describing cases of dyslexia, LDs have been viewed as stemming from CNS dysfunction—more precisely, from dysfunction of specific portions of the cerebral cortex (Doris, 1986; Huston, 1992). This long-standing presumption is being reinforced and validated by modern cognitive neuroscience. To provide a background for reviewing what is known about the etiology of LDs, some of the major processes that take place during the development of the human cerebral cortex are presented, and recent findings regarding the neurobiology of dyslexia are summarized.

Fetal brain development proceeds along a course of increasing specialization "from a few all-purpose cells into a complex organ made of billions of specialized, interconnected nerve cells called neurons" (National Institute of Mental Health [NIMH], 1993, p. 10). Neurons develop from early-forming tissue near the cerebral ventricles and then migrate in an orderly fashion to form the cortical plate and eventually the six layers or laminae of the cerebral cortex (Lyon, 1996a; Marin-Padilla, 1993). Initially, lower cortical layers are formed by the migrating neurons, and later the upper or outer layers are formed in an inside-out progression. After a few weeks of gestation, the evolving embryonic brain is divided into three primary areas or subdivisions—the hindbrain, midbrain, and forebrain. It is from the forebrain that the cerebral cortex develops. At 6 weeks, the developing brain of an embryo is almost as large as its body. At about 8 to 10 weeks, neuronal migration begins and continues until approximately the 18th to 24th week, at which time all of the neurons that will constitute the cerebral cortex have been formed and have traveled to their prescribed destinations (Lyon, 1996a; Marin-Padilla, 1993). During the remainder of fetal life and the years of infancy and early childhood, the billions of specialized neurons will continue to differentiate and to grow axons and dendritic connections, forming the complex neural networks that support human existence and behavior.

A most interesting finding from research during the last two decades is that during prenatal life and childhood, an overabundance of neurons and synaptic connections is produced. Prenatally, these neurons fire in a systematic fashion and then continue to fire postnatally in response to environmental stimulation and developing internal processes. The neurons and interconnected pathways that are activated frequently and that fire repeatedly are reinforced; they become fine-tuned, increase in speed and efficiency, and are retained. Those that are surplus, or possibly less stimulated, atrophy and are eliminated. This process of neuroconsolidation, referred to as "ontogenetic neuronal death" or "pruning," begins prenatally as soon as neuronal migration is nearing completion and continues throughout childhood. The rate of axonal growth and destruction varies in different layers of the cortex; animal research indicates that up to 50% of neuronal connections may be lost in some layers (Finlay & Miller, 1993). The "plasticity" of the brain (i.e., its ability to develop or maintain function after insult by forming new neural connections) is at its maximum during the last trimester of gestation and rapidly declines after 1 year of age (Marin-Padilla, 1993).

As a result of technological advances in brain research, knowledge about the neuro-biological correlates of LDs is expanding. That is, LDs, primarily reading disorders or dyslexia, are being linked to measurable differences in brain morphology and function. The general structure and cytoarchitecture of the brain in normal and dyslexic subjects has been studied by means of postmortem examination, computerized tomography (CT) scan, and static magnetic resonance imaging (MRI). Comparison of differences between normal readers and dyslexic readers in the specific brain regions activated and their degree of activation during performance of linguistic tasks has been accomplished with electro-encephalographic studies, including advanced brain electrical activity mapping; studies of evoked potentials; positron emission tomography (PET) and single-photon emission com-puted tomography (SPECT) scans; and functional magnetic resonance imaging (fMRI). Descriptions of these research methodologies are provided by Lyon, Newby, Recht, and Caldwell (1991), Krasuki, Horowitz, and Rumsey (1996), and Posner and Raichle (1994).

Although it is beyond the scope of this chapter to review results of the many post-mortem and neuroimaging studies of dyslexia, findings from a few selected studies are cited. Postmortem studies of the brains of individuals who experienced dyslexia and other learn-ing problems during their lifetime have revealed various disarrangements of brain archi-tecture: abnormal convolution pattern of the left parietal lobe; thinned and stretched corpus callosum; polymicrogyri (clusters of many small convulsions) in the left posterior sylvan area; neuronal ectopias (clusters of abnormally placed neurons referred to as "brain warts"); focal dysplasias (specific areas of disorganized cortical layering); many minute cellular abnormalities throughout the left hemisphere; subcortical thalamic abnormalities; and symmetry rather than normal asymmetry in the region of the planum temporale (Drake, 1968; Galaburda & Kemper, 1979; Galaburda, Sherman, Rosen, Aboitiz, & Geschwind, 1985). Most of the anomalies found were on the left side, primarily in the inferior frontal, superior temporal, and parietal regions—areas known to be important to linguistic func-tioning and reading. The brains studied exhibited no gross abnormalities or obvious struc-tural deficits; the subtle cortical and subcortical anomalies were uniquely distributed in each case (Hynd, Marshall, & Gonzalez, 1991).

Normal brains show asymmetrical development, generally larger on the left, of struc-tures implicated in language and reading (e.g., the planum temporale and the parietal–occipital cortex in the posterior region of the brain). A most striking convergent finding from many studies has been that of symmetry or even reversed asymmetry in these critical brain regions in approximately 65–75% of dyslexic subjects (Hier, LeMay, Rosenberger, & Perlo, 1978; Hynd, Semrud-Clikeman, Lorys, Novey, & Eliopulos, 1990; Larsen, Hoien, Lundberg, & Odegaard, 1990). MRI studies have shown that symmetry or reversed asym-metry is associated with general neurolinguistic deficits (as concluded by Hynd et al., 1991) and deficits in phonological processing (Larsen et al., 1990). Correlating information from CT scans with measured IQ, Rosenberger and Hier (1980) documented lower Verbal than Performance IQ in those dyslexic subjects who demonstrated symmetry or reversed asym-metry of the posterior region.

Gross-Glenn et al. (1991), utilizing PET scan technology, found that during reading tasks dyslexic subjects demonstrated relatively greater metabolic activity than control sub-jects in some brain regions (midtemporal and lingual gyri) but lower metabolic activity than controls in other regions (peri-insular cortex). Lower activation of the insular area was also implicated by Paulesu et al. (1996) in a PET study of compensated adult dyslexics whose only residual deficit was phonological processing. These researchers posit that pho-nological problems arise from disconnections between different brain areas involved in various aspects of phonological coding, and that the weak connection or disconnection may be due to a dysfunctional left insula. A number of neuroimaging studies lend preliminary support for the view that phonological processing takes place primarily in the language areas of the fronal region (Broca's area); that letter recognition occurs primarily in the occipital lobe; and that words are processed for meaning primarily in the temporal lobe (Shaywitz & Shaywitz, 1997, 1998). Additional information about neuroimaging and dyslexia is presented by Bigler et al. in Chapter 4 of this volume; for reviews, see also Rumsey (1996) and Shaywitz et al. (1996).

Taken as a whole, postmortem and neuroimaging studies indicate that dyslexia is not a unitary disorder related to dysfunction in a single region of the brain, but rather a heterogeneous disorder that involves a widely distributed aggregate of brain functions (Gross-Glenn et al., 1991; Riccio & Hynd, 1996; Rumsey, 1996). To date, this body of research provides correlational and inferential information which suggests a relationship between brain morphology/physiology and neurolinguistic processes, including dyslexia, but no causal relationship has yet been established. As discussed by Rumsey (1996), research outcomes from neuroimaging studies can be variable as a result of individual differences and the many technical and methodological challenges of this type of research. Shaywitz and Shaywitz (1997/1998) referred to an interesting study currently underway at Syracuse University. Young children with serious reading disorders are undergoing neuroimaging before and after one year of intensive reading instruction to determine whether the treatment will produce a measurable change in brain physiology. At this point, neuroimaging cannot be used as a definitive diagnostic tool in individual cases, but its use as one component of a diagnostic process is on the horizon.

Galaburda (1993) and Galaburda et al. (1985) have hypothesized that genetic predisposition is probably the main etiological factor in the cerebral asymmetry observed in many individuals with dyslexia. They have further proposed that other observed structural abnormalities are produced by genetic, immunological, or undetermined factors that alter the normal pattern of neuronal migration and cortical organization sometime during the fifth to seventh month of gestation (Hynd et al., 1991). In addition, cortical dysplasias and disarrangements of the cytoarchitecture have been associated wtih perinatal infections and fetal alcohol syndrome (Marin-Padilla, 1993). More recently, Riccio and Hynd (1996) suggested that abnormalities in the process of eliminating the excessive buildup of neurons and cortical connections (i.e., pruning) may be implicated in dyslexia. If, as has been presumed, LDs result from CNS dysfunction, anything that significantly disrupts the normal development or normal functioning of the CNS has the potential to be an etiological factor in LDs.

Environmental Factors

As indicated above, two categories of etiological factors in LDs are genetic inheritance and bioenvironmental risks or occurrences. The category of bioenvironmental events, viewed broadly, encompasses risks to the developing brain associated with prenatal environment, birth history, and postnatal environment. In comparison with genetic transmission of LDs, less is definitely known about the link between environmental factors and LDs, but it is instructive to consider the range of possibilities.

Prenatally, the developing brain appears to be protected from deficient maternal nutrition, but brain development may be affected by severe deficits in maternal nutrition if they occur before the 24th week of gestation or if essential proteins or specific micronutrients are missing (Pirozzolo & Bonnefil, 1996; Pollitt et al., 1996). Silver (1989) has stated, "Malnutrition during the first trimester can lead to a reduction in brain cell number; malnutrition during the last trimester is likely to reduce cell size rather than number" (p. 326). Deficiency in maternal thyroid hormone level has a negative impact on fetal brain development and is currently being investigated as a potential factor in LDs (An Ounce of Prevention, 1998; Research Services Committee, 1995). Immune system incompatibilities, in which maternal antibodies attack fetal brain tissue, may cause newly formed neurons to migrate to the wrong area (Galaburda, 1990; Huston, 1992). Maternal use of tobacco during pregnancy produces babies with lower birth weight, which increases the risk of developmental difficulties, including LDs (NIMH, 1993). It is well known that alcohol consumption during pregnancy may have damaging effects on the neuronal development of a fetus, leading to problems with learning, attention, memory, and problem solving. Continuous maternal alcohol consumption can lead to fetal alcohol syndrome or fetal alcohol effects, which may include mild physical anomalies, ADHD, general intellectual impairment, or subtle cognitive deficits and LDs. The duration of fetal exposure to alcohol is related to the severity of later cognitive deficits (Autti-Ramo et al., 1992).

The prenatal use of drugs, both prescribed medications and illegal substances, may affect a child's learning capabilities. The long-term effects of cocaine on a developing fetus continue to be debated (Azar, 1997); however, exposure to cocaine, especially crack cocaine, does appear to affect the proper development of the brain's sensory receptors (Hurt et al., 1995; NIMH, 1993). Although negative behavioral outcomes, including ADHD, in children are clearly associated with maternal cocaine use, the research data concerning long-term effects of cocaine on cognitive delays and learning deficits are mixed (Azar, 1997; Azuma & Chasnoff, 1993; Hurt et al., 1995). Maternal or paternal drug abuse is the most frequent source of pediatric infection resulting in AIDS or AIDS-related complex (Nicholas, Sondheimer, Willoughby, Yaffe, & Katz, 1989). Symptoms often associated with pediatric HIV/AIDS include mental retardation, cognitive deterioration, loss of developmental milestones, and delays or disorders in the acquisition of language and both gross and fine motor skills (Pirozzolo & Bonnefil, 1996).

The process of birth and birth history involve various factors that may in theory or in actuality be related to later LDs. When preterm birth deprives a fetus of the necessary time and essential environment for normal development, long-term outcomes often include mild to profound developmental delays and/or LDs (Hack et al., 1992; Saigal, Rosenbaum, Szatmari, & Campbell, 1991; Vohr et al., 1991). It is interesting to note that neuronal migration is thought to be complete at 18 to 24 weeks of gestation (as previously suggested) and that premature birth at 24 weeks is generally the earliest point at which a fetus has a chance for survival (Marin-Padilla, 1993). The continuing development of the cerebral cortex in low-birth-weight infants (weight less than 1,500 grams) is highly vulnerable to asphyxia. It is quite common to find small, medium, or large hypoxic–ischemic and/or hemorrhagic lesions in the brain after a preterm infant has experienced perinatal asphyxia (Marin-Padilla, 1993). Hypoxia–ischemia in newborns produces changes in the concentration of neurotransmitters and in protein synthesis (Finlay & Miller, 1993). The effects of these early lesions and metabolic changes on later maturation and learning continue to be studied. Long-term outcomes for low-birth-weight infants appear to be a function of both neurological/medical status and environmental risk factors related to SES and parenting style.

In addition to preterm birth, a birth history that includes hard or prolonged labor, fetal distress, anoxia, or injury from forceps delivery is a predisposing factor for neurobehavioral impairments (Pirozzolo & Bonnefil, 1996). Accordo (1980, cited by Pennington, 1991) reported a weak relationship between perinatal complications and later reading problems. Coletti (1979, cited by Mercer, 1991) found a much higher percentage of birth complications among LD subjects than among normally achieving subjects.

Insults to the brain can occur from postnatal infections and traumas such as rubella, meningitis, encephalitis, hypoxia (from cerebrovascular events, near-drowning, fires, or accidental chest compression), closed or open head injury, tumor growth and surgical resection, radiation or chemotherapy, and so on. When the resulting brain damage is significant to severe, individuals who have experienced any of the foregoing are broadly referred to as having "traumatic brain injury" and typically exhibit a variety of learning and behavioral impairments (Abayomi, Chun, & Kelly, 1990; Harding & Kleiman, 1996; Mulhern, 1996; Ryan, LaMarche, Barth, & Boll, 1996). When the resulting damage is transitory or mild there may be few if any observable sequelae. The recovering brain, through the compensatory principle of plasticity, may be able to respond with sufficient cortical reorganization to prevent overt disorders. However, the end result may be executive-function weaknesses such as ADHD, or a range of subtle cognitive and learning problems that may not be evident until years later (Allison, 1992).

Another frequently mentioned etiological factor in LDs is long-term environmental exposure to toxic substances such as lead and cadmium. Research sponsored by the National Institutes of Health has shown a connection between exposure to lead and learning difficulties in rats. Rats exposed to lead demonstrated changes in brain wave patterns concomitantly with slowing in ability to learn experimental tasks. Their learning problems persisted for weeks after their exposure to lead was terminated (NIMH, 1993). In humans, exposure to large doses of lead has been associated with mental retardation and other global impairments (Mercer, 1991). Even low-level lead exposure measured at 24 months of age has been associated with intellectual and academic performance deficits at 10 years of age (Bellinger, Stiles, & Needleman, 1992). LDs are among the developmental effects of lead toxicity (Centers for Disease Control, 1991, cited by Pipitone, 1991). The topic of lead exposure in children is further discussed by Tesman and Hills (1994).

Research that documents the critical impact of social and environmental stimulation on brain development and age-related windows of opportunity for the development of specific skills is currently receiving considerable attention in the popular media (Begley, 1996; Nash, 1997). LDs have traditionally been viewed as neurological deficits intrinsic to genetic and other biological factors within the individual and not of environmental origin. However, current research is documenting the intimate connection between environment and neuroanatomical development (Dawson & Fischer, 1994; Hutenlocher, 1991). The pervasive effects of early environmental programming on the formation and pruning of neural networks, and the theoretical relationship of this process to the occurrence of neurologically based specific LDs, constitute an area that is only beginning to be considered.

The prenatal, perinatal, and postnatal environmental factors associated with brain development and brain injury that have been presented here are best viewed as potential causes of LD, due to uncertainties and inconsistencies in the relationships among age at onset, the severity of circumstances or conditions, the degree of transient or permanent brain dysfunction, and the broad range of possible effects on learning. For example, clinical studies have documented cases in which major structural deficits, even loss of an entire brain hemisphere, result in few observable signs of LD, whereas many individuals with severe LDs have no obvious structural deficits (Bigler, 1992; Satz, 1990). In addition, confounding variables such as SES, parenting style, and early interventions mediate the degree to which a neurological abnormality will result in impaired learning. In many or most cases of LD, an environmental etiology is presumably not a factor; however, in some cases, an environmental cause is directly known or fairly certain. In other cases, the environmental contribution to etiology is cloudy, involving subtle factors that may be undocumented or unknown.

Studies have shown that an aggregate of brain functions are involved in both verbal and nonverbal learning and that LDs involve more than dysfunction within a single hemisphere. However, it is widely theorized that NLDs result primarily from right hemispheric dysfunction (i.e., from disruption or destruction of white matter fibers, which are concentrated in the right hemisphere) or from difficulties with intermodal/interhemispheric integration (James & Selz, 1997; Rourke, 1987, 1989). NLDs sometimes appear to arise *de novo*, without any known brain disease or disorder, but they are frequently observed in conjunction with developmental anomalies or environmental insults such as head injuries, poorly controlled hydrocephalus, irradiation for malignancy, congenital absence of the corpus callosum, or surgical removal of tissue from the right hemisphere. In contrast with NLDs, verbal or language-based LDs are more likley to arise from dysfunction of the left hemisphere or from intrahemispheric integration difficulties and are viewed as being more likely of genetic origin (Pennington, 1991; Rourke, 1989).

Genetic Factors

The terms "word blindness" and "dyslexia" were first used as terms for reading disability in the 1870s by German physicians. In about 1900 two British physicians, Dr. W. Pringle Morgan and Dr. James Hinshelwood, began to describe some cases of word blindness as congenital rather than acquired (Doris, 1986; Huston, 1992). From 1895 onward, a number of early workers in the field of learning disorders observed that there were often several members of the same family with similar types of reading problems; this suggested a genetic etiology. In the United States during the 1920s and 1930s, Dr. Samuel T. Orton, a neuropsychiatrist, worked extensively with children who exhibited reading and writing disorders. He also noted the frequently familial nature of these disorders and viewed them as likely to be hereditary (Huston, 1992).

In the last 40 years, experimental research has provided strong support for genetic factors in some forms of LD. The familial occurrence of reading, spelling, and writing disabilities has been investigated via several methodologies, such as study of family members and pedigree analysis, determination of concordance rates among identical and fraternal twins, comparison of linear regression in reading scores between identical and fraternal twins, and chromosomal analysis of family members.

Family Studies

The earliest widely cited family pedigree study of reading disorder, conducted by Hallgren in 1950 (cited in Pennington, 1991), consisted of a statistical analysis of dyslexia in 112 families. Among first-degree relatives (parents and siblings of an identified child), the risk for co-occurrence of this disorder was 41%, which is much higher than the usual prevalence estimates for the general population of 5–10%. Huston (1992), reporting on Hallgren's study, indicated that of the 112 families, in 90 families one parent was dyslexic; in 3 families both parents were dyslexic; and in 19 families neither parent had dyslexia. Although Hallgren's study has been criticized for methodological flaws, later studies carried out with greater technical precision, such as that of Finucci, Guthrie, Childs, Abbey, and Childs (1976, cited in DeFries, 1991), have found similar familial rates in the range of 35–45%. Finucci (1978) published a critical review of the early investigations of dyslexia and genetics.

The Colorado Family Reading Study, begun in 1973, compared the reading abilities of 125 reading-disabled children (probands) and their family members to those of 125 matched control children who were not reading-disabled and their family members. The total number of subjects in this study was 1,044, making it an extensive family study. The results clearly demonstrated that reading disorders are familial in nature. Scores for siblings of proband subjects were significantly lower than scores for siblings of control subjects on measures of both reading and symbol-processing speed. A similar pattern of significant results was observed for the parents of probands and controls. An interesting finding was that brothers of probands were significantly more reading-impaired on average than were sisters of probands. Similarly, fathers of probands were less skilled readers on average than were mothers of probands; however, the score difference between fathers and mothers was less than the score difference between male and female siblings (DeFries, 1991). Although reading disabilities have now conclusively been shown to be familial in nature, familial occurrence suggests but does not demonstrate genetic heritability. Empirical investigations to ascertain the genetic inheritance of LDs (specifically, reading disability) have included concordance studies of twins, multiple-regression studies of twins, segregation analysis studies, and chromosomal linkage studies.

Concordance Studies of Twins

Comparisons of pairs of identical and fraternal twins have been used to investigate the genetic component of reading disability in the same way that other twin studies have researched the heritability of intelligence and a variety of other personal characteristics. Many twin studies have employed a comparison of concordance rates to test for genetic etiology. A pair of twins is concordant for reading disability if both twins are reading-disabled; if just one twin is reading-disabled, the pair is discordant. Identical twins share an identical genetic makeup, while fraternal twins share about 50% of heritable variation (LaBuda & DeFries, 1990). To the extent that reading disability is genetically determined, the concordance rate for pairs of identical twins should be considerably higher than that for pairs of fraternal twins when at least one member of each identical and fraternal pair has been identified as reading-disabled.

Two of the earlier reports of concordance rates for reading disability in twins were those of Hermann (1959) and Zerbin-Rudin (1967). Both of these researchers pooled the findings of smaller previous studies, possibly with some overlap in their reporting of cases. The concordance rates reported by the two authors were nearly identical. Their combined data, as reported by Huston (1992), showed an average of 100% concordance for 29 identical twin pairs and 34% concordance for 67 fraternal twin pairs.

Due to technical differences in the method for determining concordance rates, different authors sometimes report different concordance figures for the same study; that is, some authors report "pairwise" concordance rates, and others report "probandwise" concordance rates. The first method counts each concordant twin pair one time. The latter method considers each member of a concordant pair as a separate research subject, and therefore counts each concordant pair twice. Using probandwise concordance increases the percentage of concordance for both identical and fraternal twin pairs (LaBuda & DeFries, 1990). For example, in the Zerbin-Rudin (1967) study, a pairwise concordance rate for fraternal twin pairs was 34% (12 of 34 cases), as reported by Huston (1992); however, the probandwise concordance rate for those same twin pairs was 52% (24 [12 + 12] of 46 [34 + 12]) cases, as reported by DeFries (1991).

Bakwin (1973, cited by LaBuda and DeFries, 1990) studied 31 pairs of identical and 31 pairs of fraternal twins, finding 84% pairwise concordance for identical twin males and 83% for identical twin females. Interestingly, the pairwise concordance rate for male fraternal twins was 42%, while the rate for female fraternal twins was just 8%. Bakwin also investigated the environmental factors of birth weight and birth order as predictors of reading disability, but found no significant differences between normally reading twins and reading-disabled twins on these variables.

Stevenson, Graham, Fredman, and McLoughlin (1987, cited by Thomson 1990), conducted a large-scale study of the reading and spelling abilities of 285 13-year-old twins, who were divided into several subgroups according to type and severity of skill deficiencies. In contrast to other concordance studies of twins, these authors reported relatively similar pairwise concordance rates for identical and fraternal twin pairs (32% and 21%, respectively). Their findings suggest a fairly low level of heritability for reading disorder. However, with IQ controlled for, Stevenson et al. found a strong genetic influence on spelling ability.

The most technologically sound large-scale twin study to date has been the Colorado Twin Study, begun in 1982 as part of the Colorado Reading Project. With IQ controlled for (Verbal or Performance IQ = 90 or above) and other types of selection criteria in place, the Colorado Twin Study examined reading disability in 101 pairs of identical twins and 114 pairs of fraternal twins. The pairwise concordance rate of 52% for identical twins was lower than those in most earlier studies, while the rate for fraternal twins was fairly typical at 33% (LaBuda & DeFries, 1990). Although there is some variation in the concordance figures generated by different studies, on the whole they do provide strong evidence for a genetic factor in the etiology of reading disability.

Multiple-Regression Studies of Twins

The statistical data from concordance studies are based on a simple, dichotomous variable: the presence or absence of reading disability among twins and other first-degree relatives. A more powerful statistical approach to the question of the genetic heritability of reading disability is to employ reading scores as a continuous variable. With these more robust data, a *t*-test of the significance of the difference between the reading scores of reading-disabled twins and the scores of their cotwins can be performed. Alternatively, reading scores can be established for reading-disabled twins, and then the scores of their cotwins can be examined to determine the degree to which the cotwins' scores regress toward the test mean or toward the mean of a control group (LaBuda & DeFries, 1990). To the extent that reading disability is inherited, the amount of regression to the mean should be significantly less for identical twins (whose degree of genetic relationship is 1.00) than for fraternal twins (whose degree of relationship is about .50).

As part of the Colorado Reading Project, DeFries and Fulker (1985) generated two multiple-regression models to test this hypothesis. Based on an analysis of reading data from 101 pairs of identical twins and 114 pairs of fraternal twins in which at least one member of each twin pair was reading-disabled, they found that on average the reading scores of identical twins regressed just 0.22 of a standard deviation toward the control group mean (from −2.74 to −2.52), while the scores of fraternal twins regressed 0.86 of a standard deviation (from −2.65 to −1.79). With continued study, DeFries and his colleagues have concluded that there is definitive evidence for a genetic etiology of reading disability, with inherited factors accounting for approximately 50% of the observed deficit in reading-disabled twins.

Segregation Analysis Studies

In the search for the genetic mechanisms underlying reading disability, two primary strategies have been employed: chromosomal linkage studies and segregation analysis. Working from phenotype (clinical manifestation of disability) to genotype (underlying genetic substrate of disability), segregation analysis involves testing all members of affected families for the presence of a reading disorder and then fitting the data to potential models of genetic transmission (e.g., autosomal dominant, autosomal recessive, codominant, or polygenic models). Pennington et al. (1991), after performing segregation analysis on four subject samples, found support for a major-gene model, in which dyslexia in some families is transmitted by one or more dominant or partially dominant genes. They also found support for genetic heterogeneity (i.e., multiple genetic mechanisms in the transmission of dyslexia). Further research with more sophisticated segregation analysis has also pointed toward a major-dominant-gene effect, which occurs frequently (57% of the population) and which, when present, increases an individual's liability for reading problems (Gilger, Vorecki, DeFries, & Pennington, 1994). However, this putative gene is of low penetrance, such that only 3% of individuals having one or two copies of the defective allele demonstrated reading deficits greater than 1.96 standard deviations below the population mean. Nonaffected individuals (43% of the population) with two normal alleles and no copies of the defective allele had an extremely low probability ($p = .0027$) of being classified as reading-disabled.

Linkage Analysis Studies

Working from genotype to phenotype, linkage studies have been conducted to identify the specific chromosomes and the genetic loci on those chromosomes that are associated with dyslexia. Through cytogenic studies of families in which there are a number of persons identified as dyslexic, the search for a gene or genes that may cause dyslexia can be narrowed. Smith, Pennington, Kimberling, and Ing (1990) and DeFries and Gillis (1993) have summarized the complex principles of linkage analysis, which involve investigating both the link between marker genes and the disability gene on a chromosome and the link between that chromosome and the phenotypic occurrence of reading disability.

The pioneering linkage study of Smith, Kimberling, Pennington and Lubs (1983) found evidence in some families for a link between reading disability and a marker on chromosome 15p. A later study with a larger number of subjects provided additional support for this finding (Smith et al., 1990) and further suggested that the apparent linkage was present in approximately 15–20% of families with multiple cases of reading disability.

A second possible genetic locus for reading disability in families was suggested by the observation of the co-occurrence of dyslexia and disorders of the immune system, which are coded to the human leukocyte antigen (HLA) region of chromosome 6. Subsequent research to test this hypothesis (Cardon et al., 1994) studied linkage in two independent samples, 126 sibling pairs and 50 fraternal twin pairs, in which at least one member of each pair was reading-disabled. Analyses of the reading performance of subject pairs genotyped for DNA markers localized the reading disability trait to a small region within the HLA complex of chromosome 6p.

A high incidence of reading disability is found in individuals with abnormalities in sex chromosome karyotypes; the most common of these is the 47,XXY karyotype in males (Klinefelter syndrome), occurring in approximately 1 in 700 to 1 in 1,000 births (Berkow & Fletcher, 1992; Pennington, Bender, Puck, Salbenblatt, & Robinson, 1982). Although such abnormalities are not frequent occurrences in the LD population, the strong association between some sex chromosome anomalies and reading disorders provides additional evidence for the genetic heterogeneity of reading disability.

There is evidence that reading disability per se is not inherited, but that genetic variations influence specific subskills connected to the reading process. Olson, Wise, Conners,

Rack, and Fulker (1989) found significant heritability for a phonological coding task, but not for an orthographic coding task. Pauls (1996) reported genetic linkage studies of dyslexic subjects and their family members, in which subjects were assigned to one of four research groups according to the primary deficient process evident in their reading difficulty: phonological segmentation, nonword reading, rapid naming, and single-word identification. Similar to previous findings, phonological segmentation showed linkage to the HLA region of chromosome 6. There was no evidence for a connection between word identification and chromosome 6; however, there was some evidence that the single-word identification phenotype was tied to a variation in the same portion of chromosome 15 that was first implicated by Smith et al. (1983).

Summary

In summary, family studies, concordance studies of twins, and multiple-regression studies of twins have shown that reading disabilities run in families, that they are heritable, and that the heritable component is approximately 50%. Presently, segregation analyses point to genetic transmission via the effect of a partially dominant or dominant major gene. Genetic linkage studies have provided strong evidence that in some families and subject populations studied, reading disability is linked to chromosome 6p or chromosome 15p. Both segregation analyses and linkage analyses have led to the conclusion that phenotypic reading disability is genotypically heterogeneous; that is, increased susceptibility to reading disability can be produced by multiple genetic profiles. Furthermore, preliminary evidence suggests that within a single individual, the component processes of reading may be influenced by separate genes at different loci.

SUBTYPES

Although public agencies have primarily chosen to define LD on the basis of a discrepancy between achievement and IQ-based estimates of potential achievement, this statistical definition does little to facilitate an understanding of the underlying processes that contribute to successful—and, in this case, unsuccessful—achievement. Although it has been suggested that LDs are broad, nonspecific symptoms for which causes must be identified, it has yet to be demonstrated that different causes lead to different types of LD or require different treatments.

The work of Boder (1973) and Bakker (1979) exemplifies efforts to identify and classify LDs on the basis of educational criteria. Boder (1973) described three subtypes of children with reading disabilities: (1) a "dysphonetic" group, lacking word analysis skills and having difficulty with phonetics; (2) a "dyseidetic" group, experiencing impairment in visual memory and discrimination; and (3) a mixed "dysphonetic–dyseidetic" group. The dysphonetic group included two-thirds of those identified as reading-disabled with the dyseidetic group constituting approximately 10%. Bakker (1979) described "L-type" and "P-type" dyslexias. Children with L-type dyslexia read quickly but made errors of omission, addition, and word mutilation. The P-type group tended to work slowly and to make time-consuming errors involving fragmentations and repetitions.

Among the interesting and promising attempts to define LD are studies involving multivariate analysis. These efforts to subgroup LDs find that differences between good and poor readers may reflect impairment in minor skills, such as oral word rhyming, vocabulary, discrimination of reversed figures, speed of perception for visual forms, and sequential processing (Doehring, 1968). In 1979, Petrauskas and Rourke utilized a factor-analytic method to describe the difficulties of a group of deficient readers. They found that those problems fell statistically into four subtypes: (1) primarily verbal problems; (2) primarily visual problems; (3) difficulty with conceptual flexibility and linguistic skills; and (4) no identified specific weakness. The first two groups correspond with the dysphonetic and dyseidetic groups in Boder's analysis. The third may reflect weaker intellectual skills, while the fourth may in fact confirm the long-standing clinical perception that certain children experience achievement problems that may be secondary to non-neurological factors (e.g., emotional disorder).

Mattis, French, and Rapin (1975) identified three distinct subgroups of children with LD, based upon a factor analysis. These included (1) children struggling to read as the result of language problems; (2) children with articulation and graphomotor problems affecting academic achievement; and (3) children with visual–spatial or perceptual disorder. The third group displayed better verbal than nonverbal intellectual abilities. Almost 80% of the impaired children fell into the first two groups. Denckla (1972, 1977) reported similar statistics, noting that approximately 16% of LD children experienced some type of visual–spatial or perceptual motor problem.

Thus there is a strong tendency among factor-analytic studies to find a large group of children with problems related to verbal weaknesses and a smaller but significant group with problems related to visual–perceptual weaknesses. Joschko and Rourke (1985), in an analysis of scores on the Wechsler Intelligence Scale for Children, found a clear distinction between children with learning problems stemming from verbal weaknesses and those whose problems stemmed from nonverbal weaknesses.

Satz and Morris (1981) found five distinct groups of reading-disabled children, that again fell along this verbal–nonverbal continuum. These included (1) those with language impairment; (2) those with specific language problems related to naming; (3) those with mixed global language and perceptual problems; (4) those with perceptual–motor impairment only; and (5) a group similar to that reported by Petrauskas and Rourke (1979) in which no significant impairments were identified. Some researchers have hypothesized that this last group of children simply has not experienced adequate education to develop essential achievement skills, while others, as noted earlier, suggest an emotional basis for this group's problems. Using cluster analysis of a neuropsychological battery, Phillips (1983) identified a fairly similar profile of five LD subtypes, including groups with a pattern of normal test scores, auditory processing problems, difficulty with receptive and expressive language, spatial weaknesses, or a global pattern of low test scores.

Rourke (1978) concluded that cluster-analytic studies have identified some association between learning delay and a wide variety of perceptual, linguistic, sequential, and cognitive skills. This finding is reinforced by the work of others over nearly a 40-year period (Benton, 1975). According to Swartz (1974), a pattern consisting of depressed scores on four Wechsler subtests, the "ACID" pattern (ACID is an acronym for Arithmetic, Coding, Information, and Digit Span) characterizes the weaknesses of most LD children. Although this view is held by many others and has been most recently advanced by Kaufman (1997), not all LD children display this pattern. Children who do, however, are thought to have a particularly poor prognosis for academic performance in reading, spelling, and arithmetic (Ackerman, Dykman, & Peters, 1977). Some researchers have suggested that in a population of LD children demonstrating this pattern, one subgroup experiences particularly poor auditory–verbal memory and sequencing, while a second group experiences poor visual–spatial abilities. This distinction is similar to that described by Joschko and Rourke (1985). However, Joschko and Rourke reported a further distinction in the ACID pattern by age between a younger group (5 to 8 years old) and an older group (9 to 15 years old). On the basis of an extensive neuropsychological battery, these authors found a distinct pattern of differences resulting in four subtypes (see Table 6.1). Joschko and Rourke (1985) noted that "although the ACID subtypes generated in this research do not differ significantly in terms of level of academic performance, the plots of the factor score profiles for each of the reliable subtypes indicate that they have qualitatively different ability profiles which may have practical applications" (p. 77). However, these authors noted that effective remediation has not been clearly tied to this manner of ability profiling.

The inclusion of LD among the disorders evaluated and diagnosed by the medical and mental health community has been considered an adjunct to formal psychiatric, psychological, or neuropsychological evaluation. However, as it has been recognized that LD children appear more likely than others to develop psychiatric problems, efforts have been made to refine the clinical diagnosis of learning impairments. The *Diagnostic and Statistical Manual of Mental Disorders*, fourth edition (DSM-IV; American Psychiatric Association, 1994) lists four academic skill disorders: reading disorder, mathematics disorder, disorder of written expression, and learning disorder not otherwise specified. All four diagnoses require the collection of standardized test data that indicate performance substantially below what would be expected from the individual's age, intelligence, and educational experience. According to these loosely definitive criteria, the problem must interfere with the child's academic performance or activities of daily living. The "not otherwise specified" category is intended for LDs as isolated weaknesses—for example, difficulty with spelling independent of other written language problems. The DSM-IV also contains a diagnosis of developmental coordination disorder, reflecting weak gross or fine motor skills that may interfere with academic achievement or daily living but are not due to a specific medical condition. The NLD subtype, which is not directly included as a category of learning disorder in DSM-IV, will be discussed in later sections of this chapter. Readers interested in an extensive discussion of subtypes of LD in childhood are referred to Silver and Hagin (1990).

A NEUROPSYCHOLOGICAL MODEL FOR ASSESSMENT

From the neuropsychologist's perspective, a practical or functional conceptualization of LD is of critical importance. It is the neuropsychologist's job to evaluate and transmit information to educators, vocational counselors, family members, and the affected individual in a manner that will facilitate practical understanding, increase motivation, and lead directly to intervention. Table 6.2 lists problems related to the basic skills necessary for suc-

TABLE 6.1. Performance Characteristics of Reliable ACID Subtypes

Neuropsychological measures	ACID subtypes			
	Younger subtype 2	Younger subtype 4	Older subtype 1	Older subtype 3
Tactile perceptual	Poor	Average	Average	Poor
Visual perceptual	Poor	Average	Average	Average
Auditory perceptual and language-related	Poor	Poor	Poor	Poor
Sequencing	Average	Poor	Poor	Average
Concept formation and reasoning	Average	Average	Average	Average
Motor	Poor	Average	Average	Poor
Academic	Poor	Poor	Poor	Poor

Note. "Poor" indicates a tendency for poorer test performances in comparison to the norms for the test. "Average" indicates test performance generally within one standard deviation of the normative mean. From Joschko and Rourke (1985). Copyright 1985 by The Guilford Press. Reprinted by permission.

TABLE 6.2. Problems Related to Basic Skills Necessary for Successful Academic Achievement

Skill	Problem
Reading	
Appreciation of language sounds	Language sounds don't seem very clear or distinct.
Remembering sound–symbol association	The sounds of combinations of letters are difficult to remember.
Holding together the sounds in a word	The sounds of letters are known, but it's difficult to put together the sounds in the right order to make the words during reading.
Reading fast enough	It takes too long to pronounce or understand each word.
Understanding sentences	The vocabulary or grammar is too difficult.
Understanding paragraphs or passages	It's difficult to find the main ideas and the important details, or it's difficult to understand the concepts, ideas, or facts.
Remembering while reading	Ideas don't stay in memory during reading.
Summarizing what was read	It's too difficult to decide and remember what's important, and to organize important ideas in one's own words and sentences.
Applying what was read	It's difficult to use what was read.
Enjoying reading	Reading is too much work; it's not automatic.
Spelling	
Remembering letters and sounds	It's difficult to remember that a certain combination of letters stands for a certain language sound. It's difficult to understand how sounds are different from each other.
Picturing words	It's difficult to remember how words look.
Spelling longer words	It's difficult to recall and sequence the sounds of multisyllable words.
Understanding spelling rules	It's difficult to understand what combination of letters is allowed. It is also difficult to understand the vowel rules.
Spelling words consistently each time	It's difficult to concentrate on little details.
Writing and spelling at the same time	It's difficult to write and spell at the same time. It's difficult to remember how to spell when writing words in sentences or paragraphs.
Making mixed spelling errors	It's difficult to distinguish word sounds, remember the rules, and picture words.
Writing	
Fine motor coordination	It's difficult to keep track of just where the pencil is while writing. It's difficult getting the right muscles to work together quickly and easily. It's difficult getting finger muscles in touch with memory through many different nerve connections between the hand and the brain. It's difficult getting eyes and fingers to work together.
Remembering and writing at the same time (mechanics)	It's difficult to remember punctuation, spelling, capitalization, grammar, vocabulary, letter formation, and ideas all at the same time.
Thinking about ideas and writing at the same time	It's difficult to think fast about ideas at the same time one is writing.
Planning and organizing	It's difficult thinking up something to write about or understanding what the teacher expects; deciding who will read the writing; thinking up many good ideas and writing them down; taking all the ideas and putting together the ones that belong together; knowing what ideas to put first and what ones to put second; getting rid of ideas that don't fit; making sure that things make sense; and reorganizing what has been written.

(cont.)

TABLE 6.2. (cont.)

Skill	Problem
Knowing how to translate ideas into language on paper	It's difficult to get ideas into good language when writing.

Math

Grasping the concepts	It's difficult to understand concepts that include things such as number, place value, percentage, decimals, and equations.
Remembering mathematics	Mathematics is a big memory strain. It's difficult to remember mathematical facts quickly, or to remember everything that has to be done. When one part of a math problem is finished, it's difficult to remember what to do next.
Understanding the language of mathematics	There is a lot of language (e.g., labels) in a math class, which makes it difficult keeping up with what the teacher is saying and understanding certain assignments.
Using problem-solving skills	It's difficult to think up the best way (or ways) to come up with a correct answer. It's difficult to take time to think about a solution.
Visualizing	It's difficult to see what one is able to describe in words. It's tricky to understand some concepts unless they can be put into clear pictures or images.
Remembering things in the right order	It's difficult to put things, do things, or keep things in the correct order. It's difficult to do the right steps in the right order to get the right answer.
Paying attention to detail	It's difficult to be alert and tuned in to the many little details in mathematics.
Recognizing or admitting a lack of understanding	It's difficult to recognize or admit that one does not understand or remember basic concepts in order to get the necessary help to understand new ones.

Note. Adapted from Levine (1990). Copyright 1990 by Melvin D. Levine, M.D. Educators Publishing Service, Inc. Cambridge, MA. Adapted by permission.

cessful academic achievement, beginning with the simplest and building to the more complex. These skills are hypothesized to be essential to the development of basic reading, spelling, writing, and mathematical abilities. This conceptualization is adapted from and based upon the work of developmental pediatrician Mel Levine (1990).

The consensus in current factor-analytic research is that there are two broad groups of skills necessary for efficient learning:

1. *Auditory–verbal processes.* Weaknesses in these areas result in reading disorders and other language-based learning problems.
2. *Visual–motor and perceptual processes.* Weaknesses in these areas may result in reading problems but are more likely to affect handwriting, mathematics, and certain social skills.

Tables 6.3 and 6.4 present a model for conceptualizing these skills according to rote/automatic versus conceptual levels and linguistic versus visual modalities. Table 6.3 groups categories of academic skills according to this conceptualization in a 2 × 2 grid; Table 6.4 groups specific academic and daily living skills in a similar grid.

As it has also been demonstrated that there is a significant but small group of children experiencing academic achievement problems in the absence of weaknesses in either of these sets of skills, neuropsychologists are also urged to consider the impact of other factors related to achievement: an environment conducive to learning, problems with attention and impulse control, self-concept as a learner, and other emotional (e.g., depression/anxiety) and behavioral (oppositional defiant disorder, conduct disorder) problems (Goldstein & Mather, 1998).

As Tables 6.3 and 6.4 suggest, language-based LDs are directly related to impairments in a variety of language skills, especially those related to phonological processes (Pennington, 1991). For many children, poor higher-order listening and reading comprehension results from poor lower-order rote language skills such as inability to discriminate similar sounds. Poor auditory discrimination also leads to weak phonetic decoding skills for reading. In addition, problems with verbal short-term memory are common among reading-impaired individuals. One reason is that memory requires phonological skill. Poor readers may experience problems automatically recalling letters, digits, words, or phrases individually or in exact sequence. It is also not surprising that related language-based skills such as spelling and writing are impaired in reading-disabled children. For many, spelling is even more impaired than reading (Snowling & Hulme, 1991). The majority of children with language-based LDs struggle to master basic foundational academic skills; others are capable of learning to read, but when the curriculum begins to accelerate in third or fourth grade and they must read to learn, they struggle as the result of weak conceptual linguistic skills.

Weaknesses in visual–motor skills tend to cause problems with arithmetic and handwriting, often independent of associated reading disability. Included in problems for this group of children are difficulties involving social awareness and judgment. These problems do not appear to be primarily language-based and have been referred to collectively in the neuropsychology literature as "nonverbal LD" (NLD) (Pennington, 1991; Rourke, 1989). Children with NLD have been reported to experience problems with spatial organization, attention to visual detail, and procedural skills; mathematics; problems in shifting psychological set from one operation to another; graphomotor weaknesses; poor factual memory; and poor judgment and reasoning (Rourke, 1985). It can reliably be concluded that children with NLD experience greatest deficits in visual perceptual and organizational skills, psychomotor coordination, and complex tactile perceptual abilities (Harnadek & Rourke, 1994). Finally, it is also suspected that individuals with NLD experience greater internalizing problems related to depression and anxiety than those with language-based LDs. It is unclear whether this pattern contributes to or is a consequence of NLD.

TABLE 6.3. A Model for Conceptualizing Categories of Academic Skills

Auditory–verbal	Visual–motor
Conceptual	
Verbal conceptual skills	Visual, nonverbal conceptual skills
Rote/automatic	
Auditory perception	Visual perception of symbols
Rote associational memory and retrieval	Spatial organization and nonverbal integration
Rote auditory-sequential memory	Rote visual-sequential memory and retrieval
Auditory-oral motor skills	Motor sequencing and fine motor control

Note. Adapted from table prepared by Sally Ingalls. Copyright 1991 by the Neurology, Learning and Behavior Center, Salt Lake City, Utah. Adapted by permission.

TABLE 6.4. A Model for Conceptualizing Specific Academic and Daily Living Skills

Auditory–verbal	Visual–motor
Conceptual	
Language semantics: Usual word meanings, formal definitions, antonyms, synonyms Listening comprehension: Understanding and memory of overall ideas Specificity and variety of verbal concepts for oral or written expression Verbal reasoning, logic, and problem solving	Social insight and reasoning: Understanding strategies of games, jokes, motives of others, social conventions, tact Mathematical concepts: Use of 0 in +, −, ×; place value; money equivalencies; missing elements; etc. Inferential reading comprehension: Getting the main idea, drawing conclusions Understanding relationship of historical events across time; understanding scientific concepts Structuring ideas hierarchically; outlining skills Generalization abilities Integrating material into a well-organized report
Rote/automatic	
Early speech; naming objects Auditory processing; clear enunciation of speech; pronouncing sounds or syllables in correct order Naming colors Recalling birthdate, phone number, address, etc. Saying alphabet and other lists (days, months) in order; remembering two to four-part directions Easily selecting and sequencing words with proper grammatical structure for oral or written expression Discriminating sounds, especially vowels, auditorily; blending sounds to words; distinguishing words that sound alike (e.g., mine/mind) Labeling and retrieval of letters, sounds, common syllables, sight words (b/d, her/here) Phonic spelling: Hearing the sounds in words Listening and reading comprehension involving short-term memory, especially for rote facts Mathematical labeling and retrieval: Counting sequentially, labeling numbers (e.g., 16/60), memory for +, −, ×, and ÷ facts and sequences of steps for computation (e.g., long division) Recalling names, dates, and historical facts Learning and retaining scientific terminology	Assembling puzzles and building with construction toys Social perception and awareness of environment Time sense: Doesn't ask, "Is this the last recess?" Remembering and executing correct sequence for tying shoes Easily negotiating stairs, climbing on play equipment, learning athletic skills, riding bike Executing daily living skills such as pouring without spilling, spreading a sandwich, dressing self correctly Using the correct sequence of strokes to form manuscript or cursive letters Eye–hand coordination for drawing, assembling art projects, and handwriting Directional stability for top–bottom and left–right tracking Copying from board accurately Viewing visual symbols accurately, visual discrimination, directionality, recognizing shape or form of words Spelling: Visual memory for the nonphonetic elements of words

Note. Adapted from table prepared by Sally Ingalls. Copyright 1991 by Neurology, Learning and Behavior Center, Salt Lake City, Utah. Adapted by permission.

ASSESSMENT IN THE CONTEXT OF A COMPREHENSIVE NEUROPSYCHOLOGICAL EVALUATION

A number of volumes provide thorough, in-depth models for neuropsychological assessment utilizing a myriad of tests and batteries. Interested readers are referred to Reynolds and Fletcher-Janzen (1997) and Goldstein (1997). The basic task facing the neuropsychologist is to answer questions concerning underlying neuropsychological skills essential to learning; both assets and liabilities must be identified. Screening of basic academic skills must also be completed. Due to space limitations, this section briefly reviews only the assessment of academic achievement.

In many situations, the neuropsychologist can rely upon data collected at school to provide basic achievement measures. The most widely used instrument, the Woodcock–Johnson Psycho-Educational Battery—Revised (Woodcock & Johnson, 1989), has recently been updated and will soon be published in a third edition. It offers by far the most thorough, well-developed assessment of academic skills. The Woodcock–Johnson is based on a factor-analytic model that fits well with the concepts presented in this chapter concerning the underlying neuropsychological deficits contributing to LDs. Subtest analysis often reveals patterns consistent with verbal, visual, rote, or conceptual weaknesses. A significant or severe intelligence/achievement discrepancy is the most widely used criterion for identifying LD. Although the issue of identifying high-IQ individuals with average achievement as LD continues to be controversial (Gordon & Keiser, 1998), this practice was recently affirmed by the United States Court of Appeals for the Second Circuit in the case of *Bartlett v. New York State Board of Law Examiners* (Hagin, 1998).

In the absence of a comprehensive battery such as the Woodcock, it is recommended that neuropsychologists address the collection of basic achievement data as follows:

1. *Reading.* A measure should be used to assess single-word reading, reflecting phonetic skills, and sight-word achievement. An estimate of the ability to read within context and comprehend what is read should also be obtained. Achievement tests such as the Woodcock Reading Mastery Test—Revised (Woodcock, 1987), the Gilmore Oral Reading Test (Gilmore & Gilmore, 1968), the Gray Oral Reading Test, third edition (Wiederholt & Bryant, 1992), or the Test of Reading Comprehension, third edition (Brown, Hammill, & Wiederholt, 1995) can provide clinicians with these data.

2. *Spelling.* Estimates of sight-word memory for spelling and phonetic spelling ability can be analyzed qualitatively utilizing the Wide Range Achievement Test—3 (Wilkinson, 1993) or the Test of Written Spelling, fourth edition (Larsen & Hammill, 1999).

3. *Mathematics.* The Wide Range Achievement Test—3 (Wilkinson, 1993) or the KeyMath Revised (Connoloy, 1988) can be utilized to generate observations of math concepts versus rote sequencing and rote memory mathematical skills.

4. *Written language.* Written language skills of vocabulary, thematic maturity, capacity to organize ideas, grammar, punctuation, and general execution can be assessed with the story writing task from the Test of Written Language—3 (Hammill & Larsen, 1996).

INTERVENTIONS

Since views differ regarding the nature and etiology of LD, views also differ about what constitutes appropriate and effective interventions for individuals with LD. Lyon and Moats (1988) have discussed critical issues in the instruction of LD students. Numerous authors, representing different theoretical orientations and instructional paradigms, have presented intervention methodologies developed or adapted for disabled learners. These include the psycholinguistic-process or specific-abilities approach (Johnson & Myklebust, 1967; Kirk & Kirk, 1971); behavioral approaches, including direct instruction and data-based instruction (Haring & Gentry, 1976; Lovitt, 1984; Marston & Tindal, 1995; White, 1986); cognitive approaches, including constructivism and instruction in learning strategies (Butler, 1998; Deshler & Lenz, 1989; Harris & Graham, 1994; Swanson, 1993); and neuropsychological approaches (Rourke, Fisk, & Strang, 1986; Hooper, Willis, & Stone, 1996). Mercer

(1991) and Lerner (1993) have provided lucid discussions of these instructional approaches and their application to individuals with LD. Mercer and Mercer (1993), Mather (1991), Mather and Jaffe (1992), and Lerner (1993) outline a broad array of specific teaching strategies and techniques that have been utilized successfully with atypical learners, including those with LD.

Aptitude × Treatment Interaction

As the field of LD developed, the process of individualizing instruction led to treatment approaches that emphasized aptitude × treatment interaction (ATI). ATI attempts to match different learning strengths and weaknesses to particular instructional methods. ATI theory suggests that matching treatment to LD diagnosis or subtype will produce improved outcomes (Hooper et al., 1996; Reschly & Ysseldyke, 1995). After intense and empirical scrutiny, many applications of ATI to LDs—particularly those involving training of psycholinguistic processes in isolation, and instruction based on auditory or visual modality preference—have been discredited (Hammill & Larsen, 1974; Ysseldyke & Mirkin, 1982). However, a number of researchers and practitioners in the LD field hold out the possibility that as the sophistication and specificity of LD theory and research methodology increase, ATI approaches will yet be validated for different subtypes of LD (Doris, 1993; Lyon, 1996b; Mather & Roberts, 1994; Torgesen, 1986). In discussing progress in the field of LD, Doris (1993) stated that "one wonders if the real progress will not come from disentangling groups of children from this huge conglomerate mass, rigorously specifying the nature of their difficulties, and systematically exploring appropriate educational intervention for these subgroups" (p. 112). Lyon (1996b) has suggested abandoning the general term "LD," and, along with Doris, favors specifying each type of LD individually according to definition, etiology, developmental course, identification, procedures, and treatment.

Much recent research is leading to better development of causal theories of LDs and to promising avenues of intervention for the LD subtypes or the specific information-processing weaknesses explicated by those theories. According to Torgesen (1993), "The two most completely developed current causal theories of learning disabilities are the nonverbal learning disabilities syndrome . . . and the theory of reading disabilities involving limitations in phonological processing" (p. 158).

As described earlier in this chapter, individuals with NLD have difficulty perceiving and organizing the nonverbal aspects of the physical and social environment, leading not only to academic problems (primarily in math and abstract comprehension) but also to social interaction difficulties and performance problems in activities of daily living. Since NLDs differ qualitatively from verbal LDs in the extent to which they affect total environmental adaptation, they require different intervention strategies—often strategies that are broader in scope, addressing functional skills in educational, home, and community settings. Rourke and colleagues have studied and are gradually refining an overall approach to habilitation for persons with NLD (Rourke, 1989; Rourke & Del Dotto, 1994; Strang & Rourke, 1985). Thompson (1997) provided a description of NLD from a developmental perspective and discussed appropriate intervention strategies for NLD individuals of all ages. At present, due to the complexity of outcome research with this LD subtype, the intervention approach for NLD is based on logic and longitudinal observation rather than on empirical validation.

A great deal of attention and research has been directed toward understanding phonological processing skills and their relation to the development of reading skills (Lyon,

1996b; Pennington, 1991; Shaywitz, 1996; Stanovich, 1993; Stanovich & Siegel, 1994; Torgesen, Wagner, & Rashotte, 1994; Wagner & Torgesen, 1987). A number of well-designed longitudinal studies have documented the efficacy of instruction in phonological awareness and/or phonemic analysis and synthesis for the initial development of reading skills and for improving reading in reading-deficient children (Ball & Blachman, 1988; Blachman, Ball, Black, & Tangel, 1994, cited in Lyon, 1996b; Hatcher, Hulme, & Ellis, 1994; Lundberg, Frost, & Petersen, 1988).

At the conclusion of their research report, Hatcher et al. (1994) suggested that children differ in their ability to acquire phonological competence, and they posed the question of how to facilitate acquisition of underlying phonological skills. In this critical area of instruction, research-based practices are emerging. In a recent contribution, Torgesen, Wagner, and Rashotte (1997) discuss approaches to the prevention and remediation of phonologically based reading disabilities. Research with the Auditory Discrimination in Depth program (Lindamood & Lindamood, 1969) has shown that intensive instruction led to significant gains in reading and spelling skills for 281 subjects aged 5 to 55 years (Truch, 1994). Employing a new and promising approach, Merzenich et al. (1996) acoustically modified speech to train sound discrimination abilities in children with language-based learning impairments. Subjects engaged in highly motivating discrimination tasks with speech stimuli altered by a computer algorithm, which stretched the duration or increased the volume of sound elements critical to the discrimination process. After a few weeks' instruction, children in the study markedly improved their ability to discriminate phonemes and to recognize both brief and fast sequences of speech stimuli. They also showed significant improvement in language comprehension abilities. Although accustically modified speech is a logically conceived and exciting intervention concept, experts in the field of dyslexia and LD, as reported by Travis (1996), suggest caution in regard to its potential benefits until further research data confirm its effectiveness with specific populations.

Just as well-designed research can validate intervention practices and techniques for LDs, it can also identify methods that are contraindicated for many LD students. In special education and in education as a whole, there continues a great debate about the relative merits of code-oriented versus whole-language approaches to reading instruction (Foorman, 1995). From the available research, most professionals in the field of LD have concluded that when used as the primary mode of instruction, the whole-language method is less effective than structured, explicit instruction in phonics for children with reading disabilities (Iverson & Tunmer, 1993; Liberman & Liberman, 1992; Pressley & Rankin, 1994; Shapiro, 1992; Stanovich, 1994; Torgesen et al., 1994).

A Functional Paradigm for Intervention: Factors to Consider

While efforts are intensifying to elucidate interventions for LDs based on adequate theory, subtype analysis, and research-validated practices, an empirical approach to treatment planning is still far from a reality. Practitioners must use the available research, their own experience, and informed clinical judgment to develop appropriate, practical intervention plans for individuals with LD. To guide present practice, aspects of the various theory-based paradigms for LD intervention can be combined into a functional, multidimensional, eclectic, and interactional treatment paradigm (Mercer, 1991). Consistent with such a functional paradigm, we outline a variety of factors to be considered and selectively incorporated into comprehensive LD intervention plans:

1. Multifaceted assessment is the essential first step for determining the direction and necessary components of an intervention plan. However, even the most thorough and careful assessment cannot guarantee the success of any specific intervention (Accardo, 1996).

2. A practitioner needs to weigh potential contributions from all available resources: the individual with an LD, the family, regular educators, special educators, private providers, and the community (Rourke & Del Dotto, 1994).

3. Both short-term and long-term goals should be specified and prioritized into a balanced and pragmatic intervention plan. As a treatment plan is formulated, the practitioner must consider the needs of the whole person by providing time for home and family, friendship development, leisure and recreation, and so forth (Accardo, 1996).

4. Although numerous goals may each be highly desirable, only a certain amount can be accomplished within the constraints of time and resources. The practitioner should focus on a limited number of goals with sufficient intensity to produce stable progress, rather than broadening intervention efforts to such an extent that they become fragmented and ineffective (Ellis & Friend, 1991). Over the long term, various important goals can be addressed in a timely and sequential manner. "The key to successful intervention is intensity and duration" (Cannon, 1997, p. 7).

5. Educational intervention with a strong emphasis on academic development is the primary form of treatment for most types of LD. The practitioner should select instructional goals and methodologies after interfacing a task analysis of the learner's strengths and weaknesses, including miscue analysis, with an in-depth task analysis of the skills to be taught/learned (Lerner, 1993). One-to-one clinical teaching/tutoring is usually the most effective form of instruction, with small-group instruction of students with similar needs an acceptable alternative (Cannon, 1997).

6. Specific information-processing skills need to be developed in the context of relevant curriculum and adaptive tasks, or subportions of tasks, not in isolation (Mercer, 1991).

7. As each individual's needs dictate, the practitioner should provide instruction for acquisition of lower-order rote or mechanical basic skills, and opportunities/strategies for developing higher-order concepts, comprehension, problem solving, and creative expression.

8. Varied forms of repetition should be used to teach selected items or a limited amount of curriculum material to an independent mastery level. Frequent review and reinforcement are needed to maintain skills. If important skills deteriorate or are lost, they should be relearned (Ellis & Friend, 1991).

9. The learner's innate cognitive strategies for acquiring and retaining information must be observed. As needed, the practitioner should teach specific strategies, including perceptual aids, mnemonic devices, study skills, metacognitive strategies, and compensatory strategies. Creative techniques and product modifications may be needed to assist individual students with specific problems or idiosyncratic disability characteristics.

10. The practitioner should explore the appropriateness and availability of technology, including computers and other assistive devices for enhancing instruction, guided practice, compensation, and so on (Anderson-Inman, Knox-Quinn, & Horney, 1996; Day & Edwards, 1996; Gay, 1996; Raskind, 1993; Welch & Jensen, 1990; Wissick, 1996).

11. Ecological and motivational factors, and their implications for all aspects of the treatment plan, need to be taken into consideration. Examples of such factors include instructor–student relationship, joint goal setting, structure and pacing of learning materials and activities, maintenance of high levels of on-task behavior and accurate task comple-

tion, performance feedback to students, external reinforcement, peer/social support, and the like (Brophy & Good, 1986; Christenson, Ysseldyke, & Thurlow, 1989).

12. The teaching/learning process should be approached both diagnostically (Johnson & Myklebust, 1967) and empirically (Marston & Tindal, 1995). That is, the practitioner should test, instruct, observe, retest, modify instruction, and repeat the process as necessary. With frequent tracking and charting of student performance, the nature and impact of specific LD characteristics will become clearer, and instructional approaches and procedures can be modified to maximize progress.

13. Since most individuals resist displaying incompetence for or receiving correction from their significant others, remedial instruction is best provided by expert teachers rather than by parents or family members (Pennington, 1991). Along with other contributions, parents can assist with instruction by helping students complete homework assignments that call for repetition or review, rather than by providing initial teaching (Mercer, 1991).

14. Additional evaluation and related services (central auditory processing assessment, speech and language therapy, occupational therapy, etc.) should be obtained as warranted. For many individuals with auditory–verbal LDs, speech and language therapy is an essential component of an appropriate treatment plan.

15. Any comorbid conditions (e.g., ADHD, other psychological or psychiatric disorders, social skill deficits, etc.) must be evaluated and addressed. For individuals with NLD, social deficits usually constitute an integral part of this disability; therefore, social skill development must be an integral part of the treatment plan.

16. A practitioner needs to be very cautious about encouraging parents in their pursuit of specialized or alternative treatments (e.g., sensory–motor integration training, ocular pursuit training, Irlen lenses, neurolinguistic programming, etc.). An alternative intervention should be endorsed only when the intervention would appear to be related to a particular student's core deficit and there is some likelihood of benefit. Families should be provided with information to help them avoid dubious and unproven treatments (Ingersoll & Goldstein, 1993; Silver, 1975, 1995; Worrall, 1990).

17. Over time, the individual with an LD and his or her family members should be helped to understand the specific nature of the disability in terms of learning strengths, weaknesses, and needs, so that they can comprehend the treatment program and become effective advocates in obtaining necessary services (Brinckerhoff, 1996; Roffman, Herzog, & Wershba-Gershon, 1994; Young, 1996).

18. The practitioner needs to remain informed about scientific advances in the field of LD. Intervention plans should be revamped and refined as research validates specific approaches and methodologies for treating different LD subtypes (Mercer, 1991).

In the context of current educational trends, which emphasize inclusion or mainstreaming and constructivist teaching methods (including the whole-language approach to reading), there is a tendency to view LDs as mild disabilities that can be dealt with through curricular accommodations in a regular classroom. Instead, LDs must be understood as complex phenomena, ranging from mild to severe, and it must be acknowledged that even mild LDs can have a devastating impact on the academic, emotional, and general life adjustment of affected individuals. Assessment and intervention are most effective when a person with an LD, committed family members, and highly trained professionals select from a full complement of methodologies and services to design and implement an intervention plan that is in the best interest of that individual. Common sense suggests and research is showing that severe LDs respond more slowly to treatment and require more intensive and lengthy interventions than milder LDs (Lyon, 1996b). In addition, LDs often persist and must be confronted and dealt with throughout life.

LD THROUGH THE LIFESPAN

Both clinical observation and research confirm that neurologically based specific LDs can and do affect individuals of all ages (Gajar, 1992; Mercer, 1991; White, 1992). In a position paper, the national Learning Disability Association (LDA) stated that when validly diagnosed, a specific LD is "a lifelong handicapping condition. . . . While the manifestations of the condition may change over time, the inherent condition persists" (LDA, 1990, p. 2a). Precursors of both verbal LDs and NLDs can be observed in preschoolers, although academic LDs are usually not diagnosed until school age. Diagnostic and intervention services typically peak during the elementary and secondary school years. Adult outcomes for individuals with LD are varied: As LD persists over time, it may influence a widening array of cognitive and interpersonal abilities. For most individuals who receive early and effective intervention, learning skills improve, compensation occurs, and the overt signs of LD decrease. However, the effects of LD usually continue to be experienced throughout elementary and secondary school years and into adulthood.

Preschoolers with LD

The identification of preschoolers with specific LD requires distinguishing them from children who present with a maturational lag or more generalized developmental delay; however, as Lerner (1993) has stated, "Preschool children with learning disabilities can be identified" (p. 250). Suspicion that an LD exists may be aroused by inconsistency in attainment of early developmental milestones, with better development observed in some skill areas than in others. Early speech and language delay and a family history of LD are probably the most significant risk factors for reading disability. A pattern of motor delay, social integration difficulty, and inability to understand and enjoy puzzles and other manipulative toys, in the presence of age-appropriate speech and language development, can be an early indicator of an NLD. Other developmental circumstances and medical conditions that might signal the presence of an LD in a preschool child include specific genetic syndromes, maternal alcohol or drug use, HIV infection, prematurity/low birth weight, cerebral palsy, brain tumor or infection, CNS radiation, seizure disorder, traumatic brain injury, lead poisoning, strabismus, and chronic otitis media ("Medical Diagnoses/Conditions," 1998). The presence of any risk factor for LD does not dictate its occurrence. Many children with early risk factors will not go on to demonstrate LDs, whereas other children without early developmental delays or known risk factors will later be diagnosed as LD.

Due to the variability among and rapid growth of preschoolers, appropriate evaluation is typically a complex process requiring specially trained multidisciplinary examiners; longitudinal assessment; cautious use of nondiscriminatory and technically adequate standardized measures; use of criterion-referenced developmental scales; and systematic observations of a child's skills, temperament, attention, and self-regulation in home, day care/preschool, and community settings. The final criterion for diagnosing LD in a preschooler is clinical judgment based on multidimensional assessment (Pennington, 1991). At younger ages, assessment often results in a noncategorical determination of developmental delay, rather than in a categorical LD classification.

Mercer (1991) reviewed prediction research in early identification, concluding that teacher perception, some single instruments, and some multiple-instrument batteries are acceptable predictors of risk for school failure. He also provided an annotated list of selected screening instruments and tests for identification and program planning for children from birth to age 8. Mercer reported that reliable and valid screening measures can yield a hit rate of 80–90% in identifying at-risk preschoolers and kindergarteners.

Most research studies that have attempted to predict specific LDs have employed subjects in the age range of 5 to 6 years, rather than preschoolers. However, research into reading acquisition is beginning to provide reliable predictors of reading success or failure for younger children. Cannon (1997) reported that syntactic and phonological production at 30 months of age has been shown to predict reading failure at second grade. Early determination of specific LDs or of at-risk status makes possible the provision of early interventions targeted to the specific developmental and learning needs of each identified child. A recent text edited by Blachman (1997) discusses prevention and empirically based early intervention for reading disorders.

P.L. 99-457, the Education of the Handicapped Amendments of 1986 (amending P.L. 94-142), and P.L. 102-19, the Early Childhood Amendments of 1991 (amending P.L. 101-476, IDEA), have set forth federal policies and mandates for special education services to preschoolers. Children aged 3 to 5 years with LD are now extended the same rights and protections under the law that are afforded to older children with LD. In 1991, about 3.5% of children aged 3 through 5 received early intervention services through home-based or center-based programs provided by public schools (USDE, 1991, cited by Lerner, 1993). Since in most states children can qualify for such services under a noncategorical designation of developmental delay, the number of these children with LD is not known. However, many states do use a categorical system, which includes the category of LD, for determining the eligibility of preschoolers to receive services. Federal policy does not permit any state to exclude those with specific LD from the preschool population to be served.

Adolescents with LD

Many adolescents with LD are students *at risk*. Shaywitz and Shaywitz (1994) reported that 75% of students with reading disabilities who are not identified before third grade continue to exhibit reading disabilities, scoring in the lowest quartile in ninth grade. A low level of basic skills places LD students at risk for course failure, which Wagner and Blackorby (1996) identified as one of the strongest predictors associated with becoming a school dropout. Depending on the specific study, 26% to 54% of students with LD drop out of high school compared to 8% to 33% of non-LD students. In 1986–1987, 55% of students identified as LD graduated with a regular diploma compared to a graduation rate of 71% for their nondisabled peers (USDE, 1989, cited in Spector, Decker, & Shaw, 1991). From year to year the graduation rate for LD students hovers at about 50%. Disabled students who do not attain a high school diploma do not fare as well in their postschool years in terms of postsecondary education and economic well-being as those who do (Wagner & Blackorby, 1996).

The academic and social problems encountered by adolescents with LD result from the interaction of their skills and specific disabilities with the multiple demands of their increasingly complex school environment (Ellis & Friend, 1991). Secondary education requires adolescents to demonstrate competence in gaining information from lectures, taking class notes, expressing information in writing, acquiring effective study skills, taking tests, and independently maintaining organizational consistency. These things are to be accomplished under conditions that include a larger physical plant, multiple teachers, complicated schedules, social and emotional turmoil, and less consistent adult monitoring. Although some compensated and resilient LD adolescents require fewer special interventions during junior and senior high school, others require intensive academic and social support, while still others are being diagnosed with LD for the first time. Thus, the heterogeneity among adolescents with LD dictates a continued need for child-find procedures (especially within the juvenile justice and mental health systems), diagnostic services, and a variety of appropriate interventions.

P.L. 101-476, the Individuals with Disabilities Education Act of 1990, requires special education to be made available to all disabled students, including those with LD, until they graduate from high school or until their twenty-second birthday. In addition, Section 504 of the Rehabilitation Act of 1973 (amended under Section 506 of the Rehabilitation Act Amendments of 1992) and the Americans with Disabilities Act of 1990, which are antidiscrimination laws, have provisions requiring that schools that receive any form of federal funds make reasonable accommodations for students with disabilities. LD students who do not qualify for services under IDEA may qualify for a formal classroom accommodation plan under Section 504. To safeguard students' rights, a new provision of P.L. 105-17, the Individuals with Disabilities Education Act Amendments of 1997, requires that by the age of 17, high school special education students receive training in understanding principles of self-advocacy and informed consent so that they are prepared to assume responsibility for their legal rights, which transfer to them at the age of majority.

Mercer (1991) listed five types of program services that should be available to adolescents with LD on an as need basis: (1) academic remediation, (2) supportive help with regular education courses, (3) training in learning strategies, (4) training in functional living skills including social skills, and (5) vocational/career preparation. Since there is usually insufficient time to effectively address all of an LD adolescent's needs, the relative merits of each form of intervention should be carefully considered when making programming decisions. A frequently perplexing conflict is that continued remediation of basic skills (or in some recently diagnosed cases, even initial remediation) competes for time with providing supportive help with regular courses so that students can fulfill graduation requirements. Ellis and Friend (1991) suggested guidelines to consider when attempting to resolve this dilemma. Intensive instruction in organizational and cognitive learning strategies, which has been shown to be an effective intervention for adolescents with LD, has been described by Deshler and Lenz (1989), Mercer (1991), and Spector et al. (1991). LD students who are not college-bound benefit from classes in basic skills, core curriculum, and functional living skills taught by special educators along with regular education classes for less academic subjects. College-bound students with LD typically are educated in mainstream classes with necessary accommodations such as a study skills class, note takers, taping of class lectures, taped textbooks, portable keyboards for classroom use, modified curriculum requirements, extended time limits, and alternative reporting or test-taking requirements.

Despite differences in program emphasis, all students with LD require ongoing transition services as an integral part of their secondary education. Transition services, which may include career education, vocational assessment, vocational training, job placement, or preparation for college, aid students to move smoothly from high school to postsecondary education or to employment within the community. Polloway, Patton, Epstein, and Smith (1989, cited by Mercer, 1991) suggested that the life domains of goal setting and attainment, physical and emotional health, home and family, friendships and leisure, and community participation are also appropriate targets for transition planning. Independence, responsibility, and productivity are generally agreed upon goals for adolescents to work toward.

Under the Individuals with Disabilities Education Act Amendments of 1997, initial transition planning that addresses necessary courses of study is mandated to begin no later than fourteen years of age with implementation of specific vocational training or other transition activities beginning no later than sixteen years of age. Brinckerhoff (1996) presented a detailed timetable of transition activities for students going on to higher education.

The diverse needs of adolescents with learning disabilities can be met through a combination of mainstream education, special education, and after-school or summer tutoring or therapy. Some families are financially able to provide private clinical tutoring for their LD child or placement in a full-time private school that specializes in education of students with LD. As the inclusion movement in public education moves forward, attention must be focused on the issues of instructional quality and sufficient academic support for adolescents with LD. These students benefit from less rather than more mainstreaming, unless they are prepared or supported to succeed in mainstream courses (Accardo, 1996; Wagner and Blackorby, 1996). Positive postschool outcomes for students with LD are based on their degree of in-school success regardless of where or in which program services are provided.

Postsecondary Students and Adults with LD

Adults with LD continue to be a diverse group whose needs for education, employment, a home and family, and life satisfaction are similar to those of nondisabled individuals. However, as LD persons confront these adult life tasks, they must cope with the particular challenges and limitations imposed by their disabilities.

A number of investigators have found that the cognitive patterns of adults with LD parallel those observed in LD children, with individual profiles often remaining quite consistent over time (Bruck, 1993; Gajar, 1992; Gerber et al., 1990). Although the spectrum of academic skill levels in LD adults is broad, deficits in skills such as language processing, memory, reading, writing, and mechanical arithmetic often persist (Adelman & Vogel, 1991; White, 1992). With IQ and SES controlled, Felton, Naylor, and Wood (1990) found that among adults with a childhood history of reading disability, rapid word naming, phonological awareness, and nonword reading remained core deficits. Spelling is often the most severely impaired academic skill in LD adults even among those who have successfully compensated for their reading disabilities (Adelman & Vogel, 1991; Bruck, 1993; Lefly & Pennington, 1991).

In addition to hindering educational attainment, the neuropsychological and social profiles of many adults with LD impact their ability to obtain employment and meet performance expectations on the job (Brown, 1984). In a survey by Schwarz and Taymans (1991, cited by Adelman & Vogel, 1993), 84% of LD respondents reported finding jobs through networks of family members or friends. Job training time, task organization, work production rate, and accuracy may be negatively influenced by a variety of LDs. For example, auditory processing, oral language, and nonverbal social perception deficits can interfere with following directions, communicating with customers and coworkers, and using the telephone effectively. Adelman and Vogel (1990) found that 4-year college graduates with LD commonly report work problems such as slow processing and retention of new information, requiring extra time to complete assigned work, and having to cope with perceptual deficits (e.g., reversing or transposing numbers and letters).

The LDs of some individuals, particularly those who are intellectually bright or gifted, may remain unrecognized and undiagnosed until their adult years when a disability is brought to the fore by the performance demands of college curricula or employment. Diagnosis during adult years requires comprehensive assessment of early development, medical history, cognitive abilities, academic skill levels, socioemotional adjustment, and occupational functioning, including an analysis of vocational strengths and weaknesses (Brackett & McPherson, 1996; LDA, 1990). Brackett & McPherson (1996) suggest that the IQ/achievement discrepancy model, which is currently highly controversial, is inappropriate for diagnosing LDs in adults. Once again, clinical judgment based on comprehensive assessment should be the basis for determining presence of absence of LD. Diagnostic services for adults may be obtained through mental health agencies, college counseling or study skills centers, university-affiliated hospitals, state vocational rehabilitation offices, private practitioners, or other community resources.

A valid diagnosis of specific LD may be necessary to access postsecondary educational or vocational rehabilitation programs or to receive the educational and employment accommodations available for persons with disabilities. In 1981 the Federal Rehabilitation Services Administration first included LD as one of the recognized disability categories that may qualify an individual to receive government-sponsored vocational rehabilitation services. However, the development and implementation of specific assessment and eligibility guidelines for those with LD remains an ongoing debate (Dowdy, 1992; Gajar, 1992).

The primary legislation and regulations that protect the civil rights of adults with LD are Section 506 of P.L. 102-569, the Rehabilitation Act Amendments of 1992 (amending Section 504 of P.L. 93-112, the Rehabilitation Act of 1973), and P.L. 101-336, the Americans with Disabilities Act of 1990. These statutes jointly prohibit discrimination on the basis of disability by requiring that when requested, educational institutions receiving federal funds and public service providers including licensing boards and employers make reasonable accommodations for persons with a documented LD. Lerner (1993) listed eight published guidebooks to colleges with programs or services for LD students including *A National Directory of Four-Year Colleges, Two-Year Colleges, and Post High School Training Programs for Young People with Learning Disabilities* (Fielding & Fabian-Isaacs, 1993). Appropriate academic or employment accommodations are determined on an individual basis by interfacing setting specific demands with type and severity of LD. What constitutes reasonable and appropriate accommodation is a gray area in which customary practices may or may not satisfy the intent of legal mandates. Scott (1994) discussed the process of determining reasonable academic adjustments for college students with LD. Gregg, Johnson, & McKinley (1996) presented a succinct guide covering policy, legal issues, and case law in regard to adults with LD.

Research targeting the adult LD population has yielded varied results in terms of educational and vocational outcomes and successful adjustment to adult life. In 1991–1992, 19% of LD high school students went on to vocational school, with a completion rate of 11.1%; 13.7% attended two-year colleges, with a completion rate of 2.9%, and 4.4% enrolled in a four-year college or university, with a 0.4% completion rate (Wagner, D'Amico, Marder, Newman, & Blackorby, 1992, cited in Accardo, 1996). However, with sufficient supportive resources, this rather bleak picture can be improved. As an example, the Achieve Program, an intensive support program for students with LD at Southern Illinois University, reported an 83% graduation rate for program students (Cordoni, 1989). Progressive medical schools are implementing identification and support services for medical students with LD, leading to a substantial improvement in student performance (Walters & Croen, 1993).

Despite many individual successes, most adults with LD have some vocational adjustment problems, and many are not independent or self-supporting. Employment rates range from 36% to 87%, with most studies reporting a rate above 50% (White, 1992). Unemployment, only part-time employment, jobs with lower pay and lower social status, and less job satisfaction are frequently reported (Adelman & Vogel, 1993; Gajar, 1992). Most adults with LD are employed in entry-level positions in service, fast food, laborer, production, and helper occupations; a somewhat lower percentage of LD adults than non-LD adults are employed in clerical or sales positions (White, 1992). Adults with LD surveyed within a few years after leaving high school are typically single and living with family members (Adelman & Vogel, 1991; White, 1992). Their most often self-reported concerns involved improving social relationships, obtaining career counseling, developing self-esteem, overcoming dependence, obtaining vocational training, and getting and holding a job (Chesler, 1982, cited in Mercer, 1991).

Factors that enhance positive adult outcomes for persons with LD include higher measured intelligence, higher SES, male gender, type and severity of disability, younger age at time of diagnosis (for less severe LDs), and quality of intervention (Adelman & Vogel, 1991, 1993; Hoy & Manglitz, 1996). Hoy and Manglitz (1996) indicated that adults with severe language-based LD or serious NLD tend toward poorer outcomes than those with other diagnoses or with a milder degree of disability. Successful LD students and adults take control of their lives by understanding the nature of their disabilities and needed compensations. They remain persistently goal oriented despite setbacks, spend extra time to complete tasks, seek out effective support systems, and creatively find a niche that plays to their strengths (Adelman & Vogel, 1991; McCann, 1989; Reiff, Gerber, & Ginsberg, 1994). Comprehensive reviews of information about adults with LD have been provided by Adelman and Vogel (1991); Goldstein (1997); Gregg, Hoy, and Gay (1996); Johnson and Blalock (1987); and Polloway, Smith, and Patton (1984).

SOCIOCULTURAL FACTORS

LDs are cross-cultural conditions that affect children and adults in all cultures and countries of the world. Language-based LDs are evident in cultures with a pictorial system of written language, as well as in cultures with an alphabetical system of written language (Lerner, 1993). The United States has traditionally been an ethnically and culturally diverse nation. In 1994 over 8% of U.S. residents had been born outside the country (Statistical Abstract of the United States, 1995, cited in Puente, Sol Mora, and Munoz-Cespedes, 1997) and in 1989 5.3 million children entered school speaking languages other than English (Children's Defense Fund, 1989, cited in Lopez, 1995). In some areas of the United States, the number of primary or first languages spoken by students and their families can range as high as 120 (Lerner, 1993). It is expected that the number of ethnically diverse school children in this country will continue to increase, with Hispanics becoming the largest group of ethnic minorities by the year 2025 (Statistical Abstract, 1995, cited in Puente et al., 1997). Culturally diverse students without LD may experience difficulty in academic learning as a result of many factors, such as overt culture shock, language differences, differences in cultural values and norms, delayed or disrupted schooling, loss of support from extended family members, poor health or nutrition, effects of poverty, and inappropriate instruction provided by teachers and school districts unprepared to understand or accommodate their educational needs. The problems faced by these students become even more complicated if they also experience specific LDs.

The present special education definition of LD requires the determination of intelligence and academic achievement, and lists cultural difference and economic disadvantage as exclusionary criteria. As has been well documented, the measurement of both intelligence and achievement is greatly affected by degree of language proficiency and acculturation, and is therefore highly susceptible to cultural bias (Barona & Pfeiffer, 1992; Greenfield, 1997; Olivarez, Palmer, & Guillemard, 1992; Reynolds & Kaiser, 1990; Suzuki & Valencia, 1997). Although language differences have often been cited as the major factor contributing to lower intelligence test scores for ethnically diverse students, sometimes nonverbal measures of intelligence yield even larger racial/ethnic group differences (Suzuki & Valencia, 1997). Illiteracy affects neuropsychological performance in the areas of visual–spatial and praxis abilities, as well as in the areas of language and memory abilities (Ardila & Roselli, 1989; Roselli & Ardila, 1990, 1993, cited by Puente et al., 1997). Thus the process of validly and reliably diagnosing LDs, which in and of itself is a thorny issue, becomes even more complex when culturally and linguistically diverse individuals are being assessed.

Inaccurate and biased assessment practices have been linked to overrepresentation of minority students in special education, with consequent concerns about harmful effects such as stigma and restriction of educational opportunity. Barona and Faykus (1992) found that among students referred to special education, the sociocultural variables of ethnicity and SES each made a small but significant contribution to the prediction of LD eligibility, which should not have been the case if these were truly exclusionary criteria. MacMillan (1993) has provided an instructive discussion of the interaction between identification and placement issues for minority students classified as LD and those classified as mentally retarded. Although national data from the Office of Civil Rights suggest that African American and Hispanic students are not overrepresented in the special educational category of LD (Reschly & Wilson, 1990; Reschly, 1996), regional studies have reported otherwise (Ortiz & Yates, 1983, cited by MacMillan, 1993).

Among sociocultural factors that influence learning and thus LDs, it is important to consider the stresses and educational barriers associated with low SES, poverty, and homelessness. In 1995 over 14 million children, or about 20.8% of all children in the United States, were classified as poor; this figure has risen from approximately 15% in the early 1970s (Brooks-Gunn & Duncan, 1997). Factors related to poverty include single-parent families, young or poorly educated parents, disabled parents, and belonging to an ethnic or racial minority. "Developmental patterns of children from poverty environments differ from those of middle class students" (Garcia & Ortiz, 1988, p. 6). Economic and experiential differences affect cognitive and learning styles, language and information processing, and motivational patterns. Ability and achievement appear to be more strongly affected than emotional outcomes (Brooks-Gunn & Duncan, 1997). Wallach, Wallach, Dozier, and Kaplan (1977, cited by Pennington, 1991) reported an apparently large SES effect on phoneme awareness, which is currently viewed as the most robust predictor of later reading ability (Lyon, 1996b). Although genetic inheritance and family interactional patterns differ, such that not all low-income persons are at increased risk for learning problems, SES has a well-established relationship to both intelligence test scores and levels of academic achievement. When these two constructs are being assessed in the process of diagnosing LD, specific background variables and the potential effects of low SES must be carefully weighed.

Poverty is a factor in long-term outcomes for disabled individuals. Wagner and Blackorby (1996) reported data from the National Longitudinal Transition Study of Special Education Students, which confirmed that independent of functional mental ability, gender, or ethnic background, students with mild disabilities from low-income households (including those with LD) experienced poorer postsecondary school outcomes than disabled students from higher-income households. Low-income disabled students were significantly less likely to attend postsecondary academic or vocational training programs. They were as likely to be employed as their disabled peers from wealthier families but earned less per year, possibly as a result of holding lower-level jobs. The negative effects of family poverty, especially for persons with disabilities, can be both pervasive and intergenerational.

At present there are many unanswered questions about appropriate assessment and intervention practices for culturally diverse and low-SES individuals with LD. The lack of empirically validated practices for the LD field as a whole becomes even more problematic when issues associated with cultural diversity and poverty are complicating factors.

A number of publications provide information about the psychology of diversity and offer suggestions for assisting culturally diverse individuals and their families. Harry (1992) has described the cultural perspectives of African Americans, Hispanics, Native Americans, and Asians in terms of their traditional world views, and has explored the ways in which cultural diversity influences families as they encounter the special education system. Mosley-Howard (1995) and Flanagan and Miranda (1995) discussed the concepts of culture and acculturation, the impact of culture on individuals and families, and best practices for working with culturally different students. Garcia and Ortiz (1988) have outlined detailed prereferral procedures that can be implemented to prevent inappropriate referral of language-minority students to special education. The American Psychological Association (1993) has issued guidelines for providers of psychological services to ethnic, linguistic, and culturally diverse populations. Waterman (1994) presented a comprehensive overview of both traditional and alternative strategies for assessing children for the presence of a disability, with emphasis on the relevance of particular strategies for use with minority students. Caterino (1991) set forth a step-by-step procedure for the assessment of language-minority children, with specific suggestions for assessing language dominance, cognition, academic achievement, social behavior, and emotional adjustment. Hessler (1993) has discussed using the Woodcock–Johnson Psycho-Educational Battery—Revised to assess the impact of cultural diversity on test performance, first by determining oral language proficiency in English, and second by comparing scores on Woodcock–Johnson subtests with a high degree of cultural loading to scores on subtests with a low to moderate degree of cultural loading. He also provides a case study that illustrates the process of Woodcock–Johnson test interpretation with a culturally different student. Puente et al. (1997) recently addressed the topic of neuropsychological assessment of Spanish-speaking children and youth, and Lopez (1995) reviewed best practices for school psychologists in working with bilingual children. It is the responsibility of each practitioner in the field of LD to be sensitive to cultural variables, to be cognizant of issues surrounding inadequate and biased assessment, and to seek out current best practices (however empirically limited they may be) for working with culturally diverse and low-income individuals and families.

COMORBID DISORDERS

Caron and Rutter (1991) have reviewed the concept of psychiatric comorbidity and summarized different scenarios for the existence of either true or artificial comorbidity. As discussed by Lyytinen (1995), the term "comorbidity," applied in this context, may refer to (1) the co-occurrence of two or more presumably separate neurocognitive disorders;

(2) the co-occurrence of two or more independent conditions that are mediated by a common genetic or environmental etiology; (3) conditions, possibly related, that share the same or overlapping risk factors; (4) conditions that co-occur because of the secondary effects of one disorder on the other; (5) comorbid characteristics that combine to define a meaningful syndrome; and (6) conditions that result from interactive combinations of the other five states. The frequently observed comorbid conditions associated with LDs illustrate all six types of comorbidity, although due to present empirical limitations, the specific form of comorbidity in a given instance may be questionable or undetermined. In addition, an apparent comorbidity may be a function of the current definitions of LD and the other disorders under consideration or of the diagnostic procedures used for classification, rather than representing true comorbidity. Also, it may be unclear whether a given characteristic (e.g., psychosocial deficit) is an integral part of an LD pattern or whether that characteristic constitutes an associated comorbid condition (Lyytinen, 1995).

ADHD is probably the DSM-IV diagnostic category that has the highest rate of comorbidity with LD. Among children diagnosed as LD, the reported rate of ADHD has generally ranged from 15% (Shaywitz, Fletcher, & Shaywitz, 1992, cited in Lyon, 1996b) to as high as 85% (Safer & Allen, 1976); most studies, as reported by Shaywitz and Shaywitz (1987), find a comorbidity figure between 30% and 40%. There have been conflicting views about whether LD and ADHD are independent disorders or whether they are both manifestations of the same underlying brain dysfunction. James and Selz (1997) suggested that this question has not been fully resolved because of methodological flaws in accumulated research; however, many experts have concluded that although they frequently co-occur, there is strong evidence for the separateness of LD and ADHD (Barkley, 1990; Dykman & Ackerman, 1991; Goldstein, 1997; Pennington, Grossier, & Welsh, 1993; Shaywitz, Fletcher, & Shaywitz, 1995; Silver, 1990). After reviewing several possible mechanisms for the comorbidity of ADHD with dyslexia, Pennington (1991) suggested that in most cases dyslexia leads to ADHD as a secondary symptom, but that in a small percentage of cases there may be a genetic correlation between the two disorders. In taking a new look at LD-ADHD comorbidity in twin data, Light, Pennington, Gilger, and DeFries, 1995 (cited in Lyytinen, 1995), concluded that shared genetic influences account for a substantial portion of the covariance between dyslexia and ADHD.

It is widely believed that both LD and ADHD are comorbid to a greater than average degree with other categories of psychiatric disorders, such as conduct disorder, anxiety disorders, and depression. To date, few methodologically sound studies with well-defined LD subject populations have evaluated this premise. Porter and Rourke (1985), using the Personality Inventory for Children (Wirt, Lachar, Klinedinst, & Seat, 1977), identified four distinct personality patterns or subtypes that characterized the majority of the LD children in their study. Of those classified, 44% displayed balanced, well-adjusted socio-emotional functioning; 26% exhibited marked internalizing psychological disturbances (depression, anxiety, low social skills); 13% displayed roughly normal personality functioning, but with a high degree of somatic concerns; and 17% exhibited behavioral disturbance, reflected in hyperkinetic, aggressive, and antisocial behaviors. Three studies that employed the Minnesota Multiphasic Personality Inventory (Hathaway & McKinley, 1989) to assess emotional functioning in LD adults (Balow & Blomquist, 1965; Gregg, Hoy, King, Moreland, & Jagota, 1992; Spreen, 1988, cited by Hooper & Olley, 1996) were consistent in reporting more maladjustment and serious psychopathology (e.g., depression, anxiety, social withdrawal, phobias, acting-out tendencies, disorganized thoughts, etc.) in LD adults than in their normal counterparts. In contrast, Lamm and Epstein (1992) found few differences in degree of psychopathology between individuals with LD and control subjects who were assessed via a structured rating scale. As reviewed by James and Selz (1997), the emotional consequences of LD may vary by subtype, but conflicting results have been reported. The most widely reported psychopathology–subtype linkage is the association of significant internalizing problems (including social isolation, anxiety, depression, and suicide) with NLD, or, as it is often termed, right-hemisphere-based LD (Bigler, 1989; Hooper & Olley, 1996; James & Selz, 1997; Rourke, 1989; Voeller, 1986).

"Psychosocial adjustment difficulties frequently are assumed to be the major social-emotional manifestation of learning disabilities" (Hooper & Olley, 1996, p. 170). Two of the earlier and persistent voices underscoring the need for a sociological perspective on LDs were those of Kronick (1974, 1976) and Bryan (1974, 1978, 1991). Kronick explored ways in which difficulties with attention, concentration, perception, inference, labeling of emotions, and communication of feelings interfere with identity formation, disrupt family relationships, and produce interactional dysfunction. Bryan (1991) provided a comprehensive review of research on the attitudes of LD children and adolescents toward themselves, their social competence, their communicative competence, and teachers' judgments of their school behavior. In all areas, with the exception of knowledge of social norms, LD students were described as less socially competent than their normally achieving classmates. Voeller (1986) found that children with NLD often failed to perceive social cues and thus had difficulty correctly interpreting their social environment. These NLD children tended to push and crowd their peers, to get into arguments or fights with peers, and to have difficulty maintaining friendships. They were frequently considered "strange" or "weird" by their classmates.

Adolsecents with LD are statistically at increased risk for juvenile delinquency and substance abuse, but no causal link has been established between LD and either of these conditions (Morrison & Cosden, 1997). The reported prevalence of LD among juvenile offenders generally ranges from 35% to 65%, but these figures cannot be accepted at face value due to the methodological limitations of the research. No specific prevalence figures for substance abuse among LD adolescents are presently available. The risk for both juvenile delinquency and substance abuse is increased when LD is accompanied by hyperactivity and/or conduct disorder (Morrison & Cosden, 1997).

A number of hypotheses have been proposed to account for the link between LD and juvenile delinquency or substance abuse. The most frequently offered explanations suggest the following: Low self-esteem and stresses associated with school failure may lead to delinquency or substance abuse; LD youth may be more susceptible to delinquent acts as a result of impulsivity, limited understanding of cause and effect, or poor social judgment; and young LD offenders may lack the strategic planning skills to avoid being caught or to conceal their behavior when being questioned by legal authorities. A study by Waldie and Spreen (1993) provided some support for the susceptibility hypothesis that for those who are LD, comorbid juvenile delinquency is linked to impulsivity and poor judgment. Reviews of the literature on LD, juvenile delinquency, and substance abuse are provided by Murray (1976), Lane (1980), Skaret and Wilgosh (1989), and Morrison and Cosden (1997).

After reviewing relevant research, Polloway et al. (1984) concluded that the social skill deficits observed in children with LD persist into adulthood. In a group of 93 adults diagnosed as LD at the Learning Disabilities Clinic at Northwestern University, 25% expressed concerns about social difficulties (Blalock & Johnson, 1987). Their social problems included difficulty making and keeping friends, as well as problems related to their specific disabilities (e.g., following and participating in conversational exchanges, locating addresses, dancing, playing cards or word games, writing personal notes and letters, etc.). In general, the adults with NLD experienced the greatest social problems and social isolation, but they were not always aware of their social handicaps.

The frequently cited comorbidity of psychopathology or psychosocial difficulty with LD may result from several different direct or indirect mechanisms or from a dynamic combination of mechanisms. As described by Hooper and Olley (1996), these mechanisms may include the following:

> (1) Behavioral disruption that arises directly from abnormal brain activity; (2) heightened exposure to failure, frustration, and social stigma due to associated disabilities; (3) the possible effects of brain damage or anomalous neurodevelopment on subsequent temperament and personality development; (4) adverse family reactions ranging from overprotection to scapegoating; (5) the individual's own reaction to being handicapped and its effect on his or her actual capacity to cope and compete; and (6) possible adverse effects from treatments themselves (e.g., lack of or poor treatment for specific learning problems) that may restrict normal activities and socialization. (p. 164)

Although individuals with LD are at increased risk for psychopathology and psychosocial deficits, there is wide variation in their patterns of socioemotional adjustment, and group findings do not dictate individual outcomes. The majority of children and adults with LD do not exhibit significant emotional disorders and function well in society. Morrison and Cosden (1997) view LD as constituting a risk factor that in and of itself does not predict positive or negative outcomes. They propose that other internal and environmental risk/protective factors interact with the presence of LD to mediate nonacademic outcomes such as emotional adjustment, adolescent problems (e.g., dropping out of school, juvenile delinquency, substance abuse) and adult adaptation. Although the present discussion of socioemotional development and adjustment in persons with LD has been limited in scope, Mercer (1991) and Bender (1994) provide a more extensive review of these issues.

Two additional types of comorbidity that are observed in conjunction with LDs are mentioned here. First, one diagnostic category or subtype of LD may be viewed as comorbid with another. Since reading is an essential educational tool, and since 80% of identified LD children have difficulty acquiring reading skills (Lerner, 1993), reading disability or dyslexia is often considered a child's primary deficit, with co-occurring deficits in other skill areas (e.g., mathematics or graphomotor production) considered secondary or co-morbid deficits. It is possible for two distinct LD patterns or subtypes to co-occur; for instance, deficits in phonemic awareness and processing can co-occur with deficits in visual–spatial perception and spatial organization, affecting one or more academic skill areas. However, two co-occurring academic deficits (e.g., reading disability and math disability) may actually be manifestations of a single pattern of neurocognitive deficit with a shared information-processing bottleneck that impedes acquisition of skills in both academic areas (Lyytinen, 1995). Lyytinen cites two companion articles (Ackerman & Dykman, 1995; Räsänen & Ahonen, 1995) that examine the co-occurrence of reading and mathematical disorders. Light and DeFries (1995) assessed the genetic and environmental etiologies of comorbid reading and math deficits in identical and fraternal twin pairs. Their data indicated that approximately 26% of observed reading deficit was due to genetic factors that also influenced math performance.

A final category of comorbidity involves LD patterns that are observed in association with specific disorders or genetic syndromes (e.g., Klinefelter syndrome, Turner syndrome, fragile X syndrome, Tourette disorder or syndrome, neurofibromatosis, etc.). LDs are frequent concomitants of syndromes associated with sex chromosome aberrations.

In Klinefelter syndrome (47,XXY in males), affected individuals are of normal intelligence but frequently demonstrate specific deficits in Verbal IQ, auditory processing, efficient use of language, and reading (Berkow & Fletcher, 1992). Turner syndrome (complete or partial absence of one X chromosome, usually observed in females) affects cognitive and learning processes to a variable degree. A typical phenotypic presentation involves characteristics associated with NLD, such as visual–spatial deficits, weakness in numerical and mathematical understanding, and social learning deficits (Mazzacco, 1996). Additional information about the patterns of learning abilities and disabilities that accompany specific genetic disorders is presented in other chapters of this text.

Comorbidity between LD and other neurocognitive disorders, or between LD and various forms of psychopathology, is a complex topic that is currently receiving considerable emphasis in the research literature (Lyytinen, 1995). Future investigations of comorbidity will assist practitioners to view individuals with LD from a more holistic perspective. This should result in greater intervention efforts aimed at modifying the nonacademic risk factors that impede successful long-term outcomes, and at enhancing the protective factors that facilitate such outcomes. Furthermore, explorations of comorbidity among LD categories or subtypes will contribute to the all-important process of defining more distinct and empirically defensible LD subtypes.

SUMMARY

Learning disabilities are complex phenomena that necessitate a high level of understanding and clinical expertise on the part of medical, psychological, and educational practitioners. Mather and Roberts (1994) discussed the possibility that within educational settings, the concept of specific LDs and the education of those with LD could disintegrate within an encompassing miasma of educational generalism. Standing in firm opposition to this undesirable outcome is the body of neurocognitive research that is beginning to provide scientific underpinnings to justify and direct the field of LD. To this point, the neurobiological information about the etiology of LDs is primarily correlational rather than causational in nature. However, we are beginning to understand brain/behavior relationships as researchers continue to discover anatomical and physiological correlates of LDs, identify core features of deficits, and develop meaningful clusters of subtypes. As research leads to a better understanding of the effects of environmental programming on brain development, there may come a time when LDs are defined as neurodevelopmental differences with genetic/biological and, in some cases, social/environmental roots.

It is hoped that scientific advances in LD will be translated into an increasingly sophisticated corps of practitioners who can validly diagnose LD and implement appropriate interventions. More intensive attention should be given to functional factors that affect outcomes. Through awareness campaigns, both the public and professionals can be made cognizant of how to enhance preventive and protective factors in those with significant risk for LD. Within homes and daycare settings, caregivers can be taught how to provide early brain stimulation for optimal development. Within schools, curriculum based on explicit, intensive instruction in phonics can reduce or prevent reading problems in some at-risk students. There is a critical need for more extensive teacher training that adequately prepares both regular and special educators to work effectively with identified LD students, as well as other students at risk for school failure. Revamped university coursework and in-service classes that train teachers to adopt best practices could disseminate research-validated instructional approaches from small demonstration projects into the mainstream of education. Additional topics in the evolving field of LD that need to be addressed and that will provide a broader perspective are sociocultural factors and LD, including how to improve long-term outcomes for females, and comorbidity of LD with other disorders.

Over the last fifteen years the importance of a lifespan approach for understanding LD has increased. At each stage from preschool to adulthood individuals with LD must be identified and assisted to develop the necessary skills and adaptive capacities to meet age-appropriate life tasks. With early diagnosis, effective intervention, careful vocational preparation, and necessary support services, most individuals with LD can lead fulfilling lives and make meaningful contributions to society.

REFERENCES

Abayomi, O., Chun, M. S., & Kelly, K. (1990). Cerebral calcification and learning disabilities following cranial irradiation for medulloblastoma. *Journal of the National Medical Association*, 82, 833–836.

Accardo, P. A. (1996). *The invisible disability: Understanding learning disabilities in the context of health and education* (Occasional Paper No. 11). Washington, DC: National Health and Education Consortium.

Ackerman, P. T., Dykman, R. A., & Peters, J. E. (1977). Teenage status of hyperactive and non-hyperactive learning disabled boys. *American Journal of Orthopsychiatry*, 47, 577–596.

Adelman, P. B., & Vogel, S. A. (1990). College graduates with learning disabilities: Employment attainment and career patterns. *Learning Disability Quarterly*, 12(3), 154–156.

Adelman, P. B., & Vogel, S. A. (1991). The learning-disabled adult. In B. Y. L. Wong (Ed.), *Learning about learning disabilities* (pp. 563–594). San Diego, CA: Academic Press.

Adelman, P. B., & Vogel, S. A. (1993). Issues in the employment of adults with learning disabilities. *Learning Disability Quarterly*, 16, 219–232.

Allison, M. (1992, October–November). The effects of neurologic injury on the maturing brain. *HEADLINES*, pp. 2–10.

American Psychiatric Association. (1994). *Diagnostic and statistical manual of mental disorders* (4th ed.). Washington, DC: Author.

American Psychological Association. (1993). *Guidelines for providers of psychological services to ethnic, linguistic, and culturally diverse populations*. Washington, DC: Author.

Anderson-Inman, L., Knox-Quinn, C., & Horney, M. A. (1996). Computer-based study strategies for students with learning disabilities: Individual differences associated with adoption level. *Journal of Learning Disabilities*, 29, 461–484.

An ounce of prevention is worth a pound of cure. (1998). *LDA Newsbriefs*, 33(6), 9.

Ardila, A., & Roselli, M. (1989). Neuropsychological assessment in illiterates: Visuospatial and memory abilities. *Brain and Cognition*, 11, 147–166.

Autti-Ramo, I., Korkman, M., Hilakivi-Clarke, L., Lehtonen, M., Halmesmaki, E., & Granstrom, M. L. (1992). Mental development of 2-year-old children exposed to alcohol *in utero*. *Journal of Pediatrics*, 5, 740–746.

Azar, B. (1997, December). Researchers debunk myth of the "crack baby." *APA Monitor*, p. 14.

Azuma, S. D., & Chasnoff, I. (1993). Outcome of children prenatally exposed to cocaine and other drugs: A path analysis of three-year data. *Pediatrics*, 92, 396–402.

Bakker, D. J. (1979). Hemisphere differences and reading strategies: Two dyslexias? *Bulletin of the Orton Society*, 29, 84–100.

Ball, E. W., & Blachman, B. A. (1988). Phoneme segmentation training: Effect on reading readiness. *Annals of Dyslexia*, 38, 208–225.

Balow, B., & Blomquist, M. (1965). Young adults ten to fifteen years after severe reading disability. *Elementary School Journal*, 66, 44–48.

Barkley, R. A. (1990). *Attention-deficit hyperactivity disorder: A handbook for diagnosis and treatment*. New York: Guilford Press.

Barona, A., & Faykus, S. (1992). Differential effects of sociocultural variables on special education eligibility categories. *Psychology in the Schools, 29*, 313–320.

Barona, A., & Pfeiffer, S. (1992). Effects of test administration procedures and acculturation level on achievement scores. *Journal of Psychoeducational Assessment, 10*, 124–132.

Begley, S. (1996, February 19). Your child's brain. *Newsweek*, pp. 41–45.

Bellinger, D. C., Stiles, K. M., & Needleman, H. L. (1992). Low-level lead exposure, intelligence, and academic achievement: A long-term follow-up study. *Pediatrics, 90*, 855–861.

Bender, W. N. (Ed.). (1994). Social-emotional development: The task and the challenge [Special issue]. *Learning Disability Quarterly, 17*(4).

Benton, A. L. (1975). Developmental dyslexia: Neurological aspects. In W. J. Friedlander (Ed.), *Advances in neurology* (Vol. 17, pp. 1–47). New York: Raven.

Berkow, R., & Fletcher, A. J. (Eds.). (1992). *The Merck manual of diagnosis and therapy* (16th ed.). Rahway, NJ: Merck Research Laboratories.

Bigler, E. D. (1989). On the neuropsychology of suicide. *Journal of Learning Disabilities, 22*, 180–185.

Bigler, E. D. (1992). The neurobiology and neuropsychology of adult learning disorders. *Journal of Learning Disabilities, 25*, 488–506.

Blachman, B. A. (Ed.). (1997). *Foundations of reading acquisition and dyslexia: Implications for early intervention*. Mahwah, NJ: Erlbaum.

Blalock, J. W., & Johnson, D. J. (1987). Primary concerns and group characteristics. In D. J. Johnson & J. W. Blalock (Eds.), *Adults with learning disabilities: Clinical studies* (pp. 31–45). New York: Grune & Stratton.

Boder, E. (1973). Developmental dyslexia: A diagnostic approach based on three atypical reading patterns. *Developmental Medicine and Child Neurology, 15*, 663–687.

Brackett, J., & McPherson, A. (1996). Learning disabilities diagnosis in postsecondary students: A comparison of discrepancy-based diagnostic models. In N. Gregg, C. Hoy, & A. F. Gay (Eds.), *Adults with learning disabilities: Theoretical and practical perspectives* (pp. 68–84). New York: Guilford Press.

Brinckerhoff, L. C. (1996). Making the transition to higher education: Opportunities for student empowerment. *Journal of Learning Disabilities, 29*, 118–133.

Brooks-Gunn, J., & Duncan, G. (1997). The effects of poverty on children. *The Future of Children, 7*(2), 55–71. (Available from Center for the Future of Children, 300 Second Street, Suite 102, Los Altos, CA 94022-3621)

Brophy, J., & Good, T. (1986). Teacher behavior and student achievement. In M. C. Wittrock (Ed.), *Third handbook of research on teaching* (3rd ed., pp. 328–375). New York: Macmillan.

Brown, D. (1984). Employment considerations for learning disabled adults. *Journal of Rehabilitation, 2*, 74–77, 88.

Brown, V. L., Hammill, D. D., & Wiederholt, J. L. (1995). *Test of reading comprehension* (3rd ed.) *(TORC-3)*. Austin, TX: PRO-ED.

Bruck, M. (1993). Component spelling skills of college students with childhood diagnoses of dyslexia. *Learning Disabilities Quarterly, 16*, 171–184.

Bryan, T. H. (1974). Peer popularity of learning disabled children. *Journal of Learning Disabilities, 7*, 261–268.

Bryan, T. H. (1978). Social relationships and verbal interaction of learning disabled children. *Journal of Learning Disabilities 11*, 107–115.

Bryan, T. H. (1991). Social problems and learning disabilities. In B. Y. L. Wong (Ed.), *Learning about learning disabilities* (pp. 195–229). San Diego, CA: Academic Press.

Butler, D. L. (1998). Metacognition and learning disabilities. In B.Y.L. Wong (Ed.), *Learning about learning disabilities* (2nd ed.). San Diego, CA: Academic Press.

Cannon, L. (1997). Progress and promise in research and education for individuals with learning disabilities. *LDA Newsbriefs, 32*(4), 1, 6–8.

Cardon, L. R., Smith, S. D., Fulker, D. W., Kimberling, W. J., Pennington, B. F., & DeFries, J. C. (1994). Quantitative trait locus for reading disability on chromosome 6. *Science, 266,* 276–279.

Caron, C., & Rulter, M. (1991). Comorbidity in childhood psychopathology: Concepts, issues, and research strategies. *Journal of Child Psychology and Psychiatry, 32,* 1063–1080.

Caterino, L. C. (1991). Step-by-step procedure for the assessment of language minority children. In A. Barona & E. E. Garcia (Eds.), *Children at risk: Poverty, minority status, and other issues in educational equity* (pp. 185–210). Washington, DC: National Association of School Psychologists.

Christenson, S. L., Ysseldyke, J. E., & Thurlow, M. L. (1989). Critical instructional factors for students with mild handicaps: An integrative review. *Remedial and Special Education, 10*(5), 21–31.

Connoloy, A. J. (1988). *KeyMath revised: A diagnostic inventory of essential mathematics.* Circle Pines, MN: American Guidance Service.

Cordoni, B. (1989). Broken crutches. *Their World: A Publication of the National Center for Learning Disabilities,* pp. 100–101. (Available from NCLD, 381 Park Ave., Suite 1420, New York, NY 10016)

Cruickshank, W. M., Bentzen, F. A., Ratzeburg, R. H., & Tannhauser, M. T. (1961). *A teaching method for brain-injured and hyperactive children.* Syracuse, NY: Syracuse University Press.

Dawson, G., & Fischer, K. W. (Eds.). (1994). *Human behavior and the developing brain.* New York: Guilford Press.

Day, S. L., & Edwards, B. J. (1996). Assistive technology for postsecondary students with learning disabilities. *Journal of Learning Disabilities, 29,* 486–492, 503.

DeFries, J. C. (1991). Genetics and dyslexia: An overview. In M. Snowling & M. Thomson (Eds.), *Dyslexia: Integrating theory and practice* (pp. 3–20). London: Whurr.

DeFries, J. C., & Fulker, D. W. (1985). Multiple regression analysis of twin data. *Behavior Genetics, 15*(5), 467–473.

DeFries, J. C., & Gillis, J. J. (1993). Genetics of Reading disability. In R. Plomin & G. E. McClearn (Eds.), *Nature, nurture, and psychology* (pp. 163–194). Washington, DC: American Psychological Association.

Denckla, M. B. (1972). Clinical syndromes in learning disabilities: The case for splitting versus lumping. *Journal of Learning Disabilities, 5,* 401–406.

Denckla, M. D. (1977). The neurological basis of reading disability. In F. G. Roswell & G. Natchez (Eds.), *Reading disability: A human approach to learning.* New York: Basic Books.

Deshler, D. D., & Lenz, B. K. (1989). The strategies instructional approach. *International Journal of Disability, Development and Education, 36,* 203–224.

Doehring, D. G. (1968). *Patterns of impairment in specific reading disability.* Bloomington, IN: Indiana University Press.

Doris, J. L. (1986). Learning disabilities. In S. J. Ceci (Ed.), *Handbook of cognitive, social, and neuropsychological aspects of learning disabilities* (Vol. 1, pp. 3–53). Hillsdale, NJ: Erlbaum.

Doris, J. L. (1993). Defining learning disabilities: A history of the search for consensus. In G. R. Lyon, D. B. Gray, J. F. Kavanaugh, & N. A. Krasnegor (Eds.), *Better understanding learning disabilities: New views from research and their implications for education and public policies* (pp. 97–115). Baltimore: Paul H. Brookes.

Dowdy, C. A. (1992). Identification of specific learning disabilities as a critical component in the vocational rehabilitation process. *Journal of Rehabilitation, 58*(3), 51–54.

Drake, W. E. (1968). Clinical and pathological findings in a child with a developmental learning disability. *Journal of Learning Disabilities, 1,* 486–502.

Dykman, R. A., & Ackerman, P. T. (1991). Attention deficit disorder and reading disability: Separate but often overlapping disorders. *Journal of Learning Disabilities, 24,* 96–103.

Ellis, E. S., & Friend, P. (1991). Adolescents with learning disabilities. In B. Y. L. Wong (Ed.), *Learning about learning disabilities* (pp. 505–561). San Diego, CA: Academic Press.

Felton, R. H., Naylor, C. E., & Wood, F. B. (1990). Neuropsychological profile of adult dyslexics. *Brain and Language, 39,* 485–497.

Fielding, P. M., & Fabian-Isaacs, C. (Eds.). (1993). *A national directory of four-year colleges, two-year colleges, and post high school training programs for young people with learning disabilities* (7th ed.). Tulsa, OK: Partners in Publishing.

Finlay, B. L., & Miller, B. (1993). Regressive events in early cortical maturation: Their significance for the outcome of early brain damage. In A. M. Galaburda (Ed.), *Dyslexia and development: Neurobiological aspects of extra-ordinary brains* (pp. 1–20). Cambridge, MA: Harvard University Press.

Finucci, J. M. (1978). Genetic considerations in dyslexia. In H. R. Myklebust (Ed.), *Progress in learning disabilities* (Vol. 4, pp. 41–63). New York: Grune & Stratton.

Flanagan, D. P., & Miranda, A. H. (1995). Best practices in working with culturally different families. In A. Thomas & J. Grimes (Eds.), *Best practices in school psychology—III* (3rd ed., pp. 1049–1060). Washington, DC: National Association of School Psychologists.

Foorman, B. R. (1995). Research on the great debate: Code-oriented versus whole-language approaches to reading instruction. *School Psychology Review, 24,* 376–392.

Gajar, A. (1992). Adults with learning disabilities: Current and future research priorities. *Journal of Learning Disabilities, 25,* 507–519.

Galaburda, A. M. (1990). The testosterone hypothesis: Assessment since Geschwind and Behan, 1982. *Annals of Dyslexia, 40,* 18–38.

Galaburda, A. M. (1993). Neuroanatomic basis of developmental dyslexia. *Behavioral Neurology, 11,* 161–173.

Galaburda, A. M., & Kemper, T. L. (1979). Cytoarchitectonic abnormalities in developmental dyslexia: A case study. *Annals of Neurology, 6,* 94–100.

Galaburda, A. M., Sherman, G. F., Rosen, G. D., Aboitiz, F., & Geschwind, N. (1985). Developmental dyslexia: Four consecutive patients with cortical anomalies. *Annals of Neurology, 18,* 222–233.

Garcia, S. B., & Ortiz, A. A. (1988). *Preventing inappropriate referrals of language minority student to special education* (Contract No. 300860069). Wheaton, MD: National Clearinghouse for Bilingual Education.

Gardner, R. A. (1973). *MBD: The family book about minimal brain dysfunction.* New York: Jason Aronson.

Gay, A. F. (1996). Facilitating alternative learning techniques for adults with learning disabilities through the use of technology. In N. Gregg, C. Hoy, & A. F. Gay (Eds.), *Adults with learning disabilities: Theoretical and practical perspectives* (pp. 368–392). New York: Guilford Press.

Gerber, P. J., Schneiders, C. A., Pardise, L. V., Reiff, H. B., Ginsberg, R., & Popp, P. A. (1990). Persisting problems of adults with learning disabilities: Self-reported comparisons from their school-age and adult years. *Journal of Learning Disabilities, 23,* 570–573.

Gilger, J. W., Borecki, I. B., DeFries, J. C., & Pennington, B. F. (1994). Commingling and segregation analysis of reading performance in families of normal reading probands. *Behavior Genetics, 24,* 345–355.

Gilmore, J. V., & Gilmore, E. C. (1968). *Gilmore oral reading test.* New York: Harcourt, Brace.

Goldstein, S. (1997). *Managing attention and learning disorders in late adolescence and adulthood: A guide for practitioners.* New York: Wiley.

Goldstein, S., & Mather, N. (1998). *Overcoming underachieving: An action guide to helping your child in school.* New York: Wiley.

Gordon, M., & Keiser, S. (1998). Underpinnings. In M. Gordon & S. Keiser (Eds.), *Accommodations in higher education under the Americans with Disabilities Act (ADA): A no-nonsense guide for clinicians, educators, administrators, and lawyers* (pp. 3–19). New York: Guilford Press.

Greenfield, P. M. (1997). You can't take it with you: Why ability assessments don't cross cultures. *American Psychologist, 52,* 1115–1124.

Gregg, N., Hoy, C., & Gay, A. F. (Eds.). (1996). *Adults with learning disabilities: Theoretical and practical perspectives.* New York: Guilford Press.

Gregg, N., Hoy, C., King, M., Moreland, C., & Jagota, M. (1992). The MMPI-2 profile of adults with learning disabilities in university and rehabilitation settings. *Journal of Learning Disabilities, 25,* 386–395.

Gregg, N., Johnson, Y., & McKinley, C. (1996). Learning disabilities policy and legal issues: A consumer and practitioner user-friendly guide. In N. Gregg, C. Hoy, & A. F. Gay (Eds.), *Adults with learning disabilities: Theoretical and practical perspectives* (pp. 329–367). New York: Guilford Press.

Gross-Glenn, K., Duara, R., Barker, W. W., Loewenstein, D., Chang, J. Y., Yoshii, F., Apicella, A. M., Pascal, S., Boothe, T., Sevush, S., Jallad, B. J., Nooa, L., & Lubs, H. A. (1991). Positron emission tomographic studies during serial word-reading by normal and dyslexic adults. *Journal of Clinical and Experimental Neuropsychology, 13,* 531–544.

Hack, M., Breslau, N., Aram, D., Weissman, B., Klein, N., & Borawski-Clark, E. (1992). The effect of very low birthweight and social risk on neurocognitive abilities at school age. *Journal of Developmental and Behavioral Pediatrics, 13,* 412–420.

Hagin, R. (1998). Bartlett v. New York State Board of Law Examiners: Round two. *LDA Newsbriefs, 33*(6), 3–4.

Hallahan, D. P. (Ed.). (1980). Teaching exceptional children to use cognitive strategies [Special issue]. *Exceptional Education Quarterly, 1*(1).

Hammill, D. D., & Larsen, S. C. (1974). The effectiveness of psycholinguistic training. *Exceptional Children, 41,* 5–14.

Hammill, D. D., & Larsen, S. C. (1996). *Test of written language* (3rd ed.) *(TOWL-3)*. Austin, TX: PRO-ED.

Harding, J. A., & Kleinman, M. D. (1996). Cerebrovascular disorders. In E. S. Batchelor, Jr., & R. S. Dean (Eds.), *Pediatric neuropsychology: Interfacing assessment and treatment for rehabilitation* (pp. 163–210). Needham Heights, MA: Allyn & Bacon.

Haring, N. G., & Gentry, N. D. (1976). Direct and individualized instructional procedures. In N. G. Haring & R. L. Schiefelbusch (Eds.), *Teaching special children* (pp. 72–111). New York: McGraw-Hill.

Harnadek, M. C. S., & Rourke, B. P. (1994). Principal identifying features of the syndrome of nonverbal learning disabilities in children. *Journal of Learning Disabilities, 27,* 144–154.

Harris, K. R., & Graham, S. (Eds.). (1994). Implications of constructivism for students with disabilities and students at risk: Issues and directions [Special issue]. *Journal of Special Education, 28*(3).

Harry, B. (1992). *Cultural diversity, families, and the special education system: Communication and empowerment.* New York: Teachers College Press.

Hatcher, P. J., Hulme, C., & Ellis, A. W. (1994). Ameliorating early reading failure by integrating the teaching of reading and phonological skills: The phonological linkage hypothesis. *Child Development, 65,* 41–57.

Hathaway, S., & McKinley, J. C. (1989). *The Minnesota Multiphasic Personality Inventory* (2nd ed.). Minneapolis, MN: NCS Assessments.

Hermann, K. (1959). *Reading disability: A medical study of word-blindness and related handicaps.* Springfield, IL: Charles C Thomas.

Hessler, G. L. (1993). *Use and interpretation of the Woodcock–Johnson Psycho-Educational Battery—Revised.* Dallas, TX: Riverside.

Hier, D. B., LeMay, M., Rosenberger, P. B., & Perlo, V. P. (1978). Developmental dyslexia: Evidence for a subgroup with reversal of cerebral asymmetry. *Archives of Neurology, 35,* 90–92.

Hooper, S. R., & Olley, J. G. (1996). Psychological comorbidity in adults with learning disabilities. In N. Gregg, C. Hoy, & A. F. Gay (Eds.), *Adults with learning disabilities: Theoretical and practical perspectives* (pp. 162–183). New York: Guilford Press.

Hooper, S. R., Willis, W. G., & Stone, B. H. (1996). Issues and approaches in the neuropsychological treatment of children with learning disabilities. In E. S. Batchelor, Jr., & R. S. Dean (Eds.), *Pediatric neuropsychology: Interfacing assessment and treatment for rehabilitation* (pp. 211–247). Needham Heights, MA: Allyn & Bacon.

Hoy, C., & Manglitz, E. (1996). Social and affective adjustment of adults with learning disabilities: A life-span perspective. In N. Gregg, C. Hoy, & A. F. Gay (Eds.), *Adults with learning disabilities: Theoretical and practical perspectives.* New York: Guilford Press.

Hurt, H., Brodsky, N., Betancourt, L., Braitman, L. E., Malmud, E., & Gianetta, J. (1995). Cocaine-exposed children: Follow-up at 30 months. *Journal of Developmental and Behavioral Pediatrics, 16,* 29–35.

Huston, A. M. (1992). *Understanding dyslexia: A practical approach for parents and teachers.* Lanham, MD: Madison Books.

Hutenlocher, P. (1991, September 26). *Neural plasticity.* Paper presented at the Brain Research Foundation Women's Council. University of Chicago.

Hynd, G. W., Marshall, R., & Gonzalez, J. (1991). Learning disabilities and presumed central nervous system dysfunction. *Learning Disability Quarterly, 14,* 283–296.

Hynd, G. W., Semrud-Clikeman, M., Lorys, A. R., Novey, E. S., & Eliopulos, D. (1990). Brain morphology in developmental dyslexia and attention deficit disorder/hyperactivity. *Archives of Neurology, 47,* 919–926.

Ingersoll, B. D., & Goldstein, S. (1993). *Attention deficit disorder and learning disabilities: Realities, myths, and controversial treatments.* New York: Doubleday.

Iverson, S., & Tunmer, W. E. (1993). Phonological processing skills and the Reading Recovery Program. *Journal of Educational Psychology, 85,* 112–126.

James, E. M., and Selz, M. (1997). Neuropsychological bases of common learning and behavior problems. In C. R. Reynolds & E. Fletcher-Janzen (Eds.), *Handbook of clinical child neuropsychology* (2nd ed., pp. 157–179). New York: Plenum Press.

Joschko, M., & Rourke, B. P. (1985). Neuropsychological subtypes of learning-disabled children who exhibit the ACID pattern on the WISC. In B. P. Rourke (Ed.), *Neuropsychology of learning disabilities: Essentials of subtype analysis* (pp. 65–88). New York: Guilford Press.

Johnson, D. J., & Blalock, J. W. (1987). *Adults with learning disabilities: Clinical studies.* New York: Grune & Stratton.

Johnson, D. J., & Myklebust, H. (1967). *Learning disabilities: Educational principles and practices.* New York: Grune & Stratton.

Kaufman, A. S. (1997). *Intelligent testing with the WISC-III* (4th ed.). New York: Wiley.

Kelley, D. B. (1993). Androgens and brain development: Possible contributions to developmental dyslexia. In A. M. Galaburda (Ed.), *Dyslexia and development: Neurobiological aspects of extra-ordinary brains* (pp. 21–41). Cambridge, MA: Harvard University Press.

Kenny, T., Baldwin, R., & Mackie, J. B. (1967). Incidence of minimal brain injury in adopted children. *Child Welfare, 46,* 24–29.

Keogh, B. K. (1993). Linking purpose and practice: Social-political and developmental perspectives on classification. In G. R. Lyon, D. B. Gray, J. F. Kavanaugh, & N. A. Krasnegor (Eds)., *Better understanding learning disabilities: New views from research and their implications for education and public policies* (pp. 311–323). Baltimore: Paul H. Brookes.

Kirk, S. A., & Kirk, W. D. (1971). *Psycholinguistic learning disabilities: Diagnosis and remediation.* Urbana: University of Illinois Press.

Kolata, G. (1990, August 22). Studies dispute view of dyslexia, finding girls as afflicted as boys. *The New York Times,* pp. A1, B9.

Krasuki, J., Horowitz, B., & Rumsey, J. M. (1996). A survey of functional and anatomical neuroimaging techniques. In G. R. Lyon & J. M. Rumsey (Eds.), *Neuroimaging: A window to the neurological foundations of learning and behavior in children* (pp. 25–52). Baltimore: Paul H. Brookes.

Kronick, D. (1974). Some thoughts on group identification and social needs. *Journal of Learning Disabilities, 7,* 144–147.

Kronick, D. (1976). The importance of a sociological perspective toward learning disabilities. *Journal of Learning Disabilities, 9,* 115–119.

LaBuda, M. C., & DeFries, J. C. (1990). Genetic etiology of reading disability: Evidence from a twin study. In G. T. Pavlidis (Ed.), *Perspectives on dyslexia: Vol. 1. Neurology, neuropsychology, and genetics* (pp. 47–76). New York: Wiley.

Lamm, O., & Epstein, R. (1992). Specific reading impairments: Are they to be associated with emotional difficulties? *Journal of Learning Disabilities, 25,* 605–615.

Lane, B. A. (1980). The relationship of learning disabilities to juvenile delinquency: Current status. *Journal of Learning Disabilities, 13,* 20–29.

Larsen, J. P., Hoien, T., Lundberg, I., & Odegaard, H. (1990). MRI evaluation of the size and symmetry of the planum temporale in adolescents with developmental dyslexia. *Brain and Language, 39,* 289–301.

Larsen, S. C., & Hammill, D. D. (1999). *Test of written spelling* (4th ed). (TWS-4). Austin, TX: PRO-ED.

Larsen, S. C., Parker, R. M., & Hammill, D. D. (1982). Effectiveness of psycholinguistic training: A response to Kavale. *Exceptional Children, 49,* 60–66.

Learning Disability Association (LDA). (1990). Position paper: Eligibility for services for persons with specific learning disabilities. *LDA Newsbriefs, 25*(3), 2a–8a.

Lefly, D. L., & Pennington, B. F. (1991). Spelling errors and reading fluency in compensated adult dyslexics. *Annals of Dyslexia, 41,* 143–162.

Lerner, J. W. (1993). *Learning disabilities: Theories, diagnosis, and teaching strategies* (6th ed.). Boston: Houghton Mifflin.

Levine, M. (1990). *Keeping a head in school.* Cambridge, MA: Educators Publishing Services.

Liberman, I. Y., & Liberman, A. M. (1992). Whole language versus code emphasis: Underlying assumptions and their implications for reading instruction. In P. B. Gough, L. C. Ehri, & R. Treiman (Eds.), *Reading acquisition* (pp. 343–365). Hillsdale, NJ: Erlbaum Associates.

Light, J. G., and DeFries, J. C. (1995). Comorbidity of reading and mathematics disabilities: Genetic and environmental etiologies. *Journal of Learning Disabilities, 28,* 96–106.

Lindamood, C., & Lindamood, P. (1969). *Auditory discrimination in depth.* Allen, TX: Developmental Learning Materials.

Lopez, E. C. (1995). Best practices in working with bilingual children. In A. Thomas & J. Grimes (Eds.), *Best practices in school psychology—III* (3rd ed., pp. 1111–1121). Washington, DC: National Association of School Psychologists.

Lovitt, T. C. (1984). *Tactics for teaching.* Columbus, OH: Merrill.

Lundberg, I., Frost, J., & Petersen, O. (1988). Effects of an extensive program for stimulating phonological awareness in preschool children. *Reading Research Quarterly, 23*(3), 263–283.

Lyon, G. R. (1995). Research initiatives and discoveries in learning disabilities. *Journal of Child Neurology, 10*(Suppl. 1), S120–S126.

Lyon, G. R. (1996a). Foundations of neuroanatomy and neuropsychology. In G. R. Lyon and J. M. Rumsey (Eds.), *Neuroimaging: A window to the neurological foundations of learning and behavior in children* (pp. 1–23). Baltimore: Paul H. Brookes.

Lyon, G. R. (1996b). Learning disabilities. *The Future of Children, 6*(1), 54–76. (Available from the Center for the Future of Children, 300 Second Street, Suite 102, Los Altos, CA 94022-3621)

Lyon, G. R., & Moats, L. (1988). Critical issues in the instruction of the learning disabled. *Journal of Consulting and Clinical Psychology, 56,* 830–835.

Lyon, G. R., Newby, R. E., Recht, D., & Caldwell, J. (1991). Neurospychology and learning disabilities. In B. Y. L. Wong (Ed.), *Learning about learning disabilities* (pp. 68–93). San Diego, CA: Academic Press.

Lyytinen, H. (1995). Comorbidity and developmental neurocognitive disorders [Special issue]. *Developmental Neuropsychology, 11*(3), 269–273.

MacMillan, D. L. (1993). Development of operational definitions in mental retardation: Similarities and differences with the field of learning disabilities. In G. R. Lyon, D. B. Gray, J. F. Kavanaugh, & N. A. Krasnegor (Eds.), *Better understanding learning disabilities: New views from research and their implications for education and public policies* (pp. 117–152). Baltimore: Paul H. Brookes.

Marin-Padilla, M. (1993). Pathogenesis of late-acquired leptomeningeal heterotopias and secondary cortical alterations: A Golgi study. In A. M. Galaburda (Ed.), *Dyslexia and development: Neurobiological aspects of extra-ordinary brains* (pp. 64–88). Cambridge, MA: Harvard University Press.

Marston, D., & Tindal, R. (1995). Performance monitoring. In A. Thomas & J. Grimes (Eds.), *Best practices in school psychology—III* (3rd ed., pp. 597–608). Washington, DC: National Association of School Psychologists.

Mather, N. (1991). *An instructional guide to the Woodcock–Johnson Psycho-Educational Battery—Revised.* Brandon, VT: Clinical Psychology.

Mather, N., & Jaffe, L. E. (1992). *Woodcock–Johnson Psycho-Educational Battery—Revised: Recommendations and reports.* New York: Wiley.

Mather, N., & Roberts, R. (1994). Learning disabilities: A field in danger of extinction? *Learning Disabilities Research and Practice, 9*(1), 49–58.

Mattis, S., French, J., & Rapin, I. (1975). Dyslexia in children and young adults: Three independent neuropsychological syndromes. *Developmental Medicine and Child Neurology, 17,* 150–163.

Mazzacco, M. (1996). Social and academic learning disabilities in children with identified genetic syndromes. In G. R. Lyon (Chair), *Critical discoveries in learning disabilities: A summary of findings by NIH research programs in learning disabilities.* Workshop conducted at the International Conference of the Learning Disability Association, Dallas, TX.

McCann, J. (1989). An invisible battle. *Their World: A Publication of the National Center for Learning Disabilities,* p. 104. (Available from NCLD, 381 Park Avenue, Suite, 1420, New York, NY 10016)

McElgunn, B. (1996). Critical discoveries in learning disabilities: A summary of findings by NIH research programs in learning disabilities. *LDA Newsbriefs, 31*(4), 3–4.

Medical diagnoses/conditions which might be indicators of learning disabilities. (1998). *LDA Newsbriefs, 33*(1), 8.

Mercer, C. D. (1991). *Students with learning disabilities* (4th ed.). New York: Macmillan.

Mercer, C. D., Forgnone, C., & Wolking, W. D. (1976). Definitions of learning disabilities used in the United States. *Journal of Learning Disabilities, 9,* 376–386.

Mercer, C. D., King-Sears, P., & Mercer, A. R. (1990). Learning disabilities definitions and criteria used by state education departments. *Learning Disabilities Quarterly, 13,* 141–152.

Mercer, C. D., & Mercer, A. R. (1993). *Teaching students with learning problems* (4th ed.). New York: Maxwell Macmillan.

Merzenich, M. M., Jenkins, W. M., Johnston, P., Schreiner, C., Miller, S. L., & Tallal, P. (1996). Temporal processing deficits of language learning-impaired children ameliorated by training. *Science, 271,* 77–81.

Morrison, G. M., & Cosden, M. A. (1997). Risk, resilience, and adjustment of individuals with learning disabilities. *Learning Disability Quarterly, 20,* 43–60.

Mosley-Howard, G. S. (1995). Best practices in considering the role of culture. In A. Thomas & J. Grimes (Eds.), *Best practices in school psychology—III* (3rd ed., pp. 337–345). Washington, DC: National Association of School Psychologists.

Mulhern, R. K. (1996). Intracranial tumors. In E. S. Batchelor, Jr., & R. S. Dean (Eds.), *Pediatric neuropsychology: Interfacing assessment and treatment for rehabilitation* (pp. 139–162). Needham Heights, MA: Allyn & Bacon.

Murray, C. A. (1976). *The link between learning disabilities and juvenile delinquency: Current theory and knowledge.* Washington, D.C.: American Institutes for Research in the Behavioral Sciences. (ERIC Document Reproduction Service No. ED237896)

Nash, M. (1997, February 3). Fertile minds. *Time,* pp. 48–56.

National Institute of Mental Health (NIMH). (1993). *Learning disabilities* (DHHS Publication No. ADM 93-359-181/90204). Washington, DC: U.S. Government Printing Office.

Nicholas, S. W., Sondheimer, D. L., Willoughby, A. D., Yaffe, S. L., & Katz, S. L. (1989). Human immunodeficiency virus infection in childhood, adolescence and pregnancy: A status report and national research agenda. *Pediatrics, 83,* 293–308.

Olivarez, A., Palmer, D. A., & Guillemard, L. (1992). Predictive bias with referred and nonreferred black, Hispanic, and white pupils. *Learning Disability Quarterly,* 175–186.

Olson, R. K., Wise, B., Conners, F., Rack, J., & Fulker, D. (1989). Specific deficits in component reading and language skills: Genetic and environmental influences. *Journal of Learning Disabilities, 22,* 339–348.

Paulesu, E., Frith, U., Snowling, M., Gallagher, A., Morton, J., Frackowiak, R. S. J., & Frith, C. D. (1996). Is developmental dyslexia a disconnection syndrome?: Evidence from PET scanning. *Brain, 119,* 143–157.

Pauls, D. L. (1996, March). Genetic linkage studies. In G. R. Lyon (Chair), *Critical discoveries in learning disabilities: A summary of findings by NIH research programs in learning disabilities.* Workshop conducted at the International Conference of the Learning Disability Association, Dallas, TX.

Pennington, B. F. (1991). *Diagnosing learning disorders: A neuropsychological framework.* New York: Guilford Press.

Pennington, B. F., Bender, B., Puck, M., Salbenblatt, J., & Robinson, A. (1982). Learning disabilities in children with sex chromosome anomalies. *Child Development, 53,* 1182–1192.

Pennington, B. F., Gilger, J. W., Pauls, D., Smith, S. A., Smith, S., & DeFries, J. C. (1991). Evidence for major gene transmission of developmental dyslexia. *Journal of the American Medical Association, 266,* 1527–1534.

Pennington, B. F., Grossier, D., & Welsh, M. C. (1993). Contrasting cognitive deficits in attention deficit hyperactivity disorder versus reading disability. *Developmental Psychology, 29,* 511–523.

Petrauskas, R., & Rourke, B. P. (1979). Identification of subgroups of retarded readers: A neuropsychological multivariate approach. *Journal of Clinical Neuropsychology, 1,* 17–37.

Phillips, G. W. (1983). Learning the conversation concept: A meta-analysis (Doctoral dissertation, University of Kentucky). *Dissertation Abstracts International, 44,* 1990B.

Pipitone, P. (1991, October–November). Acquired pediatric brain damage: Diverse causes. *HEAD-LINES,* p. 5.

Pirozzolo, F. J., & Bonnefil, V. (1996). Disorders appearing in the prenatal and neonatal period. In E. S. Batchelor, Jr., & R. S. Dean (Eds.), *Pediatric neuropsychology: Interfacing assessment and treatment for rehabilitation* (pp. 55–84). Needham Heights, MA: Allyn & Bacon.

Pollitt, E., Golub, M., Gorman, K., Grantham-McGregor, S., Levitsky, D., Schürch, B., Strupp, B., & Wachs, T. (1996). A reconceptualization of the effects of undernutrition on children's biological, psychological, and behavioral development. *Social Policy Report of the Society for Research in Child Development, 10*(5), 1–22.

Polloway, E. A., Smith, J. D., & Patton, J. R. (1984). Learning disabilities: An adult development perspective. *Learning Disability Quarterly, 7,* 179–186.

Porter, J. E., & Rourke, B. P. (1985). Socioemotional functioning of learning-disabled children: A subtypal analysis of personality patterns. In B. P. Rourke (Ed.), *Neuropsychology of learning disabilities: Essentials of subtype analysis* (pp. 237–251). New York: Guilford Press.

Posner, M. I., & Raichle, M. E. (1994). *Images of mind.* New York: Scientific American Library.

Pressley, M., & Rankin, J. (1994). More about whole language methods of reading instruction for students at risk for early reading failure. *Learning Disabilities Research and Practice, 9*(3), 157–168.

Puente, A. E., Sol Mora, M., & Munoz-Cespedes, J. M. (1997). Neuropsychological assessment of Spanish-speaking children and youth. In C. R. Reynolds & E. Fletcher-Janzen (Eds.), *Handbook of clinical child neuropsychology* (2nd ed., 371–386). New York: Plenum Press.

Raskind, M. (1993). Assistive technology and adults with learning disabilities: A blueprint for exploration and advancement. *Learning Disability Quarterly, 16,* 185–196.

Reiff, H. B., Gerber, P. J., & Ginsberg, R. (1994). Instructional strategies for long-term success. *Annals of Dyslexia, 44,* 270–288.

Reschly, D. J. (1996). Identification of students with disabilities. *The Future of Children, 6*(1), 40–53. (Available from Center for the Future of Children, 300 Second Street, Suite 102, Los Altos, CA 94022–3621)

Reschly, D. J., & Wilson, M. S. (1990). Cognitive processing vs. traditional intelligence: Diagnostic utility, intervention implications, and treatment validity. *School Psychology Review, 26,* 120–142.

Reschly, D. J., & Ysseldyke, J. E. (1995). School psychology a paradigm shift. In A. Thomas & J. Grimes (Eds.), *Best practices in school psychology—III* (3rd ed., pp. 17–31). Washington, DC: National Association of School Psychologists.

Research Services Committee. (1995). Thyroid function and learning disabilities: Is there a connection? *LDA Newsbriefs, 30*(4), 17.

Reynolds, C. R., & Fletcher-Janzen, E. (Eds.) (1997). *The handbook of clinical child neuropsychology* (2nd ed.). New York: Plenum.

Reynolds, C. R., & Kaiser, S. M. (1990). Bias in assessment of aptitude. In C. R. Reynold & R. W. Kamphaus (Eds.), *Handbook of psychological and educational assessment of children: Intelligence and achievement* (pp. 611–653). New York: Guilford Press.

Riccio, C. A., & Hynd, G. W. (1996). Neurobiological research specific to the adult population with learning disabilities. In N. Gregg, C. Hoy, & A. F. Gay (Eds.), *Adults with learning disabilities: Theoretical and practical perspectives* (pp. 127–143). New York: Guilford Press.

Roffman, A. J., Herzog, J. E., & Wershba-Gershon, P. M. (1994). Helping young adults understand their learning disabilities. *Journal of Learning Disabilities, 27*, 413–419.

Rosenberger, P. B., & Hier, D. B. (1980). Cerebral asymmetry and verbal intellectual deficits. *Annals of Neurology, 8*, 300–304.

Rourke, B. P. (1978). Neuropsychological research in reading retardation: A review. In A. Benton & D. Pearl (Eds), *Dyslexia: An appraisal of current knowledge* (pp. 139–172). New York: Oxford University Press.

Rourke, B. P. (Ed.). (1985). *Neuropsychology of learning disabilities: Essentials of subtype analysis.* New York: Guilford Press.

Rourke, B. P. (1987). Syndrome of nonverbal learning disabilities: The final common pathway of white-matter disease/dysfunction? *The Clinical Neuropsychologist, 1*(3), 209–234.

Rourke, B. P. (1989). *Nonverbal learning disabilities: The syndrome and the model.* New York: Guilford Press.

Rourke, B. P., & Del Dotto, J. E. (1994). *Learning disabilities: A neuropsychological perspective.* London: Sage.

Rourke, B. P., Fisk, T. L., & Strang, J. D. (1986). *Neuropsychological assessment of children: A treatment-oriented approach.* New York: Guilford Press.

Rumsey, J. M. (1996). Neuroimaging in developmental dyslexia: A review and conceptualization. In G. R. Lyon & J. M. Rumsey (Eds.), *Neuroimaging: A window to the neurological foundations of learning and behavior in children* (pp. 57–77). Baltimore: Paul H. Brookes.

Ryan, T. V., LaMarche, J. A., Barth, J. T., & Boll, T. J. (1996). Neuropsychological consequences and treatment of pediatric head trauma. In E. S. Batchelor, Jr., & R. S. Dean (Eds.), *Pediatric neuropsychology: Interfacing assessment and treatment for rehabilitation* (pp. 117–137). Needham Heights, MA: Allyn & Bacon.

Safer, D. J., & Allen, R. P. (1976). *Hyperactive children: Diagnosis and management.* Baltimore: University Park Press.

Saigal, S., Rosenbaum, P., Szatmari, P., & Campbell, D. (1991). Learning disabilities and school problems in a regional cohort of extremely low birth weight (<1000 G) children: A comparison with term controls. *Journal of Developmental and Behavioral Pediatrics, 12*, 294–300.

Satz, P. (1990). Developmental dyslexia: An etiological reformulation. In G. T. Pavlidis (Ed.), *Perspectives on dyslexia: Vol. 1. Neurology, neuropsychology, and genetics* (pp. 3–26). New York: Wiley.

Satz, P., & Morris, R. (1981). Learning disability subtypes: A review. In F. J. Priozzolo & M. C. Wittrock (Eds.), *Neuropsychological and cognitive processes in reading.* New York: Academic Press.

Schumaker, J. B., Deshler, D. D., Alley, G. R., & Warner, M. M. (1983). Toward the development of an intervention model for learning disabled adolescents: The University of Kansas Institute. *Exceptional Child Quarterly, 4*, 45–74.

Scott, S. (1994). Determining reasonable academic adjustments for college students with learning disabilities. *Journal of Learning Disabilities, 27*, 403–412.

Shapiro, H. R. (1992). Debatable issues underlying whole language philosophy: A speech pathologist's perspective. *Language, Speech, and Hearing Services in Schools, 23,* 308–311.

Shaywitz, B. A., Fletcher, J. M., & Shaywitz, S. E. (1995). Defining and classifying learning disabilities and attention deficit/hyperactive disorder. *Journal of Child Neurology, 10*(Suppl. 1), S50–S57.

Shaywitz, B. A., & Shaywitz, S. E. (1994). Measuring and analyzing change. In G. R. Lyon (Ed.), *Frames of reference for the assessment of learning disabilities: New Views on measurement issues* (pp. 29–58). Baltimore: Paul H. Brookes.

Shaywitz, S. E. (1996). Dyslexia. *Scientific American, 275*(5), 98–104.

Shaywitz, S. E., & Shaywitz, B. A, (1987). Attention deficit disorder: Current perspectives. *Pediatric Neurology, 3,* 129–135.

Shaywitz, S. E., & Shaywitz, B. A, (1997/1998). *The Yale Center for the Study of Learning and Attention Disorders: Longitudinal and neurobiological studies. Their world: A Publication of the National Center for Learning Disabilities,* pp. 27–31. (Available from NCLD, 381 Park Avenue South, Suite 1420, New York, NY 10016)

Shaywitz, S. E., Shaywitz, B. A., Fletcher, J. M., & Escobar, M. D. (1990). Prevalence of reading disability in boys and girls: Results of the Connecticut Longitudinal Study. *Journal of the American Medical Association, 264,* 998–1002.

Shaywitz, S. E., Shaywitz, B. A., Pugh, K. R., Skudlarski, P., Fulbright, R. K., Constable, R. T., Bronen, R. A., Fletcher, J. M., Liberman, A. M., Shankweiler, D. P., Katz, L., Lacadie, C., Marchione, K. E., & Gore, J. C. (1996). The neurobiology of developmental dyslexia as viewed through the lens of functional magnetic resonance imaging technology. In G. R. Lyon & J. M. Rumsey (Eds.), *Neuroimaging: A window to the neurological foundations of learning and behavior in children* (pp. 79–94). Baltimore: Paul H. Brookes.

Silver, A. A., & Hagin, R. A. (1990). *Disorders of learning in childhood.* New York: Wiley.

Silver, L. B. (1970). Frequency of adoption in children with neurological learning disability syndrome. *Journal of Learning Disability, 3,* 306–310.

Silver, L. B. (1975). Acceptable and controversial approaches to treating the child with learning disabilities. *Pediatrics, 55,* 406–415.

Silver, L. B. (1989). Frequency of adoption of children and adolescents with learning disabilities. *Journal of Learning Disabilities, 22,* 325–327.

Silver, L. B. (1990). Attention deficit-hyperactivity disorder: Is it a learning disability or a related disorder? *Journal of Learning Disabilities, 23,* 394–397.

Silver, L. B. (1995). Controversial therapies. *Journal of Child Neurology, 10*(Suppl. 1), S96–S100.

Skaret, D., & Wilgosh, L. (1989). Learning disabilities and juvenile delinquency: A casual relationship? *International Journal for the Advancement of Counselling, 12,* 113–123.

Smith, S. D., Kimberling, W. J., Pennington, B. F., & Lubs, H. A. (1983). Specific reading disability: Identification of an inherited form through linkage analysis. *Science, 219,* 1345–1347.

Smith, S. D., Pennington, B. F., Kimberling, W. J., & Ing, P. S. (1990). Genetic linkage analysis with specific dyslexia: Use of multiple markers to include and exclude possible loci. In G. T. Pavlidis (Ed.), *Perspectives on dyslexia: Vol. 1. Neurology, neuropsychology and genetics* (pp. 77–89). New York: Wiley.

Snowling, M., & Hulme, C. (1991). Speech processing and learning to spell. In W. Ellis (Ed.), *All language and the creation of literacy.* Baltimore: Orton Dyslexia Society.

Spector, S., Decker, K., & Shaw, S. F. (1991). Independence and responsibility: An LD resource room at South Windsor High School. *Intervention in School and Clinic, 26,* 248–245.

Stanovich, K. E. (1993). The construct validity of discrepancy definitions of reading disability. In G. R. Lyon, D. B. Gray, J. F. Kavanaugh, & N. A. Krasnegor (Eds.), *Better understanding learning disabilities: New views from research and their implications for education and public policies* (pp. 273–307). Baltimore: Paul H. Brookes.

Stanovich, K. E. (1994). Constructivism in reading education. *Journal of Special Education, 28,* 259–274.

Stanovich, K. E., & Siegel, L. S. (1994). Phenotypic performance profile of children with reading disabilities: A regression-based test of the phonological-core variable-difference model. *Journal of Educational Psychology, 86,* 24–53.

Strang, J. D., & Rourke, B. P. (1985). Adaptive behavior of children who exhibit specified arithmetic disabilities and associated neuropsychological deficits. In B. P. Rourke (Ed.), *Neuropsychology of learning disabilities: Essentials of subtype analysis* (pp. 302–328). New York: Guilford Press.

Strauss, A., & Lehtinen, L. (1947). *Psychopathology and education of the brain-injured child.* New York: Grune & Stratton.

Suzuki, L. A., & Valencia, R. R. (1997). Race–ethnicity and measured intelligence: Educational implications. *American Psychologist, 52,* 1103–1114.

Swanson, H. L. (1993). Learning disabilities from the perspective of cognitive psychology. In G. R. Lyon, D. B. Gray, J. F. Kavanaugh, & N. A. Krasnegor (Eds.), *Better understanding learning disabilities: New views from research and their implications for education and public policies* (pp. 199–228). Baltimore: Paul H. Brookes.

Swartz, G. A. (1974). *The language-learning system.* New York: Simon & Schuster.

Tesman, J. R., & Hills, A. (1994). Developmental effects of lead exposure in children. *Social Policy Report of the Society for Research in Child Development, 8*(3), 1–16.

Thomson, M. (1990). *Developmental dyslexia* (3rd ed.). London: Whurr.

Thompson, S. (1997). *The source for nonverbal learning disorders.* East Moline, IL: LinguiSystems.

Torgesen, J. K. (1986). Learning disabilities theory: Its current state and future prospects. *Journal of Learning Disabilities, 19*(7), 399–407.

Torgesen, J. K. (1993). Variations on theory in learning disabilities. In G. R. Lyon, D. B. Gray, J. F. Kavanaugh, & N. A. Krasnegor (Eds.), *Better understanding learning disabilities: New views from Research and their implications for education and public policies* (pp. 153–170). Baltimore: Paul H. Brookes.

Torgesen, J. K. (1998). Learning disabilities: An historical and conceptual overview. In B. Y.L. Wong (Ed.), *Learning about learning disabilities* (2nd ed., pp. 3–34). San Diego, CA: Academic Press.

Torgesen, J. K., Wagner, R. K., & Rashotte, C. A. (1994). Longitudinal studies of phonological processing and reading. *Journal of Learning Disabilities, 27,* 276–286.

Torgesen, J. K., Wagner, R. K., & Rashotte, C. A. (1997). Approaches to the prevention and remediation of phonologically based reading disabilities. In B. A. Blachman (Ed.), *Foundations of reading acquisition and dyslexia: Implications for early intervention* (pp. 287–304). Mahwah, NJ: Erlbaum.

Toth, G., & Siegel, L. S. (1994). A critical evaluation of the I.Q.–achievement discrepancy-based definitions of dyslexia. In K. P. vanden Bos, L. S. Siegel, D. J. Bakker, & D. L. Share (Eds.), *Current directions in dyslexia research* (pp. 45–70). Lisse, The Netherlands: Swets & Zeitlinger.

Travis, J. (1996). Let the games begin. *Science News, 149,* 104–106.

Truch, S. (1994). Stimulating basic reading processes using Auditory Discrimination in Depth. *Annals of Dyslexia, 44,* 60–80.

Voeller, K. K. S. (1986). Right-hemisphere deficit syndrome in children. *American Journal of Psychiatry, 143,* 1004–1009.

Vohr, B., Coll, C. G., Lobato, D., Yunis, K. A., O'Dea, C., & Oh, W. (1991). Neurodevelopmental and medical status of low-birthweight survivors of bronchopulmonary dysplasia at 10 to 12 years of age. *Developmental Medicine and Child Neurology,* 690–697.

Wagner, M. M., & Blackorby, J. (1996). Transition from high school to work or college: How special education students fare. A summary of selected findings from the National Longitudinal Transition Study of Special Education Students, emphasizing outcomes and effective interventions. *The Future of Children, 6*(1), 103–120. (Available from Center for the Future of Children, 300 Second Street, Suite 102, Los Altos, CA 94022–3621)

Wagner, R. K., & Torgesen, J. K. (1987). The nature of phonological processing and its causal role in the acquisition of reading skills. *Psychological Bulletin, 101*(2), 192–212.

Waldie, K., & Spreen, O. (1993). The relationship between learning disabilities and persisting delinquency. *Journal of Learning Disabilities, 26,* 417–423.

Walters, J. A., & Croen, L. G. (1993). An approach to meeting the needs of medical students with learning disabilities. *Teaching and Learning in Medicine, 5*(1), 29–35.

Waterman, B. B. (1994). Assessing children for the presence of a disability. *National Center for Children and Youth with Disabilities (NICHCY) News Digest, 4*(1), pp. 1–27.

Welch, M., & Jensen, J. (1990). Write, P.L.E.A.S.E.: A video-assisted strategic intervention to improve written expression of inefficient learners. *Remedial and Special Education, 12,* 37–46.

White, O. R. (1986). Precision teaching—precision learning. *Exceptional Children, 52,* 522–534.

White, W. J. (1992). The postschool adjustment of persons with learning disabilities: Current status and future projections. *Journal of Learning Disabilities, 25,* 448–456.

Wiederholt, J. L., & Bryant, B. R. (1992). *Gray Oral Reading Tests—Third Edition (GORT-3).* Austin, TX: PRO-ED.

Wilkinson, G. S. (1993). *Wide Range Achievement Test* (3rd ed.) *(WRAT-3).* Wilmington, DE: Jastak Associates.

Wirt, R. D., Lachar, D., Klinedinst, J. E., & Seat, P. D. (1977). *Multidimensional assessment of child personality: A Manual for the Personality Inventory for Children.* Los Angeles: Western Psychological Services.

Wissick, C. A. (1996). Multimedia: Enhancing instruction for students with learning disabilities. *Journal of Learning Disabilities, 29,* 494–503.

Woodcock, R. W. (1987). *The Woodcock Reading Mastery Tests—Revised.* Circle Pines, MN: American Guidance Service.

Woodcock, R. W., & Johnson, M. B. (1989). *The Woodcock–Johnson Psycho-Educational Battery—Revised.* Allen, TX: DLM Teaching Resources.

Worrall, R. S. (1990). Detecting health fraud in the field of learning disabilities. *Journal of Learning Disabilities, 23,* 207–212.

Wyngaarden, J. E. (1987). *Learning disabilities: A report to the Congress.* Washington, DC: National Institutes of Health, Interagency Committee on Learning Disabilities.

Young, G. (1996). To tell or not to tell: Self-identification, self-advocacy, and civil rights in employment and post secondary education. *LDA Newsbriefs, 31*(4), 10–11.

Ysseldyke, J. E., & Mirkin, P. K. (1982). The use of assessment information to plan instructional interventions: A review of the research. In C. R. Reynolds & T. B. Gutkin (Eds.), *The handbook of school psychology* (pp. 395–409). New York: Wiley.

Zerbin-Rudin, E. (1967). Congenital word-blindness. *Bulletin of the Orton Society, 17,* 47–55.

Zigmond, N. (1993). Learning disabilities from an educational perspective. In G. R. Lyon, D. B. Gray, J. F. Kavanaugh, & N. A. Krasnegor (Eds.), *Better understanding learning disabilities: New views from research and their implications for education and public policies* (pp. 251–272). Baltimore: Paul H. Brookes.

7

ATTENTION-DEFICIT/HYPERACTIVITY DISORDER

SAM GOLDSTEIN

The childhood cognitive and behavioral difficulties categorized as problems of inattention, impulsivity, and hyperactivity have presented a clinical challenge for neuropsychologists over the past 50 years. The symptom constellation referred to as attention deficit disorder (ADD) or, more recently, attention-deficit/hyperactivity disorder (ADHD; American Psychiatric Association [APA], 1994) has become one of the most widely researched areas in childhood and adolescence, with an increasing emphasis on research throughout the adult lifespan. Problems arising from this constellation of symptoms have constituted the most chronic childhood behavior disorder (Wender, 1975) and the largest single source of referrals to mental health centers (Barkley, 1981). More recently, it has been suggested that children with ADHD may account for as many as 40% of referrals to child guidance clinics (Barkley, 1998b). In clinic settings, males outnumber females 6:1. In epidemiological studies of community settings, the ratio is 3:1 (Barkley, 1998b). The higher clinic ratio for males has been suggested as a function of the greater prevalence of other disruptive problems, such as oppositional defiant disorder and conduct disorder, in boys with ADHD (Breen & Barkley, 1988).

Even as neuropyschologists utilize the current diagnostic criteria involving symptoms of inattention, hyperactivity, and impulsivity, an increasing amount of data suggests that for the majority of affected children impulsivity represents the core deficit (for a review, see Goldstein & Goldstein, 1998). Problems with impulsivity affect children's interactions with all areas of their environment and result in the inability to meet situational demands in an age-appropriate fashion (Routh, 1978). Children with ADHD typically experience difficulties in all aspects and situations of their lives. Their behavior is often uneven, unpredictable, and inconsistent. The almost magician-like quality of their behavior—"now you see it, now you don't"—adds additional stress for caregivers and educators. It frequently leads to the erroneous belief that these children have problems of poor motivation or limited desire, rather than neurologically based difficulties.

As early as 1979, Bellak suggested that ADHD may be a lifetime disorder. Recent research very clearly reflects the significant and pervasive impact symptoms of ADHD have on the majority of affected children as they enter their adult years (for a review, see Goldstein, 1997). It is now accepted that years of inability to meet the expectations of one's surroundings results in a long history of negative interaction with others in the environment. This in turn becomes a major force in the affected individual's emerging personality (Wender, 1979). It has been well recognized that the daily experiences of children contribute to their outcomes in adult life, with even small successes building resilience and capacity to deal with life stress (Werner, 1994). Thus neuropsychologists evaluating ADHD today must be concerned not only with the core symptoms of this disorder and their direct, immediate impact on children, but with the significant secondary impact of these problems upon children's current and future lives, as well as the lives of their family members.

Although some have argued that the problems of ADHD constitute a cultural phenomenon (Block, 1977), it is well accepted at present that ADHD is a disorder in which the severity of a child's problems results from the interaction between temperamental traits and the demands placed upon the child by the environment. ADHD very clearly reflects a biopsychosocial problem: Biology appears to set the stage, but environment may well determine level of complaints and severity. Ideus (1994) has argued that although culture makes a difference in terms of the expectations and symptoms placed upon children, children with ADHD demonstrate a fairly homogeneous set of problems. This finding has been cross-culturally confirmed by other investigators (Mann, Ikeda, Muller, & Takahshi, 1992; Tao, 1992; Gray & Sime, 1989).

It has also been argued that as the tempo of our society increases, we are seeing a greater incidence of ADHD (McNamara, 1972). There is no doubt that the reported prevalence of ADHD, based upon rates of diagnosis and medication treatment, has increased at a nearly exponential rate during the 1980s and 1990s (Safer, Sito, & Fine, 1996). However, normative data obtained for assessment tools such as the revised and third editions of the Wechsler Intelligence Scale for Children do not support the hypothesis that children are increasingly less attentive or more impulsive (Wechsler, 1974, 1989; Spring, Yellin, & Greenberg, 1976). In fact, it has been suggested that due to children's early exposure to the mass media, their capacity for sustained attention has actually increased at younger ages rather than decreased. A more likely explanation for the increase in diagnosis is the increasing community, professional, and parental awareness concerning symptoms of ADHD, which may well have led to more children's being referred, correctly identified, and offered treatment (Goldstein, 1995).

The controversy and frequent confusion concerning various aspects of ADHD may in part be the results of a tradition of viewing this disorder as a unitary phenomenon with a single cause. Voeller (1991) suggests that rather than viewing ADHD as a single behavioral abnormality with associated comorbidities, it may be better to conceptualize ADHD as a "cluster of different behavioral deficits, each with a specific neuro-substrate of varying severity occurring in variable constellations and sharing a common response to psychostimulants" (p. S4). There is no doubt, however, that the cluster of symptomatic problems constituting the diagnosis of ADHD represents a distinct disorder from other disorders of childhood and adulthood (Biederman et al., 1996; Accardo, Blondis, & Whitman, 1990). The consensus among researchers and clinicians is that the core symptoms of ADHD affect a significant minority of our population. For affected individuals, however, ADHD represents a poor fit between society's expectations and these individuals' abilities to meet those expectations. This phenomenon is distinct from other disorders of childhood and adulthood, and it can be reliably evaluated and effectively treated.

TOWARD A WORKING DEFINITION OF ADHD

Attention as a Theoretical Concept

It is likely that "attention" as a theoretical or laboratory-measured concept is quite different from the construct of "attention" as a process or processes that are disrupted in ADHD. Nonetheless, prior to a review of the currently accepted ADHD diagnostic criteria and related issues, a brief discussion of attention as a theoretical concept is valuable.

"Attention" is considered a generic term used to designate a group of hypothetical mechanisms that collectively serve a function for the organism (Mesulam, 1985). Beginning with James (1890), researchers have identified attentional processes as essential prerequisites for higher cognitive functions. Hypothetical models of the development of attention have included a stagewise model (Blondis, Snow, Stein, & Roizen, 1991), as well as a model of a maturational process similar to the maturation of other executive or intellectual skills (Hagen & Hale, 1973). Although Posner and Snyder (1975) described attention as a complex field of study, others have suggested that attentional skills can be operationally and statistically defined with some confidence (Gordon & McClure, 1983). Skinner (1953) defined attention as a functional relationship between stimuli and responses. His belief was that attention is not a thing, entity, or mental function, but is a description of a set of relations between stimuli or events and responses to them. Gibson and Radner (1979) defined attention as the ability to perceive the environment in relation to a specific goal. Posner (1987) suggested that attention may consist of automatic versus conscious aspects. Finally, Fuster (1989) provided a concept of inhibition interference in his neuropsychological model of executive function related to attention. All of these theories, as well as Titchener's (1924) description of attention as a pattern of consciousness, appear to be extensions of James's (1890) characterization of attention as bimodal. James hypothesized that attention is either passive, reflective, nonvoluntary, and effortless, or active and voluntary. James defined "sustained attention" as the active and voluntary type, which is dependent upon repeated redirection of focus toward the object of attention and upon resistance to attractions that coexist in the process.

Picano, Klusman, Hornbestel, and Moulton (1992) conducted a factor analaysis that suggested three factors for attention. The first factor accounted for 35% of the variance and involved skills related to visual–motor scanning and shifting abilities. The capacity to divide attention appeared to be key to this task. The second factor accounted for 16% of the variance and reflected immediate attention and conceptual tracking consistent with the ability to repeat digits both forward and backward. Finally, the third factor accounted for 13.5% of the variance and reflected sustained, effortful processing consistent with distractibility tasks. This breakdown is consistent with factor analyses by other investigators (Shum, MacFarland, & Bain, 1990).

From a neuropsychological perspective, the concept of attention as an executive function has gained increasing popularity. Sustained mental effort, self-regulation, planning, execution, and maintenance are considered measures of executive functioning (Daigneault, Braun, and Whitaker, 1992). Mirskey, Anthony, Duncan, Ahearn, and Kellam (1991) developed a neuropsychological model of attention involving four basic concepts: the ability to focus, execute, sustain or code, and shift. Eight traditional assessment measures of attention were used in a factor-analytic study to arrive at this model.

The Nature of ADHD Symptoms

Increasingly, there is a consensus that ADHD represents a problem of faulty performance rather than faulty input. It is not so much that affected individuals do not know what to do, but that they do not do what they know consistently. It is a problem of inconsistency rather than inability (Goldstein & Goldstein, 1992). Even in their adaptive skills, this pattern of difference between possessing a skill and using it efficiently has been well defined for individuals with ADHD (Stein, 1997).

It is important for the neuropsychologist to possess a working understanding of the *Diagnostic and Statistical Manual of Mental Disorders*, fourth edition (DSM-IV) diagnostic criteria for ADHD, a practical perception of the manner in which the symptoms affect the individual's functioning, and a diagnostic strategy. The traditional disease model is not relevant to the definition of ADHD (Ellis, 1985). ADHD is more like obesity or intelligence: Individuals differ not in having or not having the traits, but in the degree of their manifestation. ADHD symptoms are multidimensional rather than unitary (Guevremont, DuPaul, & Barkley, 1993). However, there continues to be discussion as to which dimensions represent the most clearly distinguishing deficits of the disorder. The frequency and severity of symptoms fluctuate across settings, activities, and caregivers (Tarver-Behring, Barkley, & Karlsson, 1985; Zentall, 1984). There is a general consensus, however, that symptoms of ADHD fall into two broad factors: symptoms related to the behavioral manifestation of faulty attention, and those related to hyperactivity and impulsivity. Symptoms of hyperactivity and impulsivity appear to co-occur at such a high frequency that it is difficult to separate them on a factor-analytic basis. It is also important for neuropsychologists to recognize that at times the lines blur between the symptoms and consequences of ADHD. Thus a diagnostic strategy for ADHD should include not only identifying symptoms, but a list of skills and life problems hypothesized to be directly affected by symptoms. Having the symptoms without negative consequences would in fact preclude the diagnosis of ADHD according to DSM-IV criteria.

DSM-IV Criteria for ADHD

The DSM-IV diagnostic criteria (APA, 1994) represent an effort to move forward and correct the mistaken notion that ADHD represents a unipolar disorder. The DSM-IV field studies for the ADHD diagnosis were more comprehensive and better structured than previous efforts. The DSM-IV criteria appear in Table 7.1.

Of the 276 children diagnosed with ADHD in the DSM-IV field studies, 55% had the combined type, 27% the predominantly inattentive type, and 18% the predominantly hyperactive–impulse type (Lahey et al., 1994). Fewer than half (44%) of those with the hyperactive–impulsive type of ADHD received a DSM-III diagnosis of ADD with hyperactivity; these two diagnoses, therefore, only partially overlapped. The children in the hyperactive–impulsive group had fewer symptoms of inattention than children with the combined type did. They also had fewer symptoms of hyperactive–impulsive problems, suggesting that the hyperactive–impulsive type represents a less severe variant of the disorder. The hyperactive–impulsive group contained 20% females, the combined group 12%, and the inattentive group 27%. This last statistic corresponds with neuropsychologists' perceptions that females more often demonstrate the inattentive type of ADHD. This overrepresentation has not been well explained by any theoretical model (Silverthorn, Frick, Kuper, & Ott, 1996), nor is it understood why preliminary research suggests that females with ADHD may be less likely to demonstrate deficits in executive functioning than males (Seidman et al., 1997). The hyperactive–impulsive group was also younger than the other two groups in the field studies. Moreover, they had fewer symptoms of oppositional defiant disorder or conduct disorder than those with the combined type of ADHD.

A number of researchers have demonstrated the validity of the current DSM-IV diagnostic conceptualization for ADHD, utilizing various clinical and laboratory measures. Such

TABLE 7.1. DSM-IV Criteria for Attention-Deficit/Hyperactivity Disorder (ADHD)

A. Either (1) or (2):

   (1) six or more of the following symptoms of **inattention** have persisted for at least 6 months to a degree that is maladaptive and inconsistent with developmental level:

   Inattention
   (a) often fails to give close attention to details or makes careless mistakes in schoolwork, work, or other activities
   (b) often has difficulty sustaining attention in tasks or play activities
   (c) often does not seem to listen when spoken to directly
   (d) often does not follow through on instructions and fails to finish schoolwork, chores, or duties in the workplace (not due to oppositional behavior or failure to understand instructions)
   (e) often has difficulty organizing tasks and activities
   (f) often avoids, dislikes, or is reluctant to engage in tasks that require sustained mental effort (such as schoolwork or homework)
   (g) often loses things necessary for tasks or activities (e.g., toys, school assignments, pencils, books, or tools)
   (h) is often easily distracted by extraneous stimuli
   (i) is often forgetful in daily activities

   (2) six (or more) of the following symptoms of **hyperactivity–impulsivity** have persisted for at least 6 months to a degree that is maladaptive and inconsistent with developmental level:

   Hyperactivity
   (a) often fidgets with hands or feet or squirms in seat
   (b) often leaves seat in classroom or in other situations in which remaining seated is expected
   (c) often runs about or climbs excessively in situations in which it is inappropriate (in adolescents or adults, may be limited to subjective feelings of restlessness)
   (d) often has difficulty playing or engaging in leisure activities quietly
   (e) is often "on the go" or often acts as if "driven by a motor"
   (f) often talks excessively

   Impulsivity
   (g) often blurts out answers before questions have been completed
   (h) often has difficulty awaiting turn
   (i) often interrupts or intrudes on others (e.g., butts into conversations or games)

B. Some hyperactive–impulsive or inattentive symptoms that caused impairment were present before age 7 years.

C. Some impairment from the symptoms is present in two or more settings (e.g., at school [or work] and at home).

D. There must be clear evidence of clinically significant impairment in social, academic, or occupational functioning.

E. The symptoms do not occur exclusively during the course of a Pervasive Developmental Disorder, Schizophrenia, or other Psychotic Disorder and are not better accounted for by another mental disorder (e.g., Mood Disorder, Anxiety Disorder, Dissociative Disorder, or a Personality Disorder).

Code based on type:
314.01 **Attention-Deficit/Hyperactivity Disorder, Combined Type:** if both Criteria A1 and A2 are met for the past 6 months

314.00 **Attention-Deficit/Hyperactivity Disorder, Predominantly Inattentive Type:** if Criterion A1 is met but Criterion A2 is not met for the past 6 months

314.01 **Attention Deficit/Hyperactivity Disorder, Predominantly Hyperactive–Impulsive Type:** if Criterion A2 is met but Criterion A1 is not met for the past 6 months

Coding note: For individuals (especially adolescents and adults) who currently have symptoms that no longer meet full criteria, "In Partial Remission" should be specified.

Attention-Deficit/Hyperactivity Disorder Not Otherwise Specified
This category is for disorders with prominent symptoms of inattention or hyperactivity–impulsivity that do not meet criteria for Attention-Deficit/Hyperactivity Disorder.

Note. Reprinted with permission from the *Diagnostic and Statistical Manual of Mental Disorders*, Fourth Edition. Copyright 1994 American Psychiatric Association.

research has included a full battery of neuropsychological tests (Brand, Das-Smaal, & DeJonge, 1996; Halperin et al. 1993), reversal and memory tasks (O'Neill & Douglas, 1996), and neurological evaluation (Luk, Leung, & Yuen, 1991). The general consistency of symptoms, comorbidity, and related findings among large, well-controlled clinic and epidemiological studies suggests that the conceptualization of ADHD in DSM-IV has been failry well refined. Nonetheless, these criteria continue to focus excessively on inattention as the core problem for the disorder, limiting the focus on the impact of impulsivity as the core deficit. This perpetuates a number of major misconceptions, including the notion that the inattentive type of ADHD represents a subtype of the combined disorder (Anastopoulos, Barkley, & Shelton, 1994). Increasing research suggests that it does not. It is more likely that the inattentive type represents a distinct disorder, primarily reflecting difficulty attending to repetitive, effortful tasks and problems with organization. The problems this group experiences may very well be the result of faulty skills as opposed to inconsistent or inadequate use of skills.

A Practical Definition of ADHD

In clinical settings, it is suggested that neuropsychologists apply a practical definition of ADHD as a means of translating history and test data into functional behavior. Such a process may also assist parents and educators in understanding the children they live with and educate. Such a process provides a logical framework within which to evaluate and understand the seemingly illogical pattern of behavior this group of children exhibits.

The practical definition contains five components, with the first, impulsivity, considered to be the major contributing force in shaping the other four components. These components are briefly presented below. The interested reader is referred to Goldstein and Goldstein (1998) for an extended review.

1. *Impulsivity.* Children with ADHD have difficulty thinking before they act. They do not efficiently weigh consequences before acting and do not reasonably consider the consequences of their past behavior. It is a struggle for them to follow rule-governed behavior (Barkley, 1981, 1997), due to their problems with separating experience from response, thought from emotion, and action from reaction. In the heat of the moment, their limited capacity for self-control is quickly overwhelmed by their immediate need to act.

2. *Inattention.* Children with ADHD have difficulty remaining on task and focusing their attention, in comparison to non-ADHD children of similar chronological age (APA, 1994). A more precise review of the available literature, however, suggests that their problems do not occur during highly motivating or interesting tasks, but rather when tasks are repetitive, effortful, uninteresting, and not of the children's choosing. In these circumstances the children's inability to inhibit their desire to move off this task is limited, and thus they find themselves doing anything else that appears to be more interesting or less effortful. Although this pattern is true to some extent for everyone on a dimensional basis, these children represent the extreme of what is observed.

3. *Overarousal.* Due to their lack of inhibition, children with ADHD tend to be excessively restless, overactive, and easily aroused emotionally. The speed and intensity with which they move to the extreme of their emotions are much greater than those of their same-age peers.

4. *Difficulty with gratification.* Children with ADHD, due to their lack of inhibition, require immediate, frequent, predictable, and meaningful rewards. They experience diffi-

culty working toward a long-term goal, and thus often require brief, repeated payoffs rather than a single long-term reward. They also do not appear to respond to rewards in the same manner as other children do (Haenlein & Caul, 1987); that is, rewards do not appear to be effective in changing their behavior on a long-term basis. Moreover, they appear to require more trials to consistently demonstrate mastery over behaviors that are within their repertoires. This may be the result of a faulty ability to develop a self-cueing process necessary to know what to do and when to do it. Due to their impulsivity, their behavior may remain consequentially bound.

It also appears that this group of children, because of their behavior, frequently receives more negative reinforcement than others. Thus these children are victims both of their temperaments, which make it difficult for them to persist, and of their reinforcement histories, which reinforce them for starting but often not for finishing tasks. It is important to keep in mind that these children like rewards and do not like punishments. In this respect, they are similar to everyone else. Nonetheless, over time they learn to respond to demands placed upon them by the environment when an aversive stimulus is removed contingent upon performance, rather than when they are promised a future reward.

5. *Emotions and locus of control.* Due to their impulsivity, children with ADHD often appear to be on a roller-coaster ride of emotions throughout their childhood. When they are happy, they are so happy people tell them to calm down. When they are unhappy, they are so unhappy people tell them to calm down. They may learn that emotions are not valued and often lead them into trouble. They may also be more prone to develop an external locus of control, to project blame onto others, and to be unwilling to recognize and accept the role they play in their own behavior. They appear more vulnerable to certain personality problems, especially those related to antisocial difficulty, in part because of these qualities combined with their life experiences. They may be more prone to depression as well, in part due to the lack of balance between successful and unsuccessful experiences on a day-in-and-day-out basis.

GENETICS AND OTHER ETIOLOGICAL CONSIDERATIONS

ADHD is among the most common disorders of childhood. It is estimated that it affects between 3% and 5% of the school-age population (APA, 1994), although statistics vary depending upon populations studied, thresholds, and definitional criteria. A genetic contribution to ADHD has been postulated by a number of authors (Hechtman, 1993; Rutter et al., 1990; Stevenson, 1992). The underlying genetic mechanism has recently been suggested to be associated with a single dopamine transporter gene (Cook, Stein, & Krasowski, 1995), as well as with a variation in the dopamine$_4$ (D4) receptor gene (LaHoste, Swanson, & Wigal, 1996). Furthermore, it has been suggested by some that the trait locus for reading disability on chromosome 6 identified by Cardon et al. (1994) may also be a locus for ADHD (Warren et al., 1995).

Eaves, Silberg, and Hewitt (1993) describe two complementary approaches to the genetic analysis of ADHD. The first, a dimensional approach, involves the study of a normal trait or range of activity; it assumes that ADHD constitutes one extreme of the trait or continuum. The second, a categorical approach, is based upon studying families of children who meet diagnostic criteria for ADHD; it assumes that ADHD is a discrete disorder (Faraone, Biederman, Chen, & Krifcher, 1992). It is important for neuropsychologists to recognize that dimensional approaches have been found to predict life outcome better than categorical approaches (Fergusson & Horwood, 1992).

Among investigators taking the dimensional approach, Willerman (1973) found the heritability of scores on an activity questionnaire to be 0.77 for a sample of 54 monozygotic and 39 dizygotic twin pairs. However, Goodman and Stevenson (1989) reported a heritability estimate of greater than 1.00 in a sample of 285 twin pairs. This finding appeared to be due to an extremely low dizygotic correlation. Corresponding dizygotic correlations for father and teacher reports were much higher, resulting in heritability estimates ranging from 0.48 to 0.68. A subsequent twin study by Thapar, Hervas, and McGuffin (1995), using the same three activity items used by Goodman and Stevenson, confirmed the low dizygotic correlation in maternal ratings; these authors suggested that the role of reciprocal sibling interactions may be different in dizygotic versus monozygotic twins, or that mothers may exaggerate differences between their dizygotic twins. The low dizygotic correlations may, however, be unique to these specific questions about activity level. Edelbrock, Rende, Plomin, and Thompson (1995) reported correlations (predominantly from mothers' ratings) of .86 for monozygotic twins and .29 for dizygotic twins, giving a heritability estimate of 0.66. Zahn-Waxler, Schmitz, Fulker, Robinson, and Emde (1996) obtained a very similar estimate (0.72). However, somewhat lower heritability values were obtained from fathers' and teachers' ratings, and the correlations between raters were low.

Employing the categorical or diagnostic approach, Goodman and Stevenson (1989) demonstrated a probandwise concordance rate of 51% in 39 monozygotic twin pairs and 30% in 54 dizygotic twin pairs, yielding a heritability estimate of 0.64. De Fries and Fulker (1985, 1988), utilizing a statistical method developed by Gillis, Gilger, Pennington, and De Fries (1992) estimated the heritability of ADHD as 0.91 ± 0.36 for twins participating in a research project.

The issue of phenotypic definition, as indicated by the variation in estimates of siblings' risk (53%, 25% or 17%, depending upon whether the behavior is defined as hyperactivity, ADD, or ADHD), speaks to the complexity of relating phenotype to genotype (Biederman, Faraone, Keenan, Knee, & Tsaung, 1990; Biederman, Faraone, Keenan, & Benjamin, 1992; Safer, 1973; Faraone et al., 1992). Levy, Hay, McStephen, Wood, and Waldman (1997), studying a cohort of 1,938 families with twins and siblings aged 4 to 12 years recruited from the Australian National Health and Medical Research Council Twin Registry, reported that ADHD is best viewed as the extreme of behavior that varies genetically throughout the entire population, rather than as a disorder with discrete determinants. In this study, as in others, heritability estimates for monozygotic twins were significantly higher than for dizygotic twins. As Levy et al. note, ADHD has an exceptionally high heritability compared with other behavioral disorders. These authors also reported that 82% of monozygotic twins and 38% of dizygotic twins met an eight-symptom ADHD cutoff for proband concordances.

Recent studies linking polymorphisms in the dopaminergic system to ADHD (Comings, Wu, & Chiu, 1996), and specific D4 receptor polymorphisms to dimensional aspects of impulsivity (Benjamin et al., 1996; Ebstein et al., 1996), suggest that the polymorphisms identified to date do not account for all of the relevant heritable variation. The findings of Sherman, Iacono, and McGue (1997) suggest that future molecular-genetic studies of ADHD may yield more information defining ADHD as a disorder composed of two quantitative, continuously distributed dimensions—inattention and hyperactivity–impulsivity—rather than as a homogeneous categorical disorder.

The etiology of ADHD must also be considered in relation to other genetic disorders and to teratogens. Fragile X syndrome, Turner syndrome, Tourette syndrome, neurofibromatosis, glucose 6 deficiency, phosphate dehydrogenase deficiency, sickle cell anemia, phenylketonuria, Noonan syndrome, and Williams syndrome are all chromosomal and genetic abnormalities in which attentional problems and ADHD have been reported (Hagerman, 1991). Exposure to various toxins (e.g., alcohol and cocaine exposure *in utero*, lead and vapor abuse), perinatal complications, medical problems (e.g., hypothyroidism, encephalitis), and even radiation therapy secondary to leukemia have all been reported as responsible for creating problems of inattention and impulsivity (for a review, see Goldstein & Goldstein, 1998).

Understanding the cause of ADHD from the point of view of the brain as a neurological organ has interested many researchers. Early concepts such as underarousal and overarousal (Ross & Ross, 1982) were discarded after attempts to find a physiological basis for these theories met with limited success. A model characterizing frontal lobe dysfunction as causative of ADHD was proposed by Conners and Wells (1986). Levine (1987) proposed an understanding of ADHD as a dysfunction of multiple control systems, including the vocal, sensory, associative, appetite, social, motor, behavioral, communicative, and affective control systems. Levine reviewed different etiologies affecting these various systems, and described an understanding of ADHD symptoms and treatment in relation to these systems as essential. Zametkin and Rapoport (1987), in a comprehensive review concerning the neurobiology of ADHD, observed that a large number of drug studies did not support any single hypothesis of a neurotransmitter defect. Their review of the literature and hypothetical explanations for ADHD has been updated and appears in Table 7.2.

DEVELOPMENTAL COURSE AND COMORBIDITY

Although the core problems children with ADHD experience reflect similar difficulties with impulsivity, inattention, and hyperactivity, each child's presentation is unique in terms of the manifestation of these problems and associated comorbid factors (Goldstein & Goldstein, 1998). As an increasing body of scientific data is generated concerning the developmental course and adult outcome of children with ADHD, it appears that the comorbid problems they develop predict their life outcomes better than the diagnosis of ADHD itself does. ADHD in isolation appears to best predict school struggles, difficulty meeting expectations outside the home setting, and possible mild substance abuse as an adult. However, it does not predict the significant negative emotional, behavioral, and personality outcomes that have been reported.

Infants who have been noted to have difficult temperaments do not handle changes in routines well. They exhibit a low frustration threshold and a high intensity of response (Carey, 1970; Chess & Thomas, 1986; Thomas & Chess, 1977). In follow-up studies of such infants, as many as 70% develop school problems (Terestman, 1980). These infants appear at greater risk than others of receiving a diagnosis of ADHD. It is also important to note that these difficult infants exert a significant negative impact on their developing relationships with caregivers—relationships that are critical in predicting children's life outcomes (Katz, 1997).

Although early symptoms of ADHD may be viewed as transient problems of young children, research data suggest that ignoring these signs results in the loss of valuable treatment time. At least 60–70% of children later diagnosed with ADHD could have been identified by their symptoms during the preschool years (Cohen, Sullivan, Minde, Novak, & Helwig, 1981). Young children manifesting symptoms of ADHD are more likely to present with speech and language problems (Baker & Cantwell, 1987), and to develop a wide range of behavioral problems (Cantwell, Baker, & Mattison, 1981; Cohen, Davine, & Meloche-Kelly, 1989), than are children not suffering from these symptoms. Current research cogently suggests that the comorbidity of speech and language disorders with ADHD merits

TABLE 7.2. Neuroanatomical Hypotheses of Dysfunction in ADHD

Investigator(s)	Hypothesis
Laufer & Denhoff (1957)	Diencephalic dysfunction (thalamus, hypothalamus)
Knobel, Walman, & Mason (1959)	Cortical "overfunctioning"
Satterfield & Dawson (1971)	Decreased levels of reticular activating system excitation
Wender (1971, 1972)	Decreased sensitivity in limbic areas of positive reinforcement (medial forebrain bundle, hypothalamus, norepinephrine)
Conners (1969)	Lack of "cortical inhibitory capacity"
Dykman, Ackerman, Clements, & Peters (1971)	Defect in forebrain inhibitory system over ventral formulation + diencephalon
Hunt (1987)	Locus coerulens dysfunction (hypersensitive alpha postsynaptic receptor)
Lou, Henriksson, & Bruhn (1984)	Central frontal lobes, anterolateral, posterolateral caudate region
Gorenstein & Newman (1980)	Dysfunction of medial septum, hippocampus, orbito-frontal cortex
Porrino, Lucignani, Dow-Edwards, & Sokoloff (1984)	Nucleus acumbens
Mattes (1980)	Frontal lobe
Gualtieri & Hicks (1985)	Frontal lobe
Arnold, Molinoff, & Rutledge (1977)	Nigrostriatal tract
Chelune, Ferguson, Koon, & Dickey (1986)	Frontal lobe
Hynd, Hern, Novey, & Eliopulos (1993)	Reversal of the normal left-to-right asymmetry in the caudate
Castellanos et al. (1994)	Asymmetric caudate volume with the right larger than the left
Castellanos et al. (1996)	Right hemisphere basal ganglia/frontal lobe abnormality, smallest cerebral volume, smaller right globus pallidus
Hynd et al. (1991)	Smaller total brain volume
Semrud-Clikeman et al. (1994)	Smaller corpus callosum
Filipek et al. (1997)	Smaller left total caudate, decreased frontal region
Aylward et al. (1996)	Small globus pallidus volume, particularly on the left

Note. In part from Zametkin and Rapoport (1987). Copyright 1987 by the American Academy of Child and Adolescent Psychiatry. Reprinted by permission from Lippincott Williams & Wilkins.

routine screening of children suspected of either type of problem, especially during their younger years. Children with concurrent ADHD and language disorders appear to have a much poorer prognosis than those with ADHD alone (Baker & Cantwell, 1992).

Within school settings, children with ADHD appear to be victims both of their temperaments and of their learning histories, which often involve beginning but not completing tasks. The negatively reinforcing model utilized by most educators in this circumstance tends to focus on misbehavior rather than on termination of the behavior. This may further disrupt the classroom by having a disinhibitory effect on other students. Although 25 years ago it was suggested that children with ADHD may be intellectually less competent than their peers, it appears more likely that their weak performance on intellectual tasks results from the impact of impulsivity and inattention on test-taking behavior than from an innate lack of intelligence (Barkley, 1995). Children with ADHD often underperform but may not underachieve during the elementary years. However, it has been reported that by high school at least 80% of these children fall behind in a basic academic subject requiring repetition and attention for competence, such as basic math knowledge, spelling, or written language (Barkley, 1998b; Goldstein & Goldstein, 1998). Depending upon the diagnostic criteria used, approximately 20–30% of children with ADHD also suffer from a concomitant, often language-based, learning disability (for a review, see Goldstein, 1997). Although it has been hypothesized that ADHD may prevent a child from achieving his or her academic potential (Stott, 1981), the presence of a learning disability may make a child appear more inattentive than others (McGee & Share, 1988).

In classroom settings, children with ADHD may often be more interested in tasks other than those upon which the teacher may be focusing (Douglas, 1972). This leads to significantly more nonproductive activity. Children with ADHD also demonstrate an uneven and unpredictable pattern of behavior in the classroom, which frequently leads teachers to conclude that these children are noncompliant rather than incompetent. The overall rates of negative teacher–child interactions involving normal students, interestingly, are higher in classrooms also containing children with ADHD (Campbell, Endman, & Bernfeld, 1977). According to reports, teachers are more intense and controlling when interacting with children with ADHD (Whalen, Henker, & Dotemoto, 1981). Children with ADHD have also been reported as having greater difficulty with transitions, an important aspect of school activities (Zentall, 1988).

Sociometric and play studies suggest that children with ADHD are not chosen as often by their peers to be best friends or partners in activities (Pelham & Milich, 1984). They appear to be cognizant of their difficulties—an awareness that probably precipitates lower self-esteem for children with ADHD (Glow & Glow, 1980). Moreover, they appear to experience either high-incidence, low-impact problems that result in poor social acceptance, or low-incidence, high-impact problems that result in social rejection (Pelham & Milich, 1984). In addition, these children have difficulty adapting their behavior to different situational demands (Whalen, Henker, Collins, McAuliffe & Vaux, 1979). It has been suggested that the impulsive behavioral patterns of children with ADHD are most responsible for their social difficulty; this may place those with comorbid hyperactive–impulsive problems of greater severity at even greater risk of developing social difficulties (Pelham & Bender, 1982).

Some primary symptoms of ADHD may diminish in intensity by adolescence (Weiss & Hechtman, 1979). However, most adolescents with ADHD continue to experience significant problems (Milich & Loney, 1979; for a review, see Goldstein, 1997). At least 80% of adolescents with ADHD continue to manifest symptoms consistent with ADHD. Sixty percent develop at least one additional disruptive disorder (Barkley, Fischer, Edelbrock, & Smallish, 1990b). Between 20% and 60% of adolescents with ADHD are involved in antisocial behavior, as opposed to a normal occurrence of 3–4% (Satterfield, Hoppe, & Schell, 1982). At least 50–70% of these adolescents develop oppositional defiant disorder, often during their younger years, with a significant number progressing to conduct disorder (Barkley et al., 1990b). However, the high prevalence of antisocial problems in adolescents with ADHD probably reflects the comorbidity of ADHD with other disruptive disorders, principally conduct disorder (Barkley et al., 1990b). As Barkley (1998a) succinctly points out, the preponderance of the available data suggests that while ADHD is clearly a risk factor for the development of adolescent antisocial problems, life experiences (principally factors within families) most powerfully contribute to the onset and maintenance of delinquency, conduct disorder, and subsequent young adult antisocial problems.

Older studies have reported, and it probably continues to be the trend, that as many of one-third of adolescents with ADHD are suspended from school at least once (Ackerman, Dykman, & Peters, 1977), and at least 80% fall behind 1 or more years in at least one basic academic subject (Loney, Kramer, & Milich, 1981). Adolescents with a history of ADHD also appear at greater risk of developing internalizing problems, including depression (Biederman, Faraone, Mick, & Lelon, 1995) and anxiety (Pliszka, 1992). The rates of comorbidity for ADHD and internalizing disorders have been estimated to range from 20% to 70%, with a higher incidence being reported in children and adolescents receiving diagnoses of conduct disorder.

Although adult ADHD is not the direct focus of this chapter, neuropsychologists should be aware that adults who are diagnosed with ADHD as children do not appear to be at significantly greater risk of developing serious antisocial adult problems in the absence of adolescent conduct disorder (for a review, see Goldstein & Goldstein, 1998). Nonetheless, this should not diminish our concern, given the high comorbidity of ADHD with conduct disorder. Mannuzza et al. (1991) suggested that adults with ADHD appear at greater risk than others to receive diagnoses of antisocial personality disorder and substance use problems. These authors found that in a young adult population with a history of ADHD, 43% still manifested full-blown ADHD, 32% met the diagnostic criteria for antisocial personality disorder, and 10% were drug abusers. This finding, however, contrasts with others indicating a greater risk of internalizing, marital and vocational problems as well in male and female adults diagnosed with ADHD as children (Biederman et al., 1987; Weiss & Hechtman, 1993; Rucklidge & Kaplan, 1997; Millstein, Wilens, Biederman, & Spencer, 1997).

NEUROPSYCHOLOGICAL IMPAIRMENTS

The ecological validity of laboratory tests to identify, define, and determine the severity of symptoms of ADHD has been increasingly questioned (Barkley, 1991a; Barkley & Grodzinsky, 1994). As ADHD is a disorder defined by behavior in the real world, it is not surprising that laboratory measures frequently fall short in defining and identifying symptoms of the disorder, in comparison to naturalistic observation, history, and organized report in the form of questionnaires. Nonetheless, it has been increasingly recognized that neuropsychologists take comfort in supplementing their clinical impressions with laboratory-generated, objective scores (DuPaul, Guevremont, & Barkley, 1991). It is acknowledged that these scores cannot be used alone to make the diagnosis of ADHD, but they may be helpful in the process of differential diagnosis (e.g., when is impulsivity a function of ADHD vs. other disorders?), as well as in determining severity or related prognosis in a group of individuals with ADHD (Gordon, 1995a, 1995b; Hall, Halperin, Schwartz, & Newcorn, 1997).

The development of a norm-referenced, psychometric assessment battery specifically designed for ADHD has been an elusive goal for researchers and clinicians. Thus, when one reviews the extensive literature attempting to hypothetically and objectively define specific neuropsychological impairments occurring consistently in children with ADHD, it is not surprising that no tried and true battery or specific pattern of impairment has come to light. As Levine (1992) has noted, ADHD symptoms appear to reflect "elusive entities and . . . mistaken identities." The comorbidity issue, and many tests' lack of specificity in discriminating ADHD from other disorders, further complicate this endeavor. Compromised scores may be due to a variety of causes, leading some researchers to suggest that a profile of test scores be utilized in defining and explaining neuropsychological impairments in children with ADHD (Aylward, Verhulst, & Bell, 1993). Neuropsychologists should be aware that clinic or laboratory tests alone or in combination have been found to result in classification decisions that frequently disagree with a diagnosis of ADHD based upon parent interview, history, and behavior rating scales (DuPaul, Anastopoulos, Shelton, Guevremont, & Metevia, 1992a). Furthermore, although Szatmari, Offord, Siegel, Finlayson, and Tuff (1990) report that neuropsychological tests appear to distinguish children with ADHD from those with pure anxiety or affective disorders, they may not as efficiently distinguish ADHD from other disruptive disorders. These authors concluded that neuropsychological test scores are more strongly associated with externalizing than with internalizing diagnoses. They also appear to correlate with psychiatric symptoms at school but not at home. Thus it is not surprising that Barkley (1991a) suggests that when results of standardized behavior ratings, observations, and history conflict with laboratory measures, the latter should be disregarded in favor of the former, as these are considered more ecologically valid sources of data.

A brief review of laboratory and clinical measures and their hypothesized relationship to specific neuropsychological impairments in ADHD follows:

• Continuous-performance test (CPT) scores for omission and commission errors have been found to correlate statistically with a number of errors on some paper-and-pencil tasks. Modest correlations have been found between CPT scores and direct observation of ADHD behavior in the classroom. Omission scores appear to correlate modestly with behavioral categories on the Gordon Diagnostic System. CPT performance, however, has been found to be sensitive to stimulant medication, but not always reliably so (Barkley, 1977a, 1977b, 1978; Swanson & Kinsbourne, 1979; Barkley, DuPaul, & McMurray, 1991; Barkley, Fischer, Newby, & Breen, 1988). CPT scores, particularly commission scores, may have moderate ecological validity as assessed by parent and teacher ratings of inattention and overactivity. The neuropsychologist must then question, however, whether the CPT is necessary in the primary diagnosis of ADHD if similar information can be gleaned by obtaining history and parent–teacher ratings.

• Performance on cancellation tasks, such as the Children's Checking Task (Margolis, 1972), suggests that children with ADHD differ from normal children on omission and commission errors (Brown, 1982; Aman & Turbott, 1986). They may not differ, however, from other clinical groups (Keough & Margolis, 1976). This type of measure may also be sensitive to the benefits of stimulant medication (Charles, Schain, Zelniker, & Guthrie, 1979).

• Correlations of scores on the Matching Familiar Figures Test with parent and teacher ratings of ADHD have been low to moderate, but become nonsignificant when age and intelligence are partialed out (Brown & Wynne, 1982; Fuhrman & Kendall, 1986; Milich & Kramer, 1984). Milich and Kramer (1984) suggest that the ecological validity of the Matching Familiar Figures Test as a measure of impulsivity in ADHD children appears weak.

• The Draw-a-Line Slowly Test has been used to measure impulsivity, but has not been found to discriminate children with ADHD from normal children or other clinical groups once age and IQ are controlled for (Werry, Elkind, & Reeves, 1987; deHaas & Young, 1984).

• The Cookie Delay Test (Campbell, Szumowski, Ewing, Gluck, & Breaux, 1982), based on a model developed by Golden, Montare, and Bridger (1977), has found young children with ADHD to be significantly more impulsive than others. Rapport, Tucker,

DuPaul, Merlo, and Stoner (1986) provided a similar delay-of-gratification procedure that involved much longer time delays. Ninety-four percent of the ADHD subjects, as compared to 31% of the controls, chose the immediate over the delayed task. This issue holds significance for the neuropsychologist as consequences are chosen for behavior change programs.

• The ecological validity of movement or activity level devices, such as an actometer, a stabilimetric cushion, or an activity chair, is poor (Schulman & Reisman, 1959; Tryon, 1984). The actometer can discriminate ADHD children from normal children (Luk, 1985; Tryon, 1984), but not in all cases (Barkley, DuPaul, & McMurray, 1990a; Koriath, Gualtieri, Van Bourgondien, Quade, & Werry, 1985). Unfortunately, these measurements have not correlated well with parent ratings of hyperactivity (Barkley & Ullman, 1975; Ullman, Barkley, & Brown, 1978). There may be an exception when actometer measures are taken over longer periods of time; they may then correlate better with parent and teacher behavioral reports (Stevens, Kupst, Suran, & Schulman, 1978).

• The literature indicates encouraging associations between observations of ADHD in laboratory analogue settings and naturalistic reports, beginning with the work of Hutt, Hutt, and Ounsted (1963), in which the floor of a clinical playroom was divided into grids with tape. A number of studies with similar methodology have demonstrated that children with ADHD display more grid crossings, more toy changes, and shorter durations of play with toys during free play than do normal children (Campbell et al., 1982; Pope, 1970; Routh & Schroeder, 1976; Touwen & Kalverboer, 1973). Again, however, some studies have not found differences between the ADHD groups and others (Barkley & Ullman, 1975; Koriath et al., 1985). A few studies that have attempted to correlate free play with parent ratings of hyperactivity have yielded nonsignificant results (Barkley & Ullman, 1975; Ullman et al., 1978). It is when children with ADHD in analogue settings are asked to complete directed tasks with parents that they appear to have the most problems, not in free-play situations with parents.

• Analogue measures that evaluate out-of-seat behavior, off-task behavior, inappropriate vocalization, and attention shifts during free play in restricted play settings have yielded more promising findings (Milich, 1984; Milich, Loney, & Roberts, 1986). These findings have correlated significantly with parent and teacher ratings of hyperactivity. Studies comparing ADHD, normal, and clinic control groups have found significant differences among the ADHD group, the ADHD group with aggression, purely aggressive children, and normal children (Roberts, 1990; Milich, Loney, & Landau, 1982). Barkley, McMurray, Edelbrock, and Robbins (1989) placed children in a playroom setting with a shelf full of toys and asked them to sit at a small table and complete a written math task at or below their grade level for 15 minutes. They were told not to leave their seat or to touch the toys. They were then observed. This procedure was found to discriminate ADHD children from normal children, but was inconsistent in discriminating ADHD children from other clinical groups when off-task behavior, out-of-seat behavior, vocalization, fidgeting, and playing with objects were evaluated (Barkley et al., 1989; Breen, 1989). Barkley (1991a) provides a summary of these and other measures, which is given here as Table 7.3.

Douglas (1988) has suggested that the basic information-processing capabilities of children with ADHD are intact. Thus they frequently perform adequately when exerting minimal effort, almost regardless of the task. It is when more effort is required that they experience problems. Based upon a thorough review of the then-available research literature, Douglas provided a listing of tasks during which deficits have and have not been found for populations of children with ADHD. The neuropsychologist is likely to find a qualitative pattern of performance for ADHD children, in which they perform reasonably well as

TABLE 7.3. A Summary of the Evidence for the Ecological Validity of Commonly Used Laboratory and Analogue Assessments of ADHD

Measures	Group differences from		Related to other laboratory or analogue measures	Sensitive to experimental manipulations	Related to ratings observations in home/school
	Normal	Clinical			
Attention					
Reaction time tasks	Yes	No	Yes (.70)	Yes	No
Continuous-performance tasks	Yes	No	Yes (.25–.35)	Inconsistent	Yes (.21–.51)
Children's checking task	Yes	No	Yes (.25–.73)	Yes	?
Impulsivity					
Matching familiar figures	Inconsistent	No	Yes (.25–.75)	Inconsistent	Yes (.21–.53)
Differential reinforcement of learning (DRL) tasks	Yes	?	?	No	Yes (.33–.58)
Draw-a-line-slowly	No	No	No	No	Yes (.30)
Delay of gratification	Yes	?	Yes (.74)	?	?
Activity					
Actometer	Yes	?	Yes (.17–.53)	Yes	Yes (.17–.65)
Stabilimetric cushion	Yes	Yes	?	Yes	No
Analogue behavior observations					
Free play in lab playroom	Yes	No	Yes (.42–.88)	Yes	No
Restricted play in playroom	Yes	Yes	Yes (.42–.88)	Yes	No
Restricted academic setting	Yes	Yes	Yes (.17–.47)	Yes	Yes (.17–.60)

Note. The column headed "Group differences" indicates whether evidence exists that the results on the measure have been significantly different between ADHD and normal groups or ADHD and other clinical control groups. Within the table, the term "Inconsistent" means that the evidence has been inconsistent in establishing this issue. A "?" indicates that no evidence could be found to address this issue. Correlation coefficients that appear in parentheses indicate only the magnitude of the relationship and not the direction of the relationship (positive or negative). From Barkley (1991a). Copyright 1991 by Plenum Publishing Corp. Reprinted by permission.

tasks begin, but as task complexity increases (which is characteristic of most clinical measures), their performance appears to drop off more quickly than perhaps their abilities would predict. Tables 7.4 and 7.5 summarize Douglas's findings.

Cherkes-Julkowski, Stolzenberg, and Siegal (1991) suggest that perhaps the dropoff in performance for ADHD children is a function of their inability to control focus of attention. These authors suggest that when prompts are provided during testing, children with ADHD perform significantly better. In a study evaluating children with ADHD with and without medication, compared to learning-disabled children and a group of normal controls, the greatest gains for prompts were observed in the unmedicated group with ADHD. However, practitioners should be cautioned that prompts, especially on measures designed to evaluate response inhibition, may actually test a child's ability to follow directions rather than to inhibit. Practitioners should also keep in mind that there are data suggesting that level of reinforcement during test performance may have an impact on scores as well. Devers, Bradley-Johnson, and Johnson (1994) found that a 12-point improvement in Verbal IQ scores accrued when token reinforcers followed immediately for correct responses. The impact of praise on test performance has not been

TABLE 7.4. Tasks on Which Deficits Have Been Found

Monitoring tasks and automated reaction time tasks
  Deploying continuous, careful, and sustained attention to ongoing stimuli
  Inhibiting responses to inappropriate stimuli
  Inhibiting responses at inappropriate times

Perceptual search tasks
  Conducting an organized, exhaustive, intensive, and focused search of task stimuli
  Ignoring irrelevant stimuli
  Inhibiting responses to irrelevant stimuli

Logical search tasks
  Clarifying task demands
  Generating and evaluating possible problem-solving strategies
  Generating and evaluating possible solutions
  Inhibiting premature, inadequate responses

Memory tasks
  Processing task stimuli adequately
  Generating and applying effective rehearsal strategies
  Generating and applying effective retrieval strategies

Motor control and perceptual–motor tasks
  Guiding, controlling movement
  Inhibiting inappropriate movement
  Carrying out a careful perceptual analysis of complex figures
  Drawing accurate reproduction of complex figures

Note. From Douglas (1988). Copyright 1988 by Pergamon Press. Reprinted by permission of ACPP.

systematically evaluated. Finally, Draeger, Prior, and Sanson (1986) reported a greater deterioration in ADHD children's performance on a CPT than in control children's performance when the examiner left the room. These authors suggest that even an examiner's presence acts to mitigate test performance. It may well be that some children who perform poorly on test measures under these circumstances have an application deficit rather than an ability deficit.

TABLE 7.5. Memory Tasks on Which Deficits Were Not Found

Verbal memory tasks
  Digits forward
  Digits backward
  Letters forward
  Letters ordered alphabetically
  Consonant trigrams (after filled and unfilled delay intervals)
  Word lists (12 words)
  Paired associates for related word pairs (including 45-minute delayed recall)
  Story recall

Nonverbal memory tasks
  Block series forward
  Block series backward
  Recurring figures (geometric and nonsense figures)
  Recall of visual positions along a straight line (after filled and unfilled delay intervals)
  Recall of spatial locations

Note. From Douglas (1988). Copyright 1988 by Pergamon Press. Reprinted by permission of ACPP.

EVALUATION

Due to the pervasive, multisetting nature of problems related to ADHD, and ADHD's high comorbidity with other childhood disorders, assessment for ADHD involves a thorough emotional, developmental, and behavioral evaluation. The comprehensive evaluation should collect data concerning the child's behavior at home, with friends, and at school; academic and intellectual functioning; medical status; and emotional development. Barkley (1991c) has recommended that assessment for ADHD include the use of standardized behavior rating scales, a review of laboratory measures when available, and observations in both the classroom and the clinic. Direct interviews with teachers and adults, as well as other forms of face-to-face assessment with the child, are necessary for certain specific identified problems (Goldstein & Goldstein, 1998). Within the classroom setting, off-task behavior, excessive motor activity, and negative vocalization appear to be the most visible manifestations of ADHD (DuPaul, Guevremont, & Barkley, 1992b).

It is suggested that neuropsychologists consider the following multistep process in the evaluation of ADHD:

1. A complete history must be obtained. This is not a cursory process. Sufficient time (approximately 1½ to 2 hours) should be set aside to obtain a narrative of the child's development, behavior, extended family history, family relations, and current functioning. Within the context of the interview, efforts should be made to trace a developmental course that appears to fit the picture of ADHD, as well as to identify core symptoms and those related to other childhood disorders. Obtaining thorough knowledge of the diagnostic criteria for common and uncommon (e.g., high-functioning autism) childhood internalizing and externalizing disorders should be a paramount concern for the neuropsychologist, to facilitate the identification of high- as well as low-incidence disorders.

2. Data obtained from the history should be supplemented by the completion of a number of standardized, factor-analyzed questionnaires concerning children's problems. At least two adults who interact with the child on a regular basis, ideally a parent and a teacher, should be requested to complete questionnaires. For general child assessment, the most valuable questionnaire is the Child Behavior Checklist (Achenbach & Edelbrock, 1991). This well-developed questionnaire organizes childhood behavior on a disruptive–nondisruptive continuum. Recent research indicates that the Attention Problems scale correlates well with the current two-factor DSM-IV ADHD diagnosis (Achenbach, 1996). The Conners Teacher Rating Scale—Revised (Conners, 1997), the Comprehensive Teacher's Rating Scale (Ullmann, Sleator, & Sprague, 1988), the Childhood Attention Problems Scale (Edelbrock, 1990), and the Academic Performance and ADHD Rating Scales (DuPaul, 1990) are also helpful. However, these questionnaires alone do not provide sufficient information for diagnosis; they simply provide organized reports of behavior. In other words, they describe what the observer sees, but not why it is being seen.

3. From the history and questionnaires, the neuropsychologist should be able to generate a consistent set of data and a series of hypotheses to explain the child's behavior across a variety of settings.

4. Requests should be made to review school records, including report cards and results of group achievement testing. If weak performance or learning disabilities are suspected, or if the child is already receiving special education services, the neuropsychologist should review all assessment data as well as the child's individualized education plan. Then it is proper to decide which tests and what amount of time should be used to arrive at the most accurate evaluation of the child. Neuropsychologists should keep in mind that, as

just reviewed, no specific laboratory tests for ADHD have demonstrated sufficient positive and negative predictive power to be relied on. The primary purpose of face-to-face assessment with a child should be to address issues related to the child's emotional status, self-esteem, cognitive development, and possible learning disabilities. Observation of the child's behavior during assessment may also yield clues regarding his or her interpersonal style and temperament.

5. Although a number of paper-and-pencil tasks have been used over the years in research settings to identify symptoms of ADHD, most have not lent themselves easily to clinical use. In research studies some of these tests, such as the Matching Familiar Figures Test (Kagan, 1964), appear to meet sensitivity and specificity criteria for identifying impulsive children. However, in clinical practice such instruments have not proven reliable for confirming the diagnosis of ADHD. Computerized instruments designed to measure sustained attention and the ability to inhibit impulsive responses (Conners, 1994a, 1994b; Greenberg, 1991; Gordon, 1993a, 1993b) have become increasingly popular among neuro-psychologists. However, it is important to remember that although these instruments may demonstrate high positive predictive power (e.g., if a child fails such a task, it strongly confirms the presence of symptoms related to ADHD), they possess poor negative predictive power (e.g., if a child passes a task, conclusions cannot be drawn one way or the other concerning the diagnosis). Nonetheless, many neuropsychologists rely on such instruments to provide additional data as part of the diagnostic process, rather than specifically to confirm or disconfirm the diagnosis of ADHD (Conners, 1994a). The interested reader is referred to Conners (1994b) for a thorough review of the literature concerning computerized assessment of ADHD.

TREATMENT

Treatment of ADHD must be multidisciplinary, multimodal, and maintained over a long period (Goldstein & Goldstein, 1998). By far the most effective short-term interventions for ADHD are combinations of medical, behavioral, and environmental techniques. Medication has demonstrated the ability to reduce the manipulative power of the child's behavior in eliciting certain responses from teachers, peers, and family members. Behavior management increases the salience of behaving in a way consistent with environmental expectations. The manipulation of the environment (e.g., making tasks more interesting and payoffs more valuable) reduces the risk of problems within the natural setting.

Regardless of the treatment modality employed, the basic underlying premise in managing problems of ADHD involves increasing the child's capacity to inhibit responding. This is consistent with the theoretical construct that the core problem for ADHD reflects an inability to permit sufficient time to think or respond consistently to the environment.

Medication

An extensive literature attests to the benefits of medicine, specifically stimulants, in reducing key symptoms of ADHD and thus improving daily functioning (Klein, 1987; Goldstein & Goldstein, 1998). Stimulants have consistently been reported to improve academic achievement and productivity, as well as accuracy of classwork (Douglas, Barr, O'Neil, & Britton, 1986); improved attention span, reading comprehension, and even complex problem solving have also been noted (Balthazar, Wagner, & Pelham, 1991; Pelham, 1987). Related problems, including peer interactions, peer status, and even relationships with family members, have been reported to be improved with stimulants as well (Whalen & Henker, 1991).

It has been estimated that nearly a million and a half children received medication for ADHD in 1994 in the United States alone (Williams, Lerner, & Swanson, 1994). By all accounts, the number continues to increase. Approximately 90% of children in the United States who take medication for ADHD receive stimulants, particularly methylphenidate. Other stimulants (e.g, dextroamphetamine, Adderall, pemoline, and methamphetamine), as well as the tricyclic antidepressants (e.g., imipramine, desipramine, and nortriptyline), have also been reported as beneficial for ADHD symptoms. Pemoline, however, is no longer recommended as a first-line treatment for ADHD due to associated liver problems. The antihypertensives clonidine and Tenex have also been suggested as beneficial for ADHD. In contrast, the selective serotonin reuptake inhibitors (e.g., fluoxetine, paroxetine, and sertraline) have not demonstrated an effectiveness rate much beyond that of placebo.

Because the majority of children with ADHD receive methylphenidate, it is not surprising that methylphenidate has been the primary focus of medication research. The response of children with ADHD to the administration of methylphenidate is often remarkably positive. Placebo-controlled, double-blind trials demonstrate that 75–80% of children with ADHD respond to methylphenidate, whereas only 30–40% respond to placebo (for a review, see Greenhill & Osman, 1991). Conducted in classroom settings, trials of medication have found that time spent on task, work completion, accuracy of work, and general conduct all improve dramatically. Conflicts with peers and siblings decline. Negative interactions between parents and children also decline. Although the effect of methylphenidate on academic performance has been controversial, it is generally recognized that while the quality of work may improve, the rate at which academic information is acquired may not increase dramatically for children with ADHD.

DuPaul and Rapport (1993) examined 31 children with ADHD in a double-blind, placebo-controlled trial of four doses of stimulant medication. Methylphenidate exerted a significant positive effect on classroom measures of attention and academic efficiency, to the point that these problems were no longer statistically deviant in the ADHD population. However, upon individual examination, 25% of the children with ADHD failed to demonstrate normalized levels of classroom performance; this finding suggests that although stimulant medications are beneficial, a need for ancillary interventions for the ADHD population remains.

Almost all children with ADHD who do not respond to one stimulant may derive clinical benefit in the classroom or home from another (Elia, Borcherding, Rapoport, & Keysor, 1991). What defines a "good response," however, is debatable. When a good response is defined as a reduction in cardinal symptoms of ADHD and improvement in behavior and compliance at school, at least 80% of children appropriately diagnosed with ADHD respond to medication. However, when a good response is defined by performance on a cognitive task in a laboratory setting, such as a paired-associate learning task, a great number of children with ADHD are unresponsive to stimulants (Swanson, Cantwell, Lerner, McBurnett, & Hanna, 1991).

The long-term effects of methylphenidate have been debated. Studies have demonstrated consistent short-term benefits but have not demonstrated significant long-term benefits into adulthood (for a review, see Goldstein, 1997). When outlook is measured in terms of socioeconomic status, vocation, marriage, drug addiction, or criminal behavior, minimal long-term positive effects of stimulants are demonstrated. However, the immediate short-term benefits of stimulant medication far outweigh the liabilities and thus appear to justify the continued use of these medications in the treatment of ADHD.

Educational Interventions

Zentall (1995) suggests that students with ADHD possess an active learning style, with a demonstrated need to move, talk, respond, question, choose, debate, and even provoke. Thus, in classroom settings children with ADHD do not fare well in sedentary situations. Interventions for managing ADHD in the classroom have included positive and negative contingent teacher attention, token economies, peer-mediated and group contingencies, time out, home–school contingencies, reductive techniques based on reinforcement, and cognitive-behavioral strategies (Abramowitz & O'Leary, 1991). Environmental and task modifications are also critical for classroom success for the child with ADHD. However, additional research is needed, especially in the area of school-based intervention, for adolescents with ADHD.

A review of the classroom research data dealing with ADHD in children leads to a number of general conclusions (Barkley, 1998b; Goldstein & Goldstein, 1998; Parker, 1992):

- The classroom should be organized and structured, with clear rules, a predictable schedule, and separate desks.
- Rewards should be consistent, immediate, salient, and frequent.
- A response cost reinforcement program is recommended as an integral part of the classroom.
- Feedback from teachers should be constant.
- Minor disruptions, especially those that do not bother others, should be ignored.
- Tasks should be interesting and payoffs valuable.
- Academic materials should be matched to the child's ability.
- Transition times, as well as recess and assembly, should be supervised closely.
- Teachers and parents should maintain close communication, especially in the lower grades.
- Teacher expectations should be adjusted to meet the child's behavioral and academic skill level.
- Teachers must be educated concerning the issues of ADHD in the classroom and should develop a repertoire of interventions to manage these problems effectively.

Parenting Skills

Parents must be counseled to understand that managing their child's ADHD problems at home requires accurate knowledge of the disorder and its complications. They must be consistent, predictable, and supportive of their child in daily interactions. Significant research suggests that for children facing adversity, the habitual relationships they develop with their caregivers constitute a significant positive predictor of adult outcomes (Fonagy, Steele, Steele, Higgitt, & Target, 1994; Werner, 1994).

The following guidelines are recommended when practitioners are working with parents of children with ADHD. These can be implemented on an individual basis or incorporated into an existing comprehensive parent training program such as Barkley's (1997).

- Parents must be urged to become educated consumers. They must understand ADHD thoroughly, because it will affect their child throughout his or her lifespan.
- Parents must develop an understanding of, and be able to distinguish between, problems of incompetence (nonpurposeful problems resulting from the child's ADHD) and

problems of noncompliance (purposeful problems that occur when the child does not wish to do as he or she is directed). Parents must develop a system to differentiate between these two types of problems and must possess a set of interventions for both.

• Parents must be taught to tell their child specifically what to do in a clear, operationally defined way. They must "act, not yak." They must learn to give "start" rather than "stop" commands.

• Parents must be able to provide a repertoire of appropriate reinforcers. They must work to keep a balance between positive and negative reinforcement, as well as to avoid extensive reliance on tangible rewards.

• Parents must recognize that consequences—rewards as well as punishments—must be provided quickly and consistently.

• A modified response cost program must be used in the home setting. Such a program works at school as well. This system provides a child with the ability to earn, but also the risk of losing, reinforcers for noncompliant or inappropriate behavior. The interested reader is referred to Goldstein and Goldstein (1998) for an in-depth description of structuring such a program.

• Parents must be helped to understand the forces that affect their child with ADHD. They must not personalize their child's problems, They also should be guided to avoid placing their child in situations that exacerbate ADHD problems; thus planning is critical.

• Families with a child suffering from ADHD tend to experience greater stress, more marital disharmony, and more severe emotional problems in parents. Indeed, reactions to the child's behavior have the potential to tear a family apart. Parents should do their best to anticipate and forestall potential problems.

• Parents must recognize that the relationship they develop with their child with ADHD is likely to be strained. They must take extra time to balance the scales and maintain a positive relationship. They must be urged to find enjoyable activities and to engage in these activities with their child as often as possible.

Though cognitive strategies (e.g., teaching a child to "stop, look, and listen") and various nontraditional treatments (e.g., dietary manipulation, biofeedback, etc.) are popular, they have not stood the test of scientific research and thus should not be advocated as treatments of choice for children with ADHD. The interested reader is referred to Ingersoll and Goldstein (1993) and Goldstein and Goldstein (1998) for a review of these issues.

REFERENCES

Abramowitz, A. J., & O'Leary, S. G. (1991). Behavior interventions for the classroom: Implications for students with ADHD. *School Psychology Review*, 20, 220–234.

Accardo, P. J., Blondis, T. J., & Whitman, B. Y. (1990). Disorders of attention and activity level in a referral population. *Pediatrics*, 85, 426–431.

Achenbach, T. M. (1996). Subtyping ADHD: The request for suggestions about relating empirically based assessment to DSM-IV. *ADHD Report*, 4, 5–9.

Achenbach, T. M., & Edelbrock, C. (1991). *Normative data for the Child Behavior Checklist—Revised*. Burlington: University of Vermont, Department of Psychiatry.

Ackerman, P. T., Dykman, R. A., & Peters, J. E. (1977). Teenage status of hyperactive and non-hyperactive learning disabled boys. *American Journal of Orthopsychiatry*, 47, 577–596.

Aman, M. G., & Turbott, S. H. (1986). Incidental learning, distraction, and sustained attention in hyperactive and control subjects. *Journal of Abnormal Child Psychology*, 14, 441–455.

American Psychiatric Association (APA). (1994). *Diagnostic and statistical manual of mental disorders* (4th ed.). Washington, DC: Author.

Anastopoulos, A. D., Barkley, R., & Shelton, T. (1994). The history and diagnosis of attention deficit/hyperactivity disorder. *Therapeutic Care and Education, 3,* 96–110.

Arnold, E., Molinoff, P., & Rutledge, C. (1977). The release of endogenous norepinephrine and dopamine from cerebral cortex by amphetamine. *Journal of Pharmacological Experimental Therapy, 202,* 544–557.

Aylward, E. H., Reiss, A. L., Reader, M. J., Singer, H. S., Brown, J. E., & Denckla, M. B. (1996). Basal ganglia volumes in children with attention deficit hyperactivity disorder. *Journal of Child Neurology, 11,* 112–115.

Aylward, G. P., Verhulst, S. J., & Bell, S. (1993, September). *Inter-relationships between measures of attention deficit disorders: Same scores, different reasons.* Paper presented at the meeting of the Society for Behavioral Pediatrics, Providence, RI.

Baker, L., & Cantwell, D. P. (1987). A prospective psychiatric follow-up of children with speech/language disorders. *Journal of the American Academy of Child and Adolescent Psychiatry, 26,* 546–553.

Baker, L.,& Cantwell, D. P. (1992). Attention deficit disorder and speech/language disorders. *Comprehensive Mental Health Care, 2,* 3–16.

Balthazar, M. J., Wagner, R. K., & Pelham, W. E. (1991). The specificity of the effects of stimulant medication on classroom learning-related measures of cognitive processing for attention deficit disorder children. *Journal of Abnormal Child Psychology, 19,* 35–52.

Barkley, R. A. (1977a). A review of stimulant drug research with hyperactive children. *Journal of Child Psychology and Psychiatry, 18,* 137–165.

Barkley, R.A. (1977b). The effects of methylphenidate on various measures of activity level and attention in hyperkinetic children. *Journal of Abnormal Child Psychology, 5,* 351–369.

Barkley, R. A. (1978). Recent developments in research on hyperactive children. *Journal of Pediatric Psychology, 3,* 158–163.

Barkley, R. A. (1981). *Hyperactive children: A handbook for diagnosis and treatment.* New York: Guilford Press.

Barkley, R. A. (1991a). The ecological validity of laboratory and analogue assessment methods of ADHD symptoms. *Journal of Abnormal Child Psychology, 19,* 149–178.

Barkley, R. A. (1991b). Attention-deficit hyperactivity disorder. *Psychiatric Annals, 21,* 725–733.

Barkley, R. A. (1991c). Diagnosis and assessment of attention deficit hyperactivity disorder. *Comprehensive Mental Health Care, 1,* 27–43.

Barkley, R. A. (1995). ADHD and I.Q. *ADHD Report, 3,* 1–3.

Barkley, R. A. (1997). *Defiant children: A clinician's manual for assessment and parent training* (2nd ed.). New York: Guilford Press.

Barkley, R. A. (1998a). Is ADHD an excuse for antisocial actions? *ADHD Report, 5,* 1–3.

Barkley, R. A. (1998b). *Attention-deficit hyperactivity disorder: A handbook for diagnosis and treatment* (2nd ed.). New York: Guilford Press.

Barkley, R. A., DuPaul, G. J., & McMurray, M. B. (1990a). A comprehensive evaluation of attention deficit disorder with and without hyperactivity as defined by research criteria. *Journal of Consulting and Clinical Psychology, 58,* 775–789.

Barkley, R. A., DuPaul, G. J., & McMurray, M. B. (1991). Attention deficit disorder with and without hyperactivity: Clinical response to three dose levels of methylphenidate. *Pediatrics, 87,* 519–531.

Barkley, R. A., Fischer, M., Edelbrock, C. S., & Smallish, L. (1990b). The adolescent outcome of hyperactive children diagnosed by research criteria: I. An eight year prospective follow-up study. *Journal of the American Academy of Child and Adolescent Psychiatry, 29,* 546–557.

Barkley, R. A., Fischer, M., Newby, R., & Breen, M. (1988). Development of a multi-method clinical protocol for assessing stimulant drug responses in ADHD children. *Journal of Clinical Child Psychology, 17,* 14–24.

Barkley, R. A., & Grodzinsky, G. M. (1994). Are tests of frontal lobe functions useful in a diagnosis of attention deficit disorders? *Clinical Neuropsychologists, 8,* 121–139.

Barkley, R. A., McMurray, M. B., Edelbrock, C. S., & Robbins, K. (1989). The response of aggressive and non-aggressive ADHD children to two doses of methylphenidate. *Journal of the American Academy of Child and Adolescent Psychiatry, 28,* 873–881.

Barkley, R. A., & Ullman, D. G. (1975). A comparison of objective measures of activity and distractibility in hyperactive and non-hyperactive children. *Journal of Abnormal Child Psychology, 3,* 231–244.

Bellak, L. (Ed.). (1979). *Psychiatric aspects of minimal brain dysfunction in adults.* New York: Grune & Stratton.

Benjamin, J., Li, L., Patterson, C., Greenberg, B. D., Murphy, D. L., & Hamer, D. H. (1996). Population and familial association between the D4 dopamine receptor gene and measures of novelty seeking. *Nature Genetics, 12,* 81–94.

Biederman, J., Faraone, S. V., Keenan, K., & Benjamin, J. (1992). Further evidence for family-genetic risk factors in attention deficit hyperactivity disorder: Patterns of comorbidity in probands and relatives in psychiatrically and pediatrically referred samples. *Archives of General Psychiatry, 49,* 728–738.

Biederman, J., Faraone, S. V., Keenan, K., Knee, D., & Tsuang, M. T. (1990). Family-genetic and psychosocial risk factors in DSM-III attention deficit disorders. *Journal of the American Academy of Child and Adolescent Psychiatry, 29,* 526–533.

Biederman, J., Faraone, S., Mick, E., & Lelon, E. (1995). Psychiatric comorbidity among referred juveniles with major depression: Fact or artifact? *Journal of the American Academy of Child and Adolescent Psychiatry, 34,* 579–590.

Biederman, J., Faraone, S., Mick, E., Wozniak, J., Chen, L., Ouelette, C., Marrs, A., Moore, P., Garcia, J., Mennin, D., & Lelon, E. (1996). Attention deficit hyperactivity disorder in juvenile mania: An overlooked comorbidity? *Journal of the American Academy of Child and Adolescent Psychiatry, 35,* 997–1008.

Biederman, J., Munir, K., Knee, D., Armentano, M., Autor, S., Waternaux, C., & Tsuang, M. (1987). High rate of affective disorder in probands with attention deficit disorder and in their relatives: A controlled family study. *American Journal of Psychiatry, 144,* 330–333.

Block, G. H. (1977). Hyperactivity: A cultural perspective. *Journal of Learning Disabilities, 10,* 236–240.

Blondis, T. A., Snow, J. H., Stein, M., & Roizen, N. J. (1991). Appropriate use of measures of attention and activity for the diagnosis and management of attention deficit hyperactivity disorder. In P. J. Accardo, T. A. Blondis, & B. Y. Whitman (Eds.), *Attention deficit disorders and hyperactivity in children* (pp. 85–120). New York: Marcel Dekker.

Brand, E. F., Das-Smaal, E. A., & De Jonge, B. F. (1996). Subtypes of children with attention disabilities. *Child Neuropsychology, 2,* 109–122.

Breen, M. J. (1989). ADHD girls and boys: An analysis of attentional, emotional, cognitive and family variables. *Journal of Child Psychology and Psychiatry, 30,* 711–716.

Breen, M. J., & Barkley, R. A. (1988). Child psychopathology and parenting stress in girls and boys having attention deficit disorder with hyperactivity. *Journal of Pediatric Psychology, 13,* 265–280.

Brown, R. T. (1982). A developmental analysis of the visual and auditory sustained attention and reflection–impulsivity in hyperactive and normal children. *Journal of Learning Disabilities, 15,* 353–357.

Brown, R. T., & Wynne, M. E. (1982). Correlates of teacher ratings, sustained attention, and impulsivity in hyperactive and normal boys. *Journal of Clinical Child Psychology, 11,* 262–267.

Campbell, S. B., Endman, M. W., & Bernfeld, G. (1977). A three-year follow-up of hyperactive preschoolers into elementary school. *Journal of Child Psychology and Psychiatry, 18,* 239–249.

Campbell, S. B., Szumowski, E. K., Ewing, L. J., Gluck, D. S., & Breaux, A. M. (1982). A multidimensional assessment of parent-identified behavior problem toddlers. *Journal of Abnormal Child Psychology, 10,* 569–592.

Cantwell, D. P., Baker, L., & Mattison, R. (1981). Prevalence, type and correlates of psychiatric disorder in 200 children with communication disorder. *Journal of Developmental and Behavioral Pediatrics, 2,* 131–136.

Cardon, L. R., Smith, S. D., Fulker, D. W., Kimberling, W. J., Pennington, B. F., & De Fries, J. C. (1994). Quantitative trait locus for reading disability in chromosome 6. *Science, 266,* 276–279.

Carey, W. B. (1970). A simplified method for measuring infant temperament. *Journal of Pediatrics, 77,* 188–194.

Castellanos, F. X., Giedd, J. N., Eckburg, P., Marsh, W., Kozuch, P., King, A., Hamburger, S., Ritchie, G., & Rapoport, J. (1994). Quantitative morphology of the caudate nucleus in attention deficit hyperactivity disorder. *American Journal of Psychiatry, 151,* 1791–1796.

Castellanos, F. X., Giedd, J. N., Marsh, W. L., Hamburger, S. D., Vaituzis, A. C., Dickstein, D. P., Safatti, S. E., Vauss, Y. C., Snell, J. W., Lange, N., Kaysen, D., Krain, A. L., Ritchie, G. F., Rajapaksc, J. C., & Rapoport, J. L. (1996). Quantitative brain magnetic resonance imagining in attention-deficit hyperactivity disorder. *Archives of General Psychiatry, 53,* 607–616.

Charles, L., Schain, R. J., Zelniker, T., & Guthrie, D. (1979). Effects of methylphenidate on hyperactive children's ability to sustain attention. *Pediatrics, 64,* 412–418.

Chelune, G. J., Ferguson, W., Koon, R., & Dickey, T. O. (1986). Fontal lobe disinhibition in attention deficit disorder. *Child Psychiatry and Human Development, 16,* 221–232.

Cherkes-Julkowski, M., Stolzenberg, J., & Siegal, L. (1991). Prompted cognitive testing as a diagnostic compensation for attentional deficits: The Raven Standard Progressive Matrices and attention deficit disorder. *Learning Disabilities, 2,* 1–7.

Chess, S., & Thomas, A. (1986). *Temperament in clinical practice.* New York: Guilford Press.

Cohen, N. J., Davine, M., & Meloche-Kelly, M. (1989). Prevalence of unsuspected language disorders in a child psychiatric population. *Journal of the American Academy of Child and Adolescent Psychiatry, 28,* 107–111.

Cohen, N. J., Sullivan, S., Minde, K. K., Novak, C., & Helwig, C. (1981). Evaluation of the relative effectiveness of methylphenidate and cognitive behavior modification in the treatment of kindergarten-aged hyperactive children. *Journal of Abnormal Child Psychology, 9,* 43–54.

Comings, D. E., Wu, S., & Chiu, C. (1996). Polygenic inheritance of Tourette syndrome, stuttering, attention deficit hyperactivity, conduct and oppositional defiant disorder. *American Journal of Medical Genetics, 67,* 264–288.

Conners, C. K. (1969). A teacher rating scale for use with drug studies with children. *American Journal of Psychiatry, 126,* 885–888.

Conners, C. K. (1994a). Conners Continuous Performance Test (Version 3.0) [Computer software]. Toronto: Multi-Health Systems.

Conners, C. K. (1994b). *Conners Continuous Performance Test (Version 3.0): User's manual.* Toronto: Multi-Health Systems.

Conners, C. K. (1995). *Continuous Performance Test.* North Tonawanda, NY: Multi-Health Systems.

Conners, C. K. (1997). *Conners Rating Scales—Revised.* North Tonawanda, NY: Multi-Health Systems.

Conners, C. K., & Wells, K. C. (1986). *Hyperkinetic children: A neuropsychosocial approach.* Beverly Hills, CA: Sage.

Cook, E. H., Stein, M. A., & Krasowski, M. D. (1995). Association of attention deficit disorder and the dopamine transporter gene. *American Journal of Human Genetics, 56,* 993–998.

Daigneault, S., Braun, C. M. J., & Whitaker, H. A. (1992). An empirical test of two opposing theoretical models of prefrontal function. *Brain and Cognition, 19,* 48–71.

De Fries, J. C., & Fulker, D. W. (1985). Multiple regression analysis of twin data. *Behavior Genetics, 15,* 467–473.

De Fries, J. C., & Fulker, D. W. (1988). Multiple regression analysis of twin data: Etiology of deviant scores versus individual differences. *Acta Geneticae Medicae et Gemellologiae* (Roma), *37,* 205–216.

deHaas, P. A., & Young, R. D. (1984). Attention styles of hyperactive and normal girls. *Journal of Abnormal Child Psychology, 12,* 531–546.

Devers, R., Bradley-Johnson, S., & Johnson, C. M. (1994). The effect of token reinforcement on WISC-R performance for fifth through ninth grade American Indians. *Psychological Record, 44,* 441–449.

Douglas, V. I. (1972). Stop, look and listen: The problem of sustained attention and impulse control in hyperactive and normal children. *Canadian Journal of Behavioural Science, 4,* 259–282.

Douglas, V. I. (1988). Cognitive deficits in children with attention deficit disorder with hyperactivity. In L. M. Bloomingdale & J. Sergeant (Eds.), *Attention deficit disorder: Criteria, cognition and intervention* (pp. 68–76). New York: Pergamon Press.

Douglas, V. I., Barr, R. G., O'Neil, M. E., & Britton, B. G. (1986). Short-term effects of methylphenidate on the cognitive, learning, and academic performance of children with attention deficit disorder in the laboratory and classroom. *Journal of Child Psychology and Psychiatry, 27,* 191–211.

Draeger, S., Prior, M., & Sanson, A. (1986). Visual and auditory attention performance in hyperactive children: Competence or compliance. *Journal of Abnormal Child Psychology, 14,* 411–424.

DuPaul, G. J. (1990). *Academic Performance Rating Scale and ADHD Rating Scale.* Worcester: University of Massachusetts, Department of Psychiatry.

DuPaul, G. J., Anastopoulos, A. D., Shelton, T. L., Guevremont, D. C., & Metevia, L. (1992a). Multimethod assessment of attention-deficit hyperactivity disorder: The diagnostic utility of clinic-based tests. *Journal of Clinical Child Psychology, 21,* 394–402.

DuPaul, G. J., Guevremont, D. C., & Barkley, R. A. (1991). Attention deficit hyperactivity disorder in adolescence: Critical assessment parameters. *Clinical Psychology Review, 11,* 231–245.

DuPaul, G. J., Guevremont, D. C., & Barkley, R. A. (1992b). Behavioral treatment of attention-deficit hyperactivity disorder in the classroom: The use of the attention training systems. *Behavior Modification, 16,* 204–225.

DuPaul, G. J., & Rapport, M. D. (1993). Does methylphenidate normalize the classroom performance of children with attention deficit disorder? *Journal of the American Academy of Child and Adolescent Psychiatry, 32,* 190–198.

Dykman, R. A., Ackerman, P. T., Clements, S. D., & Peters, J. E. (1971). Specific learning disabilities: An attentional deficit syndrome. In H. R. Myklebust (Ed.), *Progress in learning disabilities* (Vol. 2, pp. 56–93). New York: Grune and Stratton.

Eaves, L. J., Silberg, J. L., & Hewitt, J. K. (1993). Genes, personality and psychopathology: A latent class analysis of liability to symptoms of attention deficit hyperactivity disorder in twins. In R. Plomin & G. McClean (Eds.), *Nature, nurture and psychology* (pp. 285–303). Washington, DC: American Psychological Association.

Ebstein, E. B., Novick, O., Umansky, R., et al. (1996). Dopamine D4 receptor (D4 DR) exon III polymorphism associated with the human personality trait of novelty seeking. *Nature Genetics, 12,* 78–80.

Edelbrock, C. (1990). Childhood attention problems (CAP) scale. In R. A. Barkley (Ed.), *Attention-deficit hyperactivity disorder: A handbook for diagnosis and treatment* (pp. 320–321). New York: Guilford Press.

Edelbrock, C., Rende, R., Plomin, R., & Thompson, L. A. (1995). A twin study of competence and problem behavior in childhood and early adolescence. *Journal of Psychology and Psychiatry, 36,* 775–785.

Elia, J., Borcherding, B. G., Rapoport, J. L., & Keysor, C. S. (1991). Methylphenidate and dextroamphetamine treatments of hyperactivity: Are there true nonresponders? *Psychiatry Research, 36*(2), 141–155.

Ellis, A. W. (1985). The cognitive neuropsychology of developmental (and acquired) dyslexia: A critical survey. *Cognitive Neuropsychology, 2,* 169–205.

Faraone, S. V., Biederman, J., Chen, W. J., & Krifcher, B. (1992). Segregation analyses of attention deficit hyperactivity disorder. *Psychiatric Genetics, 2,* 257–275.

Fergusson, D. M., & Horwood, L. J. (1992). Attention deficit and reading achievement. *Journal of Child Psychology and Psychiatry, 33,* 375–385.

Filipek, P. A., Semrud-Clikeman, M., Steingard, R. J., Renshaw, P. F., Kennedy, D. N., & Biederman, J. (1997). Volumetric MRI analysis comparing subjects having attention-deficit hyperactivity disorder with normal controls. *Neurology, 48,* 589–601.

Fonagy, P., Steele, M., Steele, H., Higgitt, A., & Target, M. (1994). The Emmanuel Miller Memorial Lecture, 1992: The theory and practice of resilience. *Journal of Child Psychology and Psychiatry, 35,* 231–257.

Fuhrman, M. J., & Kendall, P. C. (1986). Cognitive tempo and behavioral adjustment in children. *Cognitive Therapy and Research, 10,* 45–50.

Fuster, J. M. (1989). A theory of prefrontal functions: The prefrontal cortex and the temporal organization of behavior. In J. M. Fuster (Ed.), *The prefrontal cortex: Anatomy, physiology, and neuropsychology of the frontal lobe* (pp. 123–164). New York: Raven Press.

Gibson, E., & Radner, N. (1979). Attention: Perceiver as performer. In G. Hale & M. Lewis (Eds.), *Attention and cognitive development* (pp. 235–267). New York: Plenum.

Gillis, J. J., Gilger, J. W., Pennington, B. F., & De Fries, J. C. (1992). Attention deficit disorders in reading disabled twins: Evidence for a genetic etiology. *Journal of Abnormal Child Psychology, 20,* 303–315.

Glow, R. A., & Glow, P. H. (1980). Peer and self-rating: Children's perception of behavior relevant to hyperkinetic impulse disorder. *Journal of Abnormal Psychology, 8,* 471–490.

Golden, M., Montare, A., & Bridger, W. (1977). Verbal control of delay behavior in two year old boys as a function of social class. *Child Development, 48,* 1107–1111.

Goldstein, S. (1995). *Understanding and managing children's classroom behavior.* New York: Wiley.

Goldstein, S. (1997). *Managing attention disorders in late adolescence and adulthood: A guide for practitioners.* New York: Wiley.

Goldstein, S., & Goldstein, M. (1992). *Why won't my child pay attention?* New York: Wiley.

Goldstein, S., & Goldstein, M. (1998). *Understanding and managing attention deficit hyperactivity disorder in children: A guide for practitioners* (2nd Ed.). New York: Wiley.

Goodman, R., & Stevenson, J. (1989). A twin study of hyperactivity: II. The aetiological role of genes, family relationships and perinatal activity. *Journal of Child Psychology and Psychiatry, 30,* 691–709.

Gordon, M. (1993a). *Clinical and research applications of the Gordon Diagnostic System: A survey of users.* DeWitt, NY: Gordon Systems.

Gordon, M. (1993b). Do computerized measures of attention have a legitimate role in ADHD evaluations? *ADHD Report, 1,* 5–6.

Gordon, M. (1995a). Certainly not a fad, but it can be over-diagnosed. *Attention, 2,* 20–22.

Gordon, M. (1995b). *How to own and operate an ADHD clinic.* DeWitt, NY: Gordon Systems.

Gordon, M., & McClure, F. D. (1983). *The objective assessment of attention deficit disorders.* Paper presented at the 91st Annual Convention of the American Psychological Association, Anaheim, CA.

Gorenstein, E. E., & Newman, J. P. (1980). Disinhibitory psychopathology: A new perspective and model for research. *Psychology Review, 87,* 301–315.

Gray, W. S., & Sime, S. (1989). *Discipline in schools (the Elton Report).* London: Her Majesty's Stationery Office.

Greenberg, L. (1991). *Test of Variables of Attention (TOVA).* St. Paul, MN: Attention Technology.

Greenhill, L. L., & Osman, B. B. (1991). *Ritalin: Theory and patient management.* New York: Mary Ann Liebert.

Gualtieri, C. T., & Hicks, R. E. (1985). Neuropharmacology of methylphenidate and a neural substitute for childhood hyperactivity. *Psychiatric Clinics of North America, 8,* 875–892.

Guevremont, D. C., DuPaul, G. J., & Barkley, R. A. (1993). Behavioral assessment of attention deficit hyperactivity disorder. In J. L. Matson (Ed.). *Handbook of hyperactivity in children* (pp. 150–168). Needham Heights, MA: Allyn & Bacon.

Haenlein, M., & Caul, W. F. (1987). Attention deficit disorder with hyperactivity: A specific hypothesis of reward dysfunction. *Journal of the American Academy of Child and Adolescent Psychiatry, 26,* 356–362.

Hagen, J. W., & Hale, G. H. (1973). The development of attention in children. In *Child psychology* (Vol. 7, pp. 117–137). Minneapolis: University of Minnesota Press.

Hagerman, R. (1991). Organic causes of ADHD. *ADD-VANCE, 3,* 4–6.

Hall, S. J., Halperin, J. M., Schwartz, S. T., & Newcorn, J. H. (1997). Behavioral and executive functions in children with attention deficit hyperactivity disorder and reading disability. *Journal of Attention Disorders, 1,* 235–247.

Halperin, J. M., Newcorn, J. H., Matier, K., Sharma, V., McKay, K. E., & Schwartz, S. (1993). Discriminant validity of attention-deficit hyperactivity disorder. *Journal of the American Academy of Child and Adolescent Psychiatry, 32,* 1038–1043.

Hechtman, L. (1993). Genetic and neurobiological aspects of attention deficit hyperactivity disorder: A review. *Journal of Psychiatric Neuroscience, 9,* 193–201.

Hunt, R. D. (1987). Treatment effects of oral and transdermal clonidine in relation to methylphenidate: An open pilot study in ADD-H. *Psychopharmacology Bulletin, 23,* 111–114.

Hutt, C., Hutt, S. J., & Ounsted, C. (1963). A method for the study of children's behavior. *Developmental Medicine and Child Neurology, 5,* 233.

Hynd, G. W., Hern, K. L., Novey, E. S., & Eliopulos, D. (1993). Attention-deficit hyperactivity disorder and asymmetry of the caudate nucleus. *Journal of Child Neurology, 8,* 339–347.

Hynd, G. W., Semrud-Clikeman, M., Lorys, A. R., Novey, E. S., Eliopulos, D., & Lyytinen, H. (1991). Corpus callosum morphology in attention-deficit hyperactivity disorder (ADHD): Morphometric analysis of MRI. *Journal of Learning Disabilities, 24,* 141–146.

Ideus, K. (1994). Cultural foundations of ADHD: A sociological analysis. *Therapeutic Care and Education, 3,* 173–192.

Ingersoll, B., & Goldstein, S. (1993). *Attention deficit disorder and learning disabilities: Myths, realities and controversial treatments.* New York: Doubleday.

James, W. (1890). *The principles of psychology.* New York: Holt.

Kagan, J. (1964). *The Matching Familiar Figures Test.* Unpublished manuscript, Harvard University.

Katz, M. (1997). *Playing a poor hand well.* New York: Norton.

Keough, B. K., & Margolis, J. S. (1976). A component analysis of attentional problems of educationally handicapped boys. *Journal of Abnormal Child Psychology, 4,* 349–359.

Klein, R. G. (1987). Pharmacotherapy of childhood hyperactivity: An update. In H. Y. Meltzer (Ed.), *Psychopharmacology: The third generation of progress* (pp. 287–301). New York: Raven Press.

Knobel, M., Walman, M. B., & Mason, E. (1959). Hyperkinesis and organicity in children. *Archives of General Psychiatry, 1,* 310–321.

Koriath, U., Gualtieri, T., Van Bourgondien, M. E., Quade, D., & Werry, J. S. (1985). Construct validity of clinical diagnosis in pediatric psychiatry: Relationship among measures. *Journal of the American Academy of Child Psychiatry, 24,* 429–436.

Lahey, B. B., Applegate, B., McBurnett, K., Biederman, J., Greenhill, L., Hynd, G., Barkley, R. A., Newcorn, J., Jensen, P., Richters, J., Garfinkel, B., Kerdyk, L., Frick, P. J., Ollendick, T., Perez, D., Hart, E. L., Waldman, I., & Shaffer, D. (1994). DSM-IV field trial for attention deficit/hyperactivity disorder in children and adolescents. *American Journal of Psychiatry, 151,* 1673–1685.

LaHoste, G. J., Swanson, J. M., & Wigal, S. B. (1996). Dopamine D4 receptor gene polymorphism is associated with attention deficit hyperactivity disorder. *Molecular Psychiatry, 1,* 121–124.

Laufer, M. W., & Denhoff, E. (1957). Hyperkinetic behavior syndrome in children. *Journal of Pediatrics, 50,* 463–474.

Levine, M. D. (1987). Attention deficit: The diversive effects of weak control systems in childhood. *Pediatric Annals, 16,* 117–130.

Levine, M.D. (1992). Commentary: Attentional disorders—elusive entities and their mistaken identities. *Journal of Child Neurology, 7,* 449–453.

Levy, F., Hay, D. A., McStephen, M., Wood, C., & Waldman, I. (1997). Attention-deficit hyperactivity disorder: A category or a continuum? Genetic analysis of a large-scale twin study. *Journal of the American Academy of Child and Adolescent Psychiatry, 36,* 737–744.

Loney, J., Kramer, J., & Milich, R. (1981). The hyperkinetic child grown up: Predictors of symptoms, delinquency and achievement at follow–up. In K. D. Gadow & J. Loney (Eds.), *Psychosocial aspects of drug treatment for hyperactivity* (pp. 86–110). Boulder, CO: Westview Press.

Lou, H. C., Henriksen, L., & Bruhn, P. (1984). Focal cerebral hypoperfusion in children with dysphasia and/or attention deficit disorder. *Archives of Neurology, 41,* 825–829.

Luk, S. (1985). Direct observation studies of hyperactive behaviors. *Journal of the American Academy of Child Psychiatry, 24,* 338–344.

Luk, S. L., Leung, P. W., & Yuen, J. (1991). Clinic observations in the assessment of pervasiveness of childhood hyperactivity. *Journal of Child Psychology and Psychiatry, 32,* 833–850.

Mann, E. M., Ikeda, Y., Mueller, C. W., & Takahshi, A. (1992). Cross cultural differences in rating hyperactive disruptive behaviors in children. *American Journal of Psychiatry, 149,* 1539–1542.

Mannuzza, S., Klein, R. G., Bonagura, N., Malloy, P., Giampino, T. L., & Addalli, K. A. (1991). Hyperactive boys almost grown up: V. Replication of psychiatric status. *Archives of General Psychiatry, 48,* 77–83.

Margolis, J. S. (1972). *Academic correlates of sustained attention.* Unpublished doctoral dissertation, University of California at Los Angeles.

Mattes, J. A. (1980). The role of frontal lobe dysfunction in childhood hyperkinesis. *Comprehensive Psychiatry, 21,* 358–369.

McGee, R., & Share, D. L. (1988). Attention deficit hyperactivity disorder and academic failure: Which comes first and what should be treated? *Journal of the American Academy of Child and Adolescent Psychiatry, 27,* 318–325.

McNamara, J. J. (1972). Hyperactivity in the apartment bound child. *Clinical Pediatrics, 11,* 371–372.

Mesulam, M. M. (1985). *Principles of behavioral neurology.* Philadelphia: F. A. Davis.

Milich, R. (1984). Cross-sectional and longitudinal observations of activity level and sustained attention in a normative sample. *Journal of Abnormal Child Psychology, 12,* 261–276.

Milich, R., & Kramer, J. (1984). Reflections on impulsivity: An empirical investigation of impulsivity as a construct. In K. Gadow & I. Bialer (Eds.), *Advances in learning and behavioral disabilities* (Vol. 3, pp. 117–150). Greenwich, CT: JAI Press.

Milich, R., & Loney, J. (1979). The role of hyperactive and aggressive symptomatology in predicting adolescent outcome among hyperactive children. *Journal of Pediatric Psychology, 4,* 93–112.

Milich, R., Loney, J., & Landau, S. (1982). The independent dimensions of hyperactivity and aggression: A validation with playroom observation data. *Journal of Abnormal Psychology, 91,* 183–198.

Milich, R., Loney, J., & Roberts, M. A. (1986). Playroom observations of activity level and sustained attention: Two-year stability. *Journal of Consulting and Clinical Psychology, 54,* 272–274.

Millstein, R. B., Wilens, T. E., Biederman, J., & Spencer, T. J. (1997). Presenting ADHD symptoms and subtypes in clinically referred adults with ADHD. *Journal of Attention Disorders, 2,* 159–166.

Mirskey, A. F., Anthony, B. J., Duncan, C. C., Ahearn, M. B., & Kellam, S. G. (1991). Analysis of the elements of attention: A neuropsychological approach. *Neuropsychology Review, 2,* 109–145.

O'Neill, M. E., & Douglas, V. I. (1996). Rehearsal strategies and recall performance with boys with and without attention deficit hyperactivity disorder. *Journal of Pediatric Psychology, 21,* 73–88.

Parker, H. C. (1992). *The ADD hyperactivity workbook for schools.* Plantation, FL: ADD Warehouse.

Pelham, W. E. (1987). What do we know about the use and effects of CNS stimulants in ADD? In J. Loney (Ed.), *The young hyperactive child: Answers to questions about diagnosis, prognosis and treatment* (pp. 99–110). New York: Haworth Press.

Pelham, W. E., & Bender, M. E. (1982). Peer relationships in hyperactive children. In K. D. Gadow & I. Bialer (Eds.), *Advances in learning and behavioral disabilities* (Vol. 1, pp. 365–436). Greenwich, CT: JAI Press.

Pelham, W. E., & Milich, R. (1984). Peer relations of children with hyperactivity/attention deficit disorder. *Journal of Learning Disabilities, 17,* 560–568.

Picano, J. J., Klusman, L. E., Hornbestel, L. K., & Moulton, J. M. (1992). Replication of three-component solution for common measures of attention in HIV seropositive males. *Archives of Clinical Neuropsychology, 7,* 271–274.

Pliszka, S. R. (1992). Comorbidity of attention-deficit hyperactivity disorder and overanxious disorder. *Journal of the American Academy of Child and Adolescent Psychiatry, 31,* 197–203.

Pope, L. (1970). Motor activity in brain-injured children. *American Journal of Orthopsychiatry, 40,* 783–794.

Porrino, L. J., Lucignani, G., Dow-Edwards, D., & Sokoloff, L. (1984). Dose dependent effects and acute amphetamine administration on functional brain metabolism in rats. *Brain Research, 307,* 311–320.

Posner, M. I. (1987). Selective attention in head injury. In H. S. Levin, J. Grafman, & H. M. Eisenberg (Eds.), *Neurobehavioral recovery from head injury* (pp. 144–157). New York: Oxford University Press.

Posner, M. I., & Snyder, C. R. (1975). Attention and cognitive control. In R. Solso (Ed.), *Information processing and cognition: The Loyola symposium* (Vol. 2, pp. 163–187). Hillsdale, NJ: Erlbaum.

Rapport, M. D., Tucker, S. B., DuPaul, G. J., Merlo, M., & Stoner, G. (1986). Hyperactivity and frustration: The influence of control over and size of rewards in delaying gratification. *Journal of Abnormal Child Psychology, 14,* 191–204.

Roberts, M. A. (1990). A behavioral observation method for differentiating hyperactive and aggressive boys. *Journal of Abnormal Child Psychology, 18,* 131–142.

Ross, D. M., & Ross, S. A. (1982). *Hyperactivity: Current issues, research and theory* (2nd ed.). New York: Wiley.

Routh, D. K. (1978). Hyperactivity. In P. R. Magrab (Ed.), *Psychological management of pediatric problems* (Vol. 2, pp. 212–247). Baltimore: University Park Press.

Routh, D. K., & Schroeder, C. S. (1976). Standardized playroom measures as indices of hyperactivity. *Journal of Abnormal Child Psychology, 4,* 199–207.

Rucklidge, J. J., & Kaplan, B. J. (1997). Psychological functioning in women identified in adulthood with ADHD. *Journal of Attention Disorders, 2,* 167–176.

Rutter, M., MacDonald, H., Lecoutier, A., Harrington, R., Bolton, P., & Bailey, A. (1990). Genetic factors in child psychiatric disorders: II. Empirical findings. *Journal of Child Psychology and Psychiatry, 31,* 39–83.

Safer, D. J. (1973). A familial factor in minimal brain dysfunction. *Behavior Genetics, 3,* 175–186.

Safer, D. J., Sito, J. M., & Fine, E. M. (1996). Increased methylphenidate usage for attention deficit disorder in the 1990's. *Pediatrics, 98,* 1084–1088.

Satterfield, J. H., & Dawson, M. E. (1971). Electrodermal correlates of hyperactivity in children. *Psychophysiology, 8,* 191–197.

Satterfield, J. H., Hoppe, C. M., & Schell, A. M. (1982). A perspective study of delinquency in 110 adolescent boys with attention deficit disorder and 88 normal adolescent boys. *American Journal of Psychiatry, 139,* 795–798.

Schulman, J. L., & Reisman, J. M. (1959). An objective measure of hyperactivity. *American Journal of Mental Deficiency, 64,* 455–456.

Seidman, L. J., Biederman, J., Faraone, S. V., Weber, W., Mennin, D., & Jones, J. (1997). A pilot study of neuropsychological functioning in girls with ADHD. *Journal of the American Academy of Child and Adolescent Psychiatry, 36,* 366–373.

Semrud-Clikeman, M., Filipek, P. A., Biederman, J., Steingard, R., Kennedy, D., Renshaw, P., &

Bekken, K. (1994). Attention deficit hyperactivity disorder: Differences in the corpus callosum by MRI morphometric analysis. *Journal of the American Academy of Child and Adolescent Psychiatry, 33,* 875–881.

Sherman, D. K., Iacono, W. G., & McGue, M. K. (1997). Attention-deficit hyperactivity disorder dimensions: A twin study of inattention and impulsivity–hyperactivity. *Journal of the American Academy of Child and Adolescent Psychiatry, 36,* 745–753.

Shum, D. H., MacFarland, K. A., & Bain, J. D. (1990). Construct validity of eight tests of attention: Comparison of normal and closed head injured samples. *Clinical Neuropsychologists, 4,* 151–162.

Silverthorn, P., Frick, P. J., Kuper, K., & Ott, J. (1996). Attention deficit hyperactivity disorder and sex: A test of two etiological models to explain the male predominance. *Journal of Clinical Child Psychology, 25,* 52–59.

Skinner, B. F. (1953). *Science and human behavior.* New York: Macmillan.

Spring, C., Yellin, A. M., & Greenberg, L. M. (1976). Effects of imipramine and methylphenidate on perceptual–motor performance of hyperactive children. *Perceptual and Motor Skills, 43,* 459–470.

Stein, M. (1997). We have tried everything and nothing works: Family-centered pediatrics and clinical problem solving. *Journal of Developmental and Behavioral Pediatrics, 18,* 114–119.

Stevens, T. M., Kupst, M. J., Suran, B. G., & Schulman, J. L. (1978). Activity level: A comparison between actometer scores and observer ratings. *Journal of Abnormal Child Psychology, 6,* 163–173.

Stevenson, J. (1992). Evidence for a genetic etiology in hyperactivity in children. *Behavior Genetics, 22,* 337–344.

Stott, D. H. (1981). Behavior disturbance and failure to learn: A study of cause and effect. *Educational Research, 23,* 163–172.

Swanson, J. M., Cantwell, D., Lerner, M., McBurnett, K., & Hanna, G. (1991). Effects of stimulant medication on learning in children with ADHD. *Journal of Learning Disabilities, 24,* 219–230.

Swanson, J. M., & Kinsbourne, M. (1979). The cognitive effects of stimulant drugs on hyperactive children. In G. A. Hale (Ed.), *Attention and cognitive development* (pp. 67–94). New York: Plenum Press.

Szatmari, P., Offord, D. R., Siegel, L. S., Finlayson, M. A., & Tuff, L. (1990). The clinical significance of neurocognitive impairments among children with psychiatric disorders: Diagnosis and situational specificity. *Journal of Child Psychology and Psychiatry and Allied Disciplines, 31,* 287–299.

Tao, K. T. (1992). Clinical comment: Hyperactivity and attention deficit disorder syndromes in China. *Journal of the American Academy of Child and Adolescent Psychiatry, 31,* 1165–1166.

Tarver-Behring, S., Barkley, R. A., & Karlsson, J. (1985). The mother–child interactions of hyperactive boys and their normal siblings. *American Journal of Orthopsychiatry, 355,* 202–209.

Terestman, N. (1980). Mood quality and intensity in nursery school children as predictors of behavior disorder. *American Journal of Orthopsychiatry, 50,* 125–138.

Thapar, A., Hervas, A., & McGuffin, P. (1995). Childhood hyperactivity scores are highly heritable and show sibling competition effects: Twin study evidence. *Behavior Genetics, 35,* 537–544.

Thomas, A., & Chess, S. (1977). *Temperament and development.* New York: Brunner/Mazel.

Titchener, E. B. (1924). *A textbook of psychology.* New York: Macmillan.

Touwen, B. C. L., & Kalverboer, A. F. (1973). Neurologic and behavioral assessment of children with minimal brain dysfunction. *Seminars in Psychiatry, 5,* 79–94.

Tryon, W. W. (1984). Principles and methods of mechanically measuring motor activity. *Behavioral Assessment, 6,* 129–140.

Ullman, D. G., Barkley, R. A., & Brown, H. W. (1978). The behavioral symptoms of hyperkinetic children who successfully responded to stimulant drug treatment. *American Journal of Orthopsychiatry, 48,* 425–437.

Ullmann, R. K., Sleator, E. K., & Sprague, R. K. (1988). *ADD-H: Comprehensive Teacher's Rating Scale* (2nd ed.). Champaign, IL: MetriTech.

Voeller, K. S. (1991). Towards a neurobiologic nosology of attention deficit hyperactivity disorder. *Journal of Child Neurology, 6*, S2–S8.

Warren, R. P., Odell, J. D., Warren, L. W., Burger, R. A., Maciulis, A., Daniels, W. W., & Torres, A. R. (1995). Reading disability, attention-deficit hyperactivity disorder and the immune system. *Science, 268*, 786–787.

Wechsler, D. (1974). *Wechsler Intelligence Scale for Children—Revised.* New York: Psychological Corporation.

Wechsler, D. (1989). *Wechsler Intelligence Scale for Children—III.* San Antonio, TX: Psychological Corporation.

Weiss, G., & Hechtman, L. (1979). The hyperactive child syndrome. *Science, 205*, 1348–1354.

Weiss, G., & Hechtman, L. (1993). *Hyperactive children grown up* (2nd ed.): *ADHD in children, adolescents, and adults.* New York: Guilford Press.

Wender, P. H. (1971). *Minimal brain dysfunction in children.* New York: Wiley.

Wender, P. H. (1972). The minimal brain dysfunction syndrome in children. *Journal of Nervous and Mental Disease, 155*, 55–71.

Wender, P. H. (1975). The minimal brain dysfunction syndrome. *Annual Review of Medicine, 26*, 45–62.

Wender, P. H. (1979). The concept of adult minimal brain dysfunction. In L. Bellak (Ed.), *Psychiatric aspects of minimal brain dysfunction in adults* (pp. 148–173). New York: Grune & Stratton.

Werner, E. E. (1994). Overcoming the odds. *Journal of Developmental and Behavioral Pediatrics, 15*, 131–136.

Werry, J. S., Elkind, G. S., & Reeves, J. C. (1987). Attention deficit, conduct, oppositional and anxiety disorders in children: III. Laboratory differences. *Journal of Abnormal Child Psychology, 15*, 409–428.

Whalen, C. K., & Henker, B. (1991). Therapies for hyperactive children: Comparisons, combinations and compromises. *Journal of Consulting and Clinical Psychology, 59*, 126–137.

Whalen, C. K., Henker, B., Collins, B., McAuliffe, S., & Vaux, A. (1979). Peer interaction in a structured communication task: Comparisons of normal and hyperactive boys and of methylphenidate (Ritalin) and placebo effects. *Child Development, 50*, 388–401.

Whalen, C. K., Henker, B., & Dotemoto, S. (1981). Teacher response to methylphenidate (Ritalin) versus placebo status of hyperactive boys in the classroom. *Child Development, 52*, 1005–1014.

Willerman, L. (1973). Activity level and hyperactivity in twins. *Child Development, 44*, 288–293.

Williams, L., Lerner, M., & Swanson, J.M. (1994). *Prevalence of office visits for ADD: Gender differences over the past five years (1990–1994).* Unpublished manuscript.

Zahn-Waxler, C., Schmitz, S., Fulker, D., Robinson, J., & Emde, R. (1996). Behavior problems in five-year-old monozygotic and dizygotic twins: Genetic and environmental influences, patterns of regulation, and internationalization of control. *Developmental Psychopathology, 8*, 103–122.

Zametkin, A. J., & Rapoport, J. L. (1987). Neurobiology of attention deficit disorder with hyperactivity: Where have we come in 50 years? *Journal of the American Academy of Child and Adolescent Psychiatry, 26*, 676–686.

Zentall, S. S. (1984). Context effects in the behavioral ratings of hyperactivity. *Journal of Abnormal Child Psychology 12*, 345–352.

Zentall, S. S. (1988). Production deficiencies in elicited language but not in the spontaneous verbalizations of hyperactive children. *Exceptional Children, 60*, 143–153.

Zentall, S. S. (1995). Modifying classroom tasks and environments. In S. Goldstein (Ed.), *Understanding and managing children's classroom behavior* (pp. 356–374). New York: Wiley.

8

GILLES DE LA TOURETTE SYNDROME

RONALD T. BROWN
CAROLYN E. IVERS

Gilles de la Tourette syndrome (Tourette syndrome, or TS) is a genetic, neuropsychiatric disorder consisting of chronic motor and verbal tics that are typically present for at least 1 year (American Psychiatric Association [APA], 1994). TS often has its origins in middle childhood (mean age 7 years), with motor tics preceding the onset of vocal tics (Lombroso et al., 1995). A "tic" refers to a recurring, stereotypical, nonrhythmic vocalization or motor movement that occurs suddenly and without warning and is of short duration (APA, 1994). Tics can be suppressed for varying periods of time, although they are frequently described by an affected individual as being irresistible. All forms of tics have been demonstrated to be exacerbated by stress. For example, Silva, Munoz, Barickman, and Friedhoff (1995) examined environmental factors associated with fluctuation of symptoms in children and adolescents with TS. Findings suggested a number of factors associated with an increase in tics, including events causing anxiety (e.g., social gatherings) and emotional trauma. Tic frequency has been observed to decrease during activities that require sustained concentration and attention, as well as during sleep. The number, frequency, severity, and type of tics may change over the course of time.

According to the APA (1994), motor and vocal tics are classified as either "simple" or "complex." Commonly observed simple motor tics include blinking of eyes, jerking of the neck, shrugging of shoulders, facial grimacing, and coughing. Typical complex motor tics consist of grooming behaviors, facial gestures, touching, jumping, stomping feet, and smelling objects. Motor tics often involve the head and other parts of the body, including the torso and upper and lower limbs. Simple vocal tics commonly include clearing of the throat, clicking, sniffing, grunting, snorting, and barking (e.g., yelps). Finally, complex vocal tics may involve the repetition of words or phrases out of context, coprolalia (use of obscenities or curse words), palilalia (repetition of one's own sounds or words), and echolalia (repetition of a recently heard sound, words, or phrases) (APA, 1994). Although blurting out curse words or obscenities (i.e., coprolalia) is frequently mentioned in connection with TS in the mass media, the incidence of this type of vocal tic is actually quite low. In a survey of 112 individuals with TS, Goldenberg, Brown, and Weiner (1994) found that only 8% of the group exhibited coprolalia, although some experts have reported higher incidences of coprolalia in patients with TS (Mansdorf, 1995).

The core features of TS include multiple motor and one or more vocal tics. Over the course of the disorder, the motor and vocal tics may appear either together or separately during different periods (APA, 1994). In order to meet diagnostic criteria, the tics must occur many times throughout the day for a period of more than 1 year. The tic symptoms may not be absent for a period of more than 3 consecutive months. Finally, the presence of the disorder must cause significant impairment in occupational, social, or emotional functioning.

In children, it has been suggested that TS is expressed as a clinical spectrum that includes a range of increasing functional impairments, suggestive of various degrees of behavioral abnormality and basal ganglia development (Kurlan, 1994). According to Kurlan, the mildest form of TS includes largely asymptomatic features in which only brain morphology is affected, whereas children suffering from moderate TS evidence school and behavioral problems and may require special education. Children with the most severe form of the disorder, who suffer from disabling symptoms, may require pharmacotherapy to function in society (Kurlan, 1994).

The prevalence of TS is estimated to be between 1 and 8 cases per 1,000 males and between 0.1 and 4 cases per 1,000 females (Peterson, Leckman, & Cohen, 1995). Thus the syndrome is clearly more prevalent in males than in females, with estimates ranging from 2:1 to 10:1 in favor of males. Differences in prevalence data have been attributed to sample populations (i.e., clinic vs. community samples), the sensitivity and specificity of the diagnostic instruments employed, and the age distribution of the population sampled (Peterson et al., 1995). The highest prevalence estimates of TS are found in those studies utilizing direct examination of individuals in outpatient psychiatric clinics; lower prevalence estimates have been obtained through surveys of community populations. Clinic-based studies are likely to overestimate the prevalence of TS, as traditional structured diagnostic interviews are not sufficiently sensitive to discriminate the presence of mild tics from overt TS. Thus these examinations are apt to yield a preponderance of false positives. In contrast, community-based investigations employing surveys for the identification of TS tend to underestimate prevalence due to an underreporting of symptoms (Peterson et al., 1995). Studies of pediatric populations yield higher prevalence estimates than their adolescent or adult counterparts (Peterson et al., 1995). The higher prevalence of the disorder in children has been attributed to a decrease in tic severity at puberty. In fact, Apter et al. (1993) have provided prevalence estimates of TS in adolescents aged 16–17 years that are strikingly similar to adult prevalence estimates.

HISTORY

The first known report of the disorder was made by Jean-Marc Itard in the early 19th century (Hyde & Weinberger, 1995). Itard presented a case history of a French noblewoman who displayed motor tics at the age of 7 years, and who subsequently developed involuntary vocalizations that consisted of screams and strange cries. Later the patient developed coprolalia and was forced to live in seclusion until her death at the age of 85. Five decades later Gilles de la Tourette, under the supervision of the eminent neurologist Jean Martin Charcot, presented a series of cases detailing the history and symptoms of several patients with the same syndrome. His early descriptions included information about the waxing and waning of multiple motor and vocal tics, the early age of onset, and the importance of genetic influences on the disorder (Sprague & Newell, 1986). The syndrome was subsequently named for Tourette.

Although TS was discovered over a century ago, the syndrome continues to be misunderstood and underdiagnosed (Sprague & Newell, 1986). Until recently, TS was considered to be a psychiatric disorder because of the patient's ability to voluntarily suppress the behaviors associated with the syndrome and the tendency of tics to be exacerbated during periods of stress. In fact, during the psychoanalytic movement in North America and Europe, a number of case studies were presented offering psychodynamic interpretations for the tics (e.g., Mahler & Rangell, 1943). Although these interpretations have generally been discounted, the content and timing of tic symptoms and their relationship to important events in individuals' lives suggest that these factors can affect the course of TS to some extent. The etiology of tic disorders remains unclear, with most tics having an organic etiology, while others may be exacerbated by psychogenic factors (Mansdorf, 1995). Over the past two decades, considerable evidence has been gathered for the organic etiology of TS. Significant advances in genetics and neuroimaging have resulted in the reclassification of the syndrome as a neurological movement disorder (Peterson et al., 1995). In support of this notion, a number of biological markers have been associated with TS.

Exciting developments in the exploration of the organic basis of TS include the discovery that neurotransmitters such as dopamine may precipitate or exacerbate the symptoms (Peterson et al., 1995). In addition, a number of provocative hypotheses have been presented to suggest significant abnormal brain morphology, particularly within the basal ganglia and limbic system. These developments have led to important treatment pathways for pharmacological interventions.

DEVELOPMENTAL COURSE

The developmental course of the symptoms of individuals with TS has been found to be quite variable. Data from longitudinal investigations have generally indicated that some children have a turbulent time during adolescence and adulthood; however, others have suggested adequate adaptation during the adult years. Nonetheless, existing longitudinal investigations designed to study the natural history of TS have revealed several general trends.

Childhood

In TS the modal onset of tics is reported to be at approximately 7 years of age, although there is a range in the emergence of symptoms from early childhood (i.e., as young as 4 years of age) to young adulthood. TS develops gradually, with one or more transient episodes of mild motor or vocal tics followed by the occurrence of more frequent and severe tics. The initial tics commonly affect the face and may include eye blinking, nose twitching, facial grimacing, biting of the lips, and (less frequently) vocalizations (Bruun, 1988). The next phase slowly pervades the entire body, starting with the head and neck, proceeding to the upper extremities, and then finally moving to the lower extremities. For vocal tics, random vocalizations may later become words and subsequently develop into phrases. Thus the development of the disorder is progressive, originally consisting of single, simple tics in one location, and gradually evolving to more complex tics in multiple regions of the body. The severity of symptoms increases and subsides in a random, cyclical pattern.

If attentional deficits are comorbid with the disorder, they typically emerge at the same time as the tics. This generally occurs by the age of 4 years. On the other hand, obsessive–compulsive symptoms, if they are present, surface after the emergence of tics. In fact, for approximately 30–60% of patients with TS, obsessive thoughts and compulsive rituals do not appear until early adolescence (Leckman, Walker, Goodman, Pauls, & Cohen, 1994).

Adolescence

Frequently there is a diminishing of symptoms during adolescence. Peterson et al. (1995) have speculated that this finding is due to adolescents' increased capacity for self-control and greater preoccupation with peer conformity. Despite the diminution of symptoms, most adolescents continue to receive pharmacotherapy to manage their tics (Peterson et al., 1995). Still, some adolescents have exacerbated levels of aggression, impulsivity, obsessions and compulsions, and severe anxiety. These symptoms may be coupled with tics that are highly complex and significantly impede daily functioning (Peterson et al., 1995). As with any severe chronic illness or disability, the tasks of adolescence may be disrupted by the presence of TS symptoms. This may occur at the family level as the adolescent attempts to assert autonomy and conform with the peer group. The adolescent with TS may also be the target of ridicule and aggression from peers.

Adulthood

The severity of TS during childhood and adolescence is generally believed to be predictive of the adult course (Bruun, 1988). That is, individuals with a mild presentation of symptoms during childhood will typically have a mild presentation during adulthood; those with more severe symptoms during childhood have a greater likelihood of continuing to have more frequent and severe tics throughout their lives. In fact, one investigation has provided important data showing that 80% of individuals with a severe course in childhood had a commensurate adult course (Bruun, 1988). Conversely, Goetz, Tanner, Stebbins, Leipzig, and Carr (1992) have noted some exceptions to these findings and reported that the severity of tics during childhood did not accurately predict the severity of tics in adulthood. Also, twin studies have documented a relationship between age of onset and the course of the disorder (e.g., Hyde, Fitzcharles, & Weinberger, 1993). Findings from these studies suggest that an early age of onset of motor or vocal tics may be the best predictor of a more severe course of the disorder.

Findings from follow-up studies of children with TS have indicated that the typical symptom display can generally be predicted by early adulthood (Bruun, 1988; Erenberg, Cruse, & Rothner, 1987). Studies also have provided encouraging data to suggest that the symptoms of concomitant behavior disorders (e.g., attention-deficit/hyperactivity disorder [ADHD], oppositional defiant disorder [ODD]) and obsessive–compulsive disorder (OCD) may respond to treatment in approximately 50% of cases (Park, Como, Cui, & Kurlan, 1993). Although data from these follow-up studies are indeed encouraging, the majority of adults with TS continue to experience symptoms that significantly affect their social, vocational, and/or emotional functioning. Although many behavioral problems (e.g., impulsivity, aggression) continue to persist well into adulthood, most adults with TS report graduating from high school (Goetz et al., 1992). Many adults with TS still require medical management of their condition (i.e., pharmacotherapy), and a small percentage of them report severe difficulties in coping with the disorder. Nonetheless, a significant number of adults with TS report successful coping with and adaptation to their disorder (Erenberg et al., 1987).

The aforementioned findings must be interpreted judiciously. As with any longitudinal investigation, many of the original subjects were not available for later examination, thus biasing the results toward higher-functioning individuals who were adherent throughout the course of the investigation. As Peterson et al. (1995) have astutely observed, having a stigmatizing developmental disorder that impairs so many areas of daily functioning is likely to leave any adult with some social and emotional challenges. An important goal of future research will be to determine specific variables associated with better adaptation for all individuals with TS, regardless of the severity of their symptomatology. Clearly, as with other chronic physical and developmental disabilities or medical conditions, symptom display or severity does not account for all of the variance in an individual's adaptation to a disability (Wallander, Varni, Babani, Banis, & Wilcox, 1989).

GENETICS AND FAMILIAL PATTERNS

TS is believed to be a familial syndrome with a genetic vulnerability. In part, this explains the expression of symptoms. The majority of individuals who are genetically predisposed to TS present with few and very mild symptoms, which may be nonspecific (i.e., obsessive–compulsive traits). In fact, in many instances these individuals do not come to the attention of health care providers. Still, a small percentage of individuals with this genetic vulnerability may present with the full phenotypic expression of the syndrome. Great variability in symptomatology exists, with environment and physiology determining the magnitude of the symptom expression. Thus the presence of the TS gene (or genes) is not believed to be sufficient to produce the overt expression of the disorder (Peterson et al., 1995).

In his original writings about the syndrome, Gilles de la Tourette posited an etiological role for genetic factors. However, subsequent to these writings, genetics were basically ignored until only recently (Peterson et al., 1995). Approximately 10 years ago, an intensive research effort began to examine the genetic and familial factors that predispose individuals to TS. The syndrome is now believed to be a part of a family of neurologically related disorders that share a common genetic origin (Hyde & Weinberger, 1995; Kidd, Prusoff, & Cohen, 1980; Pauls & Leckman, 1986).

Family Genetic Studies

Compelling data from family genetic studies have addressed the pattern of transmission of TS. In a seminal investigation, Pauls, Raymond, Stevenson, and Leckman (1991b) studied 86 TS probands and 338 of their biological relatives and compared them to controls. It was found that approximately 8% of the relatives of the TS probands met criteria for a diagnosis of the disorder. This is significantly higher than what would be expected in the general population (i.e., prevalence rates are between 3 and 5 individuals per 10,000 in community samples) (Peterson et al., 1995).

In most families, TS and chronic tic disorders are believed to have an autosomal dominant pattern of inheritance, with varying degrees of "penetrance" (i.e., the frequency of expression of the condition) (Hyde & Weinberger, 1995; Pauls & Leckman, 1986; Peterson et al., 1995). Penetrance is believed to be gender-related, with males evidencing a higher prevalence of TS when there is a family history of a multitude of tic disorders (Hyde & Weinberger, 1995). Specifically, male penetrance rates have been reported to be as high as .99, and female penetrance rates are significantly lower (up to .70) (Peterson et al., 1995). Investigators have discovered associations of maternal and paternal homozygous transmission of the gene with the phenotypic expression of the full-blown syndrome in offspring (Kurlan, 1994). Other investigators have posited a semirecessive model of inheritance for TS, in which the phenotypic expression of the disorder is contingent on whether the individual inherits one or two copies of the gene (Comings, Comings, & Knell, 1989). Furthermore, whereas some investigators propose that both quantitative and qualitative differences in the actual genotype may specifically predict phenotypic expression, others suggest that environmental factors influence the clinical expression of the disorder (Kurlan, 1994). In further support of a genetic etiology for this disorder, Kurlan (1994) has noted that even for children with mild, previously undiagnosed tics, the same condition is frequently present in other family members (see also Kurlan, Whitmore, Irvine, McDermott, & Como, 1993).

Of particular interest are the family genetic studies that have demonstrated an association between TS and other psychopathologies. Many experts have interpreted these data to suggest that variability in the phenotypic expression of a gene may be responsible for the presence of TS (Peterson et al., 1995). Stated more simply, TS may represent an extreme form of the expression of a particular gene. For example, a relationship has been shown between Tourette's and OCD, which is overrepresented in many families with TS. For females, penetrance increases when OCD is included in the phenotypic expression of the TS gene. These findings have led experts to conclude that the two disorders may have the same genotype (Hyde & Weinberger, 1995). In support of this notion, Hyde and Weinberger (1995) have pointed out that obsessive–compulsive symptoms frequently occur in patients with TS, although only a small number of these patients actually meet full diagnostic criteria for OCD. Some empirical support for a genetic association between TS and OCD has been provided by Pauls and Leckman (1986). In their investigation, structured interviews were administered to 338 biological relatives of 85 TS probands and 113 relatives of 35 subjects who served as controls. Findings indicate that the rate of OCD was higher among the relatives of TS probands than among those of controls. Pauls, Raymond, and Robertson (1991a) have also presented data demonstrating a probable genetic relationship of TS and OCD; they found that the incidence of TS and chronic tics was elevated among OCD probands and their relatives. Finally, recent data from intervention studies have suggested that individuals with a family history of OCD and TS respond differentially to neuroleptic drug therapy than do individuals who exhibit OCD without any family history of TS (McDougle, Goodman, & Price, 1990). Specifically, individuals who have a family history of TS tend to respond better to neuroleptic drug therapy.

Twin Studies

Over the years, several twin studies have been conducted to explore the role of genetic factors in the transmission and expression of TS and related disorders (for a review, see Peterson et al., 1995). The data from these studies have generally indicated that monozygotic twin pairs are highly concordant for TS and other tic disorders (Peterson et al., 1995). For example, Hyde, Aaronson, Randolph, Rickler, and Weinberger (1992) have provided data indicating a 50–90% concordance rate for tic disorders between monozygotic twins. Although fewer studies of dizygotic twin pairs have been reported in the literature, the concordance rates for TS and tic disorders are significantly lower for dizygotic twins than for monozygotic twins (Peterson et al., 1995). The significant difference in concordance rates among monozygotic and dizygotic twin pairs provides compelling evidence for a strong genetic component of tic disorders.

In at least one twin study, an association has been demonstrated between age of onset of TS and the course of the disorder. Hyde et al. (1992) studied 18 pairs of monozygotic twins in which at least one member had been diagnosed with Tourette's. While 16 sets were concordant for motor tics; the age of onset of motor tics as reported by mothers and/ or medical records was variable (range = 5 to 12 years). Interestingly, the earlier the onset of the motor tics, the more severe the course of the disorder. Furthermore, 10 of the twin pairs were concordant for vocal tics; again, the earlier the age of vocal tic onset (range = 5 to 13 years), the more severe the course of the disorder. Conclusions from this investigation are that an early age of onset of motor or vocal tics may be the best predictor of a more severe course of the disorder.

BIOLOGICAL AND NEUROPSYCHOLOGICAL MARKERS

Brain Imaging Studies and Brain Morphology

With the advent of sophisticated neuroimaging techniques and other advances in neuropathology, investigators have been able to address the hypothesized abnormal brain morphology and other cerebral dysfunctions associated with TS. As noted previously, Kurlan (1994) has suggested that TS is expressed as a clinical syndrome that includes a range of increasing functional impairments indicating various abnormalities in basal ganglia development. Because of the association of abnormalities of the basal ganglia with the presence of movement disorders, including Huntington disease and postencephalitic parkinsonism, researchers have sought to link these movement disorders with TS (Hyde & Weinberger, 1995). Interestingly, lesions of the basal ganglia have frequently been associated with a range of mood and behavioral disturbances, including depression.

Magnetic Resonance Imaging Studies

Through the use of magnetic resonance imaging (MRI) techniques, Singer et al. (1993a) studied 37 children with TS and compared them to their normally developing peers. Although significant asymmetries were observed in the children with TS, no differences between groups were noted in the size of the right or the left caudate nucleus. Hyde and Weinberger (1995) conducted analyses of the MRIs of 10 monozygotic twin pairs who ranged in age from 9 to 31 years (mean age = 16 years) and were discordant for the severity of TS but concordant for the presence of the gene. The interior right caudate nuclei were found to be smaller and the left ventricles more asymmetric in the more severely affected twins; thus the greater the asymmetry, the more severe the disorder. In further support of morphological abnormalities in individuals with TS, Peterson et al. (1993) found reductions in regional basal ganglia volumes in patients with TS as compared to controls. All of these findings lend support to the notion that the basal ganglia may be involved in the pathogenesis of TS. However, studies have provided equivocal data regarding morphological differences in individuals affected with TS relative to controls (e.g., Singer et al., 1993a). Thus, although the data derived from the MRI studies have been compelling, additional research is warranted in this area to replicate the results of available studies, given the small sample sizes and equivocal data of some investigations.

Positron Emission Tomography Studies

In recent years, the use of positron emission tomography (PET) scans has shown particular promise in identifying abnormalities of cerebral functioning in individuals with TS by delineating metabolic dysfunctions in specific regions of the brain. Evidence of changes in activity of the basal ganglia and prefrontal cortex in individuals with TS has been presented (e.g., Hyde & Weinberger, 1995). For example, Braun et al. (1995) analyzed 18 drug-free patients with TS, employing PET scans in order to evaluate the association between cerebral metabolism and complex cognitive processes, as well as the behavioral features commonly associated with TS. The data suggested that obsessions and compulsions; impulsivity; coprolalia; self-injurious behavior; and attentional, visual, and spatial dysfunction were significantly associated with increased metabolic activity in the orbitofrontal cortices. Interestingly, these behavioral and cognitive features were not associated with metabolic rates in other areas of the brain. The authors have interpreted their findings to suggest that symptoms of TS may be related to increased metabolic activity in the frontal cortex.

Electroencephalographic Studies

Another means of assessing the neurological functioning of individuals with Tourette's is through electroencephalographic (EEG) studies. Earlier data documented some neurological abnormalities on EEGs (e.g., nonspecific sharp waves and diffuse slowing) in individuals with TS. However, more recent investigations have found that EEGs do not routinely discriminate between individuals with the disorder and controls (Peterson et al., 1995).

Related to the abnormalities associated with the EEG studies have been those investigations examining EEG patterns during sleep in those diagnosed with TS (Glaze, Frost, & Jankobic, 1983). The data from EEG sleep studies have generally suggested immature arousal patterns (i.e., a dysfunction in arousal associated with the reticular activating system), which are typically seen in infants and very young children. The findings therefore suggest a developmental delay in the central nervous system (CNS) of individuals with TS. Differences in sleep disturbances between normally developing individuals and those with TS have been noted, particularly when TS is comorbid with ADHD (Allen, Singer, Brown, & Salam, 1992). For a better understanding of this phenomenon, additional studies are needed to compare the sleep patterns of groups of children diagnosed with TS without comorbid ADHD, ADHD without comorbid TS, and both of the disorders. Finally, the clinical literature frequently suggests several sleep disturbances that are associated with TS, including sleepwalking, enuresis, night terrors, and nightmares. Whether or not these disturbances are more frequent in children with TS than they are in the general population is unclear (Peterson et al., 1995).

Studies of Evoked Potentials

There has been an emerging line of research on electrophysiological functioning in children with TS compared to their normally developing peers. One such investigation has suggested an absence of the normal slow premotor movement potential in the simple motor tics of TS (Obesco, Rothwell, & Marsden, 1981). Another interesting finding is that attentional and arousal mechanisms are differentially mediated in individuals with TS, depending upon whether they have received a comorbid diagnosis of either OCD or ADHD. Other studies have attempted to investigate auditory event-related potentials in individuals with TS. Although these data are provocative, findings from these studies must be interpreted judiciously, due to their small sample sizes and the comorbidity of other psychiatric and neurological disorders with TS (Peterson et al., 1995).

Studies of Neurotransmitters

The advancement in our understanding of the pathophysiology of numerous psychiatric disorders and the neurotransmitters associated with them has led to an increased understanding of TS. For instance, the neurotransmitter dopamine has been implicated in the pathophysiology of TS (Kolb & Whitshaw, 1990). Dopamine is believed to be significant in TS because it relates to the efficacy of neuroleptics in the management of the disorder and to the notion that stimulant use may trigger or exacerbate symptoms of Tourette's. Both of these pharmacological agents are associated with dopamine receptor sites; neuroleptics block reuptake of dopamine at the synaptic cleft, while stimulants facilitate reuptake of this neurotransmitter (Kolb & Whitshaw, 1990).

Of additional interest is the proposal that the dopaminergic systems are modulated by sex steroids, and this theory has implications for explaining the gender differences in the prevalence of TS (Leckman et al., 1986). Furthermore, the course of the development of the dopaminergic systems and their receptor sites has been linked to the progression of Tourette's symptoms. Specifically, children with TS evidence the most severe presentation of the disorder during the elementary school years, when components of these systems are at their peak development. There is a sharp decline of symptoms during adolescence, when there is a decline in the activation of the dopaminergic receptor sites.

Neuropsychological Studies

Neuropsychologists have also been interested in the identification of measures that are associated with various functional impairments of the CNS. Stebbins et al. (1995) have provided compelling evidence to suggest that TS is associated with frontostriatal abnormalities. Specifically, these authors evaluated different forms of memory linked to specific brain regions in unmedicated adults with TS and in normal controls of equivalent age and education. The TS patients were found to evidence greater impairments on measures of strategic, working, and procedural memory, all of which are associated with frontostriatal functioning.

Summary

Compelling evidence has suggested that TS has a strong biological basis. The neuroimaging studies have implicated asymmetries of the basal ganglia and caudate nucleus; PET scan studies have also detected increases in metabolic activity in the frontal cortex. Sleep studies, as well as other investigations employing EEGs, have posited an arousal disturbance suggesting deficits in the reticular activating system. Finally, there is substantial support for the role of neurotransmitters (specifically, dopamine) in the development and course of TS. As is often characteristic of a new program of research, the existing studies have been limited by small sample sizes and by samples consisting of subjects with other neurological or psychiatric comorbid disorders. Attention must be devoted to the careful diagnosis of TS with systematic and observable criteria, as well as to the assessment of any comorbid disorders. Whether the neurological deficits suggested in these various investigations are associated with the presence of TS alone or of TS with other psychiatric disorders (e.g., ADHD, OCD, and ODD) is unclear. A logical next step in this research endeavor would be to compare children with various types of comorbidity to children who only meet diagnostic criteria for TS. Clearly this is an exciting time in the identification of biological markers that are associated with TS, and promising pathways await further investigation.

RISK FACTORS FOR PHENOTYPIC EXPRESSION

A number of risk factors, including biological insults and environmental stressors, have been posited to be etiological in the phenotypic expression of TS. Even as early as the 1950s, researchers have provided data to suggest an association between adverse perinatal factors and the development of TS (Pasamanick & Kawi, 1956; for a review, see Peterson et al., 1995). These investigators found that mothers of children with tics were 150% more likely to have sustained complications during pregnancy than mothers of children without tics. Later studies have provided additional support for this notion. For example, Leckman et al. (1987) found that in monozygotic twin pairs, the twin with TS had a lower birth weight than the unaffected twin. In a later investigation, stressful maternal life events during the course of pregnancy, in addition to nausea and vomiting during the first trimester, were posited as potential risk factors for the development of tic disorders in the child (Leckman et al., 1990). Friedhoff (1986) has suggested that environmental stressors may modify dopamine levels in the CNS, resulting in a teratogenic affect on the fetus. Finally, obstetrical complications have been implicated in the etiology of TS, particularly when there is injury to the basal ganglia and when there is hypoxia resulting in ischemia to vulnerable areas of the brain (B. S. Peterson, Riddle, Gore, Cohen, & Leckman, 1994).

A number of environmental risk factors have also been hypothesized to influence the course and severity of TS. These include psychosocial stressors (e.g., severe punishment or reprimands for exhibiting tic symptoms), exposure to extreme temperatures, infections, and exposure to CNS stimulants (Leckman & Cohen, 1996; Peterson et al., 1995). For example, in a recent investigation of four males ranging in age from 10 to 14 years with pediatric, infection-triggered autoimmune neuropsychiatric disorders, three of the subjects were diagnosed with TS and one with OCD (Allen, Leonard, & Swedo, 1995). Interestingly, when the children were treated with immunoglobulin, their symptoms remitted; this lends support to the notion that Tourette's may be related to an autoimmune disorder.

ASSESSMENT

Differential Diagnosis

Current psychiatric nosology conceptualizes tic disorders as one of four types: (1) Tourette's disorder (i.e., TS), (2) chronic motor or vocal tic disorder, (3) transient tic disorder, and (4) tic disorder not otherwise specified (NOS) (APA, 1994). The tic disorders may be differentiated from one another on the basis of age of onset, duration, and type of tics exhibited. Table 8.1 presents summaries of the diagnostic criteria for the four types of tic disorders.

TABLE 8.1. Summaries of DSM-IV Diagnostic Criteria for Four Types of Tic Disorders

	Tourette's disorder	Chronic motor or vocal tic disorder	Transient tic disorder	Tic disorder not otherwise specified
Type of tics	Multiple motor tics and one or more vocal tics	Single or multiple motor and/ or vocal tics, but not both	Single or multiple motor and/or vocal tics	Single or multiple motor and/or vocal tics
Age of onset	Before 18 years	Before 18 years	Before 18 years	Before or after 18 years
Duration	More than 1 year	More than 1 year	From 4 weeks to 1 year	Any time period
Frequency	Many times/day; not absent for 3 consecutive months	Many times/day; not absent for 3 consecutive months	Many times/day	Not specified
Functional impairment	Marked impairment in social competence or occupational/ academic functioning	Marked impairment in social competence or occupational/ academic functioning	Marked impairment in social competence or occupational/ academic functioning	Marked impairment in social competence or occupational/ academic functioning
Differential diagnosis	Not due to direct physiological effects of a substance or medical condition	Not due to direct physiological effects of a substance or medical condition; criteria have never been met for Tourette's disorder	Not due to direct physiological effects of a substance or medical condition; criteria have never been met for Tourette's disorder or chronic motor or vocal tic disorder	Not due to direct physiological effects of a substance or medical condition; criteria have never been met for Tourette's disorder, chronic motor or vocal tic disorder, or transient tic disorder

As is evident from Table 8.1, symptoms of each of the disorders must result in marked distress or a significant impairment in social, educational/occupational, or other important areas of functioning. In addition, symptoms may not be due to the direct physiological effects of a drug substance or to another specific neurological or medical condition (APA, 1994). Except for tic disorder NOS, diagnostic criteria mandate that onset occur prior to the age of 18 years. For both Tourette's disorder and chronic motor or vocal tic disorder, the tics must occur several times a day either daily or intermittently throughout a period of more than 1 year. In addition, during this 1-year period, it must be documented that there has never been a period of more than 3 consecutive months without tics. By contrast, for transient tic disorder, the tics must occur many times throughout the course of a day, nearly consecutively for at least 4 weeks but not longer than 12 consecutive months. For tic disorder NOS, the tics may last for less than 4 weeks. For a diagnosis of Tourette's disorder, individuals must exhibit both multiple motor tics and at least one vocal tic. To meet criteria for chronic motor or vocal tic disorder, individuals must have single or multiple motor tics or vocal tics, but *not* both. Individuals with transient tic disorder suffer from multiple vocal and/or motor tics. Finally, those who suffer from only one motor and/or one vocal tic with a duration of less than 4 weeks should receive a diagnosis of tic disorder NOS (APA, 1994).

Differential Diagnosis: Tic Disorders versus Other Disorders

Because tic disorders involve abnormal movements, these conditions must necessarily be distinguished from neurological disorders that also involve abnormal movements (e.g., Huntington disease, Wilson disease, multiple sclerosis, or head injuries) (APA, 1994). Abnormal movements may also be the result of specific drug substances (including neuroleptic medications). Furthermore, tics should be distinguished from a myriad of abnormal movement types, such as choreiform movements (i.e., dancing; irregular, nonrepetitive movements), dystonic movements (i.e., slow, twisting movements interspersed with prolonged states of muscular tension), myoclonic movements (i.e., brief, shock-like muscle contractions that may affect groups of muscles), or spasms (i.e., stereotypic, slower, and more prolonged movements involving muscles) (APA, 1994). Tics also must be distinguished from the stereotyped movements that are evidenced in pervasive developmental disorders (e.g., autistic disorder, Asperger's disorder) and in stereotypic movement disorder (i.e., more rhythmic and intentional movements with a driven quality). Moreover, tics must be discriminated from the compulsions that frequently occur in OCD. Finally, tics must be distinguished from the psychotic or very disorganized behaviors that may occur in individuals with schizophrenia.

Clinical Assessment

In diagnosing a child with a suspected tic disorder, the clinician must begin with a clarification of the presenting problem. When the presenting problem includes a mention of tics, documentation should be made of the type of tics, tic onset, and the course of tics. Leckman et al. (1989) suggest that clinicians should present a list of possible motor and vocal tics to parents, as caretakers may not reliably report tics, especially more complex ones (e.g., repeating short phrases). Parents often present a symptom profile that includes variability in the type and frequency of tics. Commonly, one tic may disappear and be replaced by another (Scahill, Ort, & Hardin, 1993a). The clinician should also ask about conditions that appear to exacerbate or attenuate tic symptoms; this will assist in selecting the appropriate diagnosis, as well as in determining appropriate treatment. For example, Scahill et al. (1993a) have noted that children taking decongestants such as ephedrine and pseudoephedrine may experience exacerbations of their tic symptoms. Moreover, it has been noted that streptococcal infections may trigger tics or obsessive–compulsive symptoms (March, Swedo, & Leonard, 1992). Parents may also report increases in tics during warmer weather (Lombroso et al., 1991). Fatigue and stress have been demonstrated to increase symptom display, while it has been noted that tics diminish during activities requiring sustained attention and effort and during periods of sleep (Scahill et al., 1993a).

Comorbidities

As noted earlier in this chapter, psychiatric comorbidities are frequently present in individuals with TS (Hyde & Weinberger, 1995). A discussion regarding comorbidity of other developmental, psychiatric, and learning disorders with TS is complicated by the fact that rates of comorbid illness occur at a greater frequency in clinic populations than in the general population (Berkson, 1946; Peterson et al., 1995). The majority of studies have been conducted in clinical settings and therefore may overrepresent the rates of psychiatric comorbidities in this population. Few epidemiological studies are available to provide clinicians with rates of comorbidities of other disorders with TS in the general population.

An additional factor to consider is that when children with TS also suffer from other internalizing or externalizing psychopathology or developmental disabilities, they are more likely to be identified and referred for treatment, due to their complex symptom display. In addition, many of these children and adolescents have failed to respond to conventional therapies and thus are referred to specialty clinics. Furthermore, Comings and Comings (1984, 1987) have pointed out that the incidence of neurological or psychiatric disorders is higher among family members of these children than in the general population. Stated more simply, parents who have psychiatric disorders place their children at greater genetic and environmental risk for multiple diagnoses.

In one of the few existing large-scale epidemiological studies, over 28,000 Israeli adolescents aged 16–17 years were surveyed (Apter et al., 1993). A high frequency of OCD was found in subjects with TS; over 42% of adolescents with TS met criteria for OCD, compared to fewer than 4% of controls (Apter et al., 1993). Interestingly, the rate of ADHD was only approximately 8% in adolescents with TS, compared to 4% of controls. The authors interpret their data to suggest that OCD is frequently part of the clinical presentation of TS, whereas ADHD is a separate entity that may serve to expedite referrals of children for assessment and treatment.

Obsessive–Compulsive Disorder

Much research has suggested that TS and OCD are associated disorders (Como, 1995; Miguel et al., 1995; Pauls, Towbin, Leckman, Zahner, & Cohen, 1986; Peterson et al., 1995; Swedo & Leonard, 1994). The data we have reviewed earlier suggest a genetic vulnerability for the expression of either TS or OCD. Family studies support the relationship between the two disorders, as there is a high incidence of OCD in families of children with TS. Furthermore, for individuals with OCD, there is a high personal incidence of TS as well as a family history of tic disorders (Peterson et al., 1995). Finally, Comings (1995) has provided a compelling argument to suggest that OCD and TS may represent different points on a wide spectrum of one neuropsychiatric disorder.

In a study of children and adolescents diagnosed with OCD, approximately 60% of patients initially referred for obsessive–compulsive traits *without* tics subsequently displayed tics at follow-up 2 to 7 years later (Leonard et al., 1992). Also, nearly 25% of these patients actually met diagnostic criteria for TS. Furthermore, children and adolescents who later met criteria for TS had an earlier onset of obsessive-compulsive symptoms than those subjects who did not develop TS (Leonard et al., 1992). Rapoport, Swedo, and Leonard (1992) have noted that males with an early onset of OCD may be at particular risk for developing tics. George, Trimble, Ring, Sallee, and Robertson (1993) found that adult patients who met diagnostic criteria for both TS and OCD were more aggressive and displayed different types of compulsions (e.g., self-damaging behaviors) than those with OCD alone. Finally, as Rapoport et al. (1992) have astutely observed, distinguishing between a compulsion and a tic may be particularly difficult, because some patients with TS also have complex behavioral rituals with their tics.

Finally, there is some evidence to suggest that TS and OCD may be two distinct syndromes that are frequently comorbid. For example, the selective serotonin reuptake inhibitors (SSRIs), which are effective in managing OCD symptoms, are not particularly efficacious in treating symptoms of TS (Swedo & Leonard, 1994). Similarly, whereas neuroleptic agents are effective in reducing tic frequency and severity, these pharmacological agents have not been found to be effective for managing the symptoms associated with OCD (Miguel et al., 1995). Furthermore, Miguel et al. (1995) have demonstrated that the onset of symptoms related to OCD without comorbid TS is preceded by cognitive phenomena (i.e., ideas, thoughts, and images) and anxiety, but not sensory phenomena (i.e., unpleasant sensations). By contrast, in TS without comorbid OCD, tics are preceded by sensory phenomena but not by cognitive phenomena or anxiety.

Attention-Deficit/Hyperactivity Disorder

Many children with TS also have problems with attention and overactivity (Knell & Comings, 1993; Peterson et al., 1995; Walkup, Scahill, & Riddle, 1995). Clinical observations suggest that TS and ADHD are frequently comorbid disorders. Indeed, some research has suggested a highly significant association between TS and ADHD. In a review of this issue, Comings (1995) has made a compelling argument to underscore the similarities of the disorders by pointing out that both ADHD and TS are associated with a range of behavioral problems and show a high frequency of externalizing behavioral disorders in relatives. Furthermore, the prevalence of attentional disorders is higher in families who have an affected member with TS than in the general population. Knell and Comings (1993) examined the first-degree relatives of 131 TS probands, employing a structured psychiatric diagnostic interview. Findings were that of the relatives of individuals with TS, more than 60% were diagnosed with attention deficit disorder (ADD) according to earlier diagnostic criteria, and over 35% had ADHD as more recently defined.

In contrast to the more overt relationship between TS and OCD, however, not all genetic studies have supported an association between TS and ADHD (Pauls et al., 1986; Peterson et al., 1995). Greater research efforts are needed to delineate the relationship between TS and ADHD more precisely. As Peterson et al. (1995) have astutely observed, attentional disorders are heterogeneous psychiatric disorders that have multiple genotypes and phenotypes. Because of this, much more research needs to be conducted to identify genes that are common to TS and ADHD. Ideally, research that identifies similar genetic pathways and biological markers will lead to viable treatment techniques that are useful for both disorders.

Peterson et al. (1995) have underscored the difficulties associated with the identification of attentional disturbances in children with TS. Specifically, Randolph, Hyde, Gold, Goldberg, and Weinberger (1993) found that more severe tic symptoms were related to greater impairments on measures of attention and impulse control in monozygotic twin pairs with TS. Thus these findings might be interpreted to suggest that because of the deleterious influence of tics on cognitive and motoric functioning, attention and impulse control are difficult to assess. A better delineation of the association between ADD and/or ADHD and TS will require precise diagnostic methodology, which is not always available in clinical settings.

Learning Disorders

Not surprisingly, the literature has identified significant comorbidity of learning disorders in children with TS (Walkup et al., 1995). These difficulties may be related either to a single factor involving impairments in executive functioning, or to a multitude of factors that may include severity of the tics, the sedative effects of neuroleptic medication, the demoralizing aspect of having a stigmatizing disorder, and the existence of comorbid disorders such as OCD and ADHD (Singer, Schuerholz, & Denckla, 1994). Many children who receive special education services have been found to have a tic disorder, with a significant percentage of challenged learners meeting diagnostic criteria for TS (Comings, Himes, & Comings, 1990; Kurlan, Whitmore, Irvine, McDermott, & Como, 1994). Although children with TS do not necessarily suffer from deficient mental abilities, several investigations have revealed specific learning disabilities in reading and mathematics (Bornstein, 1990; Burd, Kauffman, & Kerbeshain, 1992; Yeates & Bornstein, 1994).

Interestingly, some studies have found that tic severity is related to neuropsychological functioning. As noted previously, Randolph et al. (1993) found that attention, visual–spatial perception, and motoric functioning were significantly more impaired in twins with a more severe presentation of TS (i.e., a greater frequency and intensity of tic symptoms). In addition, tic severity has been associated with poorer performance on such neuropsychological measures as the Trail Making Test and the Grooved Pegboard Test (Bornstein, 1990; Yeates & Bornstein, 1994).

Other Comorbidities

Because externalizing behavior problems such as conduct disorder (CD) and ODD frequently co-occur with ADHD, they also occur in children and adolescents with TS (Comings, 1990; Comings & Comings, 1987; Erenberg, Cruse, & Rothner, 1986; Stifle, 1984). Frequent problems include lying, stealing, severe aggression, fire setting, and interpersonal problems (e.g., testing limits). In studies of children with TS, preadolescent boys and adolescent girls have been found to exhibit the greatest prevalence of symptoms related to ODD and CD (Patrick, 1995).

Dysthymic disorder and major depressive disorder have also been associated with TS in adulthood (Rapoport et al., 1992). Furthermore, childhood-onset OCD has been found to have a strong relationship with eating disorders (Whitaker, Johnson, & Shaffer, 1990). This association begs the question of whether eating disorders may be comorbid with TS as well. Because eating disorders have frequently been noted to be exclusionary criteria in the pediatric studies involving children with TS, the relationship of eating disorders to TS remains unclear. Finally, there is a high prevalence of disorders related to anxiety (i.e., phobias) in children with TS; this is not surprising, given that OCD is classified under the anxiety disorders (APA, 1994).

Measures

Factors important for consideration in the assessment of tic disorders include the frequency, intensity, suddenness, type, complexity, and location of the tics. In addition, determining the degree to which the tics interfere with individuals' daily functioning (including their speech), as well as their ability to inhibit tics in various settings, is a primary task in the assessment process (Shapiro, Shapiro, Young, & Feinberg, 1988). Moreover, severity of TS is evaluated in terms of the subjective distress of the symptoms to each individual, the amount of negative attention from others the tics yield, and the degree to which the tics cause the individual to appear unusual or peculiar (Shapiro et al., 1988). Assessment instruments available include observer (e.g., clinician) rating scales, self-report rating scales, caretaker/parent rating scales, and codings for videotaped ratings.

Observer (Clinician) Rating Scales

The Shapiro Tourette's Syndrome Severity Scale (Shapiro & Shapiro, 1984) consists of a composite rating of the severity of five factors that primarily relate to the social disabilities associated with TS. The five factors include the degree to which the tics are noticeable to others; whether they elicit comments of curiosity; whether others consider the patient unusual or bizarre; whether the tics interfere with functioning; and whether the patient is incapacitated, homebound, or hospitalized because of the tics. The ratings for the five factors are summed to yield a total that may be converted into a qualitative global severity score.

The Tourette's Syndrome Global Scale (TSGS; Harcherik, Leckman, Detler, & Cohen, 1984) is another widely used instrument completed by clinicians that has been shown to be reliable and to have adequate convergent validity. The TSGS is a multidimensional scale that requires clinicians to rate the frequency and disruption of simple and complex motor and phonic tics, as well as to rate a set of associated symptoms, including motoric restlessness, behavioral problems, and school/work impairment. Two problems with the TSGS are that it provides only a composite rating and that none of the items distinguish between simple and complex motor tics (Peterson et al., 1995).

The Yale Global Tic Severity Scale (YGTSS; Leckman et al., 1989) was designed for use by experienced clinical diagnosticians following the completion of a semistructured psychiatric interview. For this rating scale, clinicians rate the severity of motor and vocal tics along five separate dimensions, including number, frequency, intensity (i.e., the forcefulness or volume of the tic symptoms), complexity, and interference (i.e., the degree to which planned actions or speech are impeded by the tic symptoms). Each of the five dimensions of the YGTSS is anchored on a 6-point ordinal scale ranging from "none" to "always." In addition, the same scales are employed to rate both motor and vocal tics. Finally, a separate rating of impairment is included in the YGTSS, which specifically focuses on the impact that the tic disorder has had on the individual within the previous week. This includes self-perception, self-esteem, relationships with family members, social or peer relationships, and the ability to perform in an academic or occupational setting. Data collected on children, adolescents, and adults who ranged in age from

5 to 51 years have provided promising construct, convergent, and discriminant validity for this measure.

Self-Report or Caregiver/Parent Rating Scales

The Motor tic, Obsessions and compulsions, Vocal tic, Evaluation Survey (MOVES; Gaffney, Sieg, & Hellings, 1994) is a self-report rating scale for the assessment of symptoms of TS. This 16-item scale was designed to be easily and rapidly completed by children, adolescents, or adults. The MOVES generates scores on five subscales: Motor Tics, Vocal Tics, Obsessions, Compulsions, and Associated Symptoms (e.g., echolalia, echopraxia, coprolalia, and copropraxia). On this measure, subscale scores may be combined to form a Tic subscale or an Obsessive–Compulsive subscale. Data from a recent investigation have revealed that a sample of patients with TS scored significantly higher on the total scale and on all subscales than did either psychiatric or nonreferred community controls. In addition, there is ample evidence for the construct validity of the measure; the MOVES was significantly associated with a number of examiner-rated scales, including the TSGS, the Shapiro Tourette's Syndrome Severity Scale, and two scales for the assessment of obsessive and compulsive symptoms. Finally, good sensitivity and specificity have been demonstrated for the measure. The MOVES is apt to be useful for clinicians and researchers, as it is one of the few self-report scales for rating the presence and severity of TS symptoms.

Another useful instrument is the Daily Record of Treatment (Shapiro et al., 1988). This scale requires the patient and/or caretaker to rate motor, vocal, and other symptoms of TS on a daily basis throughout the course of treatment. Also recorded are the daily dosage of medication, type and severity of untoward effects, and an overall percentage of decrease in tic symptoms.

Videotaped Ratings

Shapiro et al. (1988) have employed videotaped ratings of patients during three visits that differed according to stimulus control conditions. The conditions included a computation task for eliciting motor tics, an oral reading test to assess for vocal tics, and finally a no-stimulus control for a baseline tic count. Videotaped tic counts were found to have high interrater reliability and adequate construct validity, and to be independent of other measures. Tic counts did not vary under the three stimulus conditions. The investigators interpreted their findings to suggest that the patients were well aware that they were being videotaped. However, the final tic counts were consistent with the number of tics occurring in the presence of strangers.

Rating Scale Limitations and Future Directions

Leckman et al. (1989) have cited some limitations and directions for future work pertaining to the YGTSS. These limitations appear to be applicable and useful as well for future research in the clinical assessment and self-rating of symptom severity for individuals with TS. First, Leckman et al. (1989) have noted that there may be variations in age and gender distributions for the available rating instruments. Thus future research should focus on nonreferred samples and should devote particular attention to both age and gender. Second, these ratings should be evaluated during the course of longitudinal investigations, so that the natural history of the disorder can be further assessed. Finally, the data derived from each rating scale should be compared with those from other scales, as well as with data from other techniques for assessing TS symptomatology (e.g., video-taped ratings).

PSYCHOLOGICAL FACTORS RELATED TO SYMPTOMATOLOGY AND ADJUSTMENT

As noted earlier, tic severity in TS appears to be related to an individual's level of anxiety or emotional distress following stressful life events. In fact, some have referred to tic dis-orders as "stress-sensitive" conditions (Jagger et al., 1982; Shapiro & Shapiro, 1988). Clinicians have noted that a negative cycle can be created when family members or teach-ers misunderstand tics and attempt to eliminate them through punishment or humiliation (Shapiro & Shapiro, 1988). The child then may become even more distressed because the tics are the focus of much unwanted negative attention, and therefore the tic symptoms may actually increase in severity. In the worst-case scenario, this negative cycle can lead to the most severe expression of TS and to the development of depressive symptomatology.

Research indeed has supported an association between tic severity and stressful life events (Malatesta, 1990; Silva et al., 1995; Surwillo, Shafii, & Barrett, 1978). For example, in a study of children with TS who ranged in age from 6 to 14 years, 17 environmental factors were associated with an increase in tic symptoms (Silva et al., 1995). The most commonly reported factor was anxiety or "being upset." Other factors included being fatigued, attending social gatherings, watching television, and being alone for extended periods of time. The researchers found a significant relationship between a child's reactiv-ity to these factors and the intensity (i.e., forcefulness and noticeability) of the child's motor and vocal tics. Other situations reported in the literature that are related to tic severity include beginning a new school year, waiting for test results, moving to a new residence, and family conflicts (Malatesta, 1990; Silva et al., 1995; Surwillo et al., 1978).

TREATMENT

Behavioral and Other Nonpharmacological Interventions

Over the past several years, a number of behavioral approaches have been employed in treatment outcome studies of TS, including contingency management, relaxation training, habit reversal, self-monitoring, and massed negative practice (Peterson & Azrin, 1993; A. L. Peterson, Camprise, & Azrin, 1994). Behavioral techniques to treat symptoms of TS consist of either direct approaches, in which the intervention targets the tics themselves (e.g., contingency management, habit reversal, massed negative practice), or indirect ap-proaches, in which the contingencies maintaining the tics are eliminated (e.g., relaxation training, self-monitoring) (Mansdorf, 1995). A. L. Peterson et al. (1994), in a systematic search of behavioral treatment outcome studies, identified over 50 published studies that included both tic disorders and TS. As these authors noted, the majority of these were case studies or single-subject designs. Peterson and Azrin (1993) have pointed out a number of strengths related to these studies that are likely to be instructive for future group design investigations. First, TS is a disorder that lends itself nicely to objective measures of tic rates from direct observations or videotapes. Second, unlike pharmacological studies and many psychotherapy treatment outcome trials, studies of TS have assessed measurement both in the laboratory and in the natural setting, thus providing greater ecological validation. Peterson and Azrin (1993) have pointed out, however, that follow-up studies in this area have not been widespread. Only one investigation could be located that employed a between-subjects group design to evaluate treatment efficacy for children with TS (Azrin & Peterson, 1990), and only two studies used this type of design for a sample of children with tics who did not meet diagnostic criteria for TS. A review follows of the major behavioral therapies that have been used successfully in the management of TS and tic disorders. (A few other nonpharmacological interventions are also briefly mentioned.)

Habit Reversal

"Habit reversal" is a procedure in which competing responses are employed to prevent the occurrence of tics. Incorporated within habit reversal are self-monitoring, contingency management, relaxation training, and awareness training (Peterson & Azrin, 1993). For many motor tics, a competing response might be the tensing of specific muscle groups that are counter to the tic movements. Specifically, the opposing muscles are contracted for 1–2 minutes contingent on either the emission of a tic or the urge to have a tic.

Azrin and Peterson (1988) examined the effectiveness of habit reversal as a component of a treatment package to treat three adults with a diagnosis of TS. Subjects who exhibited tics consisting of arm jerks were encouraged to push a hand down on a thigh or the stomach and to push an elbow in toward a hip. For vocal tics such as barking, coughing, throat clearing, coprolalia, and sneezing, slow, rhythmic, deep-breathing exercises were encouraged through the nose while keeping the mouth closed.

Research has demonstrated habit reversal to be efficacious in the management of individuals with TS (Azrin & Peterson, 1988, 1990; Finney, Rapoff, Hall, & Christopherson, 1983; Franco, 1981; Peterson & Azrin, 1992; Young & Montano, 1988). Furthermore, habit reversal has shown particular promise in the treatment of motor tic disorders (Azrin, Nunn, & Frantz, 1980). For studies published up to the early 1990s, habit reversal was demonstrated to reduce tics by about 90% in the home environment and 80% in the clinic setting (Peterson & Azrin, 1993). Finally, these studies revealed a reduction in vocal and motoric tics across settings and situations for children, adolescents, and adults.

Contingency Management

Rooted in the notion that behaviors are maintained by learned associations, a primary principle governing contingency management is the use of punishment to decrease undesired behaviors (i.e., tics) or rewards to increase desired behaviors. A. L. Peterson et al. (1994) reviewed over 20 case studies and single-subject designs that have employed contingency management programs to treat TS (e.g., Barr, Lovibond, & Katsaros, 1972; Browning & Stover, 1971; Doleys & Kurtz, 1974; Hollandsworth & Bausinger, 1978; Miller, 1970; Rosen & Wesner, 1973; Sand & Carlson, 1973; Schulman, 1974; Tophoff, 1973).

The majority of these investigations have employed a multimodal behavioral approach, whereby several treatment techniques have been combined to reduce tic symptoms (Peterson & Azrin, 1993; A. L. Peterson et al., 1994). Many of these studies have employed time-out procedures to reduce frequency of tics. For example, Lahey, McNees, and McNees (1973) attempted to decrease the incidence of coprolalia (i.e., obscenities) with the use of time out. However, when the contingencies were removed, the level of coprolalia returned to baseline. As part of a multimodal intervention, Azrin and Peterson (1988) described a contingency management component in which families were instructed to make positive comments when their family member exhibited a decrease in tic frequency.

Other contingency management treatments have included aversive punishments delivered by means of electric shock (Barr et al., 1972; Clark, 1966) or white noise (Doleys & Kurtz, 1974). These studies have generally reported a decrease in symptoms following the intervention. Furthermore, for those studies that included a follow-up evaluation, improvement was maintained several months after the completion of therapy (Doleys & Kurtz, 1974; Varni, Boyd, & Cataldo, 1978). However, other investigations (for a review, see Peterson & Azrin, 1993) have reported that treatment effects did not generalize. The ethical implications of such aversive techniques, including electric shock, have been seriously questioned (Peterson & Azrin, 1993), and for this reason they can no longer be considered as viable treatment options.

Peterson and Azrin (1993) have astutely observed that a major limitation of these studies is that few used positive reinforcement as an incentive for behavior change. In addition, the data yielded from these studies are confounded, as multiple behavioral treatments have been used, and no one study has examined a particular type of reinforcer (i.e., positive or negative) on specific components of the treatment. Thus future research that is able to dismantle components of treatments that are effective for managing children with TS will be a valuable contribution to this literature.

In summary, the use of punishment and time out has demonstrated some efficacy in reducing tic frequency for children with TS. Although these studies have yielded some encouraging results, they have failed to test the efficacy of each specific component of the treatment package. Moreover, generalization of these treatment effects has been decidedly disappointing. Peterson and Azrin (1993) have highly recommended the use of positive reinforcement (i.e., praise and verbal encouragement) for any child with TS. The rationale is that positive reinforcement will increase a child's motivation for self-control and also enhance treatment adherence. Peterson and Azrin (1993) have also recommended that interventions studies be designed to include various forms of positive reinforcement (e.g., praise, activities, and monetary rewards) for the absence of tics or for performing other behaviors that are incompatible with tic behaviors.

Relaxation Training

The use of relaxation techniques has been demonstrated to be a particularly promising intervention for the management of TS symptoms (Azrin & Peterson, 1988, 1990; Canavan & Powell, 1981; Franco, 1981; Friedman, 1980; Michultka, Blanchard, & Rosenblum, 1989; Peterson & Azrin, 1992; Savicki & Carlin, 1972; Thomas, Abrams, & Johnson, 1971; Tophoff, 1973; Turpin & Powell, 1984). Relaxation techniques have included progressive muscle relaxation, deep breathing, visual imagery, and self-statements of relaxation. In each of these investigations, the frequency of tics was reduced; some of the investigations actually reported tics to be nonexistent during the relaxed state. Nonetheless, despite these encouraging data, the improvements were only transitory and frequently recurred upon cessation of therapy.

As an example of this type of intervention, Peterson and Azrin (1992) evaluated the use of relaxation in the clinic setting by videotaping and counting changes in the rates of tics. They found nearly a one-third decrease in tic frequency during the relaxation exercises. In addition, Singer, Waranch, Brown, Carson, and Mellitis (1993b) evaluated a controlled double-blind trial of relaxation with children and found that it provided promising results.

The use of relaxation as a viable means of managing TS shows considerable promise. Similar to studies of contingency management techniques, the majority of relaxation studies have employed multiple intervention techniques and have failed to dismantle the various components of the treatment program (Peterson & Azrin, 1993). Given this state of affairs, more controlled trials of relaxation are warranted.

Self-Monitoring

With the use of self-monitoring, children are taught to record the occurrence of each of their tics for a particular time period. In the management of TS, case studies utilizing self-monitoring as a sole intervention procedure or as a component of an intervention have yielded encouraging results (Billings, 1978; Hutzell, Platzek, & Logue, 1974; Peterson & Azrin, 1992; Savicki & Carlin, 1972; Thomas et al., 1971). When the results of these studies were considered simultaneously, Peterson and Azrin (1993) found a reduction of 55% in tic frequency. Although the data are encouraging, treatment effects have been short-lived, with the frequency of tics increasing soon after the cessation of therapy.

As an example of this type of intervention, Carr and Bailey (1996) have reported on a brief behavior therapy protocol employing self-monitoring for a 9-year-old male with snorting and throat clearing. The behavioral intervention included self-monitoring, competing-response practice, and dissimilar-response practice. The child was provided with a hand counter and told to click the button each time he had a tic. In the competing-response practice component, the child was asked to engage in a breathing exercise for 1 minute following each tic. In the dissimilar-response practice component, the child was asked to make a fist with his left hand again for 1 minute following each tic. The tics were found to be reduced by approximately 70%, and behavior change was successfully sustained at a 1-month follow-up.

As another example, Azrin and Peterson (1990) described a multimodal treatment that included a self-awareness paradigm. This component focused on increasing the subjects' awareness of the frequency and severity of the tics, environmental factors influencing symptoms, and the specific movements involved in the tics. The subjects were asked to record the incidence of the various tics for a specific period during the day. Subsequently, subjects described the details of each tic with the use of a mirror or videotape. In addition, subjects were taught to detect any occurrence of tics and were provided with practice in self-detection at the earliest sign of a tic. Finally, subjects were taught to become more aware of situations in which tics were more frequent or severe.

Massed Negative Practice

"Massed negative practice" is a procedure in which the person is encouraged to perform the tic movement rapidly and with as much effort as possible (Peterson & Azrin, 1993). Frequently the individual is asked to perform the action for a particular period of time with brief rest periods. The underlying premise of this procedure is that the individual *tires* of performing such actions and develops reactive inhibition, thereby leading to a reduction of tics. Massed negative practice is the most widely employed behavioral procedure for the management of TS (Peterson & Azrin, 1993). A number of studies have shown a decrease in tics following massed negative practice (for a review, see Peterson & Azrin, 1993), whereas others have demonstrated little or no significant effect. Peterson and Azrin (1993) reviewed data suggesting a reduction of nearly 60% in tic behaviors following massed negative practice. However, the majority of studies have not demonstrated long-term treatment effects; others have failed to assess the long-term efficacy of this approach.

Azrin and Peterson (1989) successfully employed massed negative practice for a 9-year-old girl who suffered from an eye tic. The child was taught to engage in voluntary blinking contingent upon the tic. Findings revealed cessation of the tic after 6 weeks; follow-up data showed continued reduction in tics 2 years following the intervention.

Other Treatments

Other nonpharmacological treatments for TS described in the literature have included psychoeducational approaches, school consultation, and psychotherapy that incorporates the family system (Scahill et al., 1993a; Scahill, Walker, Lechner, & Tynan, 1993b). Another viable technique described in the clinical literature involves teaching children with TS to manage stress associated with their tic symptoms. The children are taught to make assertive responses in conditions that they perceive to be psychologically threatening. They are taught to employ such self-statements as "What if they make a remark? Words can't hurt me" (Mansdorf, 1995, p. 338). These treatments are typically most effective for managing the stigmatization of the disorder, as well as for reducing stressors that may exacerbate tic symptoms.

Summary

Behavioral interventions are particularly promising in managing tic symptoms associated with TS. Most of these behavioral techniques have shown promise for the treatment of symptoms in the short term; their long-term effectiveness remains to be demonstrated. Examining specific components of treatment has been difficult, due to the fact that the majority of studies have not been able to analyze the contribution of each behavioral technique individually. Future research will need to compare various behavioral approaches alone and in combination, to determine what the most efficacious and parsimonious treatment package should include.

Another issue is that treatment studies conducted in a controlled research environment offer optimal adherence and monitoring of behavioral techniques for both patients and clinicians. Frequently, however, when a child with TS presents to a practitioner, a host of problems may interfere with optimal behavioral management, thereby impeding adherence efforts (e.g., poor family adaptability and cohesion, emotional stressors). Thus the task of the skilled clinician becomes one of carefully assessing possible impediments to treatment. It must also be recognized that several types of behavioral therapies will need to be employed simultaneously.

Psychopharmacological Interventions

More than 70% of children and adolescents with TS have been reported to take medication for the control of symptoms associated with the disorder (Gadow, 1993). The most common psychotropic medication administered for the management of TS is haloperidol, from the neuroleptic class of drugs. Stimulants, including methylphenidate, have also been used for the management of associated symptoms (e.g., impulse control problems, attentional deficits). It is noteworthy that nearly one-half of children and adolescents with TS report a worsening of symptoms following stimulant drug therapy (Gadow, 1993). More importantly, there is a high degree of dissatisfaction with pharmacotherapy in patients with TS, due to the frequency of untoward side effects (Gadow, 1993).

Reviews indicated that as of the early 1990s, there were over 100 published articles pertaining to pharmacotherapy for individuals with TS (Peterson & Azrin, 1993). The most frequently employed medications include, in addition to haloperidol (Haldol), pimozide (Orap) and clonidine hydrochloride (Catapres). Haloperidol blocks the reuptake of dopamine at the synaptic level and has been used historically to treat schizophrenia and other psychotic disorders. In an early review of clinical trials employing haloperidol for the management of TS symptoms, Shapiro, Shapiro, Bruun, and Sweet (1977) concluded that haloperidol improved symptoms in at least three-quarters of the patients participating in these trials. In subsequent controlled trials employing haloperidol, Ross and Moldofsky (1978) assessed tics by means of direct observations or videotapes. Their data indicated that haloperidol reduced the rate of tics by approximately one-half. More recently, Shapiro et al., (1989) evaluated the efficacy of haloperidol with patient and physician ratings of improvement. Although the medication decreased tics by an average of 80%, approximately one-half of the patients reported untoward effects. In fact, a follow-up investigation revealed that one-fifth of the sample had discontinued medication prematurely, due to these unwanted side effects.

Possible adverse effects reported with haloperidol include irritability, dysphoria, apathy, overactivity, aggression, and school phobia (Campbell, Gonzalez, Ernst, Silva, & Werry, 1993). In addition, sedation, skin reactions, and photosensitivity have been noted. Finally, the use of haloperidol may result in extrapyramidal side effects; these may include acute dystonic reactions (e.g., stiffening of the neck, eyes rolled back under the lids), parkinsonian effects (e.g., drooling, tremors, lack of arm swinging when walking), akathisia (i.e., motor restlessness and pacing), akinesia (i.e., diminished gestures, movements, and speech), cardiovascular reactions, seizures, and neuroleptic malignant syndrome (a rare and life-threatening condition characterized by hyperthermia and parkinsonian symptoms).

Another neuroleptic agent that has been prescribed widely in the management of TS is pimozide, a medication that has dopamine-blocking actions similar to those of haloperidol. Similar beneficial effects have been reported as for haloperidol, including the reduction of tic rates as assessed by direct observations and videotape recordings (Ross & Moldofsky, 1978; Shapiro & Shapiro, 1984; Shapiro et al., 1989). Significant adverse effects have been reported; Shapiro and Shapiro (1984) noted untoward effects in 95% of their sample.

In recent years, clonidine has been used to manage symptoms associated with TS. This medication has been traditionally used to reduce blood pressure and heart rate. Only three double-blind placebo-controlled trials that have evaluated the efficacy of clonidine for decreasing tic symptoms could be located in the literature (Borison, Ang, Hamilton, Diamond, & Davis, 1983; Goetz et al., 1987; Leckman et al., 1991). Studies employing subjective ratings have demonstrated significant improvements, as have investigations that have included the rates of motor and vocal tics as dependent measures.

Other pharmacological agents, including tricyclic antidepressants (e.g., imipramine, desipramine) and SSRIs (e.g., sertaline, fluoxotine), have been studied in children with TS (Parraga, Kelly, Parraga, Cochran, & Maxim, 1994). These investigations have been characterized by small sample sizes, thereby making any definitive conclusions premature at this time.

As noted earlier, there is frequent comorbidity of ADHD and TS, requiring that the practitioner manage both disorders simultaneously with pharmacotherapy. Since the stimulants are employed most frequently for the treatment of symptoms associated with ADHD, this places the clinician in a dilemma, as there is some clinical evidence to suggest that stimulant medication can precipitate or exacerbate motor tics, stereotypies, or other symptoms associated with TS (for a review, see Brown, Dingle, & Dreelin, 1997). To complicate this matter further, a small percentage of children with ADHD who receive stimulant medication have been found to develop tics, although these have typically been reversible upon cessation of medication. This has resulted in greater systematic efforts to carefully study the effects of stimulant medication in children with ADHD and comorbid tic disorders.

One single-blind, placebo-controlled study examined the effects of methylphenidate on teacher ratings and observed playroom behavior in four boys diagnosed with ADHD and TS (Sverd, Gadow, & Paolicelli, 1989). Results indicated that methylphenidate produced no more tics than did the placebo condition. In fact, for each of the children, the highest dose of methylphenidate produced improved teacher ratings of tics compared to placebo treatment, even though some mild tic exacerbation was noted on the lower dose of medication. Sverd and colleagues interpreted their findings to suggest that methylphenidate alone may be safe and effective for the treatment of attentional and behavioral problems in children with TS.

Sprafkin and Gadow (1993) presented case studies in which methylphenidate appears to have increased the frequency of tics. However, upon careful analyses of the cases, the data were not convincing regarding the role of stimulants in triggering tics. Although one patient's disorder appeared to become more severe with methylphenidate, the child was found to have less severe tic symptoms with higher doses. Another patient appeared to develop TS while receiving methylphenidate, but was subsequently found to have had a preexisting undiagnosed tic disorder. Sprafkin and Gadow (1993) have emphasized the importance of careful and unbiased assessment of pretreatment symptoms, variability in symptomatology over time, and any possible link between stimulant medication and tic exacerbation.

In a controlled clinical trial investigating the effects of methylphenidate in boys diagnosed with both ADHD and TS, Gadow, Nolan, and Sverd (1992) observed these children in a classroom setting for 6 weeks. Results were that methylphenidate suppressed overactive and disruptive behavior in the classroom and physical aggression on the playground. Similar findings were reported by parents on behavioral ratings for the same children (Sverd, Gadow, Nolan, Sprafkin, & Ezor, 1992). Most importantly, methylphenidate was found to reduce the occurrence of vocal tics at school; however, no differences were found during routine assessments. Of the 11 children studied, only 1 boy experienced motor tic exacerbation.

Finally, Borcherding, Keysor, Rapoport, Elia, and Amass (1990) studied the effects of methylphenidate and dextroamphetamine, and found that abnormal movements and perseverative compulsive behaviors occurred with both medications. These abnormalities were frequently subtle and transient, and usually occurred on one medication. Only one patient had to discontinue medication due to tic severity. Based on their findings, Borcherding et al. (1990) concluded that although careful monitoring of stimulants is important, it may not be necessary to discontinue medication because of tic symptoms. Adjusting the dose or selecting another stimulant may ameliorate these manifestations.

Although the recent studies are encouraging and suggest that stimulants are an effective and safe intervention for children with ADHD and comorbid tic disorders, more clinical trials are needed to definitively determine the safety and efficacy of stimulants for this population. Families of children diagnosed with Tourette's comorbid with ADHD must be apprised of the potential of stimulants to worsen tic symptoms. If a trial of stimulants is indeed elected, careful monitoring should always be the rule.

In summary, the majority of children and adolescents who are diagnosed with TS receive at least one trial of psychotropic medication. The psychotropic drug that has been most frequently employed for the management of TS is haloperidol, which has been successful in reducing at least 50% of tic symptoms. Despite this success rate in symptom management, the potential untoward effects of haloperidol cannot be overstated. It must be used judiciously and with utmost caution. Although, the data regarding the use of stimulants in children with comorbid ADHD and TS are encouraging, much more research will need to be conducted prior to endorsing the safety of these agents for children with tic disorders. Finally, there are other pharmacological agents that may be particularly promising for use with these children (e.g., SSRIs), although no systematic controlled trials have been conducted to confirm their safety or efficacy. This is a fertile area for future investigations.

GENERAL SUMMARY AND CONCLUSIONS

Important developments have been made in the assessment and management of TS. In part, this has been due to the increase in knowledge about the natural history of the disorder throughout the lifespan. There also is compelling evidence to indicate that TS has a strong biological component, with significant abnormalities as evidenced on neuroimaging studies, physiological measures, and neuropsychological testing. The recent research on the role of dopamine in both the development and course of the disorder is an exciting new development. Finally, our increased understanding of behavioral genetics has assisted in explaining the symptom variations and comorbidity patterns in individuals with TS.

Several risk factors, including perinatal and environmental stressors, are believed to be associated with both the severity and timing of tic symptoms. Environmental risk factors have also been demonstrated to influence the course of the disorder. The interaction of biological and environmental factors as they mediate symptom display will be a fruitful area for future research. Clearly, significant variability in symptom expression is part of what has made diagnostic efforts difficult. The recent revision of the psychiatric nosology for classifying various tic disorders (APA, 1994) represents an important improvement in the assessment process. Moreover, there is increasing recognition that other psychiatric comorbidities frequently occur with TS, including OCD; ADHD, ODD, and CD; mood disorders; and learning disabilities. This makes the assessment and treatment process exceedingly complex and quite challenging for the diagnostician. Finally, important progress has been made in the construction of ratings scales and observation schedules to quantify symptoms and functional impairments so that standardized tools can be used for diagnosis. The development of reliable and valid instruments will assist in documenting treatment efficacy.

Regarding management and treatment of the disorder, behavioral approaches (including habit reversal, contingency management, relaxation training, self-monitoring, and massed negative practice) have shown particular promise in diminishing the symptoms associated with TS. Most of these treatments have been proven to be efficacious in the short term; their long-term effects have yet to be demonstrated. A decided limitation of the majority of intervention outcome studies is the failure to dismantle the various components of treatment, thereby making it difficult to determine the independent contribution of each component.

Psychopharmacology continues to be a widely employed and an important treatment option for the management of symptoms associated with TS. Unfortunately, research documenting the safety and efficacy of pharmacotherapy to treat individuals with TS has lagged behind the clinical use of various psychotropic drugs. An exception to this is some of the recent research conducted regarding the association between the use of stimulant medication and the emergence of tic symptoms. Clearly, more research efforts are needed in this area. Finally, the potential efficacy of other psychotropic agents, such as specific SSRIs, in the management of TS warrants further investigation.

The development of pharmacological and behavioral approaches in the management of TS has shown particular promise. Nonetheless, the relative efficacy of psychotropics in comparison with behavioral therapies remains unclear. Moreover, whether psychotropics potentiate the effects of behavioral therapies is an important area for future research. Finally, the evaluation of other nonpharmacological interventions, including psychoeducational approaches, school consultation, and family system therapies, will be important in managing some of the demoralizing aspects of the disorder.

Until recently, the understanding and management of TS in children and adolescents have been guided chiefly by clinical lore rather than empirical data. Important advances have been made in our understanding of the biological and genetic markers as well as the environmental stressors associated with the disorder. In addition, the accumulation of data from intervention research studies in the areas of behavioral and psychopharmacological treatments has paralleled biological research efforts. Thus a firm empirical basis is emerging to guide clinical practice.

REFERENCES

Allen, A. J., Leonard, H., & Swedo, S. (1995). Current knowledge of medications for the treatment of childhood anxiety disorders. *Journal of the American Academy of Child and Adolescent Psychiatry, 34*, 976–986.

Allen, A. J., Singer, H. S., Brown, J. E., & Salam, M. M. (1992). Sleep disorders in Tourette syndrome: A primary or related problem. *Pediatric Neurology, 8*, 275–280.

American Psychiatric Association (APA). (1994). *Diagnostic and statistical manual of mental disorders* (4th ed.). Washington, DC: Author.

Apter, A., Pauls, D. L., Bleich, A., Zohar, A. H., Kron, S., Ratzoni, G., Dycian, A., Kotler, M., Weizman, A., Gadot, N., & Cohen, D. J. (1993). An epidemiological study of Gilles de la Tourette's syndrome in Israel. *Archives of General Psychiatry, 50*, 734–738.

Azrin, N. H., Nunn, R. G., & Frantz, S. E. (1980). Habit reversal versus negative practice treatment of nailbiting. *Behaviour Research and Therapy, 18*, 281–285.

Azrin, N. H., & Peterson, A. L. (1988). Habit reversal for the treatment of Tourette syndrome. *Behaviour Research and Therapy, 26*, 347–351.

Azrin, N. H., & Peterson, A. L. (1989). Reduction of an eye tic by controlled blinking. *Behavior Therapy, 20*, 467–473.

Azrin, N. H., & Peterson, A. L. (1990). Treatment of Tourette syndrome by habit reversal: A waiting-list control group comparison. *Behavior Therapy, 21*, 305–318.

Barr, R. F., Lovibond, S. H., & Katsaros, E. (1972). Gilles de la Tourette's syndrome in a brain-damaged child. *Medical Journal of Australia, ii*, 372.

Berkson, J. B. (1946). Limitations of the application of fourfold table analysis to hospital data. *Biometrics, 2*, 47–51.

Billings, A. (1978). Self-monitoring in the treatment of tics: A single-subject analysis. *Journal of Behaviour Therapy and Experimental Psychiatry, 9*, 339–342.

Borcherding, B. G., Keysor, C. S., Rapoport, J. L., Elia, J., & Amass, J. (1990). Motor/vocal tics and compulsive behaviors on stimulant drugs. *Psychiatry Research, 33*, 83–94.

Borison, R. L., Ang, L., Hamilton, W. J., Diamond, B. I., & Davis, J. M. (1983). Treatment approaches in Gilles de la Tourette syndrome. *Brain Research Bulletin, 11*, 205–208.

Bornstein, R. A. (1990). Neuropsychological performance in children with Tourette's syndrome. *Psychiatry Research, 33*, 73–81.

Braun, A. R., Randolph, C., Stoetter, B., Mohr, E., Cox, C., Vladar, K., Sexton, R., Carson, R. E., Herscovitch, P., & Chase, T. N. (1995). The functional neuroanatomy of Tourette's syndrome: An FDG-PET study. II: Relationship between regional cerebral metabolism and associated behavioral and cognitive features of the illness. *Neuropsychopharmacology, 13*, 151–168.

Brown, R. T., Dingle, A., & Dreelin, B. (1997). Neuropsychological effects of stimulant medication on children's learning and behavior. In C. R. Reynolds & E. Fletcher-Janzen (Eds.), *Handbook of clinical child neuropsychology* (2nd ed., pp. 539–572). New York: Plenum Press.

Browning, R. M., & Stover, D. O. (1971). *Behavior modification in child treatment: An experimental and clinical approach.* Chicago: Aldine-Atherton.

Bruun, R. D. (1988). The natural history of Tourette's syndrome. In D. J. Cohen, R. D. Bruun, & J. F. Leckman (Eds.), *Tourette's syndrome and tic disorders: Clinical understanding and treatment* (pp. 21–39). New York: Wiley.

Burd, L., Kauffman, D. W., & Kerbeshain, J. (1992). Tourette syndrome and learning disabilities. *Journal of Learning Disabilities, 25,* 598–604.

Campbell, M., Gonzalez, N. M., Ernst, M., Silva, R. R., & Werry, J. S. (1993). Antipsychotics (neuroleptics). In J. S. Werry & M. G. Aman (Eds.), *Practitioner's guide to psychoactive drugs for children and adolescents* (pp. 269–296). New York: Plenum Press.

Canavan, A. G., & Powell, G. E. (1981). The efficacy of several treatments of Gilles de la Tourette's syndrome as assessed in a single case. *Behaviour Research and Therapy, 19,* 549–556.

Carr, J. E., & Bailey, J. S. (1996). A brief behavior therapy protocol for Tourette syndrome. *Behavioral Interventions, 33–40.*

Clark, D. F. (1966). Behaviour therapy of Gilles de la Tourette's syndrome. *British Journal of Psychiatry, 112,* 771–778.

Comings, D. E. (1990). Blood serotonin and tryptophan in Tourette syndrome. *American Journal of Medical Genetics, 36,* 418–430.

Comings, D. E. (1995). Tourette's syndrome: A behavioral spectrum disorder. *Behavioral Neurology of Movement Disorders, 65,* 293–303.

Comings, D. E., & Comings, B. G. (1984). Tourette syndrome and attention deficit disorder with hyperactivity—are they genetically related? *Journal of the American Academy of Child Psychiatry, 23,* 138–144.

Comings, D. E., & Comings, B. G. (1987). Hereditary agoraphobia and obsessive–compulsive behaviour in relatives of patients with Gilles de la Tourette's syndrome. *British Journal of Psychiatry, 151,* 195–199.

Comings, D. E., Comings, B. G., & Knell, E. (1989). Hypothesis: Homozygosity in Tourette syndrome. *American Journal of Medical Genetics, 34,* 413–421.

Comings, D. E., Himes, J. A., & Comings, B. G. (1990). An epidemiological study of Tourette's syndrome in a single school district. *Journal of Clinical Psychiatry, 51,* 463–469.

Como, P. G. (1995). Obsessive–compulsive disorder in Tourette's syndrome. *Behavioral Neurology of Movement Disorders, 65,* 281–291.

Doleys, D. M., & Kurtz, P. S. (1974). A behavioral treatment program for the Gilles de la Tourette syndrome. *Psychological Reports, 35,* 43–48.

Erenberg, G., Cruse, R. P., & Rothner, A. D. (1986). Tourette syndrome: An analysis of 200 pediatric and adolescent cases. *Cleveland Clinic Quarterly, 53,* 127–131.

Erenberg, G., Cruse, R. P., & Rothner, A. D. (1987). The natural history of Tourette syndrome: A follow-up study. *Annals of Neurology, 22,* 383–385.

Finney, J. W., Rapoff, M. A., Hall, C. L., & Christopherson, E. R. (1983). Replication and social validation of habit reversal treatment for tics. *Behavior Therapy, 14,* 116–126.

Franco, D. D. (1981). Habit reversal and isometric tensing with motor tics. *Dissertation Abstracts International, 42,* 3418B.

Friedhoff, A. J. (1986). Insights into the pathophysiology and pathogenesis of Gilles de la Tourette syndrome. *Revue Neurologique, 142,* 860–864.

Friedman, S. (1980). Self-control of the treatment of Gilles de la Tourette's syndrome: Case study with 18-month follow up. *Journal of Consulting and Clinical Psychology, 48,* 400–402.

Gadow, K. D. (1993). A school-based medication evaluation program. In J. L. Matson (Eds.), *Handbook of hyperactivity in children* (pp. 186–219). Needham Heights, MA: Allyn & Bacon.

Gadow, K. D., Nolan, E. E., & Sverd, J. (1992). Methylphenidate in hyperactive boys with comorbid tic disorder: II. Short-term behavioral effects in school settings. *Journal of the American Academy of Child and Adolescent Psychiatry, 31,* 462–471.

Gaffney, G. R., Sieg, K., & Hellings, J. (1994). The MOVES: A self-rating scale for Tourette's syndrome. *Journal of Child and Adolescent Psychopharmacology, 4,* 269–280.

George, M. S., Trimble, M. R., Ring, H. A., Sallee, F. R., & Robertson, M. M. (1993). Obsessions in obsessive–compulsive disorder with and without Gilles de la Tourette's syndrome. *American Journal of Psychiatry, 150,* 93–97.

Glaze, D. G., Frost, J. D., & Jankobic, J. (1983). Sleep in Gilles de la Tourette's syndrome: Disorder of arousal. *Neurology, 33,* 586–592.

Goetz, C. G., Tanner, C. M., Stebbins, G. T., Leipzig, G., & Carr, W. C. (1992). Adult tics in Gilles de la Tourette's syndrome: Description and risk factors. *Neurology, 42,* 784–788.

Goetz, C. G., Tanner, C. M., Wilson, R. S., Carroll, V. S., Como, P. G., & Shannon, K. M. K. (1987). Clonidine and Gilles de la Tourette's syndrome: Double-blind study using objective rating methods. *Annals of Neurology, 21,* 307–310.

Goldenberg, J. N., Brown, S. B., & Weiner, W. J. (1994). Coprolalia in younger patients with Gilles de la Tourette syndrome. *Movement Disorders, 9*(6), 622–625.

Harcherik, D. F., Leckman, J. F., Detler, J., & Cohen, D. J. (1984). A new instrument for clinical studies of Tourette's syndrome. *Journal of the American Academy of Child Psychiatry, 23,* 153–160.

Hollandsworth, J. G., & Bausinger, L. (1978). Unsuccessful use of massed practice in the treatment of Gilles de la Tourette syndrome. *Psychological Reports, 43,* 671–677.

Hutzell, R. R., Platzek, D., & Logue, P. E. (1974). Control of symptoms of Gilles de la Tourette's syndrome by self-monitoring. *Journal of Behavior Therapy and Experimental Psychiatry, 5,* 71–76.

Hyde, T. M., Aaronson, B. A., Randolph, C., Rickler, K. C., & Weinberger, D. R. (1992). Relationship of birth weight to the phenotypic expression of Gilles de la Tourette's syndrome in monozygotic twins. *Neurology, 42,* 652–658.

Hyde, T. M., Fitzcharles, E. K., & Weinberger, D. R. (1993). Age-related prognostic factors in the severity of illness of Tourette's syndrome in monozygotic twins. *Journal of Neuropsychiatry, 5,* 178–182.

Hyde, T. M., & Weinberger, D. R. (1995). Tourette's syndrome: A model neuropsychiatric disorder. *Journal of the American Medical Association, 239,* 498–511.

Jagger, J., Prusoff, B. A., Cohen, D. G., Kidd, K. K., Carbonari, C. M., & John, K. (1982). The epidemiology of Tourette syndrome: A pilot study. *Schizophrenia Bulletin, 8,* 267–278.

Kidd, K. K., Prusoff, B. A., & Cohen, D. J. (1980). The familial pattern of Gilles de la Tourette syndrome. *Archives of General Psychiatry, 37,* 1336–1339.

Knell, E. R., & Comings, D. E. (1993). Tourette's syndrome and attention-deficit hyperactivity disorder: Evidence for a genetic relationship. *Journal of Child Psychology and Psychiatry, 54,* 331–337.

Kolb, B., & Whitshaw, I. Q. (1990). *Fundamentals of human neuropsychology.* New York: Freeman.

Kurlan, R. (1994). Hypothesis II: Tourette's syndrome is part of a clinical spectrum that includes normal brain development. *Archives of Neurology, 51,* 1145–1150.

Kurlan, R., Whitmore, D., Irvine, C., McDermott, M. P., & Como, P. G. (1993). Tourette's syndrome in a special education population: Preliminary findings. *Neurology, 43,* 310.

Kurlan, R., Whitmore, D., Irvine, C., McDermott, M. P., & Como, P. G. (1994). Tourette's syndrome in a special education population: A pilot study involving a single school district. *Neurology, 44,* 699–702.

Lahey, B. B., McNees, M. P., & McNees, M. C. (1973). Control of an obscene "verbal tic" through time out in an elementary classroom. *Journal of Applied Behavior Analysis, 6,* 101–104.

Leckman, J. F., & Cohen, D. J. (1996). Tic disorders. In M. Lewis (Ed.), *Child and adolescent psychiatry: A comprehensive textbook* (2nd ed., pp. 622–629). Baltimore: Williams & Wilkins.

Leckman, J. F., Cohen, D. J., Price, P. A., Riddle, M. A., Minderaa, R. B., Anderson, G. M., & Pauls, D. L. (1986). The pathogenesis of Tourette Syndrome: A review of the data and hypotheses. In N. S. Shah & A. G. Donald (Eds.), *Movement disorders* (pp. 257–272). New York: Plenum Press.

Leckman, J. F., Dolnansky, E. S., Hardin, M. T., Clubb, M., Walkup, J. T., Stevenson, J., & Pauls, D. L. (1990). Perinatal factors in the expression of Tourette's syndrome: An exploratory study. *Journal of the American Academy of Child and Adolescent Psychiatry, 2,* 220–226.

Leckman, J. F., Hardin, M. T., Riddle, M. A., Stevenson, J., Ort, S. I., & Cohen, D. J. (1991). Clonidine treatment of Gilles de la Tourette's syndrome. *Archives of General Psychiatry, 48,* 324–328.

Leckman, J. F., Price, R. A., Walkup, J. T., Ort, S. I., Pauls, D. L., & Cohen, D. J. (1987). Nongenetic factors in Gilles de la Tourette syndrome. *Archives of General Psychiatry, 44,* 100.

Leckman, J. F., Riddle, M. A., Hardin, M. T., Ort, S. I., Swartz, K. L., Stevenson, J., & Cohen, D. J. (1989). The Yale Global Tic Severity Scale (YGTSS): Initial testing of a clinical-rated scale of tic severity. *Journal of the American Academy of Child and Adolescent Psychiatry, 28,* 566–573.

Leckman, J. F., Walker, D. E., Goodman, W. K., Pauls, D. L., & Cohen, D. J. (1994). "Just right" perceptions associated with compulsive behaviors in Tourette's syndrome. *American Journal of Psychiatry, 151,* 675–680.

Leonard, H. L., Lenane, M. C., Swedo, S. E., Rettew, D. C., Gershon, E. S., & Rapoport, J. L. (1992). Tics and Tourette's syndrome: A 2- to 7-year follow-up of 54 obsessive–compulsive children. *American Journal of Psychiatry, 149,* 1244–1251.

Lombroso, P. J., Mack, G., Scahill, L., King, R., & Leckman, J. F. (1991). Exacerbation of Tourette's syndrome associated with thermal stress: A family study. *Neurology, 41,* 1984–1987.

Lombroso, P. J., Scahill, L. D., Chappell, P. B., Pauls, D. L., Cohen, D. J., & Leckman, J. F. (1995). Tourette's syndrome: A multigenerational, neuropsychiatric disorder. *Behavioral Neurology of Movement Disorders, 65,* 305–318.

Mahler, M. S., & Rangell, L. (1943). A psychosomatic study of maladie des tics (Gilles de la Tourette's disease). *Psychiatric Quarterly, 17,* 579.

Malatesta, V. J. (1990). Behavioral case formulation: An experimental assessment study of transient tic disorder. *Journal of Psychopathology and Behavioral Assessment, 12,* 219–232.

Mansdorf, I. J. (1995). Tic disorders. In R. T. Ammerman & M. Hersen (Eds.), *Handbook of child behavior therapy in the psychiatric setting* (pp. 323–340). New York: Wiley.

March, J. S., Swedo, S. E., & Leonard, H. (1992). *New developments in obsessive compulsive disorders.* Abstract from the annual meeting of the American Academy of Child and Adolescent Psychiatry, Washington, DC.

McDougle, C. J., Goodman, W. K., & Price, L. M. (1990). Neuroleptic addition in fluvoxamine-refractory obsessive compulsive disorder. *American Journal of Psychiatry, 147,* 652–654.

Michultka, D. M., Blanchard, E. B., & Rosenblum, E. L. (1989). Stress management and Gilles de la Tourette's syndrome. *Biofeedback and Self-Regulation, 14,* 115–123.

Miguel, E. C., Coffey, B. J., Baer, L., Savage, C. R., Rauch, S. L., & Jenike, M. A. (1995). Phenomenology of intentional repetitive behaviors in obsessive–compulsive disorder and Tourette's disorder. *Journal of Clinical Psychiatry, 56,* 246–255.

Miller, A. L. (1970). Treatment of a child with Gilles de la Tourette's syndrome using behavior modification techniques. *Journal of Behavior Therapy and Experimental Psychiatry, 1,* 319–321.

Obesco, J. A., Rothwell, J. C., & Marsden, C. D. (1981). Simple tics in Gilles de la Tourette's syndrome are not prefaced by a normal premovement EEG potential. *Journal of Neurology, Neurosurgery and Psychiatry, 44,* 735–738.

Park, S., Como, P. G., Cui, L., & Kurlan, R. (1993). The early course of the Tourette's syndrome clinical spectrum. *Neurology, 43,* 1712–1715.

Parraga, H. C., Kelly, D. P., Parraga, M. I., Cochran, M. K., & Maxim, L. T. (1994). Combined psychostimulant and tricyclic antidepressant treatment of Tourette's syndrome and comorbid disorders in children. *Journal of Child and Adolescent Psychopharmacology, 4,* 113–122.

Pasamanick, B., & Kawi, A. (1956). A study of the association of prenatal and perinatal factors in the development of tics in children. *Journal of Pediatrics, 48,* 596.

Patrick, H. T. (1995). Convulsive tic. *Journal of the American Medical Association, 44,* 437–442.

Pauls, D. L., & Leckman, J. F. (1986). The inheritance of Gilles de la Tourette syndrome and associated behaviors: Evidence for autosomal dominant transmission. *New England Journal of Medicine, 315,* 993–997.

Pauls, D. L., Raymond, C. L., & Robertson, M. M. (1991a). The genetics of obsessive–compulsive disorder. In Y. Zohar, T. Insel, & S. Rasmussen (Eds.), *Psychobiological aspects of OCD.* New York: Springer.

Pauls, D. L., Raymond, C., Stevenson, J., & Leckman, J. F. (1991b). A family study of Gilles de la Tourette syndrome. *American Journal of Human Genetics, 48,* 154–163.

Pauls, D. L., Towbin, K. E., Leckman, J. F., Zahner, G., & Cohen, D. J. (1986). Gilles de la Tourette's syndrome and obsessive–compulsive disorder: Evidence supporting a genetic relationship. *Archives of General Psychiatry, 43,* 1180–1182.

Peterson, A. L., & Azrin, N. H. (1992). An evaluation of behavioural treatments for Tourette syndrome. *Behaviour Research and Therapy, 30,* 167–174.

Peterson, A. L., & Azrin, N. H. (1993). Behavioral and pharmacological treatments for Tourette syndrome: A review. *Applied and Preventive Psychology, 2,* 231–242.

Peterson, A. L., Campise, R. L., & Azrin, N. H. (1994). Behavioral and pharmacological treatments for tic and habit disorders. *Journal of Developmental and Behavioral Pediatrics, 15,* 430–441.

Peterson, B. S., Leckman, J. F., & Cohen, D. J. (1995). Tourette's: A genetically predisposed and environmentally specified developmental psychopathology. In D. Cicchetti & D. J. Cohen (Eds.), *Manual of developmental psychology* (pp. 213–242). New York: Wiley.

Peterson, B. S., Riddle, M. A., Cohen, D. J., Katz, L., Smith, J., & Leckman, J. F. (1993). Human basal ganglia volume asymmetries on magnetic resonance images. *Magnetic Resonance Imaging, 11,* 493–498.

Peterson, B. S., Riddle, M. A., Gore, J. C., Cohen, D. J., & Leckman, J. F. (1994). CNA T2 relaxation time asymmetries in Tourette's syndrome. *Psychiatry Research: Neuroimaging, 55,* 205–221.

Randolph, C., Hyde, T. M., Gold, J. M., Goldberg, T. E., & Weinberger, D. R. (1993). Tourette's syndrome in monozygotic twins: Relationship of tic severity to neuropsychological function. *Archives of Neurology, 50,* 725–728.

Rapoport, J. L., Swedo, S. E., & Leonard, H. L. (1992). Childhood obsessive compulsive disorder. *Journal of Clinical Psychiatry, 53,* 11–16.

Rosen, M., & Wesner, C. (1973). A behavioral approach to Tourette's syndrome. *Journal of Consulting and Clinical Psychology, 41,* 303–312.

Ross, M. S., & Moldofsky, H. (1978). A comparison of pimozide and haloperidol in the treatment of Gilles de la Tourette's syndrome. *American Journal of Psychiatry, 135,* 585–587.

Sand, P. L., & Carlson, C. (1973). Failure to establish control over tics in the Gilles de la Tourette syndrome with behavior therapy techniques. *American Journal of Psychiatry, 122,* 665–670.

Savicki, V., & Carlin, A. S. (1972). Behavioral treatment of Gilles de la Tourette's syndrome. *International Journal of Child Psychotherapy, 1,* 97–109.

Scahill, L., Ort, S. I., & Hardin, M. T. (1993a). Tourette's syndrome: Part II. Contemporary approaches to assessment and treatment. *Archives of Psychiatric Nursing, 7,* 209–216.

Scahill, L., Walker, R. D., Lechner, S. N., & Tynan, K. E. (1993b). Inpatient treatment of obsessive compulsive disorder in childhood: A case study. *Journal of Clinical Psychiatric Nursing, 6,* 5–14.

Schulman, M. (1974). Control of tics by maternal reinforcement. *Journal of Behavior Therapy and Experimental Psychiatry, 5,* 95–96.

Shapiro, A. K., & Shapiro, E. S. (1984). Controlled study of pimozide versus placebo in Tourette's syndrome. *Journal of the American Academy of Child Psychiatry, 23,* 161–173.

Shapiro, A. K., & Shapiro, E. S. (1988). Signs, symptoms, and clinical course. In D. J. Cohen, R. D. Bruun, & J. F. Leckman (Eds.), *Tourette's syndrome and tic disorders: Clinical understanding and treatment* (pp. 127–193). New York: Wiley.

Shapiro, A. K., Shapiro, E. S., Bruun, R. D., & Sweet, R. D. (Eds.). (1977). *Gilles de la Tourette syndrome.* New York: Raven Press.

Shapiro, A. K., Shapiro, E. S., Young, J. G., & Feinberg, T. E. (1988). History of Tourette and tic disorders. In A. K. Shapiro, E. S. Shapiro, J. G. Young, & T. E. Feinberg (Eds.), *Gilles de la Tourette syndrome* (2nd ed., pp. 1–27). New York: Raven Press.

Shapiro, E. S., Shapiro, A. K., Fulop, G., Hubbard, M., Mandeli, J., Nordlie, L., & Phillips, R. A. (1989). Controlled study of haloperidol, pimozide, and placebo for the treatment of Gilles de la Tourette's syndrome. *Archives of General Psychiatry, 46,* 722–730.

Silva, R. R., Munoz, D. M., Barickman, J., & Friedhoff, A. J. (1995). Environmental factors and related fluctuation of symptoms in children and adolescents with Tourette's disorder. *Journal of Child Psychology and Psychiatry, 36*, 305–312.

Singer, H. S., Reiss, A. L., Brown, J., Aylward, E. H., Shih, B., Chee, E., Harris, E. L., Reader, M. J., Chase, G. A., Bryan, N., & Denckla, M. B. (1993a). Volumetric MRI changes in basal ganglia of children with Tourette's syndrome. *Neurology, 43*, 950–956.

Singer, H. S., Schuerholz, L. J., & Denckla, M. B. (1994). Learning difficulties in children with Tourette syndrome. *Journal of Child Neurology, 10*, 58–61.

Singer, H. S., Waranch, H. R., Brown, J., Carson, K., & Mellitis, D. (1993b). *Relaxation therapy: An alternative treatment for Tourette's syndrome?* Paper presented at the meeting at the Child Neurology Society, New York.

Sprafkin, R. L., & Gadow, K. D. (1993). Four purported cases of methylphenidate induced tic exacerbation: Methodological and clinical doubts. *Journal of Child and Adolescent Psychopharmacology, 3*, 231–244.

Sprague, R. L., & Newell, K. M. (1986). *Brain and behavior relationships*. Washington, DC: American Psychological Association.

Stebbins, G. T., Singh, J., Weiner, J., Wilson, R. S., Goetz, C. G., & Gabrieli, J. D. E. (1995). Selective impairments of memory functioning in unmedicated adults with Gilles de la Tourette's syndrome. *Neuropsychology, 9*, 329–337.

Stifle, M. E. (1984). Mental health associated with Tourette's syndrome. *American Journal of Public Health, 74*, 1310–1313.

Surwillo, W. W., Shafii, M., & Barrett, C. L. (1978). Gilles de la Tourette syndrome: A 20-month study of the effects of stressful life events and haloperidol on symptom frequency. *Journal of Nervous and Mental Disease, 166*, 812–816.

Sverd, J., Gadow, K. D., Nolan, E. E., Sprafkin, J., & Ezor, S. N. (1992). Methylphenidate in hyperactive boys with comorbid tic disorder. *Advances in Neurology, 58*, 271–281.

Sverd, J., Gadow, K. D., & Paolicelli, L. M. (1989). Methylphenidate treatment of attention-deficit hyperactivity disorder in boys with Tourette's syndrome. *Journal of the American Academy of Child and Adolescent Psychiatry, 28*, 574–579.

Swedo, S. E., & Leonard, H. L. (1994). Childhood movement disorders and obsessive compulsive disorder. *Journal of Clinical Psychiatry, 55*, 32–37.

Thomas, E. J., Abrams, K. S., & Johnson, J. B. (1971). Self-monitoring and reciprocal inhibition in the modification of multiple tics of Gilles de la Tourette's syndrome. *Journal of Behavior Therapy and Experimental Psychiatry, 2*, 159–171.

Tophoff, M. (1973). Massed practice, relaxation and assertion training in the treatment of Gilles de la Tourette's syndrome. *Journal of Behavior Therapy and Experimental Psychiatry, 4*, 71–73.

Turpin, G., & Powell, G. E. (1984). Effects of massed practice and cue controlled relaxation on tic frequency in Gilles de la Tourette's syndrome. *Behaviour Research and Therapy, 22*, 165–178.

Varni, J. W., Boyd, E. F., & Cataldo, M. F. (1978). Self-monitoring, external reinforcement, and time-out procedures in the control of high rate tic behaviours in a hyperactive child. *Journal of Behavior Therapy and Experimental Psychiatry, 9*, 353–358.

Walkup, J. T., Scahill, L. D., & Riddle, M. A. (1995). Disruptive behavior, hyperactivity, and learning disabilities in children with Tourette's syndrome. *Behavioral Neurology of Movement Disorders, 65*, 259–279.

Wallander, J. L., Varni, J. W., Babani, L., Banis, H. T., & Wilcox, K. T. (1989). Family resources as resistance factors for psychological maladjustment in chronically ill and handicapped children. *Journal of Pediatric Psychology, 14*, 157–173.

Whitaker, A., Johnson, J., & Shaffer, D. (1990). Uncommon troubles in young people: Prevalence estimates of selected psychiatric disorders in a nonreferred adolescent population. *Archives of General Psychiatry, 47*, 487–496.

Yeates, K. O., & Bornstein, R. A. (1994). Attention deficit disorder and neuropsychological functioning in children with Tourette's syndrome. *Neuropsychology, 8*, 65–74.

Young, M. H., & Montano, R. T. (1988). A new hypnobehavioral method for the treatment of children with Tourette's disorder. *American Journal of Clinical Hypnosis, 31*, 97–106.

9

ANXIETY DISORDERS

STEVEN R. PLISZKA
RENE L. OLVERA

Aggression and hyperactivity are overt phenomena; the fact that these symptoms can be easily observed accounts for the high reliability of such diagnoses as attention-deficit/hyperactivity disorder (ADHD) and conduct disorder (CD). Thus the study of these disorders is simpler, and a wider body of knowledge about them has emerged. Much less is known about internalizing disorders, such as the anxiety disorders of childhood and adolescence. There remain basic disagreements over the very nomenclature used, as well as about the best methods of diagnosis and treatment. Nonetheless, anxiety disorders are quite common in young people and are often associated with significant impairments in academic and social functioning. Enough data have emerged on them to guide clinicians in treatment and to raise interesting questions for researchers to explore.

FEAR, ANXIETY, AND WORRY IN CHILDREN

Fear, anxiety, and worry are common human experiences. These terms are used interchangeably by laypersons and even by mental health professionals, yet from a research perspective they are distinct. As viewed by Matthews (1990), anxiety has physiological (increased sympathetic arousal), behavioral (withdrawal from stimuli), and cognitive (worry) components. Worry involves "rehearsing possible aversive events and outcomes, and at the same time searching for ways of avoiding them" (Silverman, La Greca, & Wasserstein, 1995, p. 672). Fear, in contrast, is viewed as a biological alarm system, preparing the individual to face a real threat in the environment. Fear involves escape from an immediate danger, while worry helps the individual to avoid future dangers that have not yet materialized. Clearly, worry may be adaptive. In clinical conditions such as ADHD or CD, there may be an abnormal lack of worry, leading to poor planning (e.g., failure to study for a test). By contrast, in anxiety disorders, worry is clearly maladaptive when possible aversive events are magnified in scope or result in defective problem solving. There is also an abnormal physiological response suggestive of increased sympathetic arousal—elevated heart rate and blood pressure, as well as neuroendocrine and immune system changes.

Klein (1994) has reviewed the developmental course of anxiety and fear in children. In infants, fears of loud noises or loss of support predominate. Fear of strangers arises next, at about 8 months of age, with separation anxiety apparent at about 12–15 months. Fears of imaginary creatures arise during early childhood, and as children enter primary school, fears about performance, health, and personal harm become more pronounced. Silverman et al. (1995) extensively studied the worries of 272 elementary school children aged 7–12 years. Children were given a structured interview that assessed worries in 14 areas: school, performance, classmates, friends, war, disasters, money, health, future events, personal harm, "little things," appearance, family, and "other." The children were asked whether they worried about each broad category, and were then asked to list specific worries within that area. Children next rated the intensity of their worry and filled out a number of standardized anxiety rating forms. One-week test–retest reliability of the interview was very good, suggesting that children in this age group are reliable reporters of their worries, at least over the short term. The average child reported about 8 worries, spanning an average of 6 of the 14 areas. The most common worries were about school, health, and personal harm, with friends and appearance ranked the lowest. European American and Hispanic girls reported more worries than boys, but African American boys had as many worries as girls. The number of worries reported by a child correlated highly with the child's self-rating on anxiety scales.

Muris, Meesters, Merckelbach, Sermon, and Zwakhalen (1998) examined anxiety in 193 nonreferred children. Sixty (31%) of the sample stated that they never worried at all. The other children reported that they worried 2 to 3 times per week with most common worries being about school, dying, getting sick, or being teased. Girls worried more than boys.

Other studies have examined anxiety in an unreferred population of children (Ialongo, Edelsohn, Werthamer-Larsson, Crockett, & Kellam, 1994). Over 1,000 first-grade children filled out the Revised Children's Manifest Anxiety Scale (RCMAS). Teacher ratings of classroom adaptive behavior, peer ratings, and achievement measures were also obtained. About 400 of these children filled out the RCMAS again 4 months later; the intraclass correlation coefficients were .64 for boys and .42 for girls, showing good stability of the anxiety scores. Children with the highest anxiety scores showed lower achievement in mathematics and reading. Interestingly, self-ratings of anxiety did not predict peer or teacher nominations for shyness. Although none of the children in the study underwent a structured interview for psychiatric disorder, the findings with regard to achievement are not consistent with the notion that anxiety in childhood is a benign phenomenon. Also, the studies reviewed above show that children can reliably rate their anxious symptoms and articulate their worries; thus greater confidence can be placed in studies that base the diagnosis of anxiety on a child's report.

COMMON ANXIETY DISORDERS IN CHILDREN AND ADOLESCENTS

Definition and Prevalence

The *Diagnostic and Statistical Manual of Mental Disorders*, fourth edition (DSM-IV; American Psychiatric Association, 1994) classifies anxiety disorders into a number of categories; only one of these, separation anxiety disorder (SAD), is listed with the diagnoses first manifested during infancy, childhood, or adolescence. Generalized anxiety disorder

(GAD) replaces DSM-III-R's overanxious disorder of childhood, and DSM-III-R's avoidant disorder of childhood is now subsumed under social phobia in DSM-IV. Children may be diagnosed with specific phobia, social phobia, GAD, panic disorder, agoraphobia, obsessive–compulsive disorder (OCD), posttraumatic stress disorder (PTSD), and acute stress disorder according to the adult criteria, though some modifications to the criteria for some disorders have been made for children. (Note that because OCD is much less common than other anxiety disorders of childhood and adolescence, and is distinct from these disorders in other ways as well, it is discussed in a separate section of this chapter. In keeping with the focus in this volume on disorders proven or believed to have a genetic basis, PTSD and acute stress disorder are not discussed further at any length.) Trained clinicians are able to diagnose these disorders reliably; kappa values in interrater reliability studies have ranged from .54 to 1.0 (Last, Hersen, Kazdin, Orvaschel, & Perrin, 1991; Anderson, Williams, McGee, & Silva, 1987; Silverman & Nelles, 1988). Epidemiological studies of the anxiety disorders in children and adolescents have yielded broadly similar results and are shown in Table 9.1. When all anxiety disorders are combined, they are always found to be the most prevalent of the childhood mental disorders, but only 22% of the families of these children had sought treatment in one study (Anderson et al., 1987). In contrast, 43% of the children who met criteria for ADHD were in treatment.

The anxiety diagnoses are rarely exclusive categories, and a given patient frequently has more than one anxiety diagnosis. Half of children with DSM-III-R overanxious disorder were also found to have SAD, particularly younger patients (Strauss, Lease, Last, & Francis, 1988). Over a quarter of SAD patients have phobias (Benjamin, Costello, & Warren, 1990). This has led to the hypothesis that the various anxiety disorders are not particularly distinct from one another (Klein, 1994). To address this issue, Last, Hersen, Kazdin, Finkelstein, and Strauss (1987a) compared clinic-referred children with DSM-III

TABLE 9.1. Prevalence Rates of Childhood and Adolescent Anxiety Disorders: Findings from Epidemiological Research

Study	Age group	Comment	SAD	GAD[a]	Specific (simple) phobia	Social phobia	Any anxiety disorder
Anderson et al. (1987)	11 years		3.5	2.9	2.4	—	—
Bird et al. (1988)	4–16 years	CGAS < 61	4.7	—	2.6	—	—
		CGAS = 61–70	2.1	—	1.3	—	—
Costello (1989)	7–11 years	CGAS < 70	4.1	4.6	9.2	1.0	—
Fergusson et al. (1993)	15 years	Youth	0.5	6.3	5.1	1.7	10.8
		Mother	0.1	2.3	1.3	0.7	3.9
Shaffer et al. (1996)	9–17 years	Parent	1.4	1.9	0.7	2.8	5.3
		Youth	1.6	2.6	1.6	2.3	7.1
		Combined[b]	3.9	5.7	2.6	5.4	13.0
Verhulst, Van der Ende, Ferdinand, & Kasius (1997)	13–18	Parent	0.6	.7	9.2	6.3	16.5
		Child	1.4	.6	4.5	3.7	10.5

Note. CGAS, Children's Global Assessment Scale.

[a]Includes DSM-III/DSM-III-R overanxious disorder.

[b]Used "either–or" method.

SAD and overanxious disorder on a number of demographic and clinical characteristics. Children with overanxious disorder were older at the time of presentation, and tended to come from families of higher socioeconomic status. Nearly a third of the sample met criteria for both overanxious disorder and SAD, and children with overanxious disorder were more likely than SAD patients to meet criteria for some other anxiety diagnoses beside SAD. For instance, 11% had avoidant disorder, while over a quarter had phobias. Despite the fact that SAD appears to have much in common phenomenologically with panic disorder, only children with overanxious disorder also met criteria for panic disorder, whereas none of the SAD patients had panic attacks. We will return to this issue when we examine family studies of anxiety disorders. Thus overanxious disorder (or GAD in DSM-IV) often overlaps with other anxiety disorders, but up to half will only have GAD without any other disorder, suggesting that this is a valid diagnostic category in children.

Comorbidity with Other Psychiatric Disorders

Strauss et al. (1988) examined the comorbidity of other nonanxious psychiatric disorders in children with DSM-III-R overanxious disorder. The pattern of comorbidity varied significantly with age. Externalizing disorders were more common in anxious children under 12 years of age than in anxious adolescents. Over a third of the preadolescent children with overanxious disorder met criteria for ADHD; 25% met criteria for oppositional defiant disorder (ODD) or CD. In contrast, there were no diagnoses of CD among the adolescents with overanxious disorder, and the rates of ADHD and ODD were only 6.3% and 9.4%, respectively. A more striking finding was that while only 17.4% of younger children with overanxious disorder met criteria for major depressive disorder, nearly half (46.9%) of the teenagers with overanxious disorder were depressed. Moreover, when children with major depressive disorder are studied, an overlap with anxiety disorders is noted. In a population of 104 prepubertal children with major depressive disorder; 41% met criteria for an anxiety disorder, with SAD being the most prevalent (32% of the sample) (Kovacs, Gatsonis, Paulauskas, & Richards, 1989). In most cases, the anxiety disorder predated the episode of major depression and persisted after the remission of the depression; this suggested that the depression and anxiety were clearly distinct from each other, rather than the anxiety's being an epiphenomenon of the depression. Angold and Costello (1993) reviewed nine epidemiological studies of childhood mental disorder which at least some of the data were obtained from children themselves. They examined the rates of depressive comorbidity with the anxiety disorders, which ranged from a low of 6.6% to a high of 69%. In most of the studies, however, only about 10–20% of the anxious children were depressed. The overlap of depression and anxiety is thus asymmetrical: While approximately a quarter of anxious children are depressed, well over half and sometimes up to 75% of children with depressive disorders have comorbid anxiety disorders. Few studies have examined the impact of the comorbid disorders on the life course, treatment response, or symptom pattern of the anxiety disorders themselves.

Comparison to Other Psychiatric Disorders

Children with anxiety disorders have been compared to children with other psychiatric disorders, primarily ADHD (attention deficit disorder [ADD] or "hyperactivity" in earlier studies) or CD (Werry, Reeves, & Elkind, 1987b). In this extensive review of such studies, the authors noted several ways in which children with anxiety disorders have been found to be different from those with externalizing disorders. Anxious children, relative to those with ADHD or CD, are more likely to be female and to be older at the onset of symptoms. Anxiety-disordered children are similar to those with ADHD alone in that they come from more intact homes with less history of parental mental illness than children with CD or comorbid ADHD and CD. Reeves, Werry, Elkind, and Zametkin (1987) compared 21 children aged 6–13 with anxiety disorders to age-matched patients with ADD or ADD and comorbid CD. These groups were also compared to an age-matched control group with no psychiatric disorder. Anxiety patients were similar to normal controls in terms of intelligence (measured with the Peabody Picture Vocabulary Test), while the ADD groups were significantly lower than controls on this variable. The male–female ratio was lower among anxiety-disordered patients. In this study, patients with ADD and CD were the most impaired of these subjects; children with anxiety disorders did not differ from controls or ADD-only patients in terms of family adversity. Anxiety-disordered children were less impaired than ADD children on school achievement testing. In the laboratory, anxious children were less active than the ADD children, and no more active than controls, while doing difficult cognitive tasks (Werry, Elkind, and Reeves, 1987a). This appears to indicate that anxiety by itself does not cause fidgeting or motor activity that can be confused with ADD/ADHD.

Family Studies and Genetics

Persons with anxiety disorders, whether adults or children, have a higher prevalence of anxiety disorders among their relatives (Last, Beidel, & Perrin, 1996). In an early study addressing this issue, the children of women with major depressive disorder were assessed for psychiatric disorders (Weissman, Leckman, Merikangas, Gammon, & Prusoff, 1984). These depressed women were divided into four groups: depression alone, depression with panic disorder, depression with GAD, and depression with agoraphobia. The children of these mothers were compared to those of a control group whose mothers had no psychiatric illness. The group of mothers with both depression and panic disorder had the most children with an anxiety disorder, relative to the other groups. Taking the opposite approach, Last, Hersen, Kazdin, Francis, and Grubb (1987b) evaluated the mothers of 58 children with DSM-III anxiety disorders. Nineteen of these children had SAD, 22 had only overanxious disorder, and 17 had both of these disorders. Mothers were interviewed not only about their current symptoms, but about any childhood history of anxiety disorder. Relative to the mothers of the normal control children, the mothers of the anxious children had a higher probability of having a lifetime anxiety disorder (83% vs. 40%). There was no specific relationship between children's SAD and maternal diagnosis: Mothers of SAD children did not have elevated rates of either childhood SAD or current panic disorder.

Last et al. (1991) later performed a more extensive family study of DSM-III-R anxiety disorders. The first- and second-degree relatives of 94 children with anxiety disorders were interviewed, as well as the relatives of 58 children with ADHD and 87 controls. There was a significantly higher rate of anxiety disorder in the relatives of anxious children (35%), compared to the relatives of ADHD children (24%) or normal controls (16%). Curiously, the female relatives of ADHD children had a higher rate of anxiety disorders than the female relatives of controls (24%). The rates of all the individual anxiety disorders wee elevated among the relatives of the anxious children relative to controls, with the exception of PTSD, which was higher in the relatives of ADHD children. The study also set out to test a major hypothesis: Is there a specific relationship between SAD and panic disorder? The two disorders are quite similar in their signs and symptoms (autonomic arousal, sense of impending doom, avoidance of phobic stimuli). Klein (1964) originally suggested that these disorders might be linked. The extensive data of Last et al. (1991) did not support such a link, however: The rates of panic disorder and SAD were elevated in the relatives of children with overanxious disorder, but not among the relatives of children with SAD. Indeed, the rate of panic disorder in the relatives of SAD children did not exceed that of the normal controls.

Aggregation in families does not prove a genetic basis for any disorder, as environmental factors may clearly be involved in the transmission from parent to child. No adoptee studies of the anxiety disorders have been performed, either in children or in adults. A number of twin studies have compared anxiety disorders in monozygotic (MZ) and dizygotic (DZ) twins, in an attempt to tease apart genetic and environmental factors. Studies have focused both on the amount of anxiety or fearfulness in the general population of twins and in twins specifically diagnosed with anxiety disorders. Stevenson, Batten, and Cherner (1992) administered the Fear Survey Schedule for Children—Revised (FSSC-R) to 175 pairs of DZ and 144 pairs of MZ twins aged 8 to 18. These twins were from the general population and had been recruited through the Twin Association Clubs in the United Kingdom. Their mean scores on the FSSC-R were typical of those for nontwin children, suggesting that twins are representative of the singleton population of children. A subgroup of these twins was identified whose scores on the FSSC-R were more than one standard deviation above the mean for the children's age; heritabilities for this extreme group (which most likely contained children with anxiety disorders) were calculated separately from those for the less anxious children. This was done to explore the possibility that the genetic factors underlying severe anxiety are different from (or more pronounced than) those underlying normal fears and worries. The heritability for the Total Fear scale was 0.29, indicating that about 29% of the variance of fearfulness can be attributed to genetics. Different effects of genetics were found according to the type of fear. Fear of Failure and Fear of Medical Procedures were not found to have any genetic component, while Fear of the Unknown and Fear of Injury and Small Animals showed the greatest genetic effects, with heritabilities of 0.46 each. Twin studies can also examine the different effects of environment, examining the effects of shared environment (which both twins experience) and nonshared environment. A example of the latter might be a case in which each twin is assigned to a different teacher throughout elementary school, making the twins' educational experience different. In the Stevenson et al. (1992) study, shared environment was found to make a significant contribution to the Fear of Failure score, while it was the nonshared environment that most influenced Fear of Medical Procedures. The latter finding is likely to be due to the fact that only one twin might become ill or injured and thus experience a painful procedure that would lead to such a fear. The influence of genetics was found to be the same in children with normal FSSC-R scores and in those with extreme scores. This suggests that the genetic factors underlying anxiety disorders are similar to those influencing normal fearfulness. It must be borne in mind, however, that this study did not assess the children for anxiety disorders.

No other twin studies of children with DSM-diagnosed anxiety disorders have been performed, but a number of genetic studies of adult anxiety disorders shed light on the issue. Torgersen (1983) found a concordance rate for panic disorder of 31% for MZ twins, as opposed to a 0% rate for DZ twins. Skre, Onstad, Torgersen, Lygren, and Kringlen (1993) also found the concordance rate for panic disorder to be significantly higher in MZ twins (42%) than in DZ twins (17%). Genetic factors appear to be much more important in panic disorder than in some of the other anxiety disorders; for example, rates of concordance for simple (i.e., specific) and social phobias were similar in MZ and DZ twins in the two studies just cited.

The genetic pattern in GAD is much less clear, and may depend on the comorbidity of major depressive disorder. Torgersen (1983) found no difference between MZ and DZ twins in the rates of GAD, while Andrews, Stewart, and Henderson (1990) found that the concordance rate in MZ twins was 1.5 times the rate in DZ twins. Torgersen (1983) excluded GAD subjects with comorbid major depression; Andrews et al. (1990) did not. Skre et al. (1993) found that all their subjects with GAD had a comorbid mood disorder. The concordance rate of GAD was higher for MZ twins (60%) than for DZ twins (14%), though the difference fell short of statistical significance. Kendler, Neale, Kessler, Heath, and Eaves (1992) also found lower rates of MZ concordance for GAD when subjects with comorbid GAD and major depression were excluded.

These results raise the possibility that the genetic influence in GAD is different, depending on whether or not a subject has a lifetime history of major depression. Torgersen (1990) has suggested that in comorbid cases, the entire genetic influence is related to the mood disorder; the GAD in these cases may be considered secondary to the depression. In contrast, GAD in patients without a lifetime history of depression may not have a genetic influence at all (Torgersen, 1983). However, Kendler et al. (1992) found that the heritability of GAD could *not* be accounted for by the occurrence of GAD only during the depressive episodes. Two subsequent studies of female twins with GAD have suggested that GAD and major depression may share genes, but that environmental factors may determine which of these disorders the individual develops (Kendler, Heath, Martin, & Eaves, 1987).

Although SAD manifests itself during childhood, there have been no twin studies of this disorder in persons under age 18. Goldsmith and Gottesman (1981) did find that at age 7, MZ twins were more similar than DZ twins in manifestations of separation distress. Studies of the genetics of SAD have used adult anxiety-disordered subjects who are asked to recall their childhood symptoms. Such a methodology is filled with pitfalls, since the subjects' acute illness may color their memories of their childhood. Silove, Manicavasagar, O'Connell, and Morris-Yates (1995) identified 200 twin pairs (aged 17–66 years; mean age = 37) in Australia. These twins were not psychiatric patients, but from the general population. They filled out numerous self-report anxiety scales, including one inquiring about SAD symptoms during their school years. The influence of genetics of SAD varied markedly by sex: For males, genetics did not contribute *at all* to the development of SAD, while genetics accounted for 41% of the variance in SAD symptom scores of females. These results, while intriguing, are need of replication in a sample of children with SAD.

To summarize the present information on the genetics of common anxiety disorders in childhood and adolescence, it appears that panic disorder shows the strongest genetic effect, with phobias having the least. General fearfulness, particularly of the unknown, danger, or injury, may also have significant genetic effects. The genetics of GAD may be related to those of mood disorder. Genetic effects of SAD may be more significant in females than in males, and it has not yet been established that there is any genetic link between SAD and panic disorder. Longitudinal studies may clarify the genetics of childhood anxiety disorders, but no methodologically sound studies have been performed. Klein (1994) reviewed nine studies of "school refusers" followed into adolescence or adulthood, in the hope of clarifying the long-term course of SAD. Unfortunately, most of the studies did not use standardized criteria for SAD or any other anxiety disorder, and their methods of diagnosis at follow-up were also highly variable. The only conclusion that can be drawn is that children with school refusal continue to have psychiatric problems at least into their teen years and often longer.

Less rigorous methodologically than prospective follow-up studies, "follow-back" studies have asked adults with anxiety disorders about their childhoods, in an attempt to establish continuity between adult and childhood disorders. In two such studies, panic disorder patients with a childhood history of anxiety problems were found to be more likely to have multiple anxiety disorders, more severe anxiety symptoms, and a stronger family history of anxiety disorders than panic disorder patients with no childhood anxiety problems (Otto, Pollack, Rosenbaum, Sachs, & Asher, 1994; Pollack et al., 1996). Patients with social phobia recalled being shy as children; those with GAD met DSM-III-R criteria for overanxious disorder as children, based on their recall of symptoms. (Of course, as noted above, children can now be considered to have GAD.) Again, it should be borne in mind that current symptomatology may have biased the patients' perceptions of their childhoods. Adults with panic disorder recalled having the full range of anxiety disorders; they did no specifically recall suffering from SAD uniquely (Pollack et al., 1996). So, again, a specific relationship between SAD and panic disorder has not yet been established.

Neurobiology

If there is a genetic component in an anxiety disorder, exactly what is inherited? How does such a trait interact with the environment to produce an anxiety disorder? Intriguing data from animal and human studies are coming together to help answer these questions. Suomi and colleagues have worked with a strain of monkeys termed "highly reactive" (Suomi, 1981, 1983, 1986). When infant monkeys are exposed to mild stressors (e.g., a novel stimulus or a brief separation from similar surroundings), a subgroup of monkeys—about 15% of the population—will show high levels of anxiety in response to these modest challenges. These monkeys also show much more marked changes in plasma cortisol than their non-reactive counterparts (Suomi, 1981). If the reactive monkeys are exposed to a prolonged separation from their mothers, they show evidence of depression, with disturbances of eating and sleeping. Such a syndrome responds to tricyclic antidepressants (Suomi, Seaman, Lewis, Delizio, & McKinney, 1978). In contrast, the nonreactive monkeys rarely develop depression after prolonged separation.

The monkeys described by Suomi (1986) appear to develop their anxiety-like traits through their genetic heritage (Scanlan, Suomi, Higley, Scallet, & Kraemer, 1982; Suomi, 1981). Nonhuman primates show anxiety-like symptoms in response to manipulations of the environment as well. Furthermore, such environmental manipulations may influence the animals' biological functioning. Coplan, Rosenblum, and Gorman (1995) have described the effect of availability of food on mother–infant monkey relationships. Mothers of infant monkeys are put into one of three environments: (1) low foraging demand (LFD), where food is easily available with minimal work; (2) high foraging demand (HFD), where the same amount of food is available as in the LFD condition, but the monkeys must work much harder to get it; and (3) variable foraging demand (VFD), where the food availability is unpredictable. It is critical to understand that the monkeys are not starved or mistreated, since all the mother monkeys learn to forage to get the calories needed for themselves and their infants. What varies is the time mothers spend socializing with the infant monkeys when foraging demands differ. In the HFD condition, a mother spends less time attending to her infant. Surprisingly, disturbances in attachment are not found in HFD or

LFD infants, but only in the VFD infants. VFD infants show depressive episodes, diminished autonomy, increased timidity, and decreased timidity; they appear quite similar to the genetically influenced highly reactive infants of Suomi (1986). Mothers in the VFD condition are less responsive to infants, even when they are physically present with them. Coplan et al. (1995) have concluded that because these infants are not grossly deprived of food or emotional stimuli, they represent a more accurate model of human anxiety disorders. They noted that VFD-reared monkeys showed a number of biological changes similar to those of adult panic patients: an exaggerated anxiety response to yohimbine (an alpha-2 antagonist that activates the noradrenergic system; see below), as well as increases in cerebrospinal fluid levels of corticotropin-releasing factor, the substance that causes the release of adrenocorticotropic hormone. This hormone in turn controls the release of cortisol.

Both the highly reactive monkeys of Suomi (1986) and the monkeys raised by mothers in the VFD condition as described by Coplan et al. (1995) resemble the "inhibited" children described by Kagan and colleagues (Kagan, Reznick, Clarke, & Snidman, 1984; Kagan, Reznick, & Snidman, 1988). Children were brought to a playroom where they interacted with an unfamiliar person or objects. About 15% of the sample showed "behavioral inhibition," defined as a long latency to speak, play, or interact with a stranger, as well as maintenance of increased proximity to the mother. Such a pattern of behavior is highly stable over time (Reznick et al., 1986). High rates of motor activity and crying in infants as young as 4 months predict behavioral inhibition at ages 9 and 14 months (Kagan & Snidman, 1991). In utero heart rates may also be a predictor of behavioral inhibition (Snidman, Kagan, & Riordan, 1995). Inhibited children show increased heart rate, pupillary dilation, salivary cortisol, and urinary norepinephrine during stressful tasks, compared to uninhibited children (Kagan, Reznick, & Snidman, 1987; Kagan et al., 1988). Inhibited children show less secure attachments to their mothers as assessed by the Strange Situation, and are rated higher than uninhibited children on the Child Behavior Checklist Internalizing scale (Manassis, Bradley, Goldberg, Hood, & Swinson, 1995).

A number of studies have shown a relationship between behavioral inhibition and both adult and child anxiety disorders (Biederman et al., 1990, 1993; Hirshfield et al., 1992; Rosenbaum et al., 1988, 1992). Children of parents with panic disorder and agoraphobia had significantly higher rates of behavioral inhibition than children of controls or children of parents with major depression (Rosenbaum et al., 1988). Conversely, children who were identified as behaviorally inhibited had an increased risk of anxiety disorders (Biederman et al., 1990), as did their parents (Rosenbaum et al., 1992). At a 3-year follow-up, children who showed the most consistent behavioral inhibition had the greatest likelihood of having an anxiety disorder; these children were also more likely to show multiple anxiety disorders (Hirshfield et al., 1992; Biederman et al., 1993). It should be emphasized that not all behaviorally inhibited children go on to develop anxiety disorders; the above-cited studies found that about 40–60% of the inhibited children were free of anxiety disorders, depending on the time of follow-up.

Behaviorally inhibited children show evidence of increased sympathetic nervous system activity (Kagan et al., 1988), which is consistent with current thinking about the pathophysiology of anxiety disorders, particularly panic disorder (Gorman, Liebowitz, Fyer, & Stein, 1989). These authors divide panic disorder into three components—the acute panic attack, anticipatory anxiety, and phobic avoidance—and suggest that each may be localized to a particular central nervous system area. Lactate infusion or carbon dioxide inhalation will induce panic attacks in over two-thirds of panic disorder patients, but only about 5% of controls (Johnson & Lydiard, 1995). Carbon dioxide stimulates the nucleus tractus solitarius of the brain stem, which activates brain stem mechanisms to increase breathing rate (hyperventilation) to return carbon dioxide levels to normal. The nucleus tractus solitarius also stimulates the nucleus paragigantocellularis (PGI), which has direct input into the locus coeruleus and strongly activates it. This causes the release of norepinephrine throughout the cerebral cortex. The PGI also projects to the spinal cord, where it activates the peripheral sympathetic nervous system (see Figure 9.1). Patients with panic disorder show increased sensitivity to noradrenergic agents. Yohimbine blocks presynaptic alpha-2 receptors, leading to increased secretion of norepinephrine. When panic disorder patients are given an intravenous infusion of this drug, they develop greater anxiety and have more frequent panic attacks relative to controls; they also develop much high levels of the main metabolite of norepinephrine in their plasma (Charney, Woods, Southwick, Krystal, & Heminger, 1990; Heninger & Charney, 1988). After successful treatment with antidepressants or benzodiazepines, these patients exhibit less activation of the noradrenergic system (Charney & Heninger, 1985). Thus Gorman et al. (1989) hypothesize that panic disorder patients have a genetic predisposition to excessive activation of both the locus coeruleus and the peripheral sympathetic nervous system.

Similar to adults with panic disorder, children and adolescents with anxiety disorders show changes in ventilatory physiology. Anxious children have larger minute ventilation, larger tidal volumes, and more variable breathing patterns (Pine et al., 1998). Recently, however, resting sympathetic nervous system activity was not found to be increased in adults with panic disorder relative to controls, nor was the sympathetic system globally activated during a panic disorder (Wilkinson et al., 1998). Thus, there may not be an abnormality in the sympathetic nervous system per se in anxious patients, but it is triggered prematurely in response to stress. Also, the growth hormone response to clonidine in anxious children did not differ from controls, although OCD children did show an exaggerated response (Sallee et al., 1998). This suggests abnormality of the central noradrenergic system in OCD but not in general anxiety. Since adults showed a blunted growth hormone response to clonidine, the study also suggests that there may not be a simple biological continuity between childhood and adolescent disorders.

The locus coeruleus sends noradrenergic projections to the hippocampus, a structure with intimate connections to the limbic system, particularly the cingulate cortex. The hippocampus has connections with both the sensory information from the outside world (see Figure 9.1) and the cingulate, as well as output to the sympathetic nervous system. Gray (1982, 1987) has outlined a theory of how this circuit is involved in anxiety. Sensory information about the current state of the world enters the hippocampus through the entorhinal cortex, where it interacts with information from the long-term memory, which is accessed through the cingulate. The hippocampus serves as a "comparator," allowing the brain to determine whether the current stimulus has been encountered before. If the memory of the stimulus is associated with danger or aversive events, the hippocampus can activate the sympathetic nervous system, producing anticipatory anxiety. In animal studies, increased activity of the locus coeruleus results in a greater release of norepinephrine into the hippocampus. This increases the probability that memory formation may occur, and according to Gray (1982), such memories are more likely to be associated with fear or anxiety. Indeed, panic disorder patients have been shown to have increased blood flow in the anterior temporal lobes, precisely where the hippocampus is located (Reiman et al., 1986, 1989). This increase is seen *before* a panic attack occurs, leading Gorman et al. (1989) to suggest that this confirms the role of these structures in anticipatory anxiety.

As noted in Figure 9.1, the dorsal raphe (source of serotonergic projections to the cortex) and the locus coeruleus strongly influence each other. Drugs affecting the seroton-

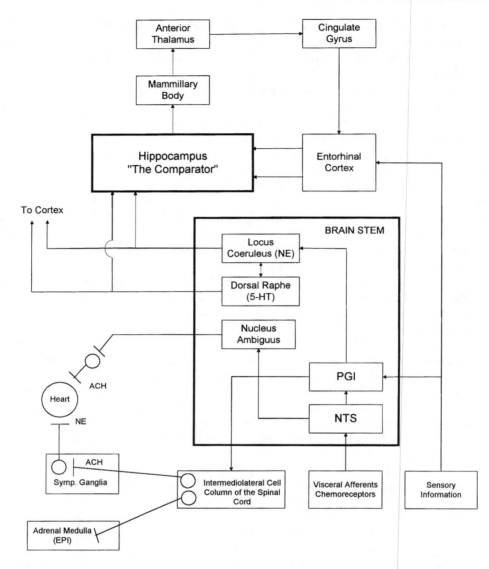

FIGURE 9.1. Neurobiology of anxiety. NE, norepinephrine; ACH, acetylcholine; EPI, epinephrine; 5-HT, serotonin; PGI, nucleus paragigantocellularis; NTS, nucleus tractus solitarius. See text for further details.

ergic system (e.g., fluoxetine and buspirone) are useful antianxiety agents, and a number of agonists of the serotonin system can induce anxiety symptoms in vulnerable subjects, though the effects are much more inconsistent than with lactate, carbon dioxide, or yohimbine (Johnson & Lydiard, 1995). It has been noted that when panic disorder patients are exposed to fenfluramine, a serotonin agonist, the anxiety response is much more gradual in onset and more sustained over time than panic attacks induced by lactate (Targum, 1992). Targum (1992) suggests that the serotonin system is more closely related to anticipatory anxiety than to the panic attack per se.

Recent findings in molecular genetics have also suggested a role for the serotonergic system in anxiety disorders (Lesch et al., 1997). Over 500 adult subjects were administered the NEO Personality Inventory, which yields a Neuroticism scale (these subjects did not necessarily have anxiety disorders). Their blood was also drawn, and genetic material was isolated from their lymphoblasts. The investigators examined the gene that codes for the promotor of the serotonin transporter. The serotonin transporter resides in the neuronal membrane and is responsible for the reuptake of serotonin after it has been released from the neuron. It thus plays a critical role in terminating the action of serotonin in the brain. The gene studied is not the one for the transporter itself, but the one for the promotor—a separate gene that is located "upstream" from the transporter gene and governs the transcription of the transporter gene. That is, the promotor is responsible for "switching on" the gene that codes for the transporter. The transporter promotor gene has been found to exist in two variants: a "normal" long variant, and a shorter variant in which 44 DNA base pairs have been deleted. The promotor transcribed rom this short variant is less efficient in "switching on" transcription of the serotonin transporter gene. In these 505 subjects, 32% had two alleles of the "long" versions (l/l); 49% were heterozygotes, having one long and one short variant (l/s); and 19% were homozygous for the short version (s/s). The l/s and s/s subjects had equally reduced expression of the serotonin transporter in their lymphocytes, relative to the l/l subjects; these subjects also rated themselves significantly higher on the Neuroticism scale of the NEO. The effects were modest; the authors calculated that the short variant accounted for 3–4% of the total variance and about 7–9% of the genetic variance of the anxiety ratings. The authors suggested that multiple genes may be involved in the development of anxiety, and that the identification of these genes may lead to the development of more specific psychopharmacological treatments. For instance, it would be of interest to compare anxiety patients with and without the short form of the promotor gene in terms of their response to serotonergic drugs.

Davidson (1992) has extensively explored the neurobiological basis of negative affect, using electroencephalographic (EEG) measures of frontal lobe activation. His work with adults showed that left anterior cerebral hemisphere activation was strongly associated with positive affect, whereas right anterior hemisphere activation was more associated with negative affect. He hypothesized that the left frontal areas of the cerebrum are part of an "approach" system, while the right frontal areas mediate "withdrawal." Furthermore, there appear to be differences between individuals at baseline in terms of asymmetry of cerebral hemisphere activation. Adults who consistently show left-sided activation in the resting state report more positive emotional responses to a pleasant film. In contrast, adults with greater right-sided activation report more intense negative feelings to a film with fearful or disgusting stimuli (Wheeler, Davidson, & Tomarken, 1993). Newborns show greater right-sided activation when a bad-tasting substance is placed on their tongues, while a good-tasting substance elicits left-sided EEG activation (Fox & Davidson, 1986). At age 10 months, infants watching a film of an actress crying or laughing show right or left activation of the anterior EEG, respectively (Davidson & Fox, 1982). Left frontal activation is found when 10-month-olds observe the approach of their mothers, while right activation is noted when a stranger approaches (Fox & Davidson, 1988). Using the criteria of Kagan et al. (1984), Davidson (1992) classified 31-month-olds into three groups of 28 subjects: inhibited, uninhibited, and a middle group. When the children were 38 months of age, EEG recordings were obtained both at rest and during several tasks. The inhibited children showed significantly more right-sided activation in the midfrontal electrodes than did the middle or uninhibited children. Uninhibited children, in contrast, showed greater left-sided activation than either of these groups. These data are striking for their consistency. Furthermore, Reiman et al (1986) found increased cerebral blood flow, primarily in the right anterior temporal cortex. Magnetic resonance imaging studies have also tended to find lesions in this area (Johnson & Lydiard, 1995).

In summary, a child may have a genetic hypersensitivity or hyperactivity of the locus coeruleus and the sympathetic nervous system. Alternatively, the child may have an inherent tendency toward right-sided anterior cerebral activation. This may be initially reflected in an inhibited temperament. The child may not progress to an anxiety disorder, however, unless the "genetic load" for this trait is unusually high, or unless environmental factors combine with such a trait to produce the anxiety disorder. It is even conceivable, in view of the studies of monkeys raised in the VFD condition, that no genetic component may be necessary to produce an anxiety disorder. Children exposed repeatedly to certain types of stressors may have their central nervous systems affected in such a way that the anxiety disorder becomes autonomous even after the stressors have been removed. (This is certainly true of PTSD, which is not discussed in this chapter, but it may be true of other anxiety disorders as well.)

Clinical Assessment

General Issues in Assessment of Anxiety

Clinicians must approach the assessment of anxiety in children with a clear sense of what "anxiety" means, for it has many definitions in both the professional and lay worlds. Just as laypeople use the term "hyperactivity" or "impulsivity" to refer to a wide range of disruptive behavior in children, so they may use the term "anxiety" to refer to any negative affect (including temper tantrums) that children display. Clinicians with a psychodynamic background may use the term "anxiety" in a manner that has nothing to do with overt symptoms. The child may be viewed as suffering from unconscious emotional conflicts, which are thought to drive such behaviors as stealing, bedwetting, or stubbornness. It may then be concluded that the underlying "anxiety" can be revealed or treated through psychotherapy. Our intent is not to debate the validity of such an approach, but to make it clear that clinicians can act at cross purposes if they do not clearly understand each other's theoretical orientations. In this chapter, "anxiety" refers only to the overt symptoms covered in the DSM-IV criteria. Reformulating externalizing symptoms as somehow arising from unrecognized or unconscious anxiety symptoms can cloud clinical judgment, since virtually any psychiatric symptoms can be viewed as "anxiety."

Clinicians should be prepared to encounter children who have both internalizing and externalizing symptoms, as Strauss et al. (1988) clearly showed that children with anxiety disorders commonly meet criteria for ADHD or ODD. This brings up the issue of dual diagnosis versus differential diagnosis. That is, when should clinicians make both types of diagnoses in a child (e.g., ADHD and GAD), and when should they attempt to discriminate between the diagnoses? A case example illustrates this problem.

C. J., a 9-year-old boy, is brought to a clinician's office because of school problems. His mother states that since kindergarten, teachers have complained that C. J. fidgets constantly, does not complete work, talks in class, and generally makes poor grades. When his current teacher works with him on a one-to-one basis, he completes his work without difficulty. He is not aggressive or antisocial, but often does not wish to go out for recess, because he says the kids are "mean." His mother states that she has trouble getting C. J. to complete tasks at home. He will not sit still at the dinner table or during homework, but is not overtly hyperactive. He has trouble sleeping and is afraid of the dark, but his mother denies that C. J. has any other symptoms. He plays normally with children in the neighborhood. C. J.'s mother and father divorced 1 year ago, and things appear to have gotten worse since then.

On clinical interview, C. J. is distracted easily. He denies depression or suicidal ideation. He says he is "dumb" because he cannot do work as well as other children. He is afraid of the dark, spiders, and tornadoes. He worries that his mother will die in a car accident.

This child presents with a mixture of attentional and anxiety symptoms. Is this a child with ADHD who has developed secondary anxiety? Is this a primary anxiety disorder, perhaps arising from the recent divorce? Is anxiety therefore interfering with the child's attention? After all, difficulty concentrating is a criterion for GAD. Is this a child with ADHD who has also developed an anxiety disorder that is completely independent of the inattention problems? The last option is frequently eschewed by mental health professionals, who prefer to have one clearly defined diagnosis or focus of treatment. Yet it is common in the health professions to treat patients with two disorders (e.g., diabetes and asthma) without attempting to seek a link between the two. Based on the information given so far, any of the above-described options is possible. How is a clinician to decide among them?

Thorough History Taking

Age at onset of symptoms, and the relationship of symptoms to life events, are often keys to making a diagnosis. In the case described above, the clinician cannot ignore the fact that the hyperactivity and inattention began in kindergarten and appear to have remained constant to the present. Because the ADHD symptoms clearly predated the divorce, it would be difficult to argue that C. J.'s inattentiveness is caused by the stress of parental separation. There is no evidence of SAD or panic disorder; there is evidence of shyness, overconcern about performance, and unrealistic fears. These may have evolved separately, well after the ADHD symptoms emerged.

Issues Related to Impairment

A simple but often overlooked fact in the diagnosis of anxiety disorders is that the anxiety symptoms must cause significant impairment of functioning. Assessing impairment of functioning is quite simple for the externalizing disorders, as academic and/or discipline problems are usually the reasons for the office visit. For the internalizing disorders, however, the symptoms may only be mentioned in passing or discovered by a clinician during the interview, as some of C. J.'s fears are in the case above. If C. J. is afraid of spiders, does this constitute a specific phobia? Not unless it prevents him from engaging in normal childhood activities. Does he refuse to play in the backyard? Will he not handle play equipment because "a spider might be on it"? Do his fears about his mother's being in a car accident interfere with his watching TV, playing with friends, or going to sleepovers? If so, they may form part of a GAD or SAD diagnosis, but if C. J. mentions them only in passing or he forgets about them in school, the clinician should not diagnose an anxiety disorder.

Parent–Child Discrepancy in Reporting Symptoms

The concordance between parent and child interviews is poor for the anxiety disorders (Klein, 1991). This means that the clinician will encounter parents who deny that their children are anxious, yet the children will report a high level of symptoms. Conversely, a parent may state that a child is anxious, yet the child denies all such symptoms when asked by the clinician. There are currently no research data to resolve the question of whether a parent or a child is the "better" reporter of anxious symptoms. Indeed, all studies of anxiety disorders have varied in the type of interview data used to make the diagnosis. Some have used a parent interview only, others have employed some combination of parent and child interviews, and still others have relied only on the child interview. Carefully designed studies are needed comparing children who meet criteria for anxiety disorder by parent report only, by child report only, and by both parent and child report. For instance, if a family history of anxiety disorder or autonomic arousal is found to be present in the child-report-only and combined-report groups, but not in the parent-report-only group, we can conclude that parent report alone is not sufficient to make a diagnosis in the child. One study has examined the problem of this discrepancy (Manassis, Mendlowitz, & Menna, 1997). Sixty-five children aged 7–12 years were diagnosed as anxious according to parent interview. The group was divided into those children who themselves endorsed anxiety and those who did not. Children who endorsed anxiety symptoms also rated themselves as more depressed; they also showed lower self-esteem. They did not, however, differ on parent or clinician measures of severity. This study would imply that there are not major differences between parent-diagnosed anxious children who endorse or deny their anxious symptoms, but further study is needed.

A parent may state that a child is "anxious" as an explanation for some behavior the parent finds troublesome (e.g., tics, hyperactivity, learning problems). Thus the real symptoms may be masked by the parent's description. For instance, a child may be failing in reading because of undiagnosed dyslexia, yet the parent reports to the clinician that the child is "too anxious" to study and avoids it. Similarly, parents may view oppositional behaviors or conduct problems as stemming from some underlying emotional problem ("We just don't know why he is acting this way!"). School refusal by a truant, oppositional child should not be confused with SAD. If a child or teen completely denies internalizing symptoms, the clinician should focus more on the disruptive behaviors, for behavior management directly aimed at these symptoms is far more likely to be successful in alleviating them. Parents who are themselves anxious or depressed are more likely to report symptoms in their children; clinicians should be aware that it may be a parent, rather than a child, who must become the focus of treatment. Conversely, a parent may not wish to reveal the family stressors that have triggered the child's anxiety. This is particularly true in the case of SAD. For example, a mother may deny that the child is afraid to leave the mother, stating only that the child "refuses to go to school." On interview with the child, the clinician may discover that the child's fear of separation is related to the fact that the mother is being beaten by her boyfriend. When dealing with anxiety disorders, the clinician must interview parent and child separately in order to untangle these issues.

"Realistic" versus "Unrealistic" Fears and Stressors

Occasionally a clinician will avoid making an anxiety disorder diagnosis because the child's fear or worry seems "appropriate" to his or her situation. For example, a child's mother develops cancer, and the child becomes worried about the mother's health. Is this not a normal response? It is a normal response only if (1) the worry does not impair functioning (it is abnormal if the child sits in school doing nothing while worrying about the mother), and (2) there is an absence of autonomic symptoms (heart racing, sweaty palms, somatic complaints). Symptoms that make a child severely uncomfortable or that impair academic or social functioning should be viewed as clinically significant.

Rating Scales, Clinical Interviews, and Psychological Tests

A number of rating scales are available for measuring childhood and adolescent anxiety. These include the RCMAS (Reynolds & Paget, 1983), the State–Trait Anxiety Inventory for Children—Modified (STAIC-M; Fox & Houston, 1983), and the FSSC-R (Ollendick, 1983). The RCMAS is a 37-item questionnaire consisting of 28 anxiety items such as "I am nervous," and 9 "lie" items such as "I am always good." The child answers "Yes" or "No" to each of the items, which are scored as 0 or 1, respectively. The Total Anxiety score can therefore range from 0 to 28. In addition, subscale scores are available for Worry/Oversensitivity, Physiological factors, and Concentration factors. Normative data are available for ages 6–18 (Reynolds & Paget, 1983). It has recently been updated with new normative data (Reynolds & Richmond, 1997). The RCMAS is simple to administer and easy for even young or cognitively impaired children to understand. The FSSC-R is an 80-item questionnaire that directly assesses children's fears about events and objects they commonly encounter. A child rates how much he or she is afraid of a particular item ("none" = 1, "some" = 2, "a lot" = 3). A Total Fear score is obtained by summing the 80 items, and an Intensity score is obtained by summing the items that are given a 3. Five factors have been found: (1) Fear of Failure, (2) Fear of the Unknown, (3) Fear of Injury and Small Animals, (4) Fear of Danger and Death, and (5) Fear of Medical Procedures. The STAIC-M has two versions; the State version assesses current symptoms, while the Trait version asks how chronic the symptom is. The STAIC-M State version has 27 items, and the Trait version has 26 items. On the State version, the child endorses the intensity of a particular anxiety symptom ("I feel [1] not scared, [2] scared, [3] very scared"). On the Trait version, the child endorses the chronicity of the symptom ("I feel scared [1] hardly ever, [2] sometimes, [3] often"). Scores are obtained by summing the ratings separately for the State and Trait versions. The language skills required for the STAIC-M are higher than those needed for the RCMAS.

How useful and reliable are these scales? All of them have acceptable test–retest reliability and correlate reasonably with other measures of anxiety (Perrin & Last, 1992), but it is unclear whether they can truly discriminate anxious children from those with other psychiatric disorders. Perrin and Last (1992) compared 105 children with anxiety disorders to nonanxious ADHD children and normal controls on all three of the measures described above. Diagnoses were established via a semistructured psychiatric interview; the interviewer was unaware of each child's scores on the rating scales. The FSSC-R did not discriminate among the three groups. Both the ADHD and anxiety disorder groups had elevated RCMAS scores relative to the controls, but did not differ from each other. The scores on the STAIC-M showed a similar pattern. Perrin and Last (1997) subsequently compared 50 children with ADHD to 72 children with anxiety disorders and 55 controls. The anxiety and ADHD groups did not differ on the number of self-reported "worries," but ADHD children were more likely to worry about friends and school, while children with anxiety worried more about separation and social evaluation by others. It is clear from these findings that anxiety scales by themselves should *never* be used to diagnose an anxiety disorder. If a child has been diagnosed by a clinical interview as having such a disorder, and also has an elevated rating scale score, the score may be used to track the success of treatment. These scales may also be used to screen for anxiety symptoms, but a full clinical interview should be carried out to confirm the presence of an anxiety disorder.

Traditionally, internalizing symptoms have been assessed via a variety of "projective" tests, such as the Rorschach and the Children's Thematic Apperception Test. The latter involves the child's telling a story about a picture he or she is shown. Such tests are widely known among educators, physicians, mental health professionals, and the lay public. Great faith is placed in their ability not only to diagnose mental disorders, but to uncover the psychological forces driving a child's inner life. Prior to acceptance of ADHD as a diagnosis qualifying children for special education, a label of "emotionally disturbed" was often procured through projective testing, even in the complete absence of overt depressive or anxiety symptoms. Gittelman (1980) extensively reviewed the use of such testing in childhood mental disorders, raising several concerns: (1) Few studies of projective tests in children control for IQ (an important variable, since these tests rely so strongly on the child's verbal expression of thoughts and feelings); (2) the tests appear able to discriminate mentally ill children from normal children, but do not appear able to discriminate among different forms of mental disorder; and (3) few studies have compared the projective test response of children from rigorously diagnosed clinical groups (e.g., ADHD vs. GAD vs. control), with the tester unaware of group membership. It is thus inappropriate to diagnose an anxiety disorder based on projective testing when the child does not meet criteria for an anxiety disorder by either parent or child clinical interview.

Pharmacotherapy

Surprisingly, despite many studies showing the effectiveness of antianxiety drugs in adults, very few well-controlled trials of these agents have been performed in children and adolescents. This makes recommendations about the precise indications for initiating drug treatment difficult. The following is an overview of the pharmacological studies performed to date.

Tricyclic Antidepressants

Several controlled trials of tricyclic antidepressants (TCAs) have been performed in children with SAD, with conflicting results. Gittelman-Klein and Klein (1970) treated 35 school refusers (aged 7–15) as part of a double-blind, placebo-controlled trial of imipramine. (All of the subjects also received a behavioral intervention.) The mean dose of imipramine was 159 mg/day. It was found that 81% of the imipramine group returned to school, as opposed to only 47% of the placebo group; the imipramine group also had significantly greater reductions in subjective anxiety. Berney et al. (1981) did not find a therapeutic effect of clomipramine in 9- to 15-year-old school refusers, but the dosages used were not adequate (40–75 mg/day). Recently, however, a number of studies have not shown TCAs to be particularly effective in SAD or school refusal. Bernstein, Garfinkel, and Borchardt (1990) randomly assigned 24 children aged 7–17 to one of three groups: placebo, imipramine, or alprazolam. By chance, the children assigned to the alprazolam group had higher baseline anxiety scores. All subjects also participated in a "school reentry plan" that involved intensive therapy and case management. Children in all three groups responded well, with increases in school attendance and decreases in anxiety. Although there was a trend for the medication groups to have a more robust reduction in anxiety, the differences were not statistically significant. Similarly, Klein, Koplewicz, and Kanner (1992) did not find that imipramine was superior to placebo in the treatment of SAD. Seventeen children (mean age 9½ years) with SAD who had not responded to behavioral intervention were randomly assigned to placebo or the TCA (the mean dose was 153 mg/day); they continued their behavioral treatment throughout the study. There was no effect of the drug on any of the behavioral or anxiety measures. There has never been a study of the use of TCAs for any childhood anxiety disorder other than SAD.

Benzodiazepines

Few studies have examined the effects of benzodiazepines in childhood or adolescence. Preliminary results from a double-blind, placebo-controlled protocol suggest that clonazepam is effective in adolescent panic disorder (Kutcher, Reiter, Gardner, & Klein, 1992), whereas two controlled trials indicate that it is ineffective in childhood GAD and SAD (Graae, Milner, Rizzotto, & Klein, 1994; Simeon et al., 1992). Thus there is no strong evidence documenting the effectiveness of benzodiazepines in childhood and adolescent anxiety disorders.

Selective Serotonin Reuptake Inhibitors

Birmaher et al. (1994) treated 30 anxious children and adolescents (mean age = 14) with an open trial of the selective serotonin reuptake inhibitor (SSRI) fluoxetine. The children (who were all nonresponders to psychotherapy) had a variety of anxiety diagnoses other than OCD; two-thirds had failed trials of TCAs. The mean dose of fluoxetine was 25.7 mg/day. Only one patient received 10 mg/day; all the others were on 20–60 mg/day. Side effects were mild and transient, and none of the subjects had any worsening of anxiety symptoms. Anxiety severity scores showed a highly significant reduction, with 56% of the patients rated as moderately or markedly improved. An open study also examined the effectiveness of fluoxetine in the treatment of childhood anxiety disorders (Fairbanks et al., 1997). Sixteen outpatients with a variety of anxiety disorders were treated with a mean dose of 0.7 mg/kg day of fluoxetine. The maximum doses were 40 mg in children under 12 and 80 mg in adolescents. All of the patients with separation anxiety disorder responded, while only 1 of the 7 patients with GAD responded. Children with multiple anxiety diagnoses required higher doses of the SSRI. No severe side effects such as agitation or suicidality were found. No double-blind placebo controlled trials of serotonin reuptake inhibitors have been performed in any childhood anxiety disorder other than OCD.

The evidence for the effectiveness of drugs in the treatment of childhood anxiety disorders is quite limited, and further studies are clearly needed. Yet the clinician will encounter situations in which pharmacological treatment is needed. These include (1) children for whom psychosocial treatment has failed after an adequate trial, and (2) children with pronounced and severe anxiety symptoms that prevent them from carrying out activities of daily living. A child or adolescent with severe SAD or panic attacks who cannot attend school is a good example; rather than waiting for psychosocial interventions to take effect, a clinician should consider a trial of imipramine or an SSRI in such a case. At present, clinicians should avoid the use of benzodiazepines unless the other agents have failed.

Psychosocial Treatments

Behavior Therapy

Behavior therapy involves a degree of exposure to the anxiety-provoking stimulus. This therapy is commonly used for specific phobias. The most widely used form of therapy is systematic desensitization, in which a child is gradually exposed to a feared stimulus. This treatment is based on Wolpe's (1958) theory of reciprocal inhibition, whereby a person produces a response that is incompatible with fear and pairs this response with a feared or phobic object. The patient continues to associate the new, pleasant response with the feared stimulus until fear is no longer provoked.

The method of systemic desensitization is well described by Drobes and Strauss (1997). The first step requires teaching the child ways to relax. These include the use of progressive muscle relaxation, engaging in a pleasurable activity, or simultaneously visualizing a pleasant stimulus. A fear hierarchy is then established. This involves the patient's describing situations or objects that are fear-provoking. The child then ranks these fear-provoking stimuli from the least to the most fearsome. Next, the child is "desensitized": The clinician has the child relax and then imagine or experience a fear-provoking stimulus. The exposure begins with the least fear-provoking stimulus and gradually progresses to the most feared stimulus. Hampe, Noble, Miller, and Barrett (1973) randomly assigned 67 phobic children to either reciprocal inhibition therapy, psychotherapy, or a waiting-list control. A significant reduction in fearfulness was found, according to parents' ratings. Children in the treatment groups improved faster and to a greater extent than the waiting-list controls. The greatest reduction in phobic behavior occurred in the first 6 weeks of treatment. The children in the 6- to 10-year-old age group displayed a faster response than those in the 11- to 15-year-old group. At a 2-year follow-up, 80% of the patients remained free of phobias.

Behavior therapy has also been used in the treatment of school refusal (Blagg & Yule, 1984). Thirty school refusers treated with behavior therapy were compared to 16 hospitalized school refusers and 20 children who were home-schooled while receiving psychodynamic psychotherapy. Children were not randomly assigned to the treatment groups. The behavior therapy began with clarification of each child's problem with both parents and teachers. Realistic fears (e.g., bullies, teacher conflicts) were dealt with. The school staff was instructed not to be punitive upon the child's return. *In vivo* flooding was then used as the parent or an appropriate escort ensured that the child attended class. The escort helped manage the child's tantrums, and if necessary, both parents or two escorts attended with the child. At a 1-year follow-up, 93% of the behavior therapy group had achieved full-time school attendance, compared with 37.5% of the hospitalized group and 10% of those treated at home. The average length of treatment was 2.53 weeks for the behavior therapy, 45.3 weeks for those hospitalized, and 72.1 weeks for those treated at home. In addition to displaying the efficacy of behavior therapy, the authors concluded that their study showed the difficulty of treating school refusers who had become accustomed to staying at home.

Behavior therapy often incorporates "modeling" as part of the therapy. Modeling involves the patient's observing another person in an anxiety-provoking situation, followed by the patient's imitating the model. Beidel and Morris (1993) describe various forms of modeling. The patient may watch a child, either filmed or in person, approach a feared object. Another method is termed "participant modeling," in which the patient is guided by the therapist or a nonanxious peer through the anxiety-provoking situation. Rao, Moely, and Lockman (1987) described the use of a modeling film in socially withdrawn preschoolers. Sixteen children were randomly assigned to either a treatment group (which viewed a film depicting social approach behavior) or a control group (which viewed a nature film of similar length). The treatment group was judged to have significantly increased social participation, compared to the nontreatment group. This behavior was maintained at a 3-week follow-up. When compared to a group of normal controls, the treated children were judged to be no different in terms of social participation at follow-up.

Contingency management relies on the basic concepts of reinforcement, punishment, and stimulus control. In anxious children, this treatment involves the use of reinforcers (i.e., praise, rewards, or tokens) when the children expose themselves to a feared stimulus, and the withholding of reinforcers for avoidance of feared stimuli. With children, it is important to be clear about the rewards and what is expected for their attainment. Contracts may be written in explicit terms to avoid disagreement. In one study, contingency management was used with 18 socially withdrawn children (Walker, Greenwood, Hops, & Todd, 1979). Three types of behavior were reinforced: (1) initiating social interactions, (2) responding to positive interactions, and (3) maintaining social interactions over time. Behaviors (nonverbal, verbal, and physical contact) were rated using a standardized system. Appropriate behavior was reinforced with tokens and praise. Children showed robust increases in social interaction, particularly when their ongoing efforts to maintain social interactions were reinforced.

Reinforced practice has been found to be effective in diminishing different fears in adults and children (Leitenburg & Callahan, 1973). This method consists of gradual repeated practice in approaching a feared stimulus, reinforcement for gains, feedback on progress, and instructions designed to arouse expectations of success. Adults using this method displayed decreased fears of heights, snakes, and shock. When verbal praise, a toy prize, and the visual reinforcer of shading a "time thermometer" were used as rewards, preschoolers increased their ability to tolerate being alone in a dark room.

Cognitive-Behavioral Therapy

Cognitive-behavioral therapy (CBT) is based on the assumption that maladaptive behaviors result from distorted cognitive structures. Zatz and Chassin (1983) found that students rated as highly anxious on the Test Anxiety Scale for Children reported numerous negative cognitions. Examples included "I must be making many mistakes," "I don't do well on tests like this," and "I'm doing worse than others." Prins (1985) found that highly anxious children used more negative self-referent cognitions before dental procedures, and that there was a strong correlation between negative self-speech and anxiety ($r = .67$, $p < .001$). Kendall (1993) theorized that childhood anxiety is based on such distortions: "Anxious children seem preoccupied with concerns about evaluations by self and others and the likelihood of severe negative consequences. They seem to misperceive characteristically the demands of the environment and routinely add stress to a variety of situations" (p. 239). CBT promotes changing negative cognitions in conjunction with using behavior therapy techniques known to decrease anxiety. Kendall's (1994) CBT approach, which requires 16–20 sessions, is summarized in Table 9.2.

These techniques were examined in a controlled study that included 30 children with DSM-III-R overanxious disorder, 8 with SAD, and 9 with avoidant disorder. After a highly structured assessment, children were randomly assigned to 16 weeks of CBT or an 8-week waiting list. Two standardized measures of anxiety (RCMAS, STAIC-M) were administered, and observations of anxious self-talk were obtained, at the end of CBT or at the end of the 8-week control period. The CBT group showed a statistically significant decline in self-ratings of anxiety as well as negative cognitions. Parents also rated the CBT-treated children significantly lower on the Child Behavior Checklist Internalizing scale. The gains in the CBT group were maintained at 1 year posttreatment. A larger randomized trial of CBT in 93 children with anxiety disorders confirmed these results and showed maintenance of the gains at 1-year follow-up (Kendall et al., 1997)

Durlak, Fuhrman, and Lampman (1991) performed a meta-analysis of research on the use of CBT for treating various childhood maladaptive behaviors, as well as anxiety, depression, and low self-esteem. About three-fourths of the studies used a combination of

TABLE 9.2. Cognitive-Behavioral Therapy (CBT) According to Kendall's Model

Session 1	Build rapport; collect information on situations that promote anxiety and on how the child responds to the anxiety.
Session 2	Teach child to identify different types of feelings.
Session 3	Rank-order anxiety-provoking situations. Help child distinguish anxiety response from other types of emotions.
Session 4	Relaxation training; give child personalized audiocassette for use outside of sessions.
Session 5	Teach child to modify self-talk (replace negative with positive) and use self-talk to reduce anxiety.
Session 6	Emphasize coping self-talk and verbal self-redirection.
Session 7	Teach child to self-evaluate and self-reward positive, nonanxious coping responses.
Session 8	Review all of the skills above.
Session 9	Have child practice skills and watch therapist model handling anxiety; use role playing to rehearse handling anxiety-provoking situations.
Sessions 10–15	Expose child to real and imagined anxiety-provoking situations. Continue practice.
Session 16	Termination issues; discuss therapy experience; encourage the child to consider how to use new coping skills in everyday life.

CBT approaches, including task-oriented problem solving, social problem solving, self-instructions, role playing, rewards, social cognition training, social skills training, and other elements. This analysis included 64 studies and found an effect size almost double in magnitude for children aged 11–13 compared to children aged 5–7, suggesting that CBT may be more effective for older children functioning at higher cognitive levels.

Not all studies of CBT in anxiety disorders have obtained positive results, however. Fox and Houston (1981) used self-instruction to treat the anxiety elicited by reciting a poem while being videotaped. Fifty-six fourth-grade children rated as having high or low trait anxiety on the STAIC-M were randomly assigned to self-instruction treatment (CBT), minimal treatment, or no treatment. Subjects in the self-instruction group were taught self-instructions that focused on reappraisal of aversive aspects of the task at hand (e.g., "Even if I don't do this correctly, nothing bad will happen"). Subjects in the minimal-treatment group focused on self-instructions concerning the impending situation (e.g., "This will just take a few minutes"). Each treatment group also watched a film of a model using similar self-statements and performing a task. The students high in trait anxiety actually displayed a worsening in signs of behavioral anxiety after cognitive treatment, compared to non-intervention matched peers. There was no difference between the minimal-treatment and no-treatment groups. CBT and an attention-control treatment were equally effective in reducing school phobia (Last, Hansen, & Franco, 1998). The highly structrued CBT approach was not superior to traditional supportive psychotherapy.

CBT has been shown to be useful in adults with panic disorder (Barlow, Craske, Cerny, & Klosko, 1989; Stanley et al., 1996). The experience with CBT in treating other anxiety syndromes in children makes it promising for the amelioration of anticipatory anxiety and avoidant behavior. Otto and Whittal (1995) note the four elements of CBT for panic disorder: (1) an informational component, in which patients are educated as to the basis of fears and the rationale for treatment; (2) somatic management skills for breathing and muscle relaxation; (3) cognitive restructuring; and (4) exposure. Ollendick (1995) reported successfully treating four adolescent outpatients with panic disorder and agoraphobia, using these CBT techniques. These patients were taught progressive muscle relaxation and breathing retraining in early sessions. Cue-controlled relaxation and applied relaxation were later taught and practiced at home. Therapist-assisted *in vivo* exposure was then employed, followed by parent-assisted exposure. Patients displayed a decrease in the frequency of panic attacks and in agoraphobic avoidance, as well as an increase in self-efficacy ratings, within 10 weeks of treatment.

Family Therapy

Although there are many case reports of family interventions in treating anxiety disorders, comparative studies are lacking. In many studies, parents work as collaborators in CBT. Parent-trained self-control instruction was used by Graziano and Mooney (1980) to decrease bedtime fears in 6- to 12-year-old children. Thirty-three families with "severely fearful children" whose symptoms had persisted for more than 18 months were studied. The treatment group consisted of instructing children to lie down and relax their muscles, having them choose and imagine a pleasant scene, and having them repeat motivational statements such "I am brave; I can take care of myself when I am in the dark." In addition, a token system was established for successful relaxation practice and time spent symptom-free at night. Parents were trained to prepare children for bed, to monitor the nightly practice of the relaxation procedures, and to award tokens when they deemed it appropriate. The treatment group displayed significantly fewer fears than the waiting-list control group. The majority of the treatment group (14 of 17 patients) improved within 2 months of treatment.

Barrett, Dadds, and Rapee (1996) incorporated family therapy and CBT in the treatment of children with DSM-IIII-R SAD, overanxious disorder, and social phobia. Seventy-nine children aged 7–14 were randomly assigned to either CBT, family therapy and CBT, or a waiting-list control. Parents in the family treatment group were trained in reinforcement strategies. Verbal praise and tangible rewards were provided when fearful situations were faced. "Planned ignoring" was used to handle anxious behavior. This strategy included listening and responding empathically at first when children complained; further complaints were followed by the parents' redirecting the children to use a coping strategy that the children had been taught in their CBT. Parents were also taught to deal with their own anxiety, to gain awareness of their anxiety responses, and to model problem-solving techniques; moreover, they were trained to improve their communication skills to improve their responses as a parenting unit. In both treatment groups (CBT and CBT plus family training), 69.8% of the children no longer met criteria for an anxiety disorder at posttreatment assessment, compared to 26.0% of waiting-list controls. At a 1-year follow-up, 95.6% of those treated with family therapy and CBT no longer met criteria for an anxiety disorder, compared to 70.3% of the children treated with CBT alone.

Psychodynamic Psychotherapy

Psychoanalytic theory views anxiety as stemming from unresolved psychosexual conflicts. Within this framework, classical psychodynamic therapy or play therapy has been the treatment of choice as a means of working through these underlying issues. Psychotherapy with anxious children is focused on providing a secure internal foundation, and has been recommended for school refusal and SAD (Bemporad, Beresin, & Rauch, 1993). The therapy may focus on symbolic play or drawings and on helping a child to accept changes in the family dynamics as a result of therapy. Anxiety may be a product of pathological relations within the family that sabotage the age-appropriate autonomy of the child; treatment therefore needs to be tailored to meet these situations. Dysfunctional family interaction patterns, such as enmeshment or parental insecurity, may have to be addressed. In some cases, parents may need to be treated for their own anxiety or mood disorders. Family therapy is recommended if numerous family issues are complicating the anxiety symptoms.

Most studies of psychoanalytic treatment do not specify diagnoses of their subjects, and thus it cannot be determined to what degree this modality is efficacious in anxiety disorders. Few studies have control groups or compare psychoanalytic treatment to other modalities of therapy.

OBSESSIVE–COMPULSIVE DISORDER

OCD is a good deal rarer than the other anxiety disorders of childhood and adolescence, yet it clearly represents an important and distinct clinical phenomenon. A survey of over 5,000 high school students revealed 18 cases of OCD, for a prevalence rate of 0.35% (Flament et al., 1988). One-third of adults with OCD report that their symptoms began during childhood (Rasmussen & Eisen, 1990). Patients with OCD may have either obsessions or compulsions, though most children will have both. Obsessions are purely mental phenomena, consisting of thoughts that are intrusive, repetitive, and clearly unwanted. Obsessions are commonly about dirt, germs, bodily waste, sex acts, or other aversive substances; they may also entail urges to hurt people close to the patient or to engage in socially inappropriate behavior. The patient does not hallucinate, and there is an absence of paranoia or thought disturbance. Compulsions consist of the performance of unwanted, repetitive physical acts such as washing hands, counting objects, checking (e.g., checking repeatedly to see that the oven is turned off), and performing meaningless rituals. The symptoms must be present for at least 6 months and must impair the patient's functioning.

No twin or adoption studies of OCD have been performed, but family studies clearly indicate an elevated rate of OCD among the first-degree relatives of both children and adults with OCD (Silverman & Nelles, 1988; Riddle et al., 1990). People with OCD and their relatives have an elevated prevalence of Tourette syndrome, suggesting a genetic link between these disorders (Pauls, Towbin, Leckman, Zahner, & Cohen, 1986; Pauls, Raymond, Stevenson, & Leckman, 1991). OCD and Tourette syndrome may be alternative expressions of the same gene; the family data are most consistent with an autosomal dominant mode of transmission (Pauls et al., 1991). Penetrance is variable, and sex may also influence the gene's expressivity. (For a fuller discussion of Tourette syndrome, see Brown & Ivers, Chapter 8, this volume.)

A fascinating "experiment of nature" has suggested the involvement of the frontal lobes and basal ganglia in OCD. Children who develop streptococcal infections occasionally develop an autoimmune response in which antibodies act against various organs. The heart (rheumatic fever) or the basal ganglia may be involved. In the latter case, Sydenham chorea may result. Swedo et al. (1989) observed that patients with Sydenham chorea have an elevated rate of OCD. These patients also have elevated levels of antineuronal antibodies in their plasma, which correlate both with OCD symptom levels and with caudate swelling on magnetic resonance scan (Swedo, Leonard, & Kiessling, 1994). These findings are also consistent with positron emission tomography data in adults with OCD. Elevated rates of glucose metabolism have been found in the frontal cortex, medio-orbital gyri, and caudate of OCD subjects (Baxter et al., 1988, 1992; Nordahl et al., 1989; Rauch et al., 1994). Children with OCD have an increase in subtle neurological and neuropsychological abnormalities, such as poor visual–spatial skills and speech prosody (March et al., 1990).

A number of studies have established the effectiveness of TCAs and SSRIs in the treatment of childhood and adolescent OCD. Forty-eight children with OCD were treated in a double-blind crossover study of clomipramine (a TCA with high potency for blocking the reuptake of serotonin) and desipramine (a TCA with little activity at the serotonin transporter) (Leonard et al., 1989). Clomipramine was clearly superior to desipramine in reducing OCD symptoms. Side effects were typical of those usually seen for TCAs—dry mouth, constipation, sedation—but children appeared to tolerate these effects better than adults.

Fluoxetine has been used in the treatment of childhood OCD with good results (Simeon, Dinicola, Ferguson, & Copping, 1990a; Simeon, Thatte, & Wiggins, 1990b). Riddle et al. (1992) performed a 20-week double-blind crossover study of fluoxetine and placebo. Fourteen children and adolescents aged 8–15 years participated, and all received a fixed dose of 20 mg of fluoxetine. Half the subjects dropped out of the study: Four had an exacerbation of OCD symptoms, one began to experience suicidal ideation, one was noncompliant, and one dropped out because of lack of response. For the remaining seven subjects, there was a highly significant effect of fluoxetine relative to placebo in reducing OCD symptoms. Total OCD symptoms fell 40% while the subjects were on fluoxetine, but remained unchanged or relapsed when placebo was administered. The use of fluvoxamine, also an SSRI, has recently been explored in the treatment of adolescent OCD (Apter et al., 1994). Fourteen inpatient adolescents (aged 13–18 years) with OCD were treated in an open trial with doses of fluvoxamine ranging from 100 to 300 mg (the mean dose was 200 mg). Many of the subjects were taking psychotropic medication for other disorders, such as Tourette syndrome or schizophrenia. After 8 weeks of fluvoxamine, OCD patients showed a significant decline in obsessive symptoms. Two patients with comorbid anorexia nervosa had a highly adverse response to the medication, showing delirium and hallucinations.

In a multicenter trial, 107 children and 80 adolescents were randomized to receive either placebo or sertraline (March et al., 1998). The starting dose of sertraline was 25 mg for children and 50 mg for adolescents, and the dose was titrated upward to a maximum of 200 mg for an 8-week trial. The mean doses for children and adolescents at the end of the study were 167 and 180 mg/day, respectively. Sertraline was superior to placebo in reducing obsessions and compulsions. Twelve of the patients discontinued the sertraline due to side effects. Insomnia, nausea, agitation, and tremor were more common in the SSRI group than in the placebo group. Overall, the drug was well tolerated by the children, with no severe side effects.

CBT has been shown to be an effective treatment for adult OCD. (March & Leonard, 1996). March (1995) examined 32 case reports of the use of CBT in children and adolescents with OCD; all but 1 showed that CBT improved OCD symptoms. No controlled trials of CBT with other forms of psychotherapy have been performed. March, Mulle, and Herbel (1994) have described the use of CBT in children with OCD. The principles are similar to those of Kendall (1994); the child moves through a highly structured series of 22 weekly sessions (see Table 9.2). Symptoms of OCD are identified, as are situations that trigger the symptoms. A "transition zone" is established—that is, a situation where the child experiences the mild onset of OCD symptoms yet is not disabled by them. These situations become the focus of exposure and response prevention, as well as anxiety management training. A manualized protocol is available from the authors.

SUMMARY

Anxiety disorders are highly heterogeneous; their causes are related to a complex interplay of genetic, medical, and environmental factors. They have not received as much research attention as have mood disorders or externalizing behavior disorders, particularly in regard to treatment. Much more study of both pharmacological and psychotherapeutic interventions is needed, in view of how common these disorders are. Anxiety disorders of youth are not benign, self-limited conditions, but are associated with significant morbidity and may herald the onset of adult anxiety and mood disorders.

REFERENCES

American Psychiatric Assocation. (1994). *Diagnostic and statistical manual of mental disorders* (4th ed.). Washington, DC: Author.

Anderson, J. C., Williams, S., McGee, R., & Silva, P. A. (1987). DSM-III disorders in preadolescent children: Prevalence in a large community sample. *Archives of General Psychiatry, 44,* 69–76.

Andrews, G., Stewart, S., & Henderson, A. S. (1990). The genetics of six neurotic disorders: A twin study. *Journal of Affective Disorders, 19,* 23–29.

Angold, A., & Costello, E. J. (1993). Depressive comorbidity in children and adolescents: Empirical, theoretical, and methodological issues. *American Journal of Psychiatry, 150,* 1779–1791.

Apter, A., Ratzoni, G., King, R. A., Weizman, A., Iancu, I., Binder, M., & Riddle, M. A. (1994). Fluvoxamine open-label treatment of adolescent inpatients with obsessive–compulsive disorder or depression. *Journal of the American Academy of Child and Adolescent Psychiatry, 33*(3), 342–348.

Barlow, D. H., Craske, M. G., Cerny, J. A., & Klosko, J. S. (1989). Behavioral treatment of panic disorder. *Behavior Therapy, 20,* 261–282.

Barrett, P. M., Dadds, M. R., & Rapee, R. M. (1996). Family treatment of childhood anxiety: A controlled trial. *Journal of Consulting and Clinical Psychology, 64*(2), 333–342.

Baxter, L. R., Schwartz, J. M., Bergman, K. S., Szuba, M. P., Guze, B. H., Mazziotta, J. C., Alazraki, A., Selin, C. E., Ferng, H., Munford, P., & Phelps, M. E. (1992). Caudate glucose metabolic rate changes with both drug and behavior therapy for obsessive–compulsive disorder. *Archives of General Psychiatry, 49*(9), 681–689.

Baxter, L. R., Schwartz, J. M., Mazziotta, J. C., Phelps, M. E., Pahl, J. J., Guze, B. H., & Fairbanks, L. (1988). Cerebral glucose metabolic rates in nondepressed patients with obsessive–compulsive disorder. *American Journal of Psychiatry, 145*(12), 1560–1563.

Beidel, D. C., & Morris, T. L. (1993). Avoidant disorder of childhood and social phobia. *Child and Adolescent Psychiatric Clinics of North America, 2*(4), 623–638.

Bemporad, J. R., Beresin, E., & Rauch, P. K. (1993). Psychodynamic theories and treatment of childhood anxiety disorders. *Child and Adolescent Psychiatric Clinics of North America, 2*(4), 763–776.

Benjamin, R. S., Costello, E. J., & Warren, M. (1990). Anxiety disorders in a pediatric sample. *Journal of Anxiety Disorders, 4,* 293–316.

Berney, T., Kolvin, I., Bhate, S. R., Garside, R. F., Jean, J., Kay, B., & Scarth, L. (1981). School phobia: A therapeutic trial with clomipramine and short-term outcome. *Journal of the American Academy of Child and Adolescent Psychiatry, 138,* 110–118.

Bernstein, G. A., Garfinkel, B. D., & Borchardt, C. M. (1990). Comparative studies of pharmacotherapy for school refusal. *Journal of the American Academy of Child and Adolescent Psychiatry, 29*(5), 773–781.

Biederman, J., Rosenbaum, J. F., Bolduc-Murphy, E. A., Faraone, S. V., Chaloff, J., Hirshfeld, D. R., & Kagan, J. (1993). A 3-year follow-up of children with and without behavioral inhibition. *Journal of the American Academy of Child and Adolescent Psychiatry, 32,* 814–821.

Biederman, J., Rosenbaum, J. F., Hirshfeld, D. R., Faraone, S. V., Bolduc, E. A., Gersten, M., Meminger, S. R., Kagan, J., Snidman, N., & Reznick, J. S. (1990). Psychiatric correlates of behavioral inhibition in young children of parents with and without psychiatric disorders. *Archives of General Psychiatry, 47,* 21–26.

Bird, H. R., Canino, G., & Rubio-Stipec, M. (1988). Estimates of prevalence of childhood maladjustment in a community survey in Puerto Rico. *Archives of General Psychiatry, 45,* 1120–1126.

Birmaher, B., Waterman, G. S., Ryan, N., Cully, M., Balach, L., Ingram, J., & Brodsky, M. (1994). Fluoxetine for childhood anxiety disorders. *Journal of the American Academy of Child and Adolescent Psychiatry, 33*(7), 993–999.

Blagg, N. R., & Yule, W. (1984). The behavioural treatment of school refusal: A comparative study. *Behaviour Research and Therapy, 22*(2), 119–127.

Charney, D. S., & Heninger, G. R. (1985). Noradrenergic function and the mechanism of action of antianxiety treatment: I. The effect of long term alprazolam treatment. *Archives of General Psychiatry, 42,* 458–467.

Charney, D. S., Woods, S. W., Southwick, S. M., Krystal, J. H., & Heninger, G. R. (1990). Noradrenergic function in panic disorder. *Journal of Clinical Psychiatry, 51*(Suppl.), 5–11.

Coplan, J. D., Rosenblum, L. A., & Gorman, J. M. (1995). Primate models of anxiety: Longitudinal perspectives. *Psychiatric Clinics of North America, 18*(4), 727–743.

Costello, E. J. (1989). Child psychiatric disorders and their correlates: A primary care pediatric sample. *Journal of the American Academy of Child and Adolescent Psychiatry, 28,* 851–855.

Davidson, R. J. (1992). Anterior asymmetry and the nature of emotion. *Brain and Cognition, 20,* 125–151.

Davidson, R. J., & Fox, N. A. (1982). Asymmetrical brain activity discriminates between positive versus negative affective stimuli in human infants. *Science, 218,* 1235–1237.

Drobes, D. J., & Strauss, C. C. (1997). Behavioral treatment of childhood anxiety disorders. *Child and Adolescent Psychiatric Clinics of North America, 6,* 779–793.

Durlak, J. A., Furhman, T., & Lampman, C. (1991). Effectiveness of cognitive-behavior therapy for maladapting children: A meta-analysis. *Psychological Bulletin, 110*(2), 204–214.

Fairbanks, J. M., Pine, D. S., Tancer, N. K., Dummit, E. S., Kentgen, L. M., Martin, Asche, B. K., & Klein, R. G. (1997). Open fluoxetine treatment of mixed anxiety disorders in children and adolescents. *Journal of Child and Adolescent Psychopharmacology, 7,* 17–29.

Fergusson, D. M., Horwood, L. J., & Lynskey, M. T. (1993). Prevalence and comorbidity of DSM-III-R diagnoses in a birth cohort of 15 year olds. *Journal of the American Academy of Child and Adolescent Psychiatry, 32,* 1127–1134.

Flament, M. F., Whitaker, A., Rapoport, J. L., Davies, M., Berg, C. Z., Kalikow, K., Sceery, W., & Shaffer, D. (1988). Obsessive compulsive disorder in adolescence: An epidemiological study. *Journal of the American Academy of Child and Adolescent Psychiatry, 27*(6), 764–771.

Fox, J. E., & Houston, B. K. (1981). Efficacy of self-instructional training for reducing children's anxiety in an evaluative situation. *Behaviour Research and Therapy, 19,* 509–515.

Fox, J. E., & Houston, B. K. (1983). Distinguishing between cognitive and somatic trait and somatic state anxiety in children. *Journal of Personality and Social Psychology, 45,* 862–870.

Fox, N. A., & Davidson, R. J. (1986). Taste-elicited changes in facial signs of emotion and the asymmetry of brain electrical activity in human newborns. *Neuropsychologia, 24,* 417–422.

Fox, N. A., & Davidson, R. J. (1988). Patterns of brain electrical activity during facial signs of emotion in ten month old infants. *Developmental Psychology, 24,* 230–236.

Gittelman, R. (1980). The role of psychological tests for differential diagnosis in child psychiatry. *Journal of the American Academy of Child Psychiatry, 19,* 413–438.

Gittelman-Klein, R., & Klein, D. F. (1970). Controlled imipramine treatment of school phobia. *Archives of General Psychiatry, 25,* 204–207.

Goldsmith, H. H., & Gottesman, I. (1981). Origins of variation in behavioral style: A longitudinal study of temperament in young twins. *Child Development, 52,* 91–103.

Gorman, J. M., Liebowitz, M. R., Fyer, A. J., & Stein, J. (1989). A neuroanatomical hypothesis for panic disorder. *American Journal of Psychiatry, 146,* 148–161.

Graae, F., Milner, J., Rizzotto, L., & Klein, R. G. (1994). Clonazepam in childhood anxiety disorders. *Journal of the American Academy of Child and Adolescent Psychiatry, 33*(3), 372–376.

Gray, J. A. (1982). *The neuropsychology of anxiety: An enquiry into the functions of the septohippocampal system.* New York: Oxford University Press.

Gray, J. A. (1987). *The psychology of fear and stress*. Cambridge, England: Cambridge University Press.

Graziano, A. M., & Mooney, K. C. (1980). Family self-control instruction for children's nighttime fear reduction. *Journal of Consulting and Clinical Psychology, 48*(2), 206–213.

Hampe, E., Noble, H., Miller, L. C., & Barrett, C. L. (1973). Phobic children one and two years posttreament. *Journal of Abnormal Psychology, 82*(3), 446–453.

Heninger, G. R., & Charney, D. S. (1988). Monoamine receptor systems and anxiety disorders. *Psychiatric Clinics of North America, 11*, 309–326.

Hirshfield, D. R., Rosenbaum, J. F., Biederman, J., Bolduc, E. A., Faraone, S. V., Snidman, N., Reznick, J. S., & Kagan, J. (1992). Stable behavioral inhibition and its association with anxiety disorder. *Journal of the American Academy of Child and Adolescent Psychiatry, 31*, 103–111.

Ialongo, N., Edelsohn, G., Werthamer-Larsson, L., Crockett, L., & Kellam, S. (1994). The significance of self-reported anxious symptoms in first-grade children. *Journal of Abnormal Child Psychology, 22*(4), 441–455.

Johnson, M. R., & Lydiard, R. B. (1995). The neurobiology of anxiety disorders. *Psychiatric Clinics of North America, 18*(4), 681–719.

Kagan, J., Reznick, J. S., Clarke, C., & Snidman, N. (1984). Behavioral inhibition to the unfamiliar. *Child Development, 55*, 2212–2225.

Kagan, J., Reznick, J. S., & Snidman, N. (1987). The physiology and psychology of behavorial inhibition in children. *Child Development, 58*, 1459–1473.

Kagan, J., Reznick, J. S., & Snidman, N. (1988). Biological basis of childhood shyness. *Science, 240*, 167–171.

Kagan, J., & Snidman, N. (1991). Infant predictors of inhibited and uninhibited profiles. *Psychological Science, 2*, 40.

Kendall, P. C. (1993). Cognitive-behavioral therapies with youth: Guiding theory, current status, and emerging developments. *Journal of Consulting and Clinical Psychology, 61*, 235–247.

Kendall, P. C. (1994). Treating anxiety disorders in children: Results of a randomized clinical trial. *Journal of Consulting and Clinical Psychology, 62*(1), 100–110.

Kendall, P. C., Flannery-Schroeder, E., Panichelli-Mindel, S. M., Southam, G., Henin, A., & Warman, M. (1997). Therapy for youths with anxiety disorders: A second randomized clinical trial. *Journal of Consulting and Clinical Psychology, 65*, 366–380.

Kendler, K. S., Heath, A. C., Martin, N. G., & Eaves, L. J. (1987). Symptoms of anxiety and symptoms of depression: Same genes, different environments? *Archives of General Psychiatry, 44*, 451–457.

Kendler, K. S., Neale, M. C., Kessler, R. C., Heath, A. C., & Eaves, L. J. (1992). Generalized anxiety disorder in women: A population-based twin study. *Archives of General Psychiatry, 49*(4), 267–272.

Klein, D. (1964). Delineation of two-drug responsive anxiety syndromes. *Psychopharmacologia, 5*, 397–408.

Klein, R. G. (1991). Parent–child agreement in clinical assessment of anxiety and other psychopathology: A review. *Journal of Anxiety Disorders, 5*, 187–198.

Klein, R. G. (1994). Anxiety disorders. In M. Rutter, E. Taylor, & L. Hersov (Eds.), *Child and adolescent psychiatry: Modern approaches* (pp. 351–374). Oxford: Blackwell Scientific.

Klein, R. G., Koplewicz, H. S., & Kanner, A. (1992). Imipramine treatment of children with separation anxiety disorder. *Journal of the American Academy of Child and Adolescent Psychiatry, 31*(1), 21–28.

Kovacs, M., Gatsonis, C., Paulauskas, S. L., & Richards, C. (1989). Depressive disorders in childhood: IV. A longitudinal study of comorbidity with a risk for anxiety disorders. *Archives of General Psychiatry, 46*, 776–782.

Kutcher, S. P., Reiter, S., Gardner, D. M., & Klein, R. G. (1992). The pharmacotherapy of anxiety disorders in children and adolescents. *Psychiatric Clinics of North America, 15*, 41–67.

Last, C. G., Beidel, D. C., & Perrin, S. (1996). Anxiety. In M. Lewis (Ed.), *Child and adolescent psychiatry: A comprehensive textbook* (pp. 291–299). Baltimore: Williams & Wilkins.

Last, C. G., Hansen, C., & Franco, N. (1998). Cognitive-behavioral treatment of school phobia. *Journal of the American Academy of Child and Adolescent Psychiatry, 37,* 404–411.

Last, C. G., Hersen, M., Kazdin, A. E., Finkelstein, R., & Strauss, C. C. (1987a). Comparison of DSM-III separation anxiety and overanxious disorders: Demographic characteristics and patterns of comorbidity. *Journal of the American Academy of Child and Adolescent Psychiatry, 26*(4), 527–531.

Last, C. G., Hersen, M., Kazdin, A. E., Francis, G., & Grubb, H. J. (1987b). Psychiatric illness in the mothers of anxious children. *American Journal of Psychiatry, 144*(12), 1580–1583.

Last, C. G., Hersen, M., Kazdin, A., Orvaschel, H., & Perrin, S. (1991). Anxiety disorders in children and their families. *Archives of General Psychiatry, 48,* 928–934.

Leitenburg, H., & Callahan, E. J. (1973). Reinforced practice and reduction of different kinds of fears in adults and children. *Behaviour Research and Therapy, 11,* 19–30.

Leonard, H. L., Swedo, S. E., Rapoport, J. L., Koby, E. V., Lenane, M. C., Cheslow, D. L., & Hamburger, S. D. (1989). Treatment of obsessive–compulsive disorder with clomipramine and desipramine in children and adolescents: A double-blind crossover comparison. *Archives of General Psychiatry, 46*(12), 1088–1092.

Lesch, K. P., Bengel, D., Heils, A., Sabol, S. Z., Greenberg, B. D., Petri, S., Benjamin, J., Muller, C. R., Hamer, D. H., & Murphy, D. L. (1997). Association of anxiety-related traits with a polymorphism in the serotonin transporter gene regulatory region. *Science, 274,* 1527–1531.

Manassis, K., Bradley, S., Goldberg, S., Hood, J., & Swinson, R. P. (1995). Behavioural inhibition, attachment and anxiety in children of mothers with anxiety disorders. *Canadian Journal of Psychiatry, 40*(2), 87–92.

Manassis, K., Mendlowitz, S., & Menna, R. (1997). Child and parent reports of childhood anxiety: Differences in coping styles. *Depression and Anxiety, 6,* 62–69.

March, J. S. (1995). Cognitive-behavioral psychotherapy for children and adolescents with OCD: A review and recommendations for treatment. *Journal of the American Academy of Child and Adolescent Psychiatry, 34,* 7–18.

March, J. S., Biederman, J., Wolkow, R., Safferman, A., Mardekian, J., Cook, E. H., Cutler, N. R., Dominguez, R., Ferguson, J., Muller, B., Riesenberg, R., Rosenthal, M., Sallee, F. R., & Wagner, K. D. (1998). Sertaline in children and adolescents with obsessive–compulsive disorder: A multicenter, randomized, controlled trial. *Journal of the American Medical Association, 280,* 1752–1756.

March, J. S., Johnston, H., Jefferson, J., Greist, J., Kobak, K., & Mazza, J. (1990). Do subtle neurological impairments predict treatment resistance in children and adolescents with obsessive–compulsive disorder? *Journal of Child and Adolescent Psychopharmacology, 1,* 133–140.

March, J. S., & Leonard, H. L. (1996). Obsessive–compulsive disorder in children and adolescents: A review of the past 10 years. *Journal of the American Academy of Child and Adolescent Psychiatry, 35*(10), 1265–1273.

March, J. S., Mulle, K., & Herbel, B. (1994). Behavioral psychotherapy for children and adolescents with obsessive–compulsive disorder: An open trial of a new protocol driven treatment package. *Journal of the American Academy of Child and Adolescent Psychiatry, 33*(3), 333–341.

Matthews, A. (1990). Why worry?: The cognitive function of anxiety. *Behaviour Research and Therapy, 28,* 455–468.

Muris, P., Meesters, C., Merckelbach, H., Sermon, A., & Zwakhalen, S. (1998). Worry in normal children. *Journal of the American Academy of Child and Adolescent Psychiatry, 37,* 703–710.

Nordahl, T. E., Benkelfat, C., Semple, W. E., Gross, M., King, A. C., & Cohen, R. M. (1989). Cerebral glucose metabolic rates in obsessive compulsive disorder. *Neuropsychopharmacology, 2*(1), 23–28.

Ollendick, T. H. (1983). Reliability and validity of the Revised Fear Survey Schedule for Children (FSSC-R). *Behaviour Research and Therapy, 21,* 685–692.

Ollendick, T. H. (1995). Cognitive behavioral treatment of panic disorder with agoraphobia in adolescents: A multiple baseline design analysis. *Behavior Therapy, 26,* 517–531.

Otto, M. W., Pollack, M. H., Rosenbaum, J. F., Sachs, G. S., & Asher, R. H. (1994). Childhood history of anxiety in adults with panic disorder: Association with anxiety sensitivity and avoidance. *Psychiatry, 1,* 288–293.

Otto, M. W., & Whittal, M. L. (1995). Cognitive-behavior therapy and the longitudinal course of panic disorder. *Psychiatric Clinics of North America, 18*(4), 803–819.

Pauls, D., Raymond, C., Stevenson, J., & Leckman, J. (1991). A family study of Gilles de la Tourette syndrome. *American Journal of Human Genetics, 48,* 154–163.

Pauls, D. L., Towbin, K. E., Leckman, J. F., Zahner, G. E., & Cohen, D. J. (1986). Gilles de la Tourette's syndrome and obsessive–compulsive disorder: Evidence supporting a genetic relationship. *Archives of General Psychiatry, 43,* 1180–1182.

Perrin, S., & Last, C. G. (1992). Do childhood anxiety measures measure anxiety? *Journal of Abnormal Child Psychology, 20,* 567–578.

Perrin, S., & Last, C. G. (1997). Worrisome thoughts in children clinically referred for anxiety disorder. *Journal of Clinical Child Psychology, 26,* 181–189.

Pine, D. S., Coplan, J. D., Papp, L. A., Klein, R. G., Martinez, J. M., Kovalenko, P., Tancer, N., Moreau, D., Dummit, E. S., Shaffer, D., Klein, D. F., & Gorman, J. M. (1988). Ventilatory physiology of children and adolescents with anxiety disorders. *Archives of General Psychiatry, 55,* 123–129.

Pollack, M. H., Otto, M. W., Sabatino, S., Majcher, D., Worthington, J. J., McArdle, E. T., & Rosenbaum, J. F. (1996). Relationship of childhood anxiety to adult panic disorder: Correlates and influence on course. *American Journal of Psychiatry, 153*(3), 376–381.

Prins, P. J. M. (1985). Self-speech and self-regulation of high- and low-anxious children in the dental situation: An interview study. *Behaviour Research and Therapy, 23*(6), 641–650.

Rao, N., Moely, B. E., & Lockman, J. J. (1987). Increasing social participation in preschool social isolates. *Journal of Clinical Child Psychology, 16*(3), 178–183.

Rasmussen, S. A., & Eisen, J. L. (1990). Epidemiology of obsessive compulsive disorder. *Journal of Clinical Psychiatry, 53*(Suppl.), 10–13.

Rauch, S. L., Jenike, M. A., Alpert, N. M., Baer, L., Breiter, H. C. R., Savage, C. R., & Fischman, A. J. (1994). Regional cerebral blood flow measured during symptom provocation in obsessive–compulsive disorder using oxygen 15-labeled carbon dioxide and positron emission tomography. *Archives of General Psychiatry, 51*(1), 62–70.

Reeves, J. C., Werry, J. S., Elkind, G. S., & Zametkin, A. (1987). Attention deficit, conduct, oppositional, and anxiety disorders in children: II. Clinical characteristics. *Journal of the American Academy of Child and Adolescent Psychiatry, 26,* 144–155.

Reiman, E. M., Raichle, M. E., Robins, E., Butler, F. K., Herscovitch, P., Fox, P., & Perlmutter, J. (1986). The application of positron emission tomography to the study of panic disorder. *American Journal of Psychiatry, 143,* 469–477.

Reiman, E. M., Raichle, M. E., Robins, E., Mintun, M. A., Fusselman, M. J., Fox, P. T., Price, J. L., & Hackman, K. A. (1989). Neuroanatomical correlates of a lactate-induced anxiety attack. *Archives of General Psychiatry, 46,* 493–500.

Reynolds, C. R., & Paget, K. D. (1983). National normative and reliability data for the Revised Children's Manifest Anxiety Scale. *School Psychology Review, 12,* 324–336.

Reynolds, C. R., & Richmond, B. O. (1997). What I think and feel: A revised measure of children's manifest anxiety. *Journal of Abnormal Child Psychology, 25,* 15–20.

Reznick, J. S., Kagan, J., Snidman, N., Gersten, M., Baak, K., & Rosenberg, A. (1986). Inhibited and uninhibited children: A follow up study. *Child Development, 57,* 660–680.

Riddle, M. A., Scahill, L., King, R. A., Hardin, M. T., Anderson, G. M., Ort, S. I., Smith, J. C., Leckman, J. F., & Cohen, D. J. (1992). Double blind crossover trial of fluoxetine and placebo in children and adolescents with obsessive compulsive disorder. *Journal of the American Academy of Child and Adolescent Psychiatry, 31*(6), 1062–1069.

Riddle, M. A., Scahill, L., King, R. A., Hardin, M. T., Towbin, K. E., Ort, S. I., Leckman, J. F., & Cohen, D. J. (1990). Obsessive compulsive disorder in children and adolescents: phenomenology and family history. *Journal of the American Academy of Child and Adolescent Psychiatry, 29*(5), 766–772.

Rosenbaum, J. F., Biederman, J., Bolduc, E. A., Hirshfeld, D. R., Faraone, S. V., & Kagan, J. (1992). Comorbidity of parental anxiety disorders as risk for childhood-onset anxiety in inhibited children. *American Journal of Psychiatry, 149*(4), 475–481.

Rosenbaum, J. F., Biederman, J., Gersten, M., Hirschfield, D. R., Meminger, S. R., Herman, J. B., Kagan, J., Reznick, J. S., & Snidman, N. (1988). Behavioral inhibition in children of parents with panic disorder and agoraphobia: A controlled study. *Archives of General Psychiatry, 45,* 463–470.

Sallee, F. R., Richman, H., Sethuraman, G., Dougherty, D., Sine, L., & Altman-Hamamdzic, S. (1998). Clonidine challenge in childhood anxiety disorder. *Journal of the American Academy of Child and Adolescent Psychiatry, 37,* 655–662.

Scanlan, J. M., Suomi, S. J., Higley, J. D., Scallet, A. S., & Kraemer, G. W. (1982). Stress and heredity in adrenocortical response in rhesus monkeys. *Society for Neuroscience Abstracts, 8,* 461.

Shaffer, D., Fisher, P., Dulcan, M. K., Davies, M., Piacentini, J., Schwab-Stone, M. E., Lahey, B. B., Bourdon, K., Jensen, P. S., Bird, H. R., Canino, G., & Regier, D. A. (1996). The NIMH Diagnostic Interview Schedule for Children Version 2.3 (DISC 2.3): Description, acceptability, prevalence rates, and performance in the Methods for the Epidemiology of Child and Adolescent Mental Disorders (MECA) study. *Journal of the American Academy of Child and Adolescent Psychiatry, 35,* 865–877.

Silove, D., Manicavasagar, V., O'Connell, D., & Morris-Yates, A. (1995). Genetic factors in early separation anxiety: Implications for the genesis of adult anxiety disorders. *Acta Psychiatrica Scandinavica, 92*(1), 17–24.

Silverman, W. K., La Greca, A. M., & Wasserstein, S. (1995). What do children worry about?: Worries and their relation to anxiety. *Child Development, 66*(3), 671–686.

Silverman, W. K., & Nelles, W. B. (1988). The Anxiety Disorders Interview Schedule for Children. *Journal of the American Academy of Child and Adolescent Psychiatry, 27,* 772–778.

Simeon, J. G., Dinicola, V. F., Ferguson, H. B., & Copping, W. (1990a). Adolescent depression: A placebo-controlled fluoxetine treatment study and follow-up. *Progress in Neuropsychopharmacology and Biological Psychiatry, 14,* 791–795.

Simeon, J. G., Ferguson, H. B., Knott, V., Roberts, N., Gautheir, B., Dubois, C., & Wiggins, D. (1992). Clinical, cognitive, and neurophysiological effects of alprazolam in children and adolescents with overanxious and avoidant disorders. *Journal of the American Academy of Child and Adolescent Psychiatry, 31*(1), 29–33.

Simeon, J. G., Thatte, S., & Wiggins, D. (1990b). Treatment of adolescent obsessive–compulsive disorder with a clomipramine–fluoxetine combination. *Psychopharmacology Bulletin, 26,* 285–290.

Skre, I., Onstad, S., Torgersen, S., Lygren, S., & Kringlen, E. (1993). A twin study of DSM-III-R anxiety disorders. *Acta Psychiatrica Scandinavica, 88,* 85–92.

Snidman, N., Kagan, J., & Riordan, L. (1995). Cardiac function and behavioral reactivity during infancy. *Psychophysiology, 32,* 199–207.

Stanley, M. A., Beck, J. G., Averill, P. M., Baldwin, L. E., Deagle, E. A., & Stadler, J. G. (1996). Patterns of change during cognitive behavioral treatment for panic disorder. *Journal of Nervous and Mental Disease, 184*(9), 567–572.

Stevenson, J., Batten, N., & Cherner, M. (1992). Fears and fearfulness in children and adolescents: A genetic analysis of twin data. *Journal of Child Psychology and Psychiatry, 33*(6), 977–985.

Strauss, C. C., Lease, C. A., Last, C. G., & Francis, G. (1988). Overanxious disorder: An examination of developmental differences. *Journal of Abnormal Child Psychology, 16,* 433–443.

Suomi, S. J. (1981). Genetic, maternal, and environmental influences on social development in rhesus monkeys. In B. Chiarelli & R. Corruccini (Eds.), *Primate behavior and sociobiology.* Berlin: Springer-Verlag.

Suomi, S. J. (1983). Social development in rhesus monkeys: Consideration of individual differences. In A. Oliverio & M. Zappella (Eds.), *The behavior of human infants.* New York: Plenum Press.

Suomi, S. J. (1986). Anxiety-like disorders in young nonhuman primates. In R. Gittelman (Ed.), *Anxiety disorders of childhood* (pp. 1–23). New York: Guilford Press.

Suomi, S. J., Seaman, S. F., Lewis, J. K., Delizio, R. D., & McKinney, W. T. (1978). Effects of imipramine treatment of separation-induced social disorders in rhesus monkeys. *Archives of General Psychiatry, 35*, 321–325.

Swedo, S. E., Leonard, H. L., & Kiessling, L. S. (1994). Speculations on antineuronal antibody-mediated neuropsychiatric disorders of childhood. *Pediatrics, 93*, 323–326.

Swedo, S. E., Rapoport, J. L., Cheslow, D. L., Leonard, H. L., Ayoub, E. M., Hosier, D. M., & Wald, E. R. (1989). High prevalence of obsessive–compulsive symptoms in patients with Sydenham's chorea. *American Journal of Psychiatry, 146*(2), 246–249.

Targum, S. D. (1992). Cortisol response during different anxiogenic challenges in panic disorder patients. *Psychoneuroendocrinology, 17*, 453–458.

Torgersen, S. (1983). Genetic factors in anxiety disorders. *Archives of General Psychiatry, 40*, 1085–1089.

Torgersen, S. (1990). Comorbidity of major depression and anxiety disorders in twin pairs. *American Journal of Psychiatry, 147*, 1199–1202.

Verhulst, F. C., Van der Ende, J., Ferdinand, R. F., & Kasius, M. C. (1997). The prevalence of DSM-III-R diagnoses in a national sample of Dutch adolescents. *Archives of General Psychiatry, 54*, 329–336.

Walker, H. M., Greenwood, C. R., Hops, H., & Todd, N. M. (1979). Differential effects of reinforcing topographic components of social interaction. *Behavior Modification, 3*(3), 291–321.

Weissman, M. M., Leckman, J. F., Merikangas, K. R., Gammon, G. D., & Prusoff, B. A. (1984). Depression and anxiety disorders in parents and children. *Archives of General Psychiatry, 41*, 845–852.

Werry, J. S., Elkind, G. S., & Reeves, J. C. (1987a). Attention deficit, conduct, oppositional, and anxiety disorders in children: III. Laboratory differences. *Journal of Abnormal Child Psychology, 15*, 409–428.

Werry, J. S., Reeves, J. C., & Elkind, G. S. (1987b). Attention deficit, conduct, oppositional, and anxiety disorders in children: I. A review of research on differentiating characteristics. *Journal of the American Academy of Child and Adolescent Psychiatry, 26*(2), 133–143.

Wheeler, R. E., Davidson, R. J., & Tomarken, A. J. (1993). Frontal brain asymmetry and emotional reactivity: A biological substrate of affective style. *Psychophysiology, 30*, 82–89.

Wilkinson, D. J. C., Thompson, J. M., Lambert, G. W., Jennings, G. L., Schwarz, S., Jefferys, D., Turner, A. G., & Esler, M. D. (1998). Sympathetic activity in patients with panic disorder at rest, under laboratory mental stress, and during panic attacks. *Archives of General Psychiatry, 55*, 511–520.

Wolpe, J. (1958). *Psychotherapy by reciprocal inhibition.* Stanford, CA: Stanford University Press.

Zatz, S., & Chassin, L. (1983). Cognitions of test-anxious children. *Journal of Consulting and Clinical Psychology, 51*(4), 526–534.

10

AUTISM AND OTHER PERVASIVE DEVELOPMENTAL DISORDERS

AMI KLIN
FRED R. VOLKMAR

The pervasive developmental disorders (PDDs) are a group of conditions that share certain core clinical features but that seem to have diverse etiologies and natural courses. The conditions have their onset in infancy or early childhood, and are characterized by typical patterns of delay and deviance affecting primarily the areas of social, affective, and communicative development. Of the various diagnostic concepts included within the overarching class of PDDs, autistic disorder (American Psychiatric Association [APA], 1994) is the best studied and is the paradigmatic condition against which other PDDs are defined. Consequently, it is discussed in greatest detail in this chapter. Other conditions within the PDD class are variably included in different diagnostic systems. Despite a recent surge of research studies on these "nonautistic" PDDs, their validity still remains controversial (Volkmar, Klin, & Cohen, 1997b).

The phenomenological definition of autism remains virtually the same as that initially formulated by Kanner (1943). However, the wide range of severity, developmental level, and natural course documented in the literature necessitated the creation of the PDD class, in order to include disorders with a presentation differing somewhat from Kanner's description of autism. The term "pervasive developmental disorder" emphasizes the pervasiveness of disturbances over a wide range of different domains (in contrast to both the relatively more circumscribed disabilities of the specific developmental disorders and the anchoring effects of cognitive deficits in primary mental retardation), and the developmental nature of the disorders affecting the normative unfolding of multiple competencies, particularly interpersonal relationships and communication.

In this chapter, we first provide a historical review of the major diagnostic concepts included in the PDD class. We then give a clinical description of autism and discuss diagnostic issues, clinical assessment, and interventions.

DIAGNOSTIC CONCEPTS

Autism

Kanner's (1943) original description of infantile autism contained detailed clinical descriptions of 11 children he had seen over a few years. Their most striking clinical feature was their pervasive lack of interest in other people, including their parents—an attitude that contrasted markedly with their all-absorbing fascination with the inanimate environment. Kanner conceptualized these cases in terms of a possible congenital disturbance affecting the children's capacity to relate emotionally to others, which resulted in marked withdrawal and social aloneness, or "autism." These children also exhibited a number of unusual developmental and behavioral features, such as a pronounced resistance to change in their environment and routines; stereotypic behaviors, including purposeless, repetitive movements; and often a specific, isolated interest and proficiency in a trivial task that was endlessly repeated, such as block constructions or puzzles. When language developed at all, it was characterized by echolalia (the echoing of another's speech), pronoun reversal, and extreme literalness. Initially, Kanner felt that infantile autism was not an early manifestation of schizophrenia; however, his use of the word "autism" suggested unintentional points of similarity. In fact, this term had previously been used to mean active withdrawal from relationships rather than an incapacity to develop them, and a rich fantasy life rather than a lack of imagination. (See Bleuler, 1916/1951.)

By adhering strictly to a description of the clinical phenomena observed, Kanner provided a remarkably enduring account of the core features of the disorder; moreover, by contrasting the limited social skills of his first patients with normative skills emerging very early in life, Kanner was careful to place his observations within a developmental context. Nevertheless, certain aspects of his 1943 report suggested false leads for research. For example, although his report emphasized the apparently congenital nature of the disorder, in his original case series he noted the unusual degrees of personal achievement of the parents and their atypical ways of interacting with their children. This observation appeared to suggest a potential role of parental psychopathology in syndrome pathogenesis. At the time, of course, there was little understanding of the potential contributions of a deviant child to disturbances in parent–child interaction (Bell & Harper, 1977). Early reports emphasized the role of experiential factors in pathogenesis, but subsequent research has shown no evidence of increased parental psychopathology (McAdoo & DeMyer, 1978) and has found that very adverse experiences early in life do not typically lead to autism (Provence & Lipton, 1962; Rutter & Bartak, 1971). Kanner also suggested that autism apparently was not associated with either mental retardation (his autistic children seemed to be particularly clever in some narrow respects) or with other "organic conditions." Again, research has established that most autistic children are also mentally retarded (Lockyer & Rutter, 1969) and that the condition can be observed in association with diverse medical conditions, such as congenital rubella (Chess, 1971) and fragile X syndrome (Watson et al., 1985). Finally, it became apparent that autistic children commonly develop seizure disorders (Volkmar & Nelson, 1990) and other neurobiological abnormalities consistent with as-yet-unspecified underlying "organic" etiology (Minshew, Sweeney, & Bauman, 1997).

The validity of the syndrome proposed by Kanner has been supported by various lines of evidence. A series of studies has consistently revealed that autism differs from childhood schizophrenia in clinical features, such as age of onset (infancy and early childhood vs. later childhood and adolescence), course (relatively unchanged vs. episodic), delusions/hallucinations (absent vs. present), impairments in social and communicative abilities (markedly more profound in autism), and family history (more frequently positive in schizo-phrenia) (Kolvin, 1971: Rutter, 1972; Volkmar, Cohen, Hoshino, Rende, & Paul, 1988b). Another series of studies has demonstrated that autism differs from developmental language disorders in the pervasiveness of the communicative deficits (in autism, the disability encompasses both verbal and nonverbal communication), as well as in social deficits (more profound in autism) and cognitive profiles (larger scatter and typical pattern in autism) (Cohen, Caparulo, & Shaywitz, 1976; Rutter, 1978b). Although autism often coexists with mental retardation, autistic children differ from children with primary mental retardation without autism in terms of pattern of scores on IQ tests (scattered vs. even), cognitive processing abilities (less symbolic in autism), and communicative and social skills (unlike the relatively even profile of skills obtained in mental retardation, autistic social dysfunction is in excess of what could be predicted from general cognitive level) (Rutter, 1978a).

Nonautistic PDDs

Childhood Disintegrative Disorder

In 1908, Theodore Heller (1930/1954), a Viennese educator, first observed six cases of children who had developed normally until 3 to 4 years of age and then exhibited marked developmental and behavioral deterioration with only minimal subsequent recovery. He named this condition "dementia infantilism"; the name of the condition was subsequently changed to "Heller syndrome," and now it is usually referred to as "childhood disintegrative disorder."

This disorder is probably extremely rare, with about 100 cases *in toto* reported in the world literature (Volkmar, 1992). Generally, the early development is entirely normal. The child progresses to the point of speaking in sentences, and then a profound developmental regression occurs; once established, the condition is behaviorally similar to autism, although the prognosis is even worse (Volkmar & Cohen, 1989). In some instances, the condition has been reported in association with a specific disease process such as a progressive neurological condition (Corbett, 1987). As a result, the disorder was not included in the third edition of the *Diagnostic and Statistical Manual of Mental Disorders* (DSM-III; APA, 1980) or in DSM-III-R (APA, 1987), on the presumption that these cases invariably reflected some other degenerative medical condition. However, it is clear that such a medical condition is observed and/or documented in only a minority of the cases (Volkmar & Rutter, 1995); accordingly, childhood disintegrative disorder has been included in both the 10th revision of the *International Classification of Diseases* (ICD-10; World Health Organization [WHO], 1992) and DSM-IV (APA, 1994).

Rett Disorder

Andreas Rett (1966) first described the syndrome now commonly referred to as "Rett disorder" or "Rett syndrome." Rett had observed two girls in a waiting room who exhibited remarkably similar patterns of deviant behavior and course of development; he subsequently identified a series of 22 cases. Although autistic-like behaviors are observed, particularly during the preschool years, this disorder differs from autism in several ways. It has been reported only in females; the more "autistic-like" phase is relatively brief; it is associated with characteristic stereotyped motor behaviors (resembling "washing" or "wringing" movements) and abnormalities in gait or trunk movement; breath-holding spells and seizures are common; and the associated mental retardation is even more severe than in autism. The early history is remarkable for initially normal early growth and development, followed (usually in the first months of life) by developmental regression, deceleration of head growth, and loss of purposeful hand movements. The apparently normal period of development is much shorter than that observed in childhood disintegrative disorder. Prevalence estimates of Rett disorder suggest that approximately 1 in 15,000 girls is affected (Trevathan & Adams, 1988). Despite the insidious regression in development and other neurological findings, the pathophysiology of the condition remains unknown (Trevathan & Naidu, 1988). The condition has been included in both ICD-10 (WHO, 1992) and DSM-IV (APA, 1994). It is discussed in greater detail by Brown and Hoadley (Chapter 20, this volume).

Asperger Disorder

In the year following Kanner's (1943) report, Hans Asperger (1944/1991), a Viennese physician, described a group of individuals who, despite adequate intellectual skills, exhibited social and behavioral peculiarities that made it difficult for them to participate in group activities and develop friendships (e.g., problems with social interaction and communication, as well as circumscribed and idiosyncratic patterns of interest). However, Asperger's description differed from Kanner's in that speech was less commonly delayed, motor deficits were more common, the onset appeared to be somewhat later, and all of the initial cases occurred in boys. Asperger also suggested that similar problems could be observed in family members, particularly fathers. Unaware of Kanner's work, Asperger coined the term "autistic psychopathy" to characterize the condition as a personality disorder.

This condition was essentially unknown in the English literature for many years. An influential review and series of case reports by Wing (1981) increased interest in the condition; since then, both the usage of the term in clinical practice and the number of case reports and case-control studies have been steadily increasing (Klin, Volkmar, & Sparrow, 1999). The commonly described clinical features of the disorder include (1) paucity of empathy; (2) naive, inappropriate, one-sided social interaction, little ability to form friendships, and consequent social isolation:(3) pedantic and monotonic speech; (4) poor nonverbal communication; (5) intense absorption in circumscribed topics such as the weather, facts about TV stations, railway tables, or maps, which are learned in rote fashion and reflect poor understanding, conveying the impression of eccentricity; and (6) clumsy and ill-coordinated movements and odd posture (Wing, 1981). Although Asperger originally reported the condition only in boys, reports of girls with the disorder have now appeared. Nevertheless, males are significantly more likely to be affected (Szatmari, Bremmer, & Nagy, 1989; Wing, 1991). Although most individuals with the condition function within the average range of intelligence, some have been reported to be mildly retarded (Wing, 1981). The apparent onset of the condition, or at least its recognition, is probably somewhat later than that of autism; this may primarily reflect the better-preserved language and cognitive abilities (Klin & Volkmar, 1997). Asperger disorder tends to be highly stable (Asperger, 1979), and the higher intellectual skills observed suggest a better outcome than is typically observed in autism (Tantam, 1991). Specific learning problems and marked discrepancies between various intellectual skills may be present (Klin, Volkmar, Sparrow, Cicchetti, & Rourke, 1995b; Ozonoff, Pennington, & Rogers, 1991).

Atypical PDD/PDD Not Otherwise Specified

The term "PDD not otherwise specified (NOS)" was used in DSM-III-R (APA, 1987) to replace the earlier term "atypical PDD"; this latter concept had unintentionally, although probably correctly, been suggestive of Rank's (1949) earlier diagnostic notion of "atypical personality development," a term also used to describe children with some (but not all) features of autism. Such children exhibit patterns of unusual sensitivities, difficulties in social interaction, and other problems suggestive of autism, without meeting full criteria for autistic disorder (Volkmar et al., 1994).

The term "PDD NOS" is problematic in several respects. The category is poorly defined, since the definition is essentially a negative one, and although the condition is probably much more common than strictly defined autism (Klin, Mayes, Volkmar, & Cohen, 1995a), research on PDD NOS has been uncommon. The lack of an explicit definition also means that the concept is used rather inconsistently: For example, some investigators equate it with Asperger disorder, while others view it as on some underlying spectrum with autism, in terms of both developmental functioning and severity of symptomatology. More commonly, the term PDD NOS has been used for children with better cognitive and communicative skills and some degree of relatedness. The most common reasons for referral in such cases include parents' concerns about the children's emotional and social development, rather than the failure to develop language, as in autism.

Over the years, children currently captured by the term PDD NOS have been characterized by numerous diagnostic labels that have been used to provide a taxonomic location and to convey the nature of their social and emotional difficulties in relating. While informal descriptions included terms such as "eccentric," "odd," "overanxious," "aloof," and "weird," formal designations included terms such as "borderline," "schizotypal," "schizoidal disorders," "atypical development," "childhood psychosis," "symbiotic states," and others (Klin et al., 1995a; Towbin, 1997). No term, however, has been fully satisfactory or broadly accepted. Moreover, though clinicians have had the sense of a category of such children, there are as yet no clearly defined diagnostic criteria that could guide systematic studies, including those on the basic validity or utility of such a grouping.

There have been several attempts to delineate subgroups within the larger PDD NOS category, involving terms such as "multiplex developmental disorder" (Cohen, Paul, & Volkmar, 1987), "childhood-onset schizophrenia" (McKenna, Gordon, & Lenane, 1994), and others related to children currently assigned by default to the PDD NOS category. Again, none of these terms is as yet operationally defined or broadly accepted. Because pathognomonic symptomatology (such as the profound social disability in autism) and profound regression (such as that seen in childhood disintegrative disorder) are lacking, it becomes very difficult for investigators to agree on specific clusters of symptoms and deficits that define specific disorders. Given the vast variability in phenomenology, careful studies of profiles of development and adjustment (including quantification of deficits and deviance) are needed in no area of childhood disorders more than in this rather amorphous PDD NOS category. Future efforts will need to take into account the fact that the pervasive early disturbances of basic developmental processes—specifically, socialization skills and the emergence of a consolidated sense of self—are likely to have a broad range of effects on multiple aspects of development, with varied manifestations (Cicchetti & Cohen, 1995).

AUTISM: CLINICAL DESCRIPTION

Onset and Characteristics of Early Development

In his original description, Kanner (1943) suggested that autism was present in the children he described from birth. Subsequent research has revealed that the condition sometimes appears within the second or third year of life, but rarely after age 3 (Short & Schopler,

1988; Volkmar, Stier, & Cohen, 1985). As discussed previously, age and type of onset have some value in the differential diagnosis of autism, although various extraneous factors may act to delay case detection (including parental perceptivity, sophistication, or denial, as well as the level of associated mental retardation in the child. Given such factors, we may refer more correctly to age of "recognition" rather than "onset" of the syndrome.

From a clinical perspective, the early recognition of autism is important, as there is some suggestion that early intervention may reduce subsequent morbidity (Simeonsson, Olley, & Rosenthal, 1987). Moreover, it is clear that developmental skills at age 5 predict subsequent outcome (Lotter, 1978a). Unfortunately, delays in case recognition remain common. For example, Siegel, Pliner, Eschler, and Elliot (1988) noted that typically 3 years elapsed between the time parents expressed concern to their child's physician and the time when a definitive diagnosis was made, usually at about age 5. Similarly, Ornitz, Guthrie, and Farley (1977) reported that 50% of the families interviewed in their study were concerned about their children at the age of 14 months, but that the median age of referral for diagnosis was 46 months—a delay of 32 months. Delays in case detection and referral reflect a lack of knowledge about autism, a dearth of readily applied screening instruments, difficulties in the use of categorical criteria, and the more general lack of awareness of mental health problems by primary health care providers.

A few lists of behavioral criteria intended to alert pediatricians to early signs of autism have been offered (e.g., Prior & Gajzago, 1974); unfortunately, their applicability is problematic, as many children with other difficulties (e.g., sensory deficits or global delay) may also present some of the delays and deviations seen in autistic children. Nevertheless, a recent study reported the successful use of a checklist completed by health care providers. This instrument consisted of normative social-cognitive behaviors (e.g., pointing, playing imaginatively) and was used for the early identification of autism among a sample including the siblings of diagnosed autistic children (Baron-Cohen, Allen, & Gillberg, 1992). Even though these results are encouraging, it seems that few if any of the children in the sample (except for the subsequently diagnosed autistic children) suffered from any degree of mental retardation or other significant physical or developmental disorder. Since other developmental disorders are far more common than autism, it remains to be established whether this checklist would be effective in preventing a great number of false positives. Despite these difficulties, and in light of recent federal mandates for extension of services to young children, the issue of early case detection and intervention is now assuming even greater importance.

Given our knowledge of the natural course of the disorder, it may be said that infants and very young autistic children exhibit the "purest" form of the condition (Volkmar & Cohen, 1988). The late detection, however, usually leaves the first 2 to 4 years of life virtually undocumented. As a result, studies of this age group are uncommon. Most studies of early development in autism rely on parental retrospection (e.g., Ornitz et al., 1977) or, less frequently, on movies or videotapes made by parents before the time of their children's diagnosis (Losche, 1990; Massie, 1978). Both of these methods have their limitations. Although parents often have concerns from the first months of a child's life, a referral usually follows later, as parents realize that the child is 18 to 24 months old and still not speaking. Parents may report concern that the child appears not to hear, although paradoxically they may also note that the child is exquisitely sensitive to certain sounds in the inanimate environment, such as the noise of the vacuum cleaner.

Similarly, the child may not respond differentially to parents, but may be particularly attached to a highly unusual object (e.g., a piece of string or a specific magazine). The young autistic child also may have interest in nonfunctional aspects of objects—their smell, taste, or reflection of light—and normal use of materials for play is typically absent. For instance, the child may prefer to spin the wheels of a toy truck continuously rather than to create a make-believe play sequence with it. Other deviant behaviors include stereotypic, motor mannerisms, such as hand flapping, twirling, and toe walking, and a preference for such activities rather than those involving social interaction. Bizarre affective responses may be observed; the child may become highly agitated if the same route or routine is not followed precisely or if an aspect of the environment is not maintained (e.g., furniture arrangement).

Initial studies of the early development of autistic children suggested that their development was erratic—characterized by lags, spurts, and uneven development across domains of functioning; "splinter skills"; and the loss of previously acquired skills. Some diagnostic systems (Ritvo & Freeman, 1978) have included unusual rates and sequences of development as criterion for the condition. Recent research confirms that there may be either islets of special ability or domains in which levels of functioning are relatively higher (Burack & Volkmar, 1992). This apparent developmental unevenness becomes more pronounced past the sensorimotor period (Losche, 1990). However, development within a given domain generally follows expected developmental sequences (Burack & Volkmar, 1992).

Social Development

The social disabilities found in autism have been consistently emphasized as important, if not the most significant central defining, features of the disorder (Kanner, 1943; Rutter, 1978a). Autistic individuals show a fundamental failure in socialization from early childhood, perhaps even from the first days or weeks of life. Unlike normally developing infants, they display a lack of reciprocity in social contact, inappropriate gaze behavior, tenuous expressions of attachment, and paucity of joint play and communicative skills (Volkmar, Carter, Grossman, & Klin, 1997a). Later in life, symptoms of social impairment persist, even in the highest-functioning individuals; they take the form of a pervasive difficulty in developing friendships, responding empathically to others, and understanding the conventions and expectations inherent in day-to-day social transactions (Volkmar & Klin, 1993).

Paradoxically, the social dysfunction has been the focus of comparatively little systematic study (Fein, Pennington, Markowitz, Braverman, & Waterhouse, 1986). Various factors appear to have contributed to this situation. One is an implicit "cognitive-primacy hypothesis" (Cairns, 1979; Rutter, 1983), or an assumption that the condition is primarily cognitive in nature; another is a lack of information on neurobiological systems related to social development (Brothers, 1989); still another is an awareness that some social skills do emerge in these children (Rutter, Greenfield, & Lockyer, 1967); and a final factor is a lack of truly operational and dimensional definitions of social deficits (Volkmar, 1987). More recently, some (primarily) experimental studies (see Baron-Cohen, 1988, for a review) have focused on different aspects of social development, including attachment behaviors, social interactions, emotional expression, symbolic play, and social cognition.

Although still very limited, the combined data from clinical observations and experimental findings indicate that the social development of young autistic children is qualitatively different from that seen in even very young infants; it differs as well from that observed in mental retardation not associated with autism (Volkmar et al., 1997a). In normative development, various perceptual, affective, and neuroregulatory mechanisms predispose young infants to engage in social interaction from very early in their lives (Cohn & Tronick, 1987; Tronick, 1980). Against this background, the social deficits of autistic infants and young children are striking. For example, the human face appears to hold little interest or to have little salience for an autistic child (Volkmar, 1987). Similarly, young autistic children appear to lack a differential preference for speech sounds (Klin, 1991, 1992). Typical forms of early nonverbal interchange are deviant. Very-early-emerging forms of "intersubjectivity" (Stern, 1985), such as the imitative games of infancy, are absent in these children. They may not seek physical comfort from parents and may be difficult to hold (Ornitz et al., 1977). Similarly, though some may exhibit differential responsiveness to familiar adults, the usual robust patterns of attachment do not develop, and autistic children may not respond differentially to their parents until the elementary school years (Mundy & Sigman, 1989).

Social interest and relatively isolated social skills may develop as autistic children enter later childhood and adolescence. However, social responsivity remains a source of considerable disability even for higher-functioning individuals; their attempts at social interaction usually fail, as a result both of their difficulties in pragmatic communication and empathy and of their failure to integrate various sources of information relevant to interaction. Normal peer relationships do not develop, and even when some social relationships do appear, these tend to be with adults rather than with peers (Volkmar et al., 1997a). In adulthood, even the highest-functioning individuals continue to exhibit significant social deficits. Such individuals are self-described "loners" who may exhibit a desire for social contact, although they are typically incapable of it (Schopler & Mesibov, 1992). In many instances, these individuals are aware of their disability; in response, they develop a number of coping strategies that usually involve learning concrete rules for mediating social interaction. An increased awareness of the disability may also result in some degree of depression (Cohen, 1991).

Communicative Development

Although autistic children may or may not exhibit problems in speech, their language, and particularly their *use* of whatever linguistic ability is available to them, are almost always deviant (Lord & Paul, 1997). About half of autistic individuals never speak; those who do speak exhibit language that is distinctive in numerous ways (Marans, 1997). Interestingly, numerous studies have revealed that in regard to the less communicative aspects of language (i.e., phonology and syntax), autistic individuals' abilities are better than those of IQ-matched controls and often comparable to those of normative samples (Fay & Mermelstein, 1982). It is in the most functional aspects of language that their degree of communicative disability is shown to be very profound. For example, autistic individuals' speech is often characterized by inappropriate use of intonational patterns and stress (Menyuk, 1978), conveying the impression of monotonic or pedantic delivery; this abnormality is also evidenced in preverbal vocal output (Ricks, 1975). Semantic difficulties are often reflected in the form of extreme literalness, as well as a paucity of conceptual words (Fay & Schuler, 1980), particularly terms that express mental states (e.g., beliefs and intentions) in others and in oneself (Tager-Flusberg, 1993). Yet the pragmatic aspects of autistic individuals' speech are the most universally dysfunctional aspects (see Baron-Cohen, 1988, for a review). Even the highest-functioning individuals tend to fail to observe the usual conventions of communication, such as turn taking, contextualization (i.e., providing background information that is not known to the interlocutor), and so forth. As a result, their conversational style may appear one-sided and sometimes incoherent.

Other phenomena commonly observed in autistic individuals' speech include pronoun reversal and both immediate and delayed echolalia (Fay & Schuler, 1980). It must be noted, however, that echolalia per se is observed in normally developing children who are acquiring language, and adaptive functions of echolalia in autistic individuals have been noted (Wetherby, Schuler, & Prizant, 1997). Finally, the language deficits in autism differ from those seen in the developmental language disorders, particularly in terms of the communicative, or functional, use of language (Cantwell, Baker, & Rutter, 1978; Lord & Paul, 1997).

Cognitive Development

One of the false leads in Kanner's (1943) original description of autism was his impression that autism apparently was not associated with mental retardation—a presumption that lasted for over two decades. This presumption was based on (1) the observation that on certain tasks of traditional IQ tests (e.g., subtests involving rote memory or visual–spatial skills), autistic children often scored within the normal or near-normal range; (2) the notion that the children's otherwise generally poor performance on IQ tests was a function of volitional noncompliance or negativism, or "untestability" (i.e., such results were due to their "autism"); and (3) the observation that some autistic children exhibited unusual "splinter skills" or islets of special ability (DeMyer, Hingtgen, & Jackson, 1981). It is now clear that when tests appropriate to the individuals' developmental level are used and supportive conditions are provided, most individuals with autism score in the mentally retarded range (Klin, Carter, & Sparrow, 1997). Subsequent research has also revealed that IQ is strongly correlated with severity of the social impairment and other aspects of the disorder (Cohen et al.,1987; Volkmar, Bregman, Cohen, Hooks, & Stevenson, 1989), and that it is a potent predictor of ultimate outcome (Lockyer & Rutter, 1969; Lotter, 1978a).

Developmental and psychological testing of infants and young children is at best a difficult procedure; in autistic children, such testing usually reveals particular difficulty with tasks requiring language, conceptual reasoning, imitation, or understanding of social conventions and events. Often nonverbal problem-solving abilities, such as those involved in matching shapes or solving inset puzzles, are closer to age-expected levels (Sigman, Ungerer, Mundy, & Sherman, 1987). Deficits in sensory–motor skills, as opposed to more symbolic or communicative skills, are more variably noted (Curcio, 1978; Morgan, Curtrer, Coplin, & Rodrigue, 1989).

A great deal of attention has been given to the cognitive profile and development of autistic children. Even though research studies date primarily from the 1960s and 1970s, particularly studies employing experimental methodologies (Hermelin & O'Connor, 1970), a comprehensive description of autistic children's cognitive abilities and disabilities could be found in Scheerer, Rothmann, and Goldstein's (1945) monograph reporting an intensive study of an "autistic savant," who was also one of the 11 children described by Kanner. Many of the experimental findings obtained in the 1960s and 1970s had been described phenomenologically in this early monograph. In contrast to Kanner's (1943) affective hypothesis, these authors proposed that the disorder affecting their patient (as well as the other 10 children reported by Kanner) was primarily a pervasive impairment of "abstract attitude" (Goldstein, 1958)—a term that corresponds to Head's (1926) impairment of "symbolic functions" in the field of traumatic aphasia. This hypothesis was described in exquisite detail by Scheerer et al., who related symptoms in the area of social, affective, communicative, cognitive, and behavioral functioning to an underlying inability to symbolize experience, and hence to profit from the flexibility afforded by conceptual (as against concrete) and generalization (as against context-specific) strategies. These ideas received much corroboration in Hermelin and O'Connor's (1970) experimental work, and were summarized and illustrated by Ricks and Wing (1975).

More recently, a new line of research has proposed that the social disabilities in autism reflect a specific, innate, and primarily cognitive incapacity to attribute mental states (e.g., beliefs, intentions, emotions) to others and oneself, and then to use these to explain and predict another person's behavior (the "theory-of-mind" hypothesis: Baron-Cohen, 1990; Leslie, 1987). This hypothesis has grown out of two lines of experimental findings: (1) Autistic children's symbolic dysfunction is not generalized, but affects a very specific cognitive capacity; and (2) this cognitive, or social-cognitive, capacity refers to the ability to conceive of other people's subjectivity, or to have a "theory of mind." This line of research is of considerable interest, as it more parsimoniously accounts for observed deficits in social interaction, communication, and play in autistic children. However, to date this theory is still limited in several important respects. First, as the postulated early manifestations of a "theory of mind" are not exhibited before 1 year of age at the very earliest, the theory does not account for the very early onset of the condition (Klin, Volkmar, & Sparrow, 1992). Second, because experiential work using this approach has tended to focus on verbal subjects, it is unclear whether the theory is applicable to lower-functioning (mute) subjects; in the same vein, higher-functioning and older autistic subjects ar often able to conceive other people's intentions cognitively, but are nevertheless unable to empathize with them (Klin & Volkmar, 1993). Third, at least some work has suggested that apparent "theory-of-mind" deficits are a function of developmental level rather than diagnostic category (Prior, Dahlstrom, & Squires, 1990).

Neurobiological Studies

Considerable evidence suggests the operation of some as-yet-unspecified neurobiological factor or factors in the pathogenesis of autism. For example, autistic children are more likely to exhibit anomalies, persistent primitive reflexes, and various neurological "soft signs"; abnormalities on electroencephalogram, computed tomography (CT), or magnetic resonance imaging (MRI); and an increased evidence of seizures (Minshew et al., 1997). As many as 25% of autistic individuals develop seizure disorders; in fact, recent work suggests that the risk of seizure is significantly increased throughout the developmental period, including infancy and early childhood (Volkmar & Nelson, 1990). There are some suggestions of reduced obstetrical and neonatal optimality (Tsai, 1987). Autism is also observed in association with a host of specific medical conditions, such as phenylketonuria, congenital rubella, tuberous sclerosis, and fragile X syndrome (Coleman, 1987); on the other hand, it is much less commonly associated with other conditions, notably Down syndrome (Bregman & Volkmar, 1988). There is now evidence of strong genetic contributions in autism (Bailey et al., 1995). For example, there is a higher-than-expected frequency of less severe developmental problems in the relatives of autistic patients. In a study of siblings, August, Stewart, and Tsai (1981) reported that the frequency of autism in siblings was nearly 3%; in other words, the frequency of autism was markedly increased over the expected prevalence in the population. Higher-than-expected rates of cognitive disorder also were present in siblings. Folstein and Piven (1991) reported that monozygotic twins are more likely than dizygotic twins to be concordant for the disorder. Other studies (e.g., Jones & Szatmari, 1988) have supported these findings, suggesting that on balance, the available data to date suggest some role of genetic factors in syndrome pathogenesis, even though a multifactorial etiology is probably very likely (Rutter, Bailey, Simonoff, & Pickles, 1997.

Despite the considerable evidence favoring some neurobiological factor or factors in the pathogenesis of autism, precise and identifiable mechanisms have yet to be specified.

Neurobiological findings vary considerably, and findings are often subtle. Neuroanatomical models of the disorder have placed the "site of lesion" at various points on the neuraxis from the brain stem and cerebellum to the cortex (Golden, 1987; Heh et al., 1989). Neurochemical findings are no clearer. For example, it is evident that as a group, autistic children exhibit elevated peripheral levels of serotonin, a central nervous system neurotransmitter; however, the significance of this observation is unclear, since the relationship of peripheral to central serotonin levels is not firmly established in individuals suffering from several other conditions that result in elevated serotonin levels (Anderson & Hoshino, 1997).

Epidemiology

Various problems pose complications for epidemiological studies: the relative infrequency of autism and associated conditions, difficulties in case identification, changes in diagnostic criteria, and the nature of definitions used. However, most studies of autism have suggested prevalence rates of between 2 and 5 cases in 10,000 children (Bryson, 1997). Most studies also suggest that autism is usually four or five times as common in males as in females; however, girls who are affected may exhibit a more severe form of the disorder, particularly in terms of having lower IQ. The significance of the observed sex difference is unclear, but it may reflect the operation of underlying genetic mechanisms (Lord & Schopler, 1987). Although Kanner (1943) initially suggested a preponderance of autism in families of higher socioeconomic status, subsequent controlled research has not confirmed this impression. In fact, autistic children come from families of all social classes (Schopler, Andrews, & Strupp, 1980) and cultures (Lotter, 1978b).

Epidemiological information on other, nonautistic PDDs is more limited (Klin & Volkmar, 1995). It does appear, however, that atypical PDD/PDD NOS is much more common than more strictly defined autism. Apparently the other PDDs are less common than autism. For example, childhood disintegrative disorder is perhaps 10 times less common than more strictly defined autism (Volkmar & Rutter, 1995).

Psychosocial Factors

Studies of parents of autistic children have suggested that they do not differ from parents of other developmentally disordered children in interactional style, in frequency of unusual personality characteristics, or in caretaking practices (DeMyer et al., 1981). The observations that autism is not often observed in other siblings, and that grossly inadequate emotional nurturing on the part of parents is associated with a different clinical presentation (APA, 1989), are also inconsistent with the notion that parents somehow "cause" autism.

On the other hand, as might be expected, the experience of having an autistic child may have a profound influence on a family (Schopler & Mesibov, 1984). The list of stressors the family must face is associated with the child's level of cognitive functioning, as well as with the severity of the social, communicative, and adaptive impairments and unusual behaviors. For example, at different points of the autistic individual's life, the parents may need to cope with the person's social and affective unresponsiveness, rigidity, and unawareness of social conventions; unusual behaviors may involve absorption in routinized and self-absorbing activities that further increase the individual's isolation and inaccessibility; when present, stereotypies, self-injurious behaviors, and limited self-sufficiency are particularly taxing for caregivers. Such stressors on parents and other family members vary over the course of an autistic child's development. Over time, different patterns of adaptation are noted, depending on such factors as personal and community resources and the availability of adequate educational and vocational services that are responsive to the child's and family's specific needs (Morgan, 1988).

Course and Prognosis

Several factors act as determinants of the course and long-term outcome of autism, particularly developmental level and communicative and adaptive functioning. Younger children more typically display the all-encompassing unrelatedness alluded to in the DSM-III (APA, 1980) criteria for autism. Although some evidence of differentiated responsiveness to parents may be observed as a child reaches the elementary school years, patterns of social interaction remain quite deviant, and the child's behavior can be quite problematic. For example, enjoyable social interaction may be restricted to circumscribed activities, such as "rough-and-tumble" or "tickling" games; if left to his or her own devices, the child may be withdrawn or absorbed with trivial aspects of the environment (e.g., puzzles). Attempts at introducing structure by placing demands on the child may lead to temper tantrums. Often some gains, such as in terms of communication and social skills, are observed during the elementary school years. During adolescence, some autistic children exhibit behavioral deterioration, and a smaller number improve (Rutter, 1970). Various interactional styles can be observed, ranging from aloof to passive to eccentric (Wing & Attwood, 1987); these styles appear to be closely related to developmental level (Volkmar et al., 1989).

Available information suggests that the outcome for autistic children is quite poor (Kanner, Rodriguez, & Ashenden, 1972), with perhaps only one-third able to achieve some degree of personal independence and self-sufficiency as adults (DeMyer et al., 1981). In general, two major factors appear predictive of ultimate outcome: the acquisition of truly communicative speech by age 5, and IQ. It is important to realize that much of the available outcome information is based on data collected during the 1960s and 1970s. During this period fewer services were available, and these often were not provided until the school years. There is some reason to hope that in the 1980s and 1990s, the mandates for earlier intervention, the tendency for earlier detection of the disorder, more intensive and early interventions (e.g., Lovaas, 1987), and the current focus on realistic life skills such as self-sufficiency and vocational training (Gerhardt & Holmes, 1997) have all improved the long-term outcome for the disorder. Research in this area remains critically needed, however.

DIAGNOSIS OF AUTISM

Categorical definitions of autism have typically emphasized four features essential for diagnosis: (1) early onset; (2) social dysfunction, including dysfunctional play; (3) communicative dysfunction; and (4) various unusual behaviors, such as stereotypies and resistance to change, which are usually subsumed under the term "insistence on sameness." Other features—for example, discrepancies in rates and sequences of development and perceptual abnormalities—are viewed less commonly as central for purposes of definition. Consistent with Rutter's (1978a) influential synthesis of Kanner's (1943) original description and subsequent research, most categorical definitions emphasize that the observed deviance in social and communicative development is not just a function of developmental level.

On the other hand, precise metrics for operationalizing this notion have not proven easy to develop. Other factors, such as range in syndrome expression, change with age, and the frequency of "autistic-like" behaviors in individuals with severe mental retardation, have all complicated the development of categorical definitions. The task of diagnosis, particularly with infants and very young children, can be very complicated.

The DSM-III (APA, 1980) definition of infantile autism was largely consistent with Rutter's (1978a) synthesis of Kanner's original description. It emphasized the early onset (less than 30 months) of all-encompassing social impairment, severe deficits in language development when speech was present, and eccentric responses to the environment. This definition proved unsatisfactory in several ways: It was most appropriate to younger and lower-functioning individuals; it failed to cover developmental changes in syndrome expression; and it did not address broader aspects of problems in communication (not just the formal aspects of language) (Volkmar & Cohen, 1988). Major revisions were made in DSM-III-R (APA, 1987).

The DSM-III-R definition of autistic disorder was intended to be more developmentally oriented and hence more inclusive of expressions of social impairment, more attuned to recent research on symbolic functioning and play in autism, and ahistorical in nature (i.e., a diagnosis could be made based on present examination only). The DSM-III-R definition consisted of a set of 16 detailed criteria grouped into three categories (deviant social development, deviant communication/play/imagination, and limited range of interests and activities). To achieve a diagnosis of autism, an individual had to exhibit at least 8 of the 16 criteria, with a minimum number of criteria specified from each category. Although age of onset was no longer a diagnostic criterion, it could be specified as before or after 36 months. Unfortunately, it appeared that the attempt to provide a greater developmental orientation resulted in an unintentionally broadened definition, so that many children, particularly those who were both young and retarded, might now inappropriately be termed "autistic" (Volkmar, Bregman, Cohen, & Cicchetti, 1988a).

In contrast to DSM-III-R, the ICD-10 (WHO, 1992) draft definition of autism produced results similar to those generated by DSM-III (if the DSM-III diagnosis was taken in its lifetime sense).The draft definition also appeared to approximate most closely the diagnosis assigned by experienced clinicians (Volkmar, Cicchetti, Bregman, & Cohen, 1992). Another difference between DSM-III-R and ICD-10 was the inclusion in ICD-10 of various other, nonautistic PDDs. The inclusion of additional disorders with some similarity to autism was meant to foster research on these conditions and made it possible to produce a somewhat more stringent definition of autism. The differences between DSM-III-R and ICD-10 were thus further emphasized, and the potential adverse effects of two markedly different official diagnostic systems were made clear (Rutter & Schopler, 1992).

As a result of the concerns about DSM-III-R and its compatibility with ICD-10, a large multisite, international field trial was undertaken (Volkmar et al., 1994). Goals of this field trial included development of a reliable and efficient diagnostic system for autism (and for other disorders that would be included within the PDD class), and achievement of a reasonable balance of sensitivity and specificity (i.e., avoiding overdiagnosis of autism in cases with severe retardation and underdiagnosis in individuals with normal IQ levels). The nature of the DSM-III-R overdiagnosis of the condition was to be established, if this indeed was the case, and various alternatives for DSM-IV (APA, 1994) were to be outlined. Issues of criterion and disorder convergence with ICD-10 in the PDD class were also to be addressed explicitly. At the same time, the important differences between ICD and DSM were noted, most notably in the ICD-10 approach of having separate guidelines for clinicians apart from research criteria (Volkmar et al., 1994).

For the DSM-IV field trial, data were collected on a sample of nearly 1,000 individuals with a diagnosis of autism or other disorders in a range of setting and sites. Cases were rated by examiners with a range of experience and professional backgrounds; cases were typically rated on the basis of contemporaneous examination and past records (not just record review). Five sites provided ratings on 100 consecutive cases over the period of a year, whereas other sites provided ratings on a smaller number of cases. Comparison cases included those in which the differential diagnosis would reasonably include autism. Certain cases, such as those with a diagnosis of a nonautistic PDD as included in ICD-10, or cases with certain characteristics (e.g., high-functioning females with autism), were intentionally oversampled. Ratings were made of DSM-III, DSM-III-R, and ICD-10 criteria, as well as of a range of potential new criteria; basic information was also obtained on each case and rater(s), with due attention to issues such as reliability of ratings.

From the results of the field trial, it did appear that the DSM-III-R definition was too broad and that it tended to overdiagnose autism in individuals with severe mental retardation. The ICD-10 approach was noted to have the best overall agreement with clinician diagnosis. Similarly, the available data provided some support for inclusion of other disorders within the PDD class.

Various alternatives for DSM-IV were outlined. In addition, from these analyses and those related to the development of ICD-10, it appeared that several of the 20 detailed ICD-10 criteria could be eliminated with minimal effect on efficiency of the definition. A decision based on both data and philosophical considerations was made to establish conceptual convergence of DSM-IV and ICD-10 definitions of autism and related PDD.

The DSM-IV definition of autistic disorder consists of 12 criteria equally divided among three clusters of symptoms (social interaction, communication/play/imagination, and limited patterns of interest and behavior) and an age-at-onset criterion; the definition is conceptually the same as that employed in ICD-10.

CLINICAL ASSESSMENT

By definition, children with autism and other PDDs have delays and deviant patterns in multiple areas of functioning; accordingly, their evaluations often require professionals with different areas of expertise, including communication, overall developmental functioning, and behavioral status. Therefore, the clinical assessment of infants and preschool children with such disorders is probably conducted most effectively by an experienced interdisciplinary team. Three fundamental considerations should guide the assessment process. It is clear that autistic children pose unusual challenges for usual assessment methods (Klin et al., 1997); hence the first consideration concerns an examiner's clinical judgment of how to obtain the most reliable measures of a child's functioning. For example, because attentional and behavioral difficulties may pose significant obstacles to the evaluation, allowances may be made for small deviations from standardized procedures, if by doing so the examiner is able to sample a wider range of the child's abilities while maintaining the general aim of the instrument used. On the other hand, the examiner should be aware that although modifications in usual procedures for administering specific tests are sometimes clinically indicated, the results thus obtained must be viewed with great caution. Given the difficulties inherent in the assessment of infants and younger children, several assessment sessions may be required.

Modifications in standard assessment procedures may be helpful to parents (Morgan, 1988); to the extent that it is possible, parents should be encouraged to observe the evaluation of their child. This procedure both helps to demystify assessment procedures and also provides a common set of observations for subsequent discussion. The rationale for specific tests and procedures, and the meaning of specific observations, can then be reviewed with parents in a more efficient fashion.

Evaluation findings should be translated into a single coherent view of the child, which in turn should give rise to a series of easily understood, detailed, concrete, realistic recommendations. Depending on the nature of the child's individual needs, the services of various professionals may be needed. If a multidisciplinary team is providing the evaluation, team members must maintain close communication with one another, to avoid fragmentation and duplication of effort. More important, the findings obtained by the different evaluators (e.g., cognitive profile, communicative functioning, clinical presentation) should be integrated with a view not only to assessing the implications of each set, but also to determining the interrelationship of all the abilities and disabilities studied. When possible, the evaluation should be sufficiently integrated that parents receive a single coherent picture of the child and his or her difficulties; a plethora of individual reports is less helpful than a longer report with input from all members of the evaluating team. Such a report also has the practical advantage of facilitating discussion among team members, who must be able to reconcile or understand apparent discrepancies in their results. When writing their reports, professionals should strive to express the implications of their findings for the child's day-to-day adaptation and learning. In this regard, technical language should be avoided as much as possible.

History

A careful history should be obtained, including information related to pregnancy and neonatal period, early development, the characteristics of development, and medical and family history. For example, was the baby very "easy" and content to be left alone? Was it hard to get a response from the child? Did the child smile responsively? Was it hard to feed the baby? Information on the nature and age of apparent onset of the condition can provide important information relevant to differential diagnosis; for example, it is important to know whether the child exhibited a prolonged period of normal development. Questions about development can sometimes be framed for parents around a specific time or well-remembered event, such as the first birthday. The history should include information about normally expected skills (early social interest, babbling and early prelinguistic communicative behaviors, motor development, etc.). The process of taking the history should convey to parents a sense that the information they provide is both helpful and welcome; this can help the clinician establish a collaborative relationship with parents. Although the child's history is best obtained during a direct interview with the parents, developmental and behavioral inventories may be mailed to the parents for them to complete prior to their visit, in order to elicit information and help them frame observations that can be further elaborated upon during the interview with the examiner's help.

Psychological Assessment

The psychological assessment aims at establishing the child's overall level of intellectual functioning, as well as describing his or her profile in terms of strengths, weaknesses, and learning style. Typically, autistic children have considerable unevenness in functioning; the evaluator should thus be aware that significant deficits in one area may not necessarily predict commensurable deficits in other areas. For example, many tests require linguistic skill and sustained attention—two abilities that children with autism frequently lack. Their failure to perform adequately on some tests may therefore reflect deficiencies in these areas rather than more general cognitive impairments. To illustrate this point, one study revealed that when the linguistic and attentional requirements for the solution of Piagetian tasks were eliminated, autistic children (aged 4 to 9) performed at levels comparable to those of normal controls (Lancy & Goldstein, 1982).

Assessment instruments should be selected with an eye to the child's apparent developmental level. For younger children or children whose intellectual skills are markedly delayed, developmental assessment instruments may be used, such as the Bayley Scales of Infant Development (Bayley, 1969), or the Uzgiris–Hunt Ordinal Scales of Psychological Development (Uzgiris & Hunt, 1975). For children with an overall mental age of 3 years or above, psychometric batteries should be used—preferably those that are less dependent on verbal abilities, such as the Kaufman Assessment Battery for Children (Kaufman & Kaufman, 1983). It is important to derive both verbal and nonverbal scores, as a discrepancy favoring the latter is often obtained. For children with nonverbal mental ages over 2 years, nonverbal tests such as the Leiter International Performance Scale (Leiter, 1948) should also be used. (See Klin et al., 1997, and Marans, 1997, for a full discussion of assessment instruments.)

In addition to framing the child's overall developmental level, the psychological assessment should provide measures of and information about the following abilities, in both the verbal and nonverbal domains: problem solving (can the child generate strategies and integrate information?); concept formation (can the child group objects by class, color, etc., or generalize knowledge from one context to another?); style of learning (can the child learn from modeling, imitation, etc.?); and memory skills (how many items of information can the child retain, and is there a difference in the child's ability to recognize inanimate [e.g., geometric] forms vs. human faces or other animate stimuli?). A measure of visual–spatial and visual–motor integration skills should also be obtained, to assess the child's sensitivity to the orientation and complexity of objects, as well as the ability to write or draw recognizable figures. A description of results should include not only quantified information, but also a judgment of how representative of the child's functioning the measure appears to be, and a description of the conditions likely to foster maximal performance on the part of the child.

Communicative Assessment

The communicative assessment aims at obtaining both quantitative and qualitative information regarding various aspects of the child's communicative skills (Marans, 1997). In contrast to some traditional practices, this assessment should include not only the formal aspects of language (articulation, vocabulary, and structure), but also, and particularly, the suprasegmental aspects of language, including intonation and inflection of voice; the use of linguistic skills for communicative purposes and other aspects of pragmatics in speech; and nonverbal forms of communication, such as gaze, gestures, or signs (Marans, 1997). Several language scales are available for very young or very low-functioning children: the Receptive–Expressive Emergent Language Scale (Bzoch & League, 1971), the Sequenced Inventory of Communicative Development (Hedrick, Prather, & Tobin, 1975), and the Reynell Developmental Language Scales (Reynell, 1969). It must be noted that in contrast to the performance of the normative population, autistic children's performance on the Peabody Picture Vocabulary Test—Revised (Dunn & Dunn, 1981) or the Expressive One Word Picture Vocabulary Test (Gardner, 1990) should be seen as reflecting receptive and expressive vocabulary only, and not as indicating language comprehension and expression abilities. This is because autistic children are typically more proficient at naming or pointing to a named picture than at communicating with or understanding another person.

For the nonverbal or primarily echolalic child, standardized tests may not be of use. In such instances, the communication specialist should employ informal means to obtain information about the child's communicative resources and prelinguistic skills. These include the child's ability to take turns, to share attention, to vocalize in a consistent fashion, and so forth. For older and higher-functioning individuals with autism, instruments such as the Clinical Evaluation of Language Fundamentals 3 (Semel, Wiig, & Secord, 1995) may include an assessment of more subtle aspects of communication, such as nonliteral utterances (e.g., metaphor and irony) and ambiguities.

Adaptive Functioning

An assessment of the child's adaptive skills or capacity for self-sufficiency is an important aspect of the comprehensive evaluation, for at least two reasons. First, such an assessment allows the clinician to obtain a representative measure of the child's functioning in real-life situations. The measures and observations obtained during the evaluation in the clinic are inherently affected by extraneous factors, such as the unfamiliarity of the environment and the adults in it, the high degree of structure introduced in order to maximize performance, and the one-to-one approach. It is therefore important to acquire information about the child's typical functioning at home and at school, so that possible discrepancies between potential performance (as measured in the clinic) and actual performance (as expressed in the child's typical environment) can be addressed. Second, several states now make eligibility for services conditional on both intellectual level (i.e., mental retardation) and adaptive level (capacity for self-sufficiency).

The most widely used assessment battery for measuring adaptive functioning is the Vineland Adaptive Behavior Scales (Sparrow, Balla, & Cicchetti, 1984). These scales include measures of Communication (receptive, expressive, and written skills), Daily Living skills (personal care, domestic chores, and functioning in the community), Socialization (interpersonal skills, play, and coping skills), and Motor functioning (both gross and fine motor skills). In addition, the Vineland contains a list of maladaptive behaviors that are thought to interfere with the individual's ability to function adaptively. The Vineland has expanded, survey, and classroom editions, depending on the objectives and level of detail required (Sparrow & Cicchetti, 1989). One useful aspect of the Vineland is the fact that all of the behaviors included in the structured interview can be incorporated immediately as objectives to be achieved within the context of intervention.

Psychiatric Examination

The psychiatric examination should include observation during more and less structured periods, such as while the child is interacting with parents and while engaged in assessment by other members of the evaluating team. Areas for observation and inquiry with parents include social development (interest in social interaction, patterns of gaze and eye contact, differential attachments, style of social interaction), communication (receptive and expressive language, nonverbal and pragmatic communication, communicative intents, echolalia), responses to the environment (motor stereotypies, idiosyncratic responses, resistance to change), and play skills (nonfunctional or idiosyncratic uses of play materials, developmental level of play). The child's capacities for self-awareness—interest in mirror image, awareness of his or her own body, and motor skills—should be observed as well. Problem behaviors that are likely to interfere with remedial programming should also be noted, such as marked aggression or problems in attention (Klin et al., 1997).

Further Consultation

For younger children, consultations with other medical professionals, such as pediatric neurologists or geneticists, may be indicated. History or examination may suggest the need for specific laboratory studies or medical procedures. For example, the presence of severe mental retardation or dysmorphic features in a child, or a family history of mental retardation, suggests the need for genetic screening and chromosome analysis (including screening for fragile X syndrome); symptoms suggestive of seizures (e.g., apparent periodic unresponsiveness) suggest the need for electroencephalograms and possible neurological consultation; and so forth. CT or MRI scans may be indicated and sometimes (although not often) reveal such disorders as tuberous sclerosis or degenerative central nervous system disease. As noted earlier, careful history of the pregnancy and neonatal period should be obtained, to ascertain possible pre- or postnatal infections such as congenital rubella. Usually the child's hearing has been tested prior to comprehensive evaluation. If this has not been done, or it was not possible to elicit the child's cooperation, alternative audiometric procedures that are independent of the child's cooperation should be adopted. In such instances, auditory brain stem evoked responses should be obtained in order to rule out sensory loss (Klin, 1993).

Although autism is associated with a number of other medical conditions, in most instances even extensive medical evaluations fail to reveal an associated medical condition. This fact suggests reasonable caution in seeking additional medical assessments. On the other hand, certain features may suggest the importance of extensive medical investigations, such as the abrupt behavioral and developmental deterioration of a child who was previously developing normally.

Differential Diagnosis

The differential diagnosis of autism and other PDDs includes language and other specific developmental disorders, mental retardation, sensory impairments (particularly deafness), and reactive attachment disorder. Usually children with language disorders do not exhibit the pattern of serious social deviance and deficit characteristic of autism; often nonverbal communicative abilities constitute an area of evident strength. In mental retardation, social and communicative skills are usually on a par with overall cognitive skills. Deaf children may exhibit some difficulties in social interaction and some repetitive activities; however, they are usually interested in social interaction and may make use of gestures for communicative purposes. Children with reactive attachment disorder have by definition experienced marked psychosocial deprivation, which results in deficits in social interaction, most notably in attachment (expressed as either withdrawal or indiscriminate friendliness). However, the quality of the social deficit is different from that in autism, and the disturbance tends to remit after an appropriately responsive and nurturing psychosocial environment is provided.

In young children, the task of differential diagnosis is complicated by the inherent difficulties posed by their early developmental level, the frequency of "autistic-like" behaviors in other conditions, and the fact that autism can be present in conjunction with deafness and with mental retardation. The issues attending diagnosis in many instances are clarified with certainty only over time and after a period of intervention. It is appropriate for the clinician to share with parents a sense of his or her degree of confidence in the diagnosis. It is also important to realize that the diagnosis may have important, if not necessarily intended, implications for a host of other purposes (e.g., educational placement and programming, and eligibility for special services in the community). It is critical that the importance of educational and other interventions be emphasized, regardless of how "classically" autistic, or low-functioning, the child appears.

INTERVENTIONS

Despite strong claims by partisans of particular treatment approaches and much dedicated effort that has gone into their implementation, no treatment has been demonstrated to produce major alterations in the natural history of the syndrome (Rutter, 1985; Ward, 1970). In the absence of a definitive cure, there are a thousand treatments. Essentially every conceivable treatment has been utilized for autism, including somatic treatments, drug therapy, psychotherapy, behavior modification, nutritional treatments, and educational interventions (DeMyer et al., 1981; Rutter, 1985). With the exception of a few areas (notably behavior modification and pharmacological intervention, and to a lesser extent educational intervention), most proposed interventions have not been studied rigorously. Consequently, it has been difficult to assess treatment effects systematically.

Unfortunately, short-term changes readily occur when treaters and/or evaluators are aware of the hypothesis under study; in addition, short-term changes may be neither sustained nor clinically meaningful. In other instances, particularly in regard to reports of treatment efficacy based on a single case, it may be unclear whether the individual was actually autistic and what factor or factors were responsible for improvement. The observation that at least a few autistic individuals achieve relatively good outcomes is gratifying, but it also complicates the interpretation of single-case studies. To compound the problem further, probably there is no "untreated" autistic child; by the time the diagnosis is definitively made, parents have often tried multiple interventions.

Although there is scant evidence that autism can be "cured," improvement in several aspects of a child's presentation and specific behaviors may be achieved. Simeonsson et al. (1987) reviewed four comprehensive studies of early intervention for autistic children. The authors concluded that the critical factors in successful programs included structured behavioral treatment, parental involvement, treatment at an early age, intensive intervention, and focus on generalization of skills to new settings. Other lines of evidence have suggested the importance of appropriate, intensive educational interventions to foster the acquisition of basic social, cognitive, communicative, and adaptive skills (Olley & Stevenson, 1989; Prizant, Schuler, Wetherby, & Rydell, 1997; Schuler, Prizant, & Wetherby, 1997), which are in turn related to outcome. Behavior modification techniques can be quite helpful. Early and continuous intervention is highly desirable; some reports (Lovaas, 1987) have suggested marked improvement following early, intensive intervention. Educational programs should be highly structured (Rutter & Bartak, 1973) and oriented to the individual needs of the child. Intervention programs should be comprehensive and include the services of various professionals, including special educators, speech pathologists, and occupational therapists. Parental involvement should be encouraged in order to enhance consistency in approaches at home and at school, and to facilitate generalization of skills across settings. Professionals should work with parents to obtain appropriate educational placement and help them become aware of other community resources, such as respite care. Forthcoming federal mandates for provision of remedial services from birth on will increase the availability of services, we hope.

During the 1950s, it was common for professionals to recommend that parents consider institutionalization for severely disabled children. This practice led to the isolation and segregation of children with severe developmental disabilities, and thus many such individuals were prevented from reaching their full potential. An awareness of these issues has produced a marked shift in social policy: Most state agencies now attempt to maintain children in their families and communities, although, unfortunately, many necessary services may not be provided. A similar issue has arisen with regard to the integration of autistic children into regular classroom settings. The rationale for this approach is based on a strongly held philosophical stance (i.e., that special educational settings are, by their nature, inferior and discriminatory), as well as on a small body of empirical research (Charlop, Schreiman, & Tryon, 1983) suggesting that autistic children can indeed learn from their normally developing peers. Given the nature of social deficits in autism, there is considerable reason to worry that autistic children may not be as able as mentally retarded, nonautistic children to profit from such an approach. When various alternative educational placements are being considered, the individual needs of the child should be paramount.

In general, pharmacological interventions with infants and young autistic children are probably best avoided. The best-studied agents, the tranquilizers, have some utility in selected cases and in regard to specific maladaptive behaviors, but their many side effects (particularly sedation) may prove problematic (Campbell, Anderson, Green, & Deutsch, 1987). These agents may be indicated in some situations; typically, however, they are given to older children, and even then at the lowest effective dose for the shortest period of time. The efficacy of other pharmacological agents has not been clearly established (McDougle, 1997).

Many nontraditional treatments are available. In discussing such treatments with parents, it is helpful for the clinician to explore the rationale for the proposed treatment, the evidence (if any) of efficacy, and its potential cost (in both financial and human terms) to the child and the family (Klin & Cohen, 1994). Treatments that are minimally disruptive of the child's educational program and that pose little apparent risk to the child are of less concern than those that entail considerable disruption of the child's educational program or the family's life.

CONCLUSION

Considerable progress in the understanding of the nature of autism and related disorders has been made over the past 50 years. Given the early onset of the condition, it is somewhat paradoxical that our knowledge of autism in infants and very young children remains limited in important respects. Our knowledge of the other PDDs is even more meager. Although it now appears that these conditions arise as a result of some insult to the developing central nervous system, precise and testable pathophysiological mechanisms have not been identified yet.

Nevertheless, autism remains one of the most studied early childhood disorders. Although much of the biological research to date has been unavailing, continued advances in the neurosciences make elucidation of brain pathobiology more likely. The neurosciences can be put to their best use if the current limits of our knowledge concerning phenotype, neurobiology, and etiology are clearly understood. Advances in the understanding of the psychology of autism—within and across individuals, as well as along behavioral dimensions and with respect to categorical issues—should serve to better direct and organize the biological research. Such advances plus the recent nosological efforts will, it is hoped, result in a better understanding of the syndrome pathogenesis, which in turn may finally translate into interventions. However, such integration of different lines of research and treatment approaches requires an appreciation of the complexity of the clinical phenomena and the enormous range of each of the salient dimensions. In the process of elucidating such a complex disorder, affecting the child's basic capacities for socialization, it is likely that a great deal of light will be shed on the intricacies of every child's development.

REFERENCES

American Psychiatric Association (APA). (1980). *Diagnostic and statistical manual of mental disorders* (3rd ed.). Washington, DC: Author.

American Psychiatric Association (APA). (1987). *Diagnostic and statistical manual of mental disorders* (3rd ed., rev.). Washington, DC: Author.

American Psychiatric Association (APA). (1989). *Treatment of psychiatric disorders.* Washington, DC: Author.

American Psychiatric Association (APA). (1994). *Diagnostic and statistical manual of mental disorders* (4th ed.). Washington, DC: Author.

Anderson, G. M., & Hoshino, Y. (1997). Neurochemical studies of autism. In D. J. Cohen & F. R. Volkmar (Eds.), *Handbook of autism and pervasive developmental disorders* (pp. 325–343). New York: Wiley.

Asperger, H. (1979). Problems of infantile autism. *Communication, 13,* 1–12.

Asperger, H. (1991). Autistic psychopathy in childhood. In U. Frith (Ed.), *Autism and Asperger syndrome* (pp. 37–92). Cambridge, England: Cambridge University Press. (Original work published 1944)

August, G. J., Stewart, M. A., & Tsai, L. (1981). The incidence of cognitive disabilities in the siblings of autistic children. *British Journal of Psychiatry, 138,* 416–422.

Bailey, A., LeCouteur, A., Gottesman, I., Bolton, P., Simonoff, E., Yuzda, E., & Rutter, M. (1995). Autism as a strongly genetic disorder: Evidence from a British twin study. *Psychological Medicine, 25*(1), 63–77.

Baron-Cohen, S. (1988). Social and pragmatic deficits in autism: Cognitive or affective? *Journal of Autism and Developmental Disorders, 3,* 379–402.

Baron-Cohen, S. (1990). Autism: A specific cognitive disorder of "mind-blindness." *International Journal of Psychiatry, 2,* 81–90.

Baron-Cohen, S., Allen, J., & Gillberg, C. (1992). Can autism be detected at 18 months?: The needle, the haystack, and the CHAT. *British Journal of Psychiatry, 161,* 839–843.

Bayley, N. (1969). *Bayley Scales of Infant Development.* New York: Psychological Corporation.

Bleuler, E. (1951). *Dementia praecox or the group of schizophrenias* (Monograph Series on Schizophrenia No. 1., J. Zinkin, Trans.). New York: International Universities Press. (Original work published 1916)

Bregman, J. D., & Volkmar, F. R. (1988). Autistic social dysfunction and Down syndrome. *Journal of the American Academy of Child and Adolescent Psychiatry, 27,* 440–441.

Brothers, L. (1989). A biological perspective on empathy. *American Journal of Psychiatry, 146,* 10–19.

Bryson, S. E. (1997). Epidemiology of autism: Overview and issues outstanding. In F. R. Volkmar & D. J. Cohen (Eds.), *Handbook of autism and pervasive developmental disorders* (2nd ed., pp. 41–46). New York: Wiley.

Burack, J., & Volkmar, F. R. (1992). Development of low- and high-functioning autistic children. *Journal of Child Psychology and Psychiatry, 33,* 607–616.

Bzoch, K., & League, R. (1971). *Receptive–Expressive Emergent Language Scale.* Gainesville, FL: Language Educational Division, Computer Management Corporation.

Cairns, R. B. (1979). *Social development: The origins and plasticity of interchanges.* San Francisco: Freeman.

Campbell, M., Anderson, L. T., Green, W. H., & Deutsch, S. I. (1987). Psychopharmacology. In D. Cohen & A. Donnellan (Eds.), *Handbook of autism and pervasive developmental disorders* (pp. 545–565). New York: Wiley.

Cantwell, D., Baker, L., & Rutter, M. (1978). A comparative study of infantile autism and specific developmental receptive language disorder: IV. Analysis of syntax and language function. *Journal of Child Psychology and Psychiatry, 19,* 351–362.

Charlop, M. J., Schreiman, L., & Tryon, A. D. (1983). Learning through observations: The effects of peer modeling on acquisition and generalization in autistic children. *Journal of Abnormal Child Psychology, 11,* 355–366.

Chess, S. (1971). Autism in children with congenital rubella. *Journal of Autism and Childhood Schizophrenia, 1,* 33–47.

Cicchetti, D. V. & Cohen, D. J. (Eds.). (1995). *Developmental psychopathology.* New York: Wiley.

Cohen, D. J. (1991). Finding meaning in one's self and others: Clinical studies of children with autism and Tourette syndrome. In F. Kessel, M. Bornstein, & A. Sameroff (Eds.), *Contemporary constructions of the child: Essays in Honor of William Kessen* (pp. 159–175). Hillsdale, NJ: Erlbaum.

Cohen, D. J., Caparulo, B., & Shaywitz, B. (1976). Primary childhood aphasia and childhood autism. *Journal of the American Academy of Child and Adolescent Psychiatry, 15,* 604–645.

Cohen, D. J., Paul, R., & Volkmar, F. R. (1987). Issues in the classification of pervasive developmental disorders and associated conditions. In D.J. Cohen & A. Donnellan (Eds.), *Handbook of autism and pervasive developmental disorders* (pp. 20–40). New York: Wiley.

Cohn, J. F., & Tronick, E.Z. (1987). The sequence of dyadic states at 3, 6, and 9 months. *Developmental Psychology, 23,* 68–77.

Coleman, M. (1987). The search for neurobiological subgroups in autism. In E. Schopler & G. Mesibov (Eds.), *Neurobiological issues in autism* (pp. 163–179). New York: Plenum Press.

Corbett, J. (1987). Development, disintegration, and dementia. *Journal of Mental Deficiency Research, 31,* 349–356.

Curcio, F. (1978). Sensorimotor functioning and communication in mute autistic children. *Journal of Autism and Developmental Disorders, 8,* 292–305.

DeMyer, M. K., Hingtgen, J. N., & Jackson, R. K. (1981). Infantile autism reviewed: A decade of research. *Schizophrenia Bulletin, 7,* 388–451.

Dunn, L., & Dunn, L. (1981). *Peabody Picture Vocabulary Test—Revised.* Circle Pines, MN: American Guidance Service.

Fay, D., & Mermelstein, R. (1982). Language in infantile autism. In S. Rosenberg (Ed.). *Handbook of applied psycholinguistics* (pp. 112–131). Hillsdale, NJ: Erlbaum.

Fay, W., & Schuler, A. L. (1980). *Emerging language in autistic children.* Baltimore: University Park Press.

Fein, D., Pennington, B., Markowitz, P., Braverman, M., & Waterhouse, L. (1986). Towards a neuropsychological model of infantile autism: Are the social deficits primary? *Journal of the American Academy of Child Psychiatry, 25,* 198–212.

Folstein, S., & Piven, J. (1991). Etiology of autism: Genetic influences. *Pediatrics, 87*(5), 767–773.

Gardner, M. (1990). *Expressive One Word Picture Vocabulary Test.* Los Angeles: Western Psychological Services.

Gerhardt, P. F., & Holmes, D. L. (1997). Employment: Options and issues for adolescents and adults with autism. In D. J. Cohen & F. R. Volkmar (Eds.), *Handbook of autism and pervasive developmental disorders* (pp. 650–664). New York: Wiley.

Golden, G. (1987). Neurobiologcal functioning. In D. J. Cohen & A. Donnellan (Eds.), *Handbook of autism and pervasive developmental disorders* (pp. 133–147). New York: Wiley.

Goldstein, K. (1948). *Language and language disturbances.* New York: Grune & Stratton.

Head, H. (1926). *Aphasia and kindred disorders of speech.* Cambridge, England: Cambridge University Press.

Hedrick, D., Prather, F., & Tobin, A. (1975). *Sequenced Inventory of Communicative Development.* Seattle: University of Washington Press.

Heh, C. W., Smith, R., Wu, J., Hazlett, E., Russell, A., Asarnow, R., Tanguay, P., & Buchsbaum, M. S. (1989). Positron emission tomography of the cerebellum in autism. *American Journal of Psychiatry, 146*(2), 242–245.

Heller, T. (1954). About dementia infantilism (translation). *Journal of Nervous and Mental Disease, 119,* 471–477. (Original work published 1930)

Hermelin, B., & O'Connor, N. (1970). *Psychological experiments with autistic children.* New York: Pergamon Press.

Jones, M. G., & Szatmari, P. (1988). Stoppage rules and genetic studies of autism. *Journal of Autism and Developmental Disorders, 18,* 31–40.

Kanner, L. (1943). Autistic disturbances of affective contact. *Nervous Child, 2,* 217–250.

Kanner, L., Rodriguez, A., & Ashenden, B. (1972). How far can autistic children go in matters of social adaptation? *Journal of Autism and Childhood Schizophrenia, 2,* 9–33.

Kaufman, A. S., & Kaufman, N. L. (1983). *K-ABC: Kaufman Assessment Battery for Children.* Circle Pines, MN: American Guidance Service.

Klin, A. (1991). Young autistic children's listening preference in regard to speech: A possible characterization of the symptom of social withdrawal. *Journal of Autism and Developmental Disorders, 21,* 29–42.

Klin, A. (1992). Listening preferences in regard to speech in four children with developmental disabilities. *Journal of Child Psychology and Psychiatry, 33,* 763–769.

Klin, A. (1993). Auditory brainstem responses in autism: Brainstem dysfunction or peripheral hearing loss? *Journal of Autism and Developmental Disorders, 23,* 15–35.

Klin, A. (1994). Asperger syndrome. *Child and Adolescent Psychiatric Clinics of North America, 3,* 131–148.

Klin, A., Carter, A., & Sparrow, S. S. (1997). Psychological assessment. In F. R. Volkmar & D. J. Cohen (Eds.), *Handbook of autism and pervasive developmental disorders* (2nd ed., pp. 418–427). New York: Wiley.

Klin, A., & Cohen, D. J. (1994). The immorality of not knowing: The ethical imperative to conduct research in child psychiatry. In Y. Hattab (Ed.), *Ethics in child psychiatry* (pp. 217–232). Jerusalem: Gefen.

Klin, A., Mayes, L. C., Volkmar, F. R., & Cohen, D. J. (1995a). Multiplex developmental disorder. *Journal of Developmental and Behavioral Pediatrics, 16*(3), S7–S11.

Klin, A., & Volkmar, F. R. (1993). The development of individuals with autism: Implications for the theory of mind hypothesis. In S. Baron-Cohen, H. Tager-Flusberg, & D. J. Cohen (Eds.), *Understanding other minds: Perspectives from autism* (pp. 317–336). Oxford: Oxford University Press.

Klin, A., & Volkmar, F. R. (1995). Autism and the pervasive developmental disorders. *Child and Adolescent Psychiatric Clinics of North America, 4*(3), 617–630.

Klin, A., & Volkmar, F. R. (1997). Asperger's syndrome. In D. J. Cohen & F. R. Volkmar (Eds.), *Handbook of autism and pervasive developmental disorders* (2nd ed., pp. 94–122). New York: Wiley.

Klin, A., Volkmar, F. R., & Sparrow, S. S. (1992). Autistic social dysfunction: Some limitations of the theory of mind hypothesis. *Journal of Child Psychology and Psychiatry, 33*, 861–876.

Klin, A., Volkmar, F. R., & Sparrow, S. S. (Eds.) (1999). *Asperger's syndrome.* Manuscript in preparation for Guilford Press.

Klin, A., Volkmar, F. R., Sparrow, S. S., Cicchetti, D. V., & Rourke, B. P. (1995b). Validity and neuropsychological characterization of Asperger syndrome. *Journal of Child Psychology and Psychiatry, 36*(7), 1127–1140.

Kolvin, I. (1971). Studies in the childhood psychoses: I. Diagnostic criteria and classification. *British Journal of Psychiatry, 118*, 381–384.

Lancy, D. F., & Goldstein, G. I. (1982). The use of nonverbal Piagetian tasks to assess the cognitive development of autistic children. *Child Development, 53*, 1233–1241.

Leiter, R. G. (1948). *Leiter International Performance Scale.* Chicago: Stoelting.

Leslie, A. M. (1987). Pretense and representation: The origins of "theory of mind." *Psychological Review, 94*, 412–426.

Lockyer, L., & Rutter, M. (1969). A five to fifteen year follow-up study of infantile psychosis: III. Psychological aspects. *British Journal of Psychiatry, 115*, 865–882.

Lord, C., & Paul, R. (1997). Language and communication in autism. In F. R. Volkmar & D. J. Cohen (Eds.), *Handbook of autism and pervasive developmental disorders* (2nd ed., pp. 195–225). New York: Wiley.

Lord, C., & Schopler, E. (1987). Neurobiological implications of sex differences in autism. In E. Schopler & G. Mesibov (Eds.), *Neurobiological issues in autism* (pp. 192–212). New York: Plenum Press.

Losche, G. (1990). Sensorimotor and action development in autistic children from infancy to early childhood. *Journal of Child Psychology and Psychiatry, 31*, 749–761.

Lotter, V. (1978a). Follow-up studies. In M. Rutter & E. Schopler (Eds.), *Autism: A reappraisal of concepts and treatment* (pp. 148–161). New York: Plenum Press.

Lotter, V. (1978b). Childhood autism in Africa. *Journal of Child Psychology and Psychiatry, 19*, 231–244.

Lovaas, O. I. (1987). Behavioral treatment and normal educational and intellectual functioning in young autistic children. *Journal of Consulting and Clinical Psychology, 55*, 3–9.

Marans, W. D. (1997). Communication assessment. In F. R. Volkmar & D. J. Cohen (Eds.), *Handbook of autism and pervasive developmental disorders* (2nd ed., pp. 427–447). New York: Wiley.

Massie, H. N. (1978). Blind ratings of mother–infant interaction in home movies of prepsychotic and normal infants. *American Journal of Psychiatry, 135*, 1271–1374.

McAdoo, W. G., & DeMyer, M. Y. (1978). Personality characteristics of parents. In M. Rutter & E. Schopler (Eds.), *Autism: A reappraisal of concepts and treatment* (pp. 192–201). New York: Plenum Press.

McDougle, C. J. (1997). Psychopharmacology. In F. R. Volkmar & D. J. Cohen (Eds.), *Handbook of autism and pervasive developmental disorders* (2nd ed., pp. 707–729). New York: Wiley.

McKenna, K., Gordon, C. T., & Lenane, M. (1994). Looking for childhood-onset schizophrenia: The first 71 cases screened. *Journal of the American Academy of Child and Adolescent Psychiatry, 33*, 636–644.

Menyuk, P. (1978). Language: What's wrong and why. In M. Rutter & E. Schopler (Eds.), *Autism: A reappraisal of concepts and treatment* (pp. 77–90). New York: Plenum Press.

Minshew, N. J., Sweeney, J. A., & Bauman, M. L. (1997). Neurological aspects of autism. In F. R. Volkmar & D. J. Cohen (Eds.), *Handbook of autism and pervasive developmental disorders* (2nd ed., pp. 344–369). New York: Wiley.

Morgan, S. (1988). The autistic child and family functioning: A developmental–family systems perspective. *Journal of Autism and Developmental Disorders, 18*, 263–280.

Morgan, S., Curtrer, P. S., Coplin, J. W., & Rodrigue, J. R. (1989). Do autistic children differ from retarded and normal children in Piagetian sensorimotor functioning? *Journal of Child Psychology and Psychiatry, 30*, 857–864.

Mundy, P., & Sigman, M. (1989). Specifying the nature of the social impairment in autism. In G. Dawson (Ed.), *Autism: Nature, diagnosis, and treatment* (pp. 54–71). New York: Guilford Press.

Olley, J. G., & Stevenson, S. E. (1989). Preschool curriculum for children with autism: Addressing early social skills. In G. Dawson (Ed.), *Autism: Nature, diagnosis, and treatment* (pp. 346–366). New York: Guilford Press.

Ornitz, E. M., Guthrie, D., & Farley, A. H. (1977). Early development of autistic children. *Journal of Autism and Childhood Schizophrenia, 7,* 207–229.

Ozonoff, S., Pennington, B. F., & Rogers, S. J. (1991). Executive function deficits in high-functioning autistic individuals: Relationship to theory of mind. *Journal of Child Psychology and Psychiatry, 32*(7), 1081–1105.

Prior, M., Dahlstrom, B., & Squires, T. (1990). Autistic children's knowledge of thinking and feeling states in other people. *Journal of Child Psychology and Psychiatry, 31,* 587–601.

Prior, M., & Gajzago, C. (1974). Recognition of early signs of autism. *Medical Journal of Australia, 2*(5), 183.

Prizant, B. M., Schuler, A. L., Wetherby, A., & Rydell, P. (1997). Enhancing language and communication development: Language approaches. In D. J. Cohen & F. R. Volkmar (Eds.), *Handbook of autism and pervasive developmental disorders* (pp. 572–605). New York: Wiley.

Provence, S., & Lipton, R. C. (1962). *Infants in institutions.* New York: International Universities Press.

Rank, B. (1949). Adaptation of the psychoanalytic technique for the treatment of young children with atypical development. *American Journal of Orthopsychiatry, 19,* 130–139.

Rett, A. (1966). Uber ein eigenartiges hirntophisces Syndrome bei Hyperammonie im Kindersalter. *Wein Medizinische Wochenschrift, 118,* 723–726.

Reynell, J. (1969). *Developmental Language Scales.* Windsor, England: National Foundation for Educational Research.

Ricks, D. M. (1975). Vocal communication in preverbal normal and autistic children. In N. O'Connor (Ed.), *Language, cognitive deficits and retardation* (pp. 101–125). London: Butterworth.

Ricks, D. M., & Wing, L. (1975). Language, communication, and the use of symbols in normal and autistic children. *Journal of Autism and Childhood Schizophrenia, 5,* 191–221.

Ritvo, E. R., & Freeman, B. J. (1978). National Society for Autistic Children definition of the syndrome of autism. *Journal of Autism and Developmental Disorders, 8,* 162–169.

Rutter, M. (1970). *Autistic children: Infancy to adulthood. Seminars in Psychiatry, 2,* 435–450.

Rutter, M. (1972). Childhood schizophrenia reconsidered. *Journal of Autism and Childhood Schizophrenia, 2,* 315–338.

Rutter, M. (1978a). Diagnosis and definitions of childhood autism. *Journal of Autism and Childhood Schizophrenia, 8*(2), 139–161.

Rutter, M. (1978b). Language disorder and infantile autism. In M. Rutter & E. Schopler (Eds.), *Autism: A reappraisal of concepts and treatment* (pp. 48–61). New York: Plenum Press.

Rutter, M. (1983). Cognitive deficits in the pathogenesis of autism. *Journal of Child Psychology and Psychiatry, 24,* 513–531.

Rutter, M. (1985). The treatment of autistic children. *Journal of Child Psychology and Psychiatry, 26*(2), 193–214.

Rutter, M., Bailey, A., Simonoff, E., & Pickles, A. (1997). Genetic influences and autism. In F. R. Volkmar & D. J. Cohen (Eds.), *Handbook of autism and pervasive developmental disorders* (2nd ed., pp. 370–387). New York: Wiley.

Rutter, M., & Bartak, L. (1971). Causes of infantile autism: Some considerations from recent research. *Journal of Autism and Childhood Schizophrenia, 1*(1), 20–32.

Rutter, M., & Bartak, L. (1973). Special educational treatment of autistic children: A comparative study. II. Follow-up findings and implications for services. *Journal of Child Psychology and Psychiatry, 14,* 241–270.

Rutter, M., Greenfield, D., & Lockyer, L. (1967). A five to fifteen year follow-up of infantile psychosis: II. Social and behavioral outcome. *British Journal of Psychiatry, 113,* 1183–1189.

Rutter, M., & Schopler, E. (1992). Classification of pervasive developmental disorders: Some concepts and practical considerations. *Journal of Autism and Developmental Disorders, 22,* 459–482.

Scheerer, M., Rothmann, E., & Goldstein, K. (1945). A case of "idiot savant": An experimental study of personality organization. *Psychological Monographs, 58*(4).

Schopler, E., Andrews, C. E., & Strupp, K. (1980). Do autistic children come from upper-middle-class parents? *Journal of Autism and Developmental Disorders, 10,* 91–103.

Schopler, E., & Mesibov, G. (1984). *The effects of autism on the family.* New York: Plenum Press.

Schopler, E., & Mesibov, G. (1992). *High-functioning individuals with autism.* New York: Plenum Press.

Schuler, A. L., Prizant, B. M., & Wetherby, A. M. (1997). Enhancing language and communication development: Prelinguistic approaches. In D. J. Cohen & F. R. Volkmar (Eds.), *Handbook of autism and pervasive developmental disorders* (pp. 539–571). New York: Wiley.

Semel, E., Wiig, E., & Secord, W. (1995). *Clinical Evaluation of Language Fundamentals 3.* San Antonio, TX: Psychological Corporation.

Short, A. B., & Schopler, E. (1988). Factors relating to age of onset in autism. *Journal of Autism and Developmental Disorders, 18,* 207–216.

Siegel, B., Pliner, C., Eschler, J., & Elliot, G. R. (1988). How autistic children are diagnosed: Difficulties in identification of children with multiple developmental delays. *Journal of Developmental and Behavioral Pediatrics, 9,* 199–204.

Sigman, M., Ungerer, J. A., Mundy, P., & Sherman, T. (1987). Cognition in autistic children. In D. J. Cohen & A. M. Donnellan (Eds.), *Handbook of autism and pervasive developmental disorders* (pp. 103–120). New York: Wiley.

Simeonsson, R. J., Olley, J. G., & Rosenthal, S. L. (1987). Early intervention for children with autism. In M. J. Guralnick & F. C. Bennett (Eds.), *The effectiveness of early intervention for at-risk and handicapped children.* New York: Academic Press.

Sparrow, S., Balla, D., & Cicchetti, D. (1984). *Vineland Adaptive Behavior Scales.* Circle Pines, MN: American Guidance Service.

Sparrow, S. S., & Cicchetti, D. V. (1989). The Vineland Adaptive Behavior Scales. In C. S. Newmark (Ed.), *Major psychological assessment instruments* (Vol. 2, pp. 248–272). Boston: Allyn & Bacon.

Stern, D. (1985). *The interpersonal world of the human infant.* New York: Basic Books.

Szatmari, P., Bremner, R., & Nagy, J. N. (1989). Asperger's syndrome: A review of clinical features. *Canadian Journal of Psychiatry, 34*(6), 554–560.

Tager-Flusberg, H. (1993). What language reveals about the understanding of mind in children with autism. In S. Baron-Cohen, H. Tager-Flusberg, & D. J. Cohen (Eds.), *Understanding other minds: Perspectives from autism* (pp. 138–157). Oxford: Oxford University Press.

Tantam, D. (1991). Asperger syndrome in adulthood. In U. Frith (Ed.), *Autism and Asperger syndrome* (pp. 147–183). Cambridge, England: Cambridge University Press.

Towbin, K. E. (1997). Pervasive developmental disorder not otherwise specified. In F.R. Volkmar & D. J. Cohen (Eds.), *Handbook of autism and pervasive developmental disorders* (2nd ed., pp. 123–147). New York: Wiley.

Trevathan, E., & Adams, M. J. (1988). The epidemiology and public health significance of Rett syndrome. *Journal of Child Neurology, 3*(Suppl.), S17–S20.

Trevathan, E., & Naidu, S. (1988). The clinical recognition and differential diagnosis of Rett syndrome. *Journal of Child Neurology, 3*(Suppl.), S6–S16.

Tronick, E. (1980). The primacy of social skills in infancy. In D. B. Sawing, R. C. Hawkins, L. Olzenski Waker, & J. H. Penticuff (Eds.), *Exceptional infant: Vol. 4. Psychosocial risks in infant–environmental transactions* (pp. 82–103). New York: Brunner/Mazel.

Tsai, L. Y. (1987). Pre-, peri-, and neonatal factors in autism. In E. Schopler & G. B. Mesibov (Eds.), *Neurobiological issues in autism* (pp. 180–191). New York: Plenum Press.

Uzgiris, I. C., & Hunt, J. M. (1975). *Assessment in infancy: Ordinal Scales of Psychological Development.* Urbana: University of Illinois Press.

Volkmar, F. R. (1987). Social development. In D. J. Cohen & A. Donnellan (Eds.), *Handbook of autism and pervasive developmental disorders* (pp. 41–60). New York: Wiley.

Volkmar, F. R. (1992). Childhood disintegrative disorder: Issues for DSM-IV. *Journal of Autism and Developmental Disorders, 22*, 625–642.

Volkmar, F. R., Bregman, J., Cohen, D. J., & Cicchetti, D.V. (1988a). DSM-III and DSM-III-R diagnoses of autism. *American Journal of Psychiatry, 145,* 1404–1408.

Volkmar, F. R., Bregman, J., Cohen, D. J., Hooks, M., & Stevenson, J. (1989). An examination of social typologies in autism. *Journal of the American Academy of Child and Adolescent Psychiatry, 28,* 82–86.

Volkmar, F. R., Carter, A., Grossman, J., & Klin, A. (1997a). Social development in autism. In F. R. Volkmar and D. J. Cohen (Eds.), *Handbook of autism and pervasive developmental disorders* (2nd ed., pp. 173–194). New York: Wiley.

Volkmar, F. R., Cicchetti, D. V., Bregman, J., & Cohen, D. J. (1992). Three diagnostic systems for autism: DSM-III, DSM-III-R, and ICD-10. *Journal of Autism and Developmental Disorders, 22,* 483–492.

Volkmar, F. R., & Cohen, D. J. (1988). Diagnosis of pervasive developmental disorders. In B. Lahey & A. Kazdin (Eds.), *Advances in clinical child psychology* (Vol. 2, pp. 249–284). New York: Plenum Press.

Volkmar, F. R., & Cohen, D. J. (1989). Disintegrative disorder or "late onset" autism. *Journal of Child Psychology and Psychiatry, 30,* 717–724.

Volkmar, F. R., Cohen, D. J., Hoshino, Y., Rende, R., & Paul, R. (1988b). Phenomenology and classification of the childhood psychoses. *Psychological Medicine, 18,* 191–201.

Volkmar, F. R., & Klin, A. (1993). Social development in autism: Historical and clinical perspectives. In S. Baron-Cohen, H. Tager-Flusberg, & D. J. Cohen (Eds.), *Understanding other minds: Perspectives from autism* (pp. 40–48). Oxford: Oxford University Press.

Volkmar, F. R., Klin, A., & Cohen, D. J. (1997b). Diagnosis and classification of autism and related conditions: Consensus and issues. In F. R. Volkmar & D. J. Cohen (Eds.), *Handbook of autism and pervasive developmental disorders* (2nd ed., pp. 4–50). New York: Wiley.

Volkmar, F. R., Klin, A., Siegel, B., Szatmari, P., Lord, C., Campbell, M., Freeman, B. J., Cicchetti, D. V., Rutter, M., Kline, W., Buitelaar, J., Hattab, Y., Fombonne, E., Fuentes, J., Werry, J., Stone, W., Kerbeshian, J., Hoshino, Y., Bregman, J., Loveland, K., Szymanski, L., & Towbin, K. (1994). DSM-IV autism/pervasive developmental disorder field trial. *American Journal of Psychiatry, 151,* 1361–1367

Volkmar, F. R., & Nelson, D. S. (1990). Seizure disorders in autism. *Journal of the American Academy of Child and Adolescent Psychiatry, 29,* 127–129.

Volkmar, F. R., & Rutter, M. (1995). Childhood disintegrative disorder: Results of the DSM-IV autism field trial. *Journal of the American Academy of Child and Adolescent Psychiatry, 34,* 1092–1095.

Volkmar, F. R., Stier, D. M., & Cohen, D. J. (1985). Age of recognition of pervasive developmental disorder. *American Journal of Psychiatry, 142,* 1450–1452.

Ward, A. J. (1970). Early infantile autism: Diagnosis, etiology and treatment. *Psychological Bulletin, 73,* 350–362.

Watson, M. S., Leckman, J. R., Annex, B., Breg, W. R., Boles, D., Volkmar, F. R., Cohen, D. J., & Carter, C. (1985). Fragile X in a survey of 75 autistic males. *New England Journal of Medicine, 310*(22), 1462.

Wetherby, A., Schuler, A. L., & Prizant, B. M. (1997). Enhancing language and communication development: Theoretical foundations. In F. R. Volkmar & D. J. Cohen (Eds.), *Handbook of autism and pervasive developmental disorders* (2nd ed., pp. 513–538). New York: Wiley.

Wing, L. (1981). Asperger's syndrome: A clinical account. *Psychological Medicine, 11,* 115–130.

Wing, L. (1991). The relationship between Asperger's syndrome and Kanner's autism. In U. Frith (Ed.), *Autism and Asperger syndrome* (pp. 93–121). Cambridge, England: Cambridge University Press.

Wing, L., & Attwood, A. (1987). Syndromes of autism and atypical development. In D. J. Cohen & A. M. Donnellan (Eds.), *Handbook of autism and pervasive developmental disorders* (pp. 3–19). New York: Wiley.

World Health Organization (WHO). (1992, May). *International Classification of Diseases* (10th rev.): *Chapter 5. Mental and behavioral disorders (including disorders of psychological development). Diagnostic criteria for research (draft for field trials).* Unpublished manuscript.

PART III

Disorders with Broader-Spectrum Effects

11

TURNER SYNDROME

M. PAIGE POWELL
TIMOTHY SCHULTE

Turner syndrome (TS) is one of the most widely known and examined chromosomal abnormalities in females (White, 1994). The syndrome—which is characterized by extremely short stature; a lack of spontaneous development of secondary sexual characteristics, with accompanying infertility; a broad chest; webbed neck; and a myriad of skeletal, renal, and cardiac abnormalities—was first identified in 1938 by Henry H. Turner. It is also referred to in the literature as monsomy X, and gonadal dysgenesis (45,X or 45,X0). In 1959, Ford, Jones, Polani, de Almeida, and Briggs were able to identify the genetic abnormality associated with the syndrome: They linked it with a loss of or an abnormality in one of the two X chromosomes present in females. This defect of the X chromosome can lead to a large number of physical, neuropsychological, and emotional sequelae.

ETIOLOGY

TS occurs in approximately 1 out of every 2,000 to 3,000 live births of female children (Jones, 1988; Orten, 1990; Orten & Orten, 1992; Ross, 1990). However, the actual conception rate for TS is much higher, and it is estimated that only 1% of pregnancies with female fetuses with TS chromosomal abnormalities actually result in live births; the other 99% of the fetuses are spontaneously aborted (Jones, 1988; Temple & Carney, 1993). TS is found across all racial and ethnic groups (Rovet, 1995). In order to understand the chromosomal abnormalities that lead to TS, it is important to understand normal chromosomal patterns.

After conception, the normally developing fetus has 46 chromosomes, which carry the inherited genetic information from the parents. The fetus receives 22 chromosomes from each parent, and an X chromosome from the mother and either an X or a Y chromosome from the father, resulting in 46 chromosomes (23 pairs) in a normal fetus. If the fetus receives an X chromosome from each parent, the child will be female (46,XX). If the fetus receives a Y chromosome from the father, the child will be male (46,XY). Each cell in a person contains exactly the same genetic information, except for the egg cells or the sperm cells. TS occurs when there is an absence of or abnormality in the X chromosome, the sex chromosome, from either parent.

In the case of TS, a number of chromosomal abnormalities can result in the syndrome. The first identified, and most common, form of TS is referred to in the literature as "pure" TS (Jones, 1988; Temple & Carney, 1993). This is referred to as 45,X0, indicating that there is an absence of one of the X chromosomes that the fetus should have received from a parent, usually the paternal chromosome (Jones, 1988). Females with this form of TS have only one X chromosome. Approximately 50% of cases of TS have this genotype. The second most common form of TS is "mosaicism," which occurs in 30–40% of cases. In mosaicism, the cell division that replicates the chromosomes fails to replicate the genetic material completely, and some cells contain a slightly different set of chromosomal material. Mosaicism can occur in females with 45,X0 or in females with the normal chromosomal pattern of 46,XX. Other types of abnormalities occur less frequently; these include a partial deletion of one arm of the X chromosome, or a duplication of one arm of the X chromosome with the loss of the other arm (Jones, 1988; Temple & Carney, 1993). The chromosomal abnormality is thought to occur during the division of the sex cell of the parent, and there does not appear to be a significant maternal age factor (Jones, 1988).

CLINICAL PRESENTATION

Physical Manifestations

There are many physical abnormalities present with TS. These physical problems vary across clients and vary depending on the chromosomal abnormality present. The most obvious and common physical characteristics of TS include extremely short stature, often between 4 feet, 6 inches and 4 feet, 10 inches (Jones, 1988); a short, webbed neck; a broad chest with broadly spaced nipples; cubitus valgus (i.e., an unusual carrying angle for the elbows); a short forth or fifth metacarpal or metatarsal; and a lack of development of secondary sexual characteristics, such as enlarged breasts and pubic hair. The lack of development of secondary sexual characteristics occurs due to ovarian (gonadal) dysgenesis. During the fetal stage of development and after birth, there is a massive loss of oocytes or egg cells (ovarian dysgenesis), which results in a lack of development of the ovaries. This results not only in a failure to develop secondary sexual characteristics, but, for the vast majority of women with TS, in infertility (Jones, 1988).

Girls and women with TS have a wide variety of other skeletal and facial abnormalities, including scoliosis (curvature of the spine), a narrow and high-arched palate, ptosis (drooping eyelids), strabismus, a low posterior hairline, low and rotated ears, and inner-ear defects resulting in recurrent ear infections and hearing problems. Other observable symptoms include hypoplastic or underdeveloped nails, increase in pigmented moles, and lymphedema (swelling of the hands and feet). Finally, serious medical problems can be found in heart defects such as coarctation (narrowing) of the aorta, and in kidney problems (e.g., horseshoe kidney, double or cleft renal pelvis). Further medical complications can include high blood pressure, obesity, diabetes mellitus, Hashimoto thyroiditis, cataracts, and arthritis (Jones, 1988). There is evidence that people with the "pure" form of TS, the 45,X0 type, are likely to have more malformations than people with the mosaic or other forms of TS (Jones, 1988). The common physical manifestations, with their relative percentage of occurrence, are listed in Table 11.1.

TABLE 11.1. Common Physical Characteristics of TS, with Percentage of Occurrence

Characteristic	Percentage
Short stature	100
Ovarian dysgenesis	90
Lymphedema	80
Broad chest with widely spaced nipples	80
Prominent ears	80
Narrow palate	80
Low posterior hairline	80
Small mandible	70
Cubitus valgus	70
Hypoplastic nails	70
Knee anomalies	60
Kidney malformations	60
Webbed neck	50
Short fourth metarcapal/metatarsal	50
Bone dysplasia	50
Excessive pigmented nevi	50

Note. Adapted from Jones (1988). Copyright 1988 by W. B. Saunders Co. Adapted by permission.

For most girls and women with TS, diagnosis of TS has typically occurred during late adolescence. The referral for a genetic evaluation is usually precipitated by the fact that a young woman has failed to begin puberty (Rovet, 1993). Because of the late diagnosis, many children and adults with TS have not received the appropriate medical, psychological, or educational intervention (Rovet, 1993). However, the diagnosis of TS is beginning to occur earlier, during infancy and early childhood (Mathiesen, Reilly, & Skuse, 1992), allowing children to receive appropriate intervention earlier.

Neuropsychological and Psychoeducational Manifestations

Neuropsychological Manifestations

For many years after the discovery of the syndrome, it was widely believed that women with TS were frequently mentally retarded, and this still occasionally continues to be reported (Orten & Orten, 1992). Research has shown that this is not the case, and that girls and women with TS have Verbal IQ (VIQ) score distributions similar to those of the general population (Bender, Puck, Salbenblatt, & Robinson, 1984; Garron, 1977; Lewandowski, Costenbader, & Richman, 1984; McCauley, Ito, & Kay, 1986a; McCauley, Kay, Ito, & Treder, 1987; Money, 1963; Money & Alexander, 1966; Rovet, 1990; Rovet & Netley, 1982; Shaffer, 1962; Waber, 1979). However, the Performance IQ (PIQ) scores tend to be somewhat lower than VIQ scores in women with TS, and these lower-than-expected PIQ scores may result in lower global IQ scores (Rovet, 1995). The lower PIQ scores on the Wechsler scales are due to difficulties in tasks that require visual–spatial processing.

Shaffer (1962) was the first researcher to suggest the presence of a specific cognitive profile for TS. His study documented that women with TS had an average PIQ that was, on average, approximately 19 points lower than their VIQ. The pattern of VIQ scores higher than PIQ scores has been consistently documented in the literature (Bender et al., 1984; Buckley, 1971; Downey et al., 1991; Garron, 1977; Lewandowski et al., 1984; McCauley et al., 1986a, 1987; Money, 1963; Money & Alexander, 1966; Pennington et al., 1985; Rovet, 1990; Rovet & Netley, 1982; Shaffer, 1962; Waber, 1979). The degree of difference between VIQ and PIQ has varied from study to study (see Table 11.2; Lewandowski, 1985; Lewandowski et al., 1984; McGlone, 1985; Netley & Rovet, 1982; Shaffer, 1962). Overall IQ scores for females with TS have covered the full range of normal IQs (Temple & Carney, 1993).

Despite the consistent finding that PIQ is lower than VIQ in most girls and women with TS, a homogeneous cognitive profile has not been documented for females with TS (Rovet, 1990). However, a number of deficits on specific subtests of intelligence scales have been reported. The Wechsler scales have been the assessment instruments most widely used in studying the neuropsychological aspects of TS (see "Assessment," below). In the first study to examine the neuropsychological manifestations of TS (Shaffer, 1962), Verbal Comprehension was found to be high, with poor scores on Performance subtests requiring perceptual organization (Block Design and Object Assembly) and freedom from distractibility (Arithmetic and Digit Span). These findings have been confirmed across the literature. Studies that have found specific Wechsler Performance subtest deficits in women and girls with TS, compared to control subjects, are listed in Table 11.3. Only subtests that were found to be deficient in at least two studies are included in the table.

Although the literature has been clear and consistent regarding the findings of deficiencies in nonverbal, visual–spatial areas in TS, it has been less clear about the exact nature and cause of the deficits. Across studies, a wide variety of deficits have been noted. The most widely reported deficits are visual–spatial processing deficits (Downey et al., 1991; Money, 1993; Robinson et al., 1986; Rovet, 1993; Rovet & Netley, 1982; Temple & Carney, 1995). Other specific deficits that have been reported include problems with visual memory (Alexander & Money, 1966; Downey et al., 1991; Lewandowski, 1985; Lewandowski et al., 1984), deficits in visual constructional skills (Downey et al., 1991; McCauley et al., 1987; Robinson et al., 1986; Temple & Carney, 1995), difficulties with Arithmetic (Buchanan, Paulovic, & Rovet, 1998; Downey et al., 1991; Garron, 1977; Money & Alexander, 1966; Shaffer, 1962), and deficits in working memory (Berch, 1996; Buchanan et al., 1998). The cognitive deficits that have been identified in TS do appear to continue across the lifespan (Downey et al., 1991; Garron, 1977).

Many studies have attempted to identify the actual area of dysfunction within the brain that leads to the typical cognitive deficits seen with TS. Currently there are two theories with some empirical support. Both of these theories revolve around the issue of lateralization of the brain. The human brain has two hemispheres, left and right, each of which is responsible for certain cognitive tasks (i.e., the brain is lateralized). The left hemisphere is thought to be responsible for language and symbolic operations. The right

TABLE 11.2. Differences in VIQ and PIQ across Studies

Study	VIQ–PIQ difference
Shaffer (1962)	18 to 19 points
Netley & Rovet (1982)	11.91 points
Rovet & Netley (1982)	12.20 to 14.74 points
Lewandowski et al. (1984)	21 points
McGlone (1985)	12.5 points
Pennington et al. (1985)	8 points
Downey et al. (1991)	12.8 points
Shucard et al. (1992)	3.8 points

TABLE 11.3. Wechsler Performance Scale Subtest Weaknesses

Study	Arithmetic	Digit span	Object asembly	Block design	Digit symbol
Dellantonio et al. (1984)			×	×	×
Downey et al. (1991)	×	×	×	×	×
Lewandowski et al. (1984)			×	×	
Money (1963, 1964)	×	×	×	×	
Rovet (1993)		×		×	
Shucard et al. (1992)			×	×	
Temple & Carney (1995)			×		

hemisphere is thought to be responsible for nonverbal information processing (Watson, 1981).

The first theory regarding dysfunction within the brain and lateralization in TS is that women and girls with TS have generalized, diffuse right-hemispheric dysfunction (Dellantonio et al., 1984; Kolb & Heaton, 1975; Rovet, 1995; Rovet & Netley, 1981; Shucard, Shucard, Clopper, & Schachter, 1992; Silbert, Wolff, & Lilienthal, 1977). This makes intuitive sense in view of the findings that women and girls with TS tend to have intact verbal skills (left hemisphere) and difficulties with nonverbal, visual–spatial tasks (right hemisphere). Little physical evidence has been obtained through the use of computed tomography scans or electroencephalography to support specific abnormalities (Nielsen, Nyborg, & Dahl, 1977; Rovet, 1995); however, Shucard et al. (1992) did find electrophysical evidence to support right-hemispheric abnormality.

The second theory suggests that there is a lack of, or failure in, development of normal lateralization of the brain in people with TS. Rovet (1990) found that people with TS used their left hemispheres more than normal controls did when processing nonverbal information. Rovet concluded that this suggests that the left hemisphere is compensating for a weaker right hemisphere, resulting in a lack of normal lateralization of the brain.

Psychoeducational Manifestations

Given the various neuropsychological deficits found with TS—specifically, difficulties with visual–spatial, visual–motor, and memory tasks—it is not surprising that educational difficulties are also associated with TS. The most common learning problem for girls with TS is in the area of mathematics. Many authors have reported that TS is associated with poorer performance on the Arithmetic subtests of the Wechsler scales (Downey et al., 1991; Garron, 1977; Money & Alexander, 1966; Shaffer, 1962). In addition, girls with TS have been found to score an average of 2 years behind grade level on mathematics achievement tests (Rovet, 1995). Mazzocco (1998) and Siegel, Clopper, and Stabler (1998) found relatively low achievement in mathematics. Rovet (1995) reported that the mathematics problems appear to be more related to the conceptual/factual area than to the actual computational area. She also reported that older girls are more likely to have a mathematics disability than younger girls, probably due to the fact that math becomes more conceptual and relies more on memory skills as children progress through school. In addition, Rovet reported that spelling and reading skills appear to remain intact; some girls may experience difficulty with reading decoding skills, but not comprehension skills. Finally, Rovet (1993) noted that reading disabilities at times coexist with the mathematics disabilities in TS, but that they have not been found to occur alone.

A growing body of literature has begun to compare children with TS to children who have nonverbal learning disabilities (NLDs) (Rovet, 1995; Williams, Richman, & Yarbrough, 1992). Children with NLDs are a subgroup of learning-disabled children who have particular difficulty with visual perceptual skills. These skill deficits result in difficulties with mathematics, nonverbal reasoning, and socialization (Strang & Rourke, 1983). There is also a VIQ-PIQ discrepancy in NLDs, with VIQ being higher than PIQ. NLDs are most common in children who have identifiable brain disorders such as neurofibromatosis, head injuries, or loss or absence of brain tissue, as well as in children who have undergone radiation treatment for cancer (Rourke, 1985).

Correlations between Phenotype and Neuropsychological and Educational Deficits

As with the physical features associated with TS, there appears to be extensive heterogeneity in the neuropsychological deficits associated with TS. Several studies have examined the impact of phenotype (i.e., 45,X0 vs. mosaicism) on these deficits. As a rule, it has been found that TS subjects with the mosaic form of TS tend to have fewer cognitive and visual–spatial difficulties than girls with the "pure" form of TS (Bender, Linden, & Robinson, 1994; El Abd, Turk, & Hill, 1995; Rovet & Ireland, 1994; Temple & Carney, 1993).

Psychosocial Aspects

Over the past 20 years, an increasing amount of attention has been given to the psychosocial aspects of TS. Overall, research has found that girls and women with TS tend to have fewer severe mental disorders than those found in the general population of females. Women with TS are less likely to experience the "positive" symptomatology of psychopathology, such as acting-out behaviors, suicidal ideation, and alcohol/drug use. However, they do appear to experience more of the "negative" symptomatology of psychopathology, such as a lack of emotional reactivity and few or poor relationships with peers and other intimates (Downey, Ehrhardt, Gruen, Bell, & Morishima, 1989). Other personality characteristics that have been commonly associated with TS have included high stress tolerance, unassertiveness, overcompliance, and a lack of emotional maturity (Baekgaard, Nyborg, & Nielsen, 1978; Downey et al., 1989; Higurashi et al., 1986; McCauley et al., 1986a; McCauley, Ross, Kushner, & Culter, 1995; McCauley, Sybert, & Ehrhardt, 1986b; Nielsen et al., 1977).

Issues in Childhood and Adolescence

The three major psychosocial areas of concern for girls with TS are the areas of self-esteem, peer relationships, and social isolation—areas that appear to be highly interrelated. Across studies, girls with TS have been found to have low self-esteem (McCauley et al., 1986a, 1995; Perheentupa et al., 1974). Among the major sources contributing to a child's sense of self-worth are the child's interactions with others, especially peers and family members. Major differences in appearance, such as short stature and the other physical anomalies associated with TS, can have a lasting impact on a developing child's sense of self and self-worth. Short children are often teased and bullied by peers at school, which may adversely affect their self-esteem (Skuse, 1987), and this appears to be a major problem for girls with TS (McCauley et al., 1986a). A child with TS, who may be less assertive than her peers (Skuse, 1987), may have greater difficulty in handling the teasing in a proactive manner. In addition, because children are often treated according to the age they appear to be rather than their actual chronological age, a child or adolescent with TS may experience the added burden of being treated like a much younger child and not having the behavioral expectations that would correspond to her chronological age (Alley, 1983). This again will set her apart from her peers and have an impact upon self-esteem. Furthermore, it has been found that for girls with TS, the greater the number of physical anomalies, the lower the self-esteem (El Abd et al., 1995). Finally, difficulties with motor coordination and hearing difficulties due to inner-ear abnormalities may affect self-esteem as well (El Abd et al., 1995).

Academic difficulties can also result in lowered self-esteem in children. There is a vast literature base examining the impact of learning disabilities on the development of a child's self-esteem and feelings of self-worth (Taylor, 1989). The psychosocial problems that are evident in children with learning disabilities, such as poor task motivation, poor social skills, externalizing behaviors, depression, and somatic complaints, may continue into adulthood (Jorm, Share, Matthews, & Maclean, 1986).

As girls with TS grow older, the delay in the onset of puberty may further decrease their self-esteem during adolescence (Skuse, 1987). There has been some evidence to suggest that girls with TS have average self-esteem until puberty, at which time they begin to fall behind their peers physically and socially, and their self-esteem decreases. As they fall behind, they begin to withdraw and are viewed as socially immature (Perheentupa et al., 1974). Problems with social isolation and poor peer relations are reported across the literature (Nielsen et al., 1977; Rovet, 1993; Skuse, 1987). As girls are teased for their physical abnormalities, including short stature, they may withdraw from peer interactions. Poor peer relations may also be due to hormonal deficits. As puberty is delayed, children with TS fail to go through the hormonal changes of adolescence and may be seen as emotionally immature as well as physically immature (Skuse, 1987). They may prefer to be with children younger than themselves (McCauley et al., 1995; Rovet & Ireland, 1994). Social difficulties may also be related to the visual–spatial processing problems associated with TS, because children with these difficulties, including girls with TS, often have problems with understanding the social cues and facial expressions of others (affective discrimination) (McCauley et al., 1987; Waber, 1979).

Other psychosocial difficulties that have been associated with TS are behavior problems. Skuse, Cave, O'Herlihy, and South (1998) found that a large number of the adolescent girls in their study exhibited adjustment problems in areas such as somatic symptoms, anxiety, and social immaturity. Sonis et al. (1983) found that parents of girls with TS reported more behavior problems for their daughters than did parents of girls in a non-TS control group. The parents of the TS group reported that their daughters were experiencing poor peer relationships, immaturity, and poor attention skills. In an effort to rule out short stature as the cause for the problems that girls with TS experience, McCauley et al. (1986a) compared the TS subjects with girls of short stature. The results of that study indicated that girls with TS had more behavior problems and poorer peer relationships than their constitutionally short counterparts. The girls were reported by parents and teachers to be socially immature and to have many problems associated with externalizing behavior, such as impulsivity, overactivity, and poor attention span. Rovet (1995) also found more "hyperactivity" among girls with TS. Rovet and Ireland (1994) found that girls with TS tended to score lower on measures of social competence and higher on measures of general behavior problems. These behavior problems were most noticeable in the areas of social relationships, attention problems, immaturity, hyperactivity, and anxiety. In addition, girls with TS were found to experience more problems in school. These problems do appear to increase across childhood (Skuse, 1987).

Finally, there have also been reports of a connection between the occurrence of anorexia nervosa in adolescents and adults with TS and the advent of hormone therapy (Kron, Katz, Gorzynski, & Weiner, 1977; Muhs & Lieberz, 1993; Taipale, Niittymaki, & Nevalainen, 1982). This appears to be related to the onset of sexual development and to anxiety caused by the new sexual feelings that occur. It is believed that the development of anorexia nervosa in TS subjects who have begun hormonal treatment has an etiology similar to that in normal girls (Muhs & Lieberz, 1993; Taipale et al., 1982). It has also been attributed to a distorted body image caused by a combination of the normal "stocky" body build associated with TS and the perceptual deficits that exist with TS (Darby, Garfinkel, Vale, Kirwan, & Brown, 1981).

Issues in Adulthood

Like the cognitive aspects of TS, many of the psychosocial difficulties reported in children with TS continue into adulthood. Women with TS have also been found to experience difficulties with self-esteem (McCauley et al., 1986b; Pavlidis, McCauley, & Sybert, 1995). The impaired development of secondary sexual characteristics and the subsequent infertility often contribute to low self-esteem in adults with TS (Skuse, 1987; El Abd et al., 1995; Pavlidis et al., 1995). In addition, women with TS may continue to be less emotionally mature and continue to experience poor, or a low number of, peer relationships (Nielsen et al., 1977).

As reported above, children with TS may tend to be more hyperactive than their same-age peers (McCauley et al., 1986a; Rovet, 1995; Rovet & Ireland, 1994; Sonis et al., 1983); however, adults with TS may have lower levels of activity than expected (Downey et al., 1989; Higurashi et al., 1986; Money & Mittenthal, 1970; Pavlidis et al., 1995; Rovet, 1995). The reason for this difference is not readily discernible. In addition, adult women with TS may be likely to experience mild depressive symptomatology. However, there does not appear to be a consistent pattern of psychological problems, nor does there seem to be an increase in the frequency of psychological problems over that seen in the general population (Money & Mittenthal, 1970; Shaffer, 1962). In addition, Orten and Orten (1992) found that women with TS reported that they were satisfied with their lives and happy. Women with TS do appear to be less independent of their parents and less likely to marry or live with partners than the general population (Nielsen et al., 1977; Nielsen & Stradiot, 1987; Orten & Orten, 1992).

Given the reported perceptual and educational problems associated with TS, another area of potential concern is the educational and occupational achievement of adults with TS. Despite the findings that the perceptual and educational difficulties found in childhood continue into adulthood (Garron, 1977; Nielsen & Stradiot, 1987), women with TS have been found to perform at an average or above-average level academically and to be gainfully employed in a wide variety of occupations (Nielsen et al., 1977; Nielsen & Stradiot, 1987; Orten & Orten, 1992).

Despite the delay in or lack of development of secondary sexual characteristics, it does appear that women with TS have a strong female gender identity (Ehrhardt, Greenberg, & Money, 1970; Money & Mittenthal, 1970). However, women with TS may be less sexually active than average (Pavlidis et al., 1995). They also report less interest in sexual relationships (Downey et al., 1989) Even with this lack of sexual activity, and maybe because of the lack of interest in sexual relationships, women with TS report moderate to high levels of sexual satisfaction (Pavlidis et al., 1995). However, higher sexual satisfaction was associated with higher frequency of sexual intercourse and a higher health status. Raboch, Kobilkova, Horejsi, Starka, and Raboch (1987) have hypothesized that the lower levels of interest in sex may be related to lower levels of sexual hormones. They also found that once women with TS were in stable, good relationships, any differences in interest and participation in sexual relationships disappeared.

Health status appears to be significantly related to a number of psychosocial issues for adults with TS. Pavlidis et al. (1995) found that health status was associated with higher self-esteem and greater sexual satisfaction

Correlations between Phenotype and Psychosocial Problems

Again, as with physical manifestations and neuropsychological manifestations, there is a wide homogeneity in psychosocial difficulties. These also appear to be related to phenotype. Children and adults with the mosaicism phenotype appear to have fewer behavioral difficulties than other forms of TS (Pasaro Mendez, Fernandez, Goyanes, & Mendez, 1994; Rovet & Ireland, 1994; Temple & Carney, 1993).

Families

At this writing, there has been only one study examining the reactions of parents to the diagnosis of TS in their daughters (Faust, Rosenfeld, Wilson, Durham & Vardopoulos, 1995). This study found that mothers of girls with TS made a better psychological adjustment to the diagnosis of TS if they utilized a more problem-focused than emotion-focused coping style. Mothers who used an emotion-focused coping style, specifically wishful thinking, experienced more depressive symptomatology than mothers who were more problem-focused. In addition, the administration of growth hormone and the children's subsequent growth in stature had a very powerful impact on the adjustment of the mothers, with less depression being found in mothers whose daughters were receiving growth hormone. The study also found that neither coping styles nor the administration of growth hormone seemed related to reports of depressive symptomatology in fathers.

Parents of girls with TS are likely to experience a significant amount of stress; this appears to surround issues of communicating about their daughters' needs to school personnel, setting up and supervising peer relationships, and attempting to normalize their children's appearance (Williams, 1995). In addition, parents of TS girls are very likely to take charge in an effort to prevent or to solve problems for their daughters (Williams, 1995). This infantilizing of their daughters can have a negative impact on the girls' development (Nielsen & Stradiot, 1987).

In a study of the level of psychopathology found with TS subjects, Money and Mittenthal (1970) concluded that it was highly related to the presence of psychopathology in the subjects' parents. In addition, they found that the relationship between a daughter and her parents had an impact on the development of psychopathology: Having parents who were rejecting or overprotective was more likely to lead to a poor psychosocial outcome in a daughter. Nielsen et al. (1977) also concluded that psychopathology was more likely to be related to difficulties within a family than to TS itself. It is unclear whether the psychopathology in the parents in this study predated the diagnosis of TS in the daughters or was a result of the strain of having a child with a chronic illness.

ASSESSMENT

Given the wide variety of difficulties that may be associated with TS, every child with this syndrome must be provided with a thorough psychoeducational evaluation. It is critical that psychoeducational problems be identified and remediated early in a child's academic career (Rovet, 1993). In order to assess for all of the possible sequelae of TS, it is important to develop a comprehensive battery. This battery should include, at a minimum, measures of intelligence, achievement (including instruments designed for intense assessment of mathematics and reading), nonverbal (visual perceptual) skills, memory, and personality. In addition to the areas listed above, assessment utilizing the traditional neuropsychological batteries, the Halstead–Reitan (Reitan & Wolfson, 1985) and the Luria–Nebraska (Golden, Purish, & Hammeke, 1985), may be useful. The following is not intended to be a thorough examination of all possible instruments for assessment in these areas.

Cognitive Measures

The first area of importance in the assessment of a child with TS is an examination of the child's current intellectual abilities. Given the wide number of studies that have utilized the Wechsler scales, they would appear to be the instruments of choice (Downey et al., 1991; Lewandowski et al., 1984; McCauley et al., 1995; Netley & Rovet, 1982; Pennington et al., 1985; Rovet, 1993; Rovet & Netley, 1982; Temple & Carney, 1993, 1995; Williams, 1994). The Wechsler scales provide a VIQ score, a PIQ score, a Full Scale IQ score, and several factor-analytic scores (Verbal Comprehension, Perceptual Organization, and Freedom from Distractibility scores), all of which can be helpful in diagnosing cognitive deficits in people with TS. All of the Wechsler scales have excellent reliability and validity. The Wechsler Preschool and Primary Scale of Intelligence—Revised (WPPSI-R; Wechsler, 1989) covers children aged 4 years, 0 months to 6 years, 6 months. The third edition of the Wechsler Intelligence Scale for Children (WISC-III; Wechsler, 1991) measures cognitive abilities in children aged 6 years, 0 months to 16 years, 11 months. The third edition of the Wechsler Adult Intelligence Scale (WAIS-III; Wechsler, 1997) is used to evaluated people aged 16 years, 0 months to 74 years, 11 months.

In addition to the Wechsler scales, other cognitive measures may also prove helpful in evaluating people with TS. The fourth edition of the Stanford–Binet Intelligence Scale (Thorndike, Hagen, & Sattler, 1986) yields a composite score and area scores in Verbal Reasoning, Abstract/Visual Reasoning, Quantitative Reasoning, and Short-Term Memory. These scores can provide critical information for the assessment and remediation of people with TS. The Stanford–Binet measures cognitive abilities in people aged 2 years, 0 months to 23 years, 11 months. For very young children, the Bayley Scales of Infant Development (Bayley, 1969), the Denver Developmental Screening Test—Revised (Frankenburg, Dodds, Fandal, Kazuk, & Cohr, 1975) and the Learning Acquisition Profile—D (LAP-D; LeMay, Griffen, & Sanford, 1992) can also provide useful information. The Bayley scales are appropriate for children aged 2 months to 2 years, 6 months; they provide a Mental Developmental Index and a Psychomotor Developmental Index. The Denver is appropriate for children from birth through 6 years of age and yields scores in four domains: Personal–Social, Fine Motor, Language, and Gross Motor. The LAP-D assesses four major areas: Fine Motor, Cognitive, Language, and Gross Motor skills. It is appropriate for children aged 2 years, 6 months to 6 years.

Achievement Measures

Academic achievement is another critical area for assessment in TS. It is critical for learning disabilities to be diagnosed so that appropriate interventions can be implemented. Given the likelihood of academic problems, especially in the area of mathematics, it is very important to obtain a thorough educational evaluation. Instruments of choice may include the Woodcock–Johnson Psycho-Educational Battery—Revised (Woodcock & Johnson, 1989), the Wechsler Individual Achievement Test (WIAT; Wechsler, 1992), the Peabody Individual Achievement Test—Revised (PIAT-R; Markwardt, 1989) and the Kaufman Tests of Educational Achievement (K-TEA; Kaufman & Kaufman, 1985).

The Woodcock–Johnson contains 27 tests that are divided into three batteries: the Tests of Cognitive Ability, the Tests of Achievement, and the Tests of Interest Level. The first two batteries are of particular interest in the assessment of people with TS, because they yield useful cluster scores. The cognitive battery yields a Broad Cognitive score and scores for Verbal Ability, Reasoning, Perceptual Speed, Memory, Reading Aptitude, Mathematics Aptitude, Written Language Aptitude, and Knowledge Aptitude. The achievement battery yields cluster scores in Reading, Mathematics, Written Language, Knowledge, and Skills. The Woodcock–Johnson is appropriate for people aged 2 years, 0 months to 79 years.

The WIAT consists of eight subtests that yield standard scores for Reading, Mathematics, Language, and Writing, as well as a Total composite score. There are norms available for children aged 5 years, 0 months to 19 years, 11 months. The PIAT-R is normed for children 5 years, 0 months to 18 years, 11 months. It has seven subtests and yields composite Reading and Total scores. The K-TEA is appropriate for people aged 6 years through 18 years and yields scores in the areas of Reading Decoding, Reading Comprehension, Mathematics Application, Mathematics Computation, and Spelling.

In addition to the broad achievement measures mentioned above, more specialized instruments may be of use in diagnosing learning disabilities and designing intervention strategies. The KeyMath Diagnostic Arithmetic Test—Revised (Connolly, 1988) provides very specific information regarding areas of deficiency in mathematics (content, operations, and applications). Specific reading tests, such as the third edition of the Gray Oral Reading Tests (Wiederholt & Bryant, 1992), measure rate, accuracy, and comprehension.

Visual Perceptual Measures

Because people with TS may exhibit a variety of visual perceptual problems, it is important to obtain a broad range of assessment in this area. Visual perceptual instruments can be divided into a number of areas. The first area is visual perceptual or gestalt integration. The Woodcock–Johnson cognitive battery, specifically the spatial relations and visual matching subtests, may be helpful. The Embedded Figures Test (10 years and up) and the Children's Embedded Figures Test (5 to 10 years of age) (Witkin, Oltman, Raskin, & Karp, 1971) can also be used to assess visual perceptual integration. Finally, the Test of Visual Perceptual Skills (Nonmotor)—Revised (Gardner, 1996) can be used. Visual–spatial skills can be measured with Benton's Line Orientation Task (Benton, Varney, & de Hamshef, 1978) or the Raven Colored Progressive Matrices (Raven, Court, & Raven, 1977). There are a number of instruments designed to assess visual constructional skills, including the Bender Visual Motor Gestalt Test (Koppitz, 1969), the Beery–Buktenica Developmental Test of Visual Motor Integration—Revised (Beery, 1997), the Benton Visual Retention

Test—Revised (Benton, 1963), the Draw-a-Person Test (Harris, 1963), and the Block Design and Object Assembly subtests of the WPPSI-R, WISC-III, and WAIS-III (Wechsler, 1989, 1991, 1997). In addition, the Visual Aural Digit Span Test (Koppitz, 1977) can be used with children aged 5 years, 6 months to 12 years for measuring the processing of aural and visual stimuli, sequencing, and recall.

Memory Measures

The Wide Range Assessment of Memory and Learning (WRAML; Sheslow & Adams, 1990) and the Test of Memory and Learning (TOMAL; Reynolds & Bigler, 1994) can be used to evaluate memory in children. The WRAML is normed for children 5 years to 17 years of age and yields four basic scores: Verbal Memory, Visual Memory, Learning, and Delayed Recall. The TOMAL is normed for children 5 years, 0 months, 0 days to 19 years, 11 months, 30 days. The standard battery includes 10 subtests and yields four main scores: Verbal Memory Index, Nonverbal Memory Index, Composite Memory Index and Delayed Recall Index. The TOMAL also includes five supplementary tests that yield the following supplementary scores when a more detailed view is needed: Sequential Recall Index, Free Recall Index, Associative Recall Index, Learning Index, and Attention/Concentration Index.

Personality Measures

Assessment of psychological adjustment is very important in evaluating a child with TS. Personality measures can be divided into three general categories: parent/teacher reports, child self-reports, and projective measures. In each of these categories, it is essential to assess psychological symptomatology, self-esteem, and social skills that may require clinical attention.

Parent and teacher report measures can include general instruments, such as the Behavior Assessment System for Children (BASC; Reynolds & Kamphaus, 1992) or the Child Behavior Checklist (CBCL; Achenbach, 1992). The BASC has a stratified sample that is based on height, and thus may be most appropriate for the assessment of girls with TS. The assessment should also include measures designed to assess for more specific problems, such as the Conners Rating Scales for Children (Conners, 1990), the Attention Deficit Disorders Evaluation Scale (McCarney, 1989), and the Social Skills Rating System (Gresham & Elliot, 1990).

Self-report measures can also include instruments designed to assess more general psychopathology, such as the BASC (Reynolds & Kamphaus, 1992), the Youth Self-Report of the CBCL (Achenbach, 1991), the Minnesota Multiphasic Personality Inventory—Adolescent (Butcher et al., 1992) and the Millon Adolescent Personality Inventory (Millon, Green, & Meagher, 1982). Specific instruments for depressive symptomatology, such as the Children's Depression Inventory (Kovacs, 1992) or the Reynolds Adolescent Depression Scale (Reynolds, 1986); for anxiety, such as the Revised Children's Manifest Anxiety Scale (Reynolds & Richmond, 1985); and for self-esteem, such as the Piers–Harris Children's Self-Concept Scale (Piers, 1984), may be important.

Finally, projective measures may aid in the assessment of some children. Instruments that can be used include the Rorschach Psychodiagnostic (Rorschach, 1942) and the Roberts Apperception Test for Children (McArthur & Roberts, 1987). These instruments can provide information regarding information-processing and coping styles.

INTERVENTIONS

Intervention for children and adults with TS is critical for a positive life outcome. A girl or woman with TS is at risk for the development of a wide range of sequelae. The clinical needs of the TS patient fall across four areas: medical, social, academic, and sexual issues (Mullins, Lynch, Orten, & Youll, 1991).

Medical Interventions

Because a wide variety of medical problems can occur with TS, it is critical that regular medical care be obtained (Mullins et al., 1991; Orten, 1990; Orten & Orten, 1994; Rovet, 1995). It is also critical that the girl or woman with TS and her family receive accurate and sensitive medical information (Orten, 1990). Medical intervention with TS can take many different forms. The most common medical intervention is supportive therapy. This includes growth hormone therapy to stimulate growth and thus to increase adult height, and estrogen replacement therapy to stimulate the development of secondary sexual characteristics and healthy bones and tissue. With early and timely use of estrogen and growth hormone, most girls with TS can be brought to normal height (Rosenfeld et al., 1992). This can have a critical impact on the development of self-esteem in these children. If the teasing that begins when a child with TS begins to lag behind her peers can be avoided by helping the child reach her developmental/physical milestones on time, self-esteem may be spared (Orten, 1990; Orten & Orten, 1994; Perheentupa et al., 1974).

Many other medical interventions can improve the quality of a TS patient's life. With recent advances in fertility interventions, such as *in vitro* fertilization with a donor egg, pregnancy is now a possibility for some women with TS and their partners. Surgical interventions may be necessary as a result of cardiac and renal abnormalities, ptosis, strabismus, and inner-ear defects. In addition, speech or hearing interventions may be necessary for girls with high-arched palates or hearing loss due to inner-ear defects (Rovet, 1995).

Psychosocial Interventions

As the review above has shown, girls and women with TS can experience a wide variety of psychosocial problems. For our purposes here, these difficulties are divided into two categories. The first area for attention is the treatment of issues of concern associated with the diagnosis of TS. The second area is the treatment of specific symptomatology.

Issues of Concern in TS

One of the first issues that people diagnosed with TS have to cope with is the diagnosis of a chronic syndrome with wide-ranging ramifications. Persons who are diagnosed with a chronic, lifelong illness must adapt to both the physical and psychological sequelae of the illness, as well as the fact that their life and potentially their view of self has been altered. Russo (1986) and Varni and Wallander (1988) discuss the need for people with chronic illnesses to address the specific stressors that affect their lives and to develop positive coping strategies to deal with these stressors. Positive adjustments lead to resilience, and poor adjustment leads to vulnerability to stressors (Varni & Wallander, 1988). Self-esteem issues are often involved in this adjustment. Both a person with TS and her family members will have many emotional reactions at the time of diagnosis, and these reactions are similar to those experienced when any major medical condition is diagnosed (Orten & Orten, 1994). According to Orten and Orten, these reactions can fall into four categories.

The first category of adjustment is the need to resolve "the personal meaning of TS" (Orten & Orten, 1994, p. 241). The age at diagnosis will have an impact on the initial issues involved in obtaining personal meaning. For younger children, the main issues may revolve around medical aspects of the syndrome and potential medical interventions (treatments, hospitalizations, and the like). During the teenage years, issues may include "being different" from others and the physical anomalies the patients may have. For late adolescents and adults, issues surrounding fertility and parenthood may arise. Coming to terms with these issues may be complicated by the severity of the medical problems that a girl or woman faces. The impact of the diagnosis can also be mediated by the parents' reactions to the diagnosis (Orten & Orten, 1994).

A second category of adjustment is coping with the reactions of others, especially reactions to the patients' short stature. Teasing about short stature often begins during the elementary school years. If growth hormone therapy is initiated at the appropriate times, this problem may be avoided. However, girls with TS may also be teased about other physical abnormalities. For adult women, short stature and youthful appearance can cause difficulties in the workplace. Teaching ways to cope and deal with teasing and potential discrimination in a positive and helpful manner is a critical part of intervention for girls and women with TS (Orten & Orten, 1994).

Deciding whether and, if so, when to tell others about the diagnosis is another issue of particular concern to girls and women with TS. For children, one form this question may take is whether or not to inform the school about the diagnosis. As with any medical or psychological problem, informing the school can lead to positive outcomes, such as greater understanding of and more accommodations to the special needs of the child; however, it can also result in the child's being stigmatized and treated differently in a negative way. The decision to inform or not to inform the school is one that needs to be made jointly by the treatment team, the parents, and the child if she is mature enough to participate in the decision (Orten & Orten, 1994).

Whether or not to tell dating partners or potential intimate relationships about TS is a question that is often faced in adulthood. Issues surrounding fertility and parenthood again become critical. These issues can have an impact on a partner as well as a woman with TS.

A final area that girls and women have to deal with when coming to terms with TS are the physical problems and their impact on lifestyle and quality of life. Often this involves grieving for lost abilities. It is important for girls and women to understand the potential medical and cognitive implications of TS, and to deal with these on a day-to-day basis.

One of the major mediating factors in coping with stress is perceived social support (Varni, 1987; Varni, Rubinfeld, Talbot, & Setoguchi, 1989). Because of this, a support group model for intervention may be very appropriate. Support groups, with members who face similar issues, can provide reassurance, information, and advice. Psychoeducational models often meet the needs and desires of participants in TS support groups (Mullins et al., 1991). Attention to family members and to their coping with the diagnosis and sequelae of TS is also important, because families can be a major source of support for some girls and women (Mullins et al., 1991; Orten & Orten, 1994). A survey by Orten and Orten (1992) found that a large number of parents were provided with incomplete and pessimistic medical explanations at the time of diagnosis, and that the parents were very dissatisfied (and at times angry) with the explanations that they were given. Thus one of the first areas of intervention with families is to assure that they receive accurate and adequate medical, psychological, and developmental information regarding TS (Orten, 1990). (Table 11.4 lists a number of sources for such information.) In addition, good family communication is important in helping girls and women with TS cope with issues surrounding it. Finally, individual therapy may be important for some girls and women at various stages of their lives.

Other Specific Psychosocial Symptomatology

As mentioned above, there are several areas of potential psychosocial symptomatology for girls and women with TS. The first is the area of social skills. Most interventions in this area have been cognitive-behavioral in nature. Target behaviors have included increasing the rate of social interaction, enhancing prosocial skills, and decreasing antisocial or aggressive behaviors. Interventions have included social problem-solving training, anger coping training, coaching, and behavioral rehearsal. These interventions can take place in individual therapy or groups (Dodge, 1989). The second major area of concern is the symptomatology of hyperactivity and inattention in some girls with TS. The most common treatment approaches for these problems are cognitive-behavioral and psychopharmacological or a combination of the two (Barkley, 1989). The National Cooperation Growth Study supported the need for a combination of educational, behavioral, and medical treatment (Siegel et al., 1998).

TABLE 11.4. Sources for Information on TS

Turner's Syndrome Society of the United States
1313 Southeast 5th Street
Suite 327
Minneapolis, MN 55414
(800) 365-9944
http://www.turner-syndrome-us-org

This is a nonprofit organization with the following mission: to increase public awareness, to increase understanding of the people who are affected by TS, to provide a forum for those affected by TS to become acquainted with one another, and to provide an opportunity for interaction between health care professionals and those affected by TS. The society sponsors a conference each year and offers a number of publications on TS.

World Wide Web resources
    http://www.eden.com/~ploof/turners — A Web site that is written by a parent
    http://www.icondata.com/health/pedbase/files/turnersy.htm — A Web site with clinical information about TS from a pediatric data base
    http://www.ami-med.com/peds/scr/000379sc.htm — Clinical description of TS
    http://www.endo-society.org/pubaffai/factshee/turner.htm — Fact sheet on TS

On-line newsgroups of interest
    alt.support.turner-syndrom — TS support group
    alt.support.short — Support group for short men and women
    alt.infertility — Infertility support group
    misc.health.infertility — Infertility support group

Academic Interventions

Early intervention is critical in helping children with learning disabilities. The first issues of concern when implementing academic interventions are the individual needs of each child. Some children will require placement in a special education program, while others may benefit from tutoring alone. It is also important to make sure that the expectations for each child are developmentally appropriate and follow a developmental sequence. In addition, interventions work best when parents and the school work as a team with the child to deal with the special needs of the child. Finally, it is very helpful to utilize areas of strength to remediate or circumvent areas of weakness. This is one of the reasons why a thorough educational assessment is important. Although there are a wide variety of intervention models for working with children with special academic needs, it is most critical that the intervention "fit" a child with TS and her personal strengths and weaknesses.

The only formal study that has examined an academic intervention with girls with TS was conducted by Williams et al. (1992). In that study, the girls with TS were compared to children with NLDs, and an intervention commonly used with NLD children—cognitive behavior modification or strategy training (Meichenbaum, 1985)—was utilized with girls with TS. The intervention included the use of verbal mediation skills for planning and executing a learning task. This allowed the TS subjects to use a well-developed skill area, their verbal skills, to help them learn ways of performing a nonverbal task. The results of this study showed a significant improvement in spatial task performance in both the TS group and the NLD group following the cognitive behavior modification training. This suggests that girls with TS may be responsive to remediation of their educational deficits.

SUMMARY AND CONCLUSIONS

TS, a chromosomal abnormality that affects only females, can result in a myriad of life-long physical/medical, psychosocial, and educational problems. The type and severity of the problems may vary widely across patients. However, there are some hallmark symptoms associated with the syndrome; these include short stature, failure to develop secondary sexual characteristics at puberty, infertility, visual perceptual difficulties, academic problems with mathematics, and social skill difficulties. Many of the physical/medical problems can be dealt with through supportive therapy, including hormone replacement therapy. Special attention should be given to the psychosocial sequelae of the syndrome, and appropriate therapeutic interventions should be undertaken. Finally, early and appropriate intervention is critical for continued academic success. With the proper support, encouragement, and interventions, girls and women with TS can live long, productive, and happy lives.

REFERENCES

Achenbach, T. M. (1991). *Manual for the youth self-report and 1991 profile*. Burlington: University of Vermont, Department of Psychiatry.

Achenbach, T. M. (1992). *Manual for the Child Behavior Checklist/2–3 and 1992 Profile*. Burlington: University of Vermont, Department of Psychiatry.

Alexander, D., & Money, J. (1966). Turner's syndrome and Gerstmann's syndrome: Neuropsychological comparisons. *Neuropsychologica, 4*, 265–273.

Alley, T. R. (1983). Growth produced changes in body shape and size as determinants of perceived age and adult caregiving. *Child Development, 54,* 241–248.

Baekgaard, W., Nyborg, H., & Nielsen, J. (1978). Neuroticism and extroversion in Turner's syndrome. *Journal of Abnormal Psychology, 87,* 583–586.

Barkley, R. A. (1989). Attention deficit-hyperactivity disorder. In E. J. Mash & R. A. Barkley (Eds.), *Treatment of childhood disorders* (pp. 39–72). New York: Guilford Press.

Bayley, N. (1969). *Bayley Scales of Infant Development.* New York: Psychological Corporation.

Beery, K. E. (1997). *The Beery–Buktenica Developmental Test of Visual Motor Integration* (4th ed.). Cleveland, OH: Modern Curriculum Press.

Bender, B. G., Linden, M. G., & Robinson, A. (1994). Neurocognitive and psychosocial phenotypes associated with Turner syndrome. In S. H. Broman & J. Grafman (Eds.), *Atypical cognitive deficits in developmental disorders* (pp. 197–216). Hillsdale, NJ: Erlbaum.

Bender, B. G., Puck, M., Salbenblatt, J., & Robinson, A. (1984). Cognitive development of unselected girls with complete and partial X monosomy. *Pediatrics, 73,.175–182.*

Benton, A. L. (1963). *Benton Visual Retention Test—Revised.* New York: Psychological Corporation.

Benton, A. L., Varney, N. R., & de Hamshef, K. (1978). Visuo-spatial judgment: A clinical test. *Archives of Neurology, 35,* 364–367.

Berch, D. B. (1996). Memory. In J. Rovet (Ed.), *Turner Syndrome across the lifespan* (pp. 140–145). Toronto: Klein Graphics.

Buchanan, L., Pavlovic, J., & Rovet J. (1998). A reexamination of the visuospatial definition of Turner syndrome: Contributions of working memory. *Developmental Psychology, 14,* 341–367.

Buckley, F. (1971). Preliminary report on intelligence quotient scores of patients with Turner's syndrome: A replication study. *British Journal of Psychiatry, 119,* 513–514.

Butcher, J. N., Williams, C. L., Graham, J. R., Archer, R. P., Tellegen, A., Ben-Porath, S., & Kaemmer, B. (1992). *Minnesota Multiphasic Personality Inventory—Adolescent (MMPI-A): Manual for administration, scoring, and interpretation.* Minneapolis: University of Minnesota Press.

Conners, C. K. (1990). *The Conners Rating Scales for Children.* North Tonawanda, NY: Multi-Health Systems.

Connolly, A. J. (1988). *The KeyMath Diagnostic Arithmetic Test—Revised.* Circle Pines, MN: American Guidance Service.

Darby, P. L., Garfinkel, P. E., Vale, J. M., Kirwan, P. J., & Brown, G. M. (1981). Anorexia nervosa and "Turner syndrome": Cause or coincidence? *Psychological Medicine, 11,* 141–145.

Dellantonio, A., Lis, A., Saviolo, N., Rigon, F., & Tenconi, R. (1984). Spatial performance and hemispheric specialization in the Turner syndrome. *Acta Medica Auxologica, 16,* 193–203.

Dodge, K. A. (1989). Problems in social relationships. In E. J. Mash & R. A. Barkley (Eds.), *Treatment of childhood disorders* (pp. 222–244). New York: Guilford Press.

Downey, J., Ehrhardt, A., Gruen, R., Bell, J., & Morishima, A. (1989). Psychopathology and social functioning in women with Turner syndrome. *Journal of Nervous and Mental Disease, 177,* 191–200.

Downey, J., Elkin, E. J., Ehrhardt, A. A., Meyer-Bahlburg, H. F. L., Ball, J. J., & Morishima, A. (1991). Cognitive ability and everyday functioning in women with Turner syndrome. *Journal of Learning Disabilities, 24,* 32–39.

Ehrhardt, A. A., Greenberg, N., & Money, J. (1970). Female gender identity and absence of fetal hormones: Turner's syndrome. *Johns Hopkins Medical Journal, 126,* 142–155.

El Abd, S., Turk, J., & Hill, P. (1995). Annotation: Psychological characteristics of Turner syndrome. *Journal of Child Psychiatry, 36,* 1109–1125.

Faust, J., Rosenfeld, R. G., Wilson, D., Durham, L., & Vardopoulos, C. C. (1995). Prediction of depression in parents of Turner syndrome adolescents as a function of growth hormones, family conflict, and coping style. *Journal of Developmental and Physical Disabilities, 7,* 221–233.

Ford, C. E., Jones, K. W., Polani, P. E., de Almeida, J. C., & Briggs, J. H. (1959). A sex chromosome anomaly in a case of gonadal dysgenesis (Turner's syndrome). *Lancet, i,* 711–713.

Frankenburg, W. K., Dodds, J. B., Fandal, A. W., Kazuk, E. & Cohr, M. (1975). *The Denver Developmental Screening Test—Revised.* Denver, CO: Denver Developmental Materials.

Gardner, M. F. (1996). *The Test of Visual Perceptual Skills (Nonmotor)—Revised*. Burlingame, CA: Psychological and Educational Publishing.

Garron, D. C. (1977). Intelligence among persons with Turner's syndrome. *Behavior Genetics, 7,* 105–127.

Golden, C. J., Purisch, A. D., & Hammeke, T. A. (1988). *Luria–Nebraska Neuropsychological Battery: Form I and II Manual*. Los Angeles: Western Psychological Services.

Gresham, F. M., & Elliott, S. N. (1990). *Social Skills Rating System (SSRS) Manual*. Circle Pines, MN: American Guidance Service.

Harris, D. B. (1963). *Good Enough–Harris Drawing Test*. Beverly Hills, CA: Western Psychological Services.

Higurashi, M., Kawai, H., Segawa, M., IiJima, K., Ikeda, Y., Tanaka, F., Egi, S., & Kamashita, S. (1986). Growth, psychological characteristics, and sleep wakefulness cycle of children with sex chromosome abnormalities. *March of Dimes Birth Defects Foundation: Original Article Series, 22,* 251–275.

Jones, K. L. (1988). XO syndrome (Turner syndrome). In *Smith's recognizable patterns of human malformation* (pp. 74–79). Philadelphia: Saunders.

Jorm, A. F., Share, D. L., Matthews, R., & Maclean, R. (1986). Behavior problems in specific reading retarded and general reading backward children: A longitudinal study. *Journal of Child Psychology and Psychiatry, 27,* 33–43.

Kaufman, A. S., & Kaufman, N. G. (1985). *Kaufman Tests of Educational Achievement*. Circle Pines, MN: American Guidance Service.

Kolb, J. E., & Heaton, R. K. (1975). Lateralized neurologic deficits and psychopathology in a Turner syndrome patient. *Archives of General Psychiatry, 32,* 1198–1200.

Koppitz, E. M. (1969). *The Bender Visual Motor Gestalt Test*. New York: Grune & Stratton.

Koppitz, E. M. (1977). *The Visual Aural Digit Span Test*. New York: Grune & Stratton.

Kovacs, M. (1992). *The Children's Depression Inventory*. North Tonawanda, NY: Multi-Health Systems.

Kron, L., Katz, J. L., Gorzynski, G., & Weiner, H. (1977). Anorexia nervosa and gonadal dysgenesis. *Archives of General Psychiatry, 34,* 332–335.

LeMay, D. W., Griffen, P. M., & Sanford, A. R. (1992). *Learning Acquisition Profile—D*. Lewisville, NC: Kaplan Press.

Lewandowski, L. J. (1985). Clinical syndromes among the learning disabled. *Journal of Learning Disabilities, 18,* 177–178.

Lewandowski, L. J., Costenbader, V., & Richman, R. (1984). Neuropsychological aspects of Turner syndrome. *International Journal of Clinical Neuropsychology, 7,* 144–147.

Markwardt, F. C. (1989). *The Peabody Individual Achievement Test—Revised*. Circle Pines, MN: American Guidance Service.

Mathiesen, B., Reilly, S., & Skuse, D. (1992). Oral–motor dysfunction and feeding disorders in infants with Turner syndrome. *Developmental Medicine and Child Neurology, 34,* 141–149.

Mazzocco, M. M. (1998). A process approach to describing mathematics difficulties in girls with Turner syndrome. *Pediatrics, 102,* 492–494.

McArthur, D. S., & Roberts, G. E. (1987). *Roberts Apperception Test for Children: Manual*. Los Angeles: Western Psychological Services.

McCarney, S. B. (1989). *The Attention Deficit Disorders Evaluation Scale*. Columbus, MO: Hawthorne Educational Services.

McCauley, E., Ito, J., & Kay, T. (1986a). Psychosocial functioning in girls with the Turner syndrome and short stature. *Journal of the American Academy of Child Psychiatry, 25,* 105–112.

McCauley, E., Kay, T., Ito, J., & Treder, R. (1987). The Turner syndrome: Cognitive deficits, affective discrimination, and behavior problems. *Child Development, 58,* 464–473.

McCauley, E., Ross, R., Kushner, H., & Culter, G. (1995). Self-esteem and behavior in girls with Turner syndrome. *Journal of Developmental and Behavioral Pediatrics, 16,* 82–88.

McCauley, E., Sybert, V. P., & Ehrhardt, A. A. (1986b). Psychosocial adjustment of adult women with Turner syndrome. *Clinical Genetics, 29,* 284–290.

McGlone, J. (1985). Can spatial deficits in Turner's syndrome be explained by focal CNS dysfunction or atypical speech lateralization? *Journal of Clinical and Experimental Neuropsychology,* 7, 375–394.

Meichenbaum, D. (1985). Teaching thinking: A cognitive-behavioral perspective. In S. F. Chipman, J. W. Segal, & R. Glaser (Eds.), *Thinking and learning skills: Vol. 2. Research and open questions* (pp. 407–426). Hillsdale, NJ: Erlbaum.

Millon, T., Green, C. J., & Meagher, R. B. (1982). *The Millon Adolescent Personality Inventory manual.* Minneapolis, MN: National Computer Systems.

Money, J. (1963). Cytogenetic and psychosexual incongruities with a note on space–form blindness. *American Journal of Psychiatry,* 119, 820–827.

Money, J. (1964). Two cytogenetic syndromes: Psychologic comparisons. I. Intelligence and specific factor quotients. *Journal of Psychiatric Research,* 2, 223–231.

Money, J. (1993). Specific neurocognitive impairments associated with Turner (45,X) and Klinefelter (47,XXY) syndromes: A review. *Social Biology,* 40, 147–151.

Money, J., & Alexander, D. (1966). Turner's syndrome: Further demonstration of the presence of specific cognitional deficiencies. *Journal of Medical Genetics,* 3, 47–48.

Money, J., & Mittenthal, S. (1970). Lack of personality pathology in Turner's syndrome: Relations to cytogenetics, hormones, and physique. *Behavior Genetics,* 1, 43–56.

Muhs, A., & Lieberz, K. (1993). Anorexia nervosa and Turner's syndrome. *Psychopathology,* 26, 29–40.

Mullins, L. L., Lynch, J., Orten, J., & Youll, L. K. (1991). Developing a program to assist Turner's syndrome patients and families. *Social Work in Health Care,* 16, 69–79.

Netley, C., & Rovet, J. (1982). Atypical hemispheric lateralization in Turner syndrome subjects. *Cortex,* 18, 377–384.

Nielsen, J., Nyborg, H., & Dahl, G. (1977). Turner's syndrome: A psychiatric–psychological study of 45 women with Turner's syndrome. *Acta Jutlandica,* 45 (Monograph).

Nielsen, J., & Stradiot, M. (1987). Transcultural study of Turner's syndrome. *Clinical Genetics,* 32, 260–270.

Orten, J. D., & Orten, J. L. (1992). Achievement among women with Turner's syndrome. *Families in Society: The Journal of Contemporary Human Services,* 73, 424–431.

Orten, J. L. (1990). Coming up short: The physical, cognitive and social effects of Turner's syndrome. *Health and Social Work,* 7, 100–106.

Orten, J. L., & Orten, J. D. (1994). Women with Turner's syndrome: Helping them reach their full potential. *Disability and Society,* 9, 239–248.

Pasaro Mendez, E. J., Fernandez, R. M., Goyanes, V., & Mendez, J. (1994). Turner's syndrome: A behavioral and cytogenetic study. *Journal of Genetic Psychology,* 154, 433–447.

Pavlidis, K., McCauley, E., & Sybert, V. P. (1995). Psychosocial and sexual functioning in women with Turner syndrome. *Clinical Genetics,* 47, 85–89.

Pennington, B. F., Heaton, R. K., Karzmark, P., Pendleton, M. G., Lehman, R., & Shucard, D. W. (1985). The neuropsychological phenotype in Turner syndrome. *Cortex,* 21, 391–404.

Perheentupa, J., Lenko, H. L., Nevalainen, I., Nittymaki, M., Soderheim, A., & Taipale, V. (1974). Hormone therapy in Turner's syndrome: Growth and psychological aspects. *Growth and Developmental Endocrinology,* 5, 121–127.

Pidcock, F. S. (1984). Intellectual functioning in Turner's syndrome. *Developmental Medicine and Child Neurology,* 26, 539–545.

Piers, E. V. (1984). *The Piers–Harris Children's Self-Concept Scale.* Los Angeles: Western Psychological Services.

Raboch, J., Kobilkova, J., Horejsi, J., Starka, L., & Raboch, J. (1987). Sexual development and life of women with gonadal dysgenesis. *Journal of Sex and Marital Therapy,* 13, 117–126.

Raven, J. C., Court, J. H., & Raven, J. (1977). *The coloured progressive matrices.* London: H. K. Lewis.

Reitan, R. M., & Wolfson, D. (1985). *The Halstead–Reitan Neuropsychological Test Battery: Theory and clinical interpretation.* Tucson, AZ: Neuropsychology Press.

Reynolds, C. R., & Bigler, E. D. (1994). *The Test of Memory and Learning.* Austin, TX: Pro-Ed.

Reynolds, C. R. & Kamphaus, R. W. (1992). *The Behavior Assessment System for Children*. Circle Pines, MN: American Guidance Service.

Reynolds, C. R., & Richmond, B. O. (1985). *The Revised Children's Manifest Anxiety Scale*. Los Angeles: Western Psychological Services.

Reynolds, W. R. (1986). *Reynolds Adolescent Depression Scale*. Odessa, FL: Psychological Assessment Resources.

Robinson, A., Bender, B., Borelli, J., Puck, M., Salbenblatt, J., & Winter, J. (1986). Sex chromosomal aneuploidy: Prospective and longitudinal studies. In S. Ratliffe & N. Paul (Eds.), *Prospective studies on children with sex chromosome aneuploidy* (pp. 23–73). New York: Alan R. Liss.

Rorschach, H. (1942). *The Rorschach Psychodiagnostic: A diagnostic test based on perception*. Bern: Huber.

Rosenfeld, R., Franke, J., Artie, K., Brase, J. A., Bursteen, S., Cara, J., Chernausek, S., Gotlin, R., Krintze, J., Lippe, B., Mahoney, P., Moore, W., Salnger, P., & Johnson, A. (1992). Six year results of a randomized prospective trial of human growth hormone and oxandrolone in Turner's syndrome. *Journal of Pediatrics*, 121, 49–55.

Ross, J. L. (1990). Disorders of the sex chromosomes: Medical overview. In C. S. Holmes (Ed.), *Psychoneuroendocrinology: Brain, behavior and hormonal interactions* (pp. 127–137). New York: Springer-Verlag.

Rourke, B. P. (Ed.). (1985). *Neuropsychology of learning disabilities: Essentials of subtype analysis*. New York: Guilford Press.

Rovet, J. (1990). The cognitive and neuropsychological characteristics of children with Turner syndrome. In D. Berch & B. Bender (Eds.), *Sex chromosome abnormalities and human behvior: Psychological studies* (pp. 38–77). Boulder, CO: Westview Press.

Rovet, J. (1993). The psychoeducational characteristics of children with Turner syndrome. *Journal of Learning Disabilities*, 26, 333–341.

Rovet, J. (1995). Turner syndrome. In B. P. Rourke (Ed.), *Syndrome of nonverbal learning disabilities: Neurodevelopmental manifestations* (pp. 351–371). New York: Guilford Press.

Rovet, J., & Ireland, L. (1994). The behavioral phenotype of children with Turner syndrome. *Journal of Pediatric Psychology*, 19, 779–790.

Rovet, J., & Netley, C. (1981). Turner syndrome in a pair of dizygotic twins: A single case study. *Behavior Genetics*, 11, 65–72

Rovet, J., & Netley, C. (1982). Processing deficits in Turner's syndrome. *Developmental Psychology*, 18, 77–94.

Russo, D. C. (1986). Chronicity and normalcy as the psychological basis for research and treatment in chronic disease in children. In N. A. Krasnegor, J. D. Arasteh, & M. F. Cataldo (Eds.), *Child health behavior: A behavioral pediatrics approach* (pp. 521–536). New York: Wiley.

Shaffer, J. (1962). A specific cognitive deficit observed in gonadal aplasia (Turner's syndrome). *Journal of Clinical Psychology*, 18, 403–406.

Sheslow, D., & Adams, W. (1990). *The Wide Range Assessment of Memory and Learning*. Wilmington, DE: Wide Range.

Shucard, D. W., Shucard, J. L., Clopper, R. R., & Schachter, M. (1992). Electrophysiological and neuropsychological indices of cognitive processing deficits in Turner syndrome. *Developmental Neuropsychology*, 8, 299–323.

Siegel, P. T., Clopper, R., & Stabler, B. (1998). The psychological consequences of Turner syndrome and review of the National Cooperative Growth Study psychological substudy. *Pediatrics*, 102, 488–491.

Silbert, A., Wolff, P., & Lilienthal, J. (1977). Spatial and temporal processing in patients with Turner's syndrome. *Behavior Genetics*, 7, 11–21.

Skuse, D. (1987). Annotation: The psychological consequences of being small. *Journal of Child Psychology and Psychiatry*, 28, 641–650.

Skuse, D. H., Cave, S., O'Herlihy, A., & South, R. (1998). Quality of life in children with Turner syndrome: Parent, teacher, and individual perspectives. In D. Drotar et al. (Eds.), *Measuring health related quality of life in children and adolescents: Implications for research and practice.* Mahwah, NJ: Lawrence Erlbaum.

Sonis, W. A., Levine-Ross, J., Blue, J., Cutler, G. B., Loriaux, P. L., & Klein, R. P. (1983, October). *Hyperactivity and Turner's syndrome.* Paper presented at the American Academy of Child Psychiatry Meetings, San Francisco, CA.

Strang, J. D., & Rourke, B. P. (1983). Concept formation of non-verbal reasoning abilities of children who exhibit specific academic problems with arithmetic. *Journal of Clinical Child Psychology, 12,* 33–39.

Taipale, V., Niittymaki, M., & Nevelainen, I. (1982). Turner's syndrome and anorexia nervosa symptoms. *Acta Paedopsychiatrica, 48,* 231–238.

Taylor, H. G. (1989). Learning disabilities. In E. J. Mash & R. A. Barkley (Eds.), *Treatment of childhood disorders* (pp. 437–480). New York: Guilford Press.

Temple, C. M., & Carney, R. A. (1993). Intellectual functioning of children with Turner syndrome: A comparison of behavioural phenotypes. *Developmental Medicine and Child Neurology, 35,* 691–698.

Temple, C. M., & Carney, R. A. (1995). Patterns of spatial functioning in Turner's syndrome. *Cortex, 31,* 109–118.

Thorndike, R. C., Hagen, E. P., & Sattler, J. M. (1986). *The Stanford–Binet Intelligence Scale* (4th ed.). Chicago: Riverside.

Turner, H. H. (1938). A syndrome of infantilism, congenital webbed neck, and cubitus valgus. *Endocrinology, 23,* 566–574.

Varni, J. W., Rubinfeld, L. A., Talbot, D., & Setoguchi, Y. (1989). Stress, social support, and depressive symptomatology in children with congenital/acquired limb deficiencies. *Journal of Developmental and Behavioral Pediatrics, 10,* 13–16.

Varni, J. W., & Wallander, J. C. (1988). Pediatric chronic disabilities: Hemophilia and spina bifida as examples. In D. K. Routh (Ed.), *Handbook of pediatric psychology* (pp. 190–221). New York: Guilford Press.

Waber, D. (1979). Neuropsychological aspects of Turner syndrome. *Developmental Medicine and Child Neurology, 21,* 58–70.

Watson, W. C. (1981). *Physiological psychology: An introduction.* Boston: Houghton Mifflin.

Wechsler, D. (1989). *Wechsler Preschool and Primary Scale of Intelligence—Revised.* New York: Psychological Corporation.

Wechsler, D. (1991). *Wechsler Intelligence Scale for Children* (3rd ed.). New York: Psychological Corporation.

Wechsler, D. (1992). *Wechsler Individual Achievement Test.* New York: Psychological Corporation.

Wechsler, D. (1997). *Wechsler Adult Intelligence Scale* (3rd ed.). New York: Psychological Corporation.

White, B. J. (1994). The Turner syndrome: Origin, cytogenetic variants, and factors influencing the phenotype. In S. H. Broman & J. Grafman (Eds.), *Atypical cognitive deficits in developmental disorders* (pp. 183–195). Hillsdale, NJ: Erlbaum.

Wiederholt, J. L., & Bryant, B. R. (1992). *The Gray Oral Reading Test* (3rd ed.). Austin, TX: Pro-Ed.

Williams, J. K. (1994). Behavioral characteristics of children with Turner syndrome and children with learning disabilities. *Western Journal of Nursing Research, 19,* 26–39.

Williams, J. K. (1995). Parenting a daughter with precocious puberty or Turner syndrome. *Journal of Pediatric Health Care, 9,* 109–114.

Williams, J. K., Richman, L. C., & Yarbrough, D. B. (1992). Comparison of visual–spatial performance strategy training in children with Turner syndrome and learning disabilities. *Journal of Learning Disabilities, 25,* 658–663.

Witkin, H., Oltman, P., Raskin, E., & Karp, S. (1971). Embedded figure test and children's embedded figure test. Palo Alto, CA: Consulting Psychologists Press.

Woodcock, R. W., & Johnson, M. B. (1989). *Woodcock–Johnson Psycho-Educational Battery—Revised.* Allen, TX: DLM Teaching Resources.

12

FRAGILE X SYNDROME

RANDI J. HAGERMAN
MEGAN E. LAMPE

Fragile X syndrome (FXS) causes a broad spectrum of involvement, ranging from learning disabilities and emotional problems to more significant intellectual deficits (including mental retardation). It is caused by a genetic mutation in the fragile X mental retardation 1 (FMR1) gene, which was discovered in 1991 (Verkerk et al., 1991; Yu et al., 1991; Oberlé et al., 1991; Bell et al., 1991). Before the discovery of FMR1, individuals were diagnosed with FXS by cytogenetic testing, which demonstrated a fragile site on the bottom end of the X chromosome at Xq27.3. Sutherland, a researcher in Australia, discovered that the detecting presence of the fragile site was dependent on the utilization of a folic-acid-deficient tissue culture medium, and he reported this discovery in 1977. Subsequently, all during the 1980s, individuals were diagnosed with FXS when cytogenetic testing demonstrated the fragile site. Because the fragile site only occurs in individuals who are significantly affected by FXS (mainly individuals with mental retardation), cytogenetic testing is not effective in identifying individuals who are carriers of FXS. Nonretarded individuals with FXS (i.e., individuals with just emotional or learning problems) are sometimes cytogenetically negative, and unaffected carriers almost always obtain negative results on chromosome testing. With the discovery of the FMR1 gene, DNA testing became available; this specifically shows the mutation at FMR1, and therefore is a much more effective test for FXS. DNA testing identifies all carrier individuals, in addition to individuals who are affected by FXS. Not only is the DNA test more precise and inclusive in identifying individuals with FXS, but the test is considerably less expensive (at this writing, approximately $250) than cytogenetic testing (approximately $600). Patients who have a positive family history of FXS but who previously tested negative through cytogenetic testing should be reevaluated with DNA testing.

The mutation that causes FXS is a trinucleotide expansion (cytosine–guanine–guanine, or CGG) at the upper end of the FMR1 gene. In normal individuals, there are between 6 and 54 repetitive CGG sequences, and the FMR1 gene works normally, producing FMR1 protein (FMRP) (Pieretti et al., 1991; Imbert, Feng, Nelson, Warren, & Mandel, 1998). The repetitive CGG sequence normally remains stable from one generation to the next.

In carrier individuals, there is a "premutation," or an expansion of the CGG repeat number to more than 50 but less than 200 (Pieretti et al., 1991; Warren & Ashley, 1995). Individuals who are carriers of the premutation are intellectually unaffected but may have emotional problems related to their carrier state, such as anxiety and depression (Reiss, Freund, Abrams, Boehm, & Kazazian, 1993; Sobesky, Porter, Pennington, & Hagerman, 1995; Hagerman, 1996a; Franke, Maier, Iwers, Hautzinger, & Froster, 1996). Most women who have children with FXS are premutation carriers who have normal IQs.

Individuals who are intellectually affected by FXS have a full mutation, which is defined by a CGG repeat number of more than 230, in addition to methylation of the FMR1 gene, which silences the production of FMRP (Pieretti et al., 1991; Brown, 1996; Oostra, 1996). It is the absence of or a deficiency in FMRP that causes FXS, including the physical, cognitive, and behavioral characteristics associated with the disorder.

PREVALENCE

Numerous studies have been done to determine the prevalence of FXS, not only in the general population but among mentally retarded and autistic individuals (Wahlstrom, Gillberg, Gustavson, & Holmgren, 1986; Webb, Bundey, Thake, & Todd, 1986; Turner, Robinson, Laing, & Purvis-Smith, 1986; Hagerman et al., 1994b; Sherman, 1996; Turner, Webb, Wake, & Robinson, 1996). Cytogenetic testing indicated that approximately 1 in 1,250 males and 1 in 2,500 females in the general population were mentally retarded as a result of FXS (Webb et al., 1986). Subsequent studies using DNA, however, have demonstrated a lower prevalence for mental retardation caused by FXS in Australia, at approximately 1 per 4,000 males in the general population (Turner et al., 1996). In addition, DNA testing has demonstrated that the prevalence of individuals with the premutation is higher than previously thought. One research group has found that 1 in 259 females (Rousseau, Rouillard, Morel, Khandjian, & Morgan, 1995) and 1 in approximately 700 males (Rousseau, Morel, Rouillard, Khandjian, & Morgan, 1996) in the general population are carriers of the premutation.

FXS is the most common inherited cause of mental retardation known, and it represents approximately 30% of all X-linked forms of mental retardation (Sherman, 1996). Approximately 2–3% of males with mental retardation of unknown etiology have FXS (Slaney et al., 1995). Therefore, individuals who present with mental retardation of unknown etiology should be tested for FXS. Likewise, individuals with autism of unknown etiology should also be tested, because approximately 6% of males with autism have FXS (Brown et al., 1986). Furthermore, the majority of males with FXS have autistic-like features, including hand biting, hand flapping, perseverative speech, and self-stimulating behaviors (Hagerman 1996a).

There have been no complete studies to show any significant differences among ethnic groups in the prevalence of FXS. A relatively high prevalence of FXS in Finland and Tunisia suggests a "founder effect"—that is, the presence of a carrier in the original founding population for these areas (Zhong et al., 1996; Eichler & Nelson, 1996).

INHERITANCE

The expansion from a premutation to a full mutation only occurs when the FMR1 gene is passed on to the next generation through a female. When the gene passes from a male with the premutation, he will pass on the premutation to all of his daughters, because the sperm in males with FXS has only the premutation (Reyniers et al., 1993). Therefore, whether a male has a full mutation, a mosaic pattern (premutation in some cells and full mutation in others), or a premutation, he will only pass the premutation on to his daughters. A female, however, can pass either the premutation or the full mutation on to her children. The greater the CGG repeat number in a carrier female, the greater the chance of expansion to a full mutation in the next generation (Cronister, 1996). If a female has more than 100 CGG repeats and she passes the X chromosome with the mutation on to her child, it will expand to a full mutation 100% of the time in the next generation. Since females have two X chromosomes, the risk of passing the mutation on to the next generation is 50% with each pregnancy. A carrier mother can therefore have affected daughters as well as affected sons.

In contrast, a male will pass on the premutation to all of his daughters but none of his sons. His sons will receive the Y chromosome and therefore will be unaffected by FXS. Daughters who receive the mutation from their fathers have a high risk of producing retarded children in the next generation. Therefore, once the diagnosis of FXS is made, it is essential to have genetic counseling so that all individuals in the family who are at risk to be carriers of or affected by FXS can subsequently undergo DNA testing and review their risk of passing the mutation on to the next generation (Cronister, 1996).

It is imperative for families to understand the inheritance pattern of FXS. Family members should be well informed of the dynamics of inheritance, so that relatives who are reluctant to have testing will be inclined to do so. Figure 12.1 shows a family pedigree that demonstrates the change in CGG repeats through four generations.

PHYSICAL, BEHAVIORAL, AND COGNITIVE PHENOTYPE

Physical Phenotype

Young children with FXS usually present with language and motor delays, hypotonia, and hyperactivity. The typical physical features of FXS may not be present in early childhood,

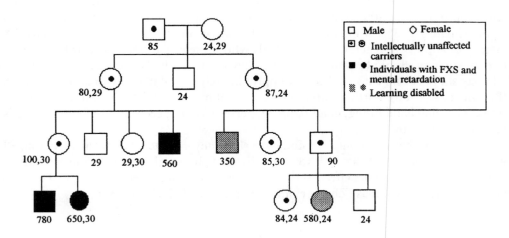

FIGURE 12.1. A pedigree of a family affected by FXS. The numbers represent the CGG repeat numbers at FMR1 in each X chromosome. Note that the male with 350 repeats has an unmethylated full mutation; he is not mentally retarded, but does have learning disabilities. The female with 650 repeats has a full mutation and is mentally retarded, whereas the female with 580 repeats also has a full mutation, but has learning disabilities and is not mentally retarded.

so it is important not to dismiss a diagnosis of FXS solely because of a lack of these physical features (see Figure 12.2). Physical features of FXS include prominent ears, long face, hyperextensible finger joints, double-jointed thumbs, flat feet, soft skin, and a high-arched palate (Hagerman, 1996a). Most of these features can be seen in the general population, and children with FXS do not typically look dysmorphic or unusual. On occasion, ears can be dramatically prominent, with a cupping in the upper part of the ear. Among females, we typically only see the classic physical features in females with a full mutation. Female carriers are less likely to present with typical physical features. For males, macroorchidism (i.e., large testicles) is also part of the physical phenotype, but it is usually not present until adolescence (Lachiewicz & Dawson, 1994). In adolescence or adulthood, the testicular volume may be two to three times normal size, although this is also not always recognized in a physical examination (Butler et al., 1991; Hagerman, 1996a).

In our clinic, we use a Physical Index (PI) to assess the number of physical features that present in each patient with FXS (see Table 12.1). The PI score (1 point for each feature) correlates with the degree of involvement in the DNA and the level of FMRP measured in the blood (Tassone et al., 1999). Although the PI is a good indicator of typical FXS features, it should be considered in conjunction with other behavioral and cognitive characteristics. Many of the physical features in FXS are considered part of a connective tissue dysplasia (Opitz, Westphal, & Daniel, 1984; Hagerman, 1996a). The high frequency of otitis media difficulties in early childhood is probably related to the connective tissue problems, in that the eustachian tube is very collapsable, trapping fluid in the middle ear. The connective tissue problems on occasion lead to other medical complications, such as hernias, scoliosis, and mitral valve prolapse (Hagerman, 1996a).

Growth abnormalities also may occur in FXS. Young patients often have a large head circumference, and on occasion more significant overgrowth in height and weight (deVries et al., 1993, 1995). In puberty, however, the growth velocity may be slowed, and short stature is not uncommon in adulthood (Loesch, Huggins, & Hoang, 1995).

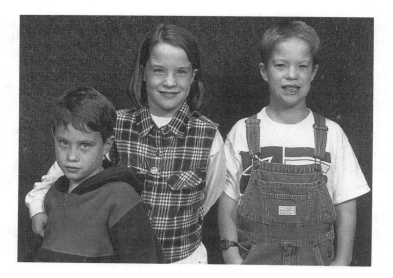

FIGURE 12.2. These siblings all have the full mutation of FXS. Although they do not display typical physical features of FXS, they do present with characteristic behavioral features of FXS (see text). Photograph used by permission of the children's parents.

TABLE 12.1. Typical Physical and Behavioral Features of FXS

Physical Index (PI)	Behavioral Index (BI)
Long ears	Poor eye contact
Prominent ears	Tactile defensiveness
Long face	Hand flapping
Single palmar crease	Hand biting
Cardiac murmur or click	Perseveration
Hand calluses	Hyperactivity
Flat feet	Diagnosis of attention-deficit/hyperactivity disorder (ADHD)
Hyperextensible finger joints	Violent outbursts
Double-jointed thumbs	Tantrums
High-arched palate	Shyness or social anxiety

Note. These indices are used in our clinic to assess physical and behavioral characteristics of patients with FXS.

Behavioral Phenotype

Behavioral features of FXS include an extremely short attention span, impulsivity, and hyperactivity, as well as hypersensitivity to visual, auditory, tactile, and olfactory stimuli (Belser & Sudhalter, 1995; Hagerman, 1996a). Children with FXS often have difficulty in crowds and with loud noises, because their hypersensitivity and hyperarousal lead to tantrums. They may also overreact to some smells. In addition, children with FXS may experience tactile defensiveness to such an extent that they pull away from light touch, and tags in clothes or textures of materials can be irritating. Children with FXS are easily hyperaroused and may present with tantrums on a daily basis and aggression on occasion. These types of behaviors usually occur when a child is overwhelmed. Transitions—even going from the car into the house—can be difficult for children with FXS. Behavioral interventions and therapy, as described later, can be helpful in alleviating the intensity of some of these behaviors.

Perseveration is a typical communicative and behavioral feature in FXS. Children may repeat a certain activity (e.g., stacking toys, spinning objects, flushing the toilet, or watching the same video) over and over again. Perseveration is also present in speech—not only in repeating the same phrase, but in talking about the same subject continually. Mumbling, echolalia, cluttered speech, and self-talk (i.e., carrying on a conversation with oneself, often using different vocal tones) are all commonly seen in FXS (Abbeduto & Hagerman, 1997).

Autistic-like features are also common in children with FXS, including hand flapping, hand biting, toe walking, poor eye contact, tactile sensitivity, shyness, and social anxiety. Children with FXS typically do not have a pervasive lack of interest in social interactions. Indeed, they are usually interested in social interactions, but they usually demonstrate avoidance behavior that relates to their oversensitivity to sensory input (Cohen et al., 1991; Cohen, 1995; Belser & Sudhalter, 1995). Because of the autistic-like features in FXS, several studies have screened autistic populations for the fragile X chromosome or the FMR1 mutation (Brown et al., 1986; Cohen et al., 1989). Overall, approximately 6% of males with autism are positive for FXS. In addition, studies comparing males with FXS and IQ-matched controls have demonstrated differences in the profile of *Diagnostic and Statistical Manual of Mental Disorders*, third edition, revised (DSM-III-R) features of autism in each group (Reiss & Freund, 1990, 1991). Overall, approximately 15% of males with FXS have been found to fulfill the DSM-III-R criteria for autism (Hagerman, 1996a; Reiss &

Freund, 1991; Baumgardner, Reiss, Freund, & Abrams, 1995). Therefore, all individuals with autism of unknown etiology should be tested at this time with DNA studies for FXS.

In our clinic, we use a Behavioral Index (BI) to measure the number of typical FXS behaviors each patient displays (see Table 12.1). The overall BI score correlates with the patient's degree of FXS involvement as reflected by DNA studies and FMRP levels (Tassone et al., 1999).

Cognitive and Neuroanatomical Phenotype

The majority of males with FXS have mental retardation; females are less affected by FXS because they have two X chromosomes, and although the full mutation may be present on one of the X chromosomes, the other is normal and is producing FMRP. All females inactivate one of their X chromosomes, and an activation ratio (AR), which can be calculated from the DNA studies, represents the percentage of cells with the normal X chromosome as the active chromosome (Rousseau, Heitz, Oberlé, & Mandel, 1991; Taylor et al., 1994; Abrams et al., 1994). The AR has been found to correlate with the IQ (Abrams et al., 1994; Riddle et al., 1998), although deVries et al. (1996) have found a correlation with the Performance IQ and not the Verbal IQ. Strengths in verbal memory have been documented in both males and females affected by FXS (Freund & Reiss, 1991; Mazzocco, Pennington, & Hagerman, 1993; Sobesky, Pennington, Porter, Hull, & Hagerman, 1994). Sobesky, Taylor, Pennington, Riddle, and Hagerman (1996) have found that the AR correlates more strongly with deficits in executive functioning than with the overall IQ in nonretarded females with FXS. Approximately 50–70% of females with the full mutation have intellectual deficits in the borderline or mildly retarded range (deVries et al., 1996). Females with normal IQ but with the full mutation usually demonstrate learning disabilities, including attentional and organizational problems and math difficulties. Approximately 70% of nonretarded women with the full mutation have deficits in executive functioning, which are perhaps causal to their difficulties with organization and attention (Mazzocco et al., 1993; Sobesky et al., 1996). Their behavior is often impulsive, and they can be tangential in their speech, as well as mood-labile. Young girls with the full mutation usually demonstrate significant shyness and social anxiety. In a controlled study by Freund, Reiss, and Abrams (1993), the majority of girls demonstrated avoidant personality disorder or an anxiety disorder; in this respect, they were significantly different from IQ-matched controls. On occasion the social withdrawal and anxiety may lead to quieter language and even selective mutism in school, but usually not at home (Hagerman, 1996a).

Studies of neuroanatomical changes in FXS have helped to increase our understanding of the neurobehavioral phenotype of FXS. In general, the brain is larger in patients with FXS than in controls (Shapiro et al., 1995), and certain parts of the brain are generally larger in patients with FXS than in age- and IQ-matched controls (Abrams & Reiss, 1995). Studies by Reiss and colleagues (Reiss, Patel, Kumar, & Freund, 1988; Reiss, Aylward, Freund, Joshi, & Bryan, 1991a; Reiss, Freund, Tseng, & Joshi, 1991b; Reiss, Lee, & Freund, 1994; Reiss, Abrams, Greenlaw, Freund, & Denckla, 1995) demonstrated a larger hippocampus, caudate, thalamus, and lateral ventricles, but a smaller posterior cerebellar vermis. This last finding appears to relate to the sensory integration problems, since the cerebellar vermis is important for processing sensory stimuli and motor coordination. The findings of a larger hippocampus could be important for the hyperarousal and disinhibition in individuals with FXS, in addition to their excellent memory for events and locations. The enlarged caudate may relate to the problems with executive functioning or frontal deficits that are found in females with FXS, in addition to attention-deficit/hyperactivity disorder (ADHD), which is also present in both males and females.

PHENOTYPIC ILLUSTRATIONS

Case 1

M. P., a boy aged 4 years, 3 months, was diagnosed with FXS by FMR1 testing. He has a full mutation that is fully methylated. M. P. was born after a normal pregnancy, and his birth weight was 8 pounds, 14 ounces. He did well in the newborn period, although his developmental milestones were mildly delayed. He sat at 10 months and walked at 15 months. At present, he does not yet speak in phrases but can use approximately 10 to 15 words. M. P. began to flap and bite his hands in his first year. His father called him "little butterfly" because of his hand flapping. M. P. also chews excessively on things, has poor eye contact, and has problems with perseveration. He is easily overstimulated and has a high activity level, as well as impulsivity and distractibility. In addition, tantrums are a problem for M. P., although he is not physically aggressive. He has difficulty with transitions and becomes easily overwhelmed.

Like many children with FXS, M. P. has had recurrent otitis media infections. Pressure equalizing (PE) tubes were used to help alleviate this problem. His height is at the 75th percentile for his age, and both his weight and head circumference are at the 95th percentile for his age. M. P. has visually prominent ears as well as ear cupping, but his face is not long. He has a high-arched palate, along with hyperextensible joints and double-jointed thumbs. In addition, his hands display a single palmar crease. His cardiac examination is normal, with no click or murmur, and he has flat feet.

M. P.'s cognitive abilities have been assessed with the Bayley Scales of Infant Development and the Vineland Adaptive Behavior Scales. On the Bayley, M. P. is performing at a developmental level between 23 and 25 months. His mother describes him as difficult to motivate; she notes that he mainly enjoys watching videos and/or eating. On the Vineland, his Adaptive Behavior Composite score is 51, which is typical of a child 21–22 months of age. His other Vineland scores are as follows: Communication, 52; Daily Living Skills, 55; Socialization, 66; and Motor Skills, 49. M. P. has not yet been able to complete the Kaufman Assessment Battery for Children (K-ABC) because of significant attention and concentration problems in addition to language deficits.

Case 2

J. P. is a boy aged 4 years, 6 months who has FXS and has also been diagnosed as autistic. DNA testing demonstrates that J. P. has a full mutation that is fully methylated, and he has no detectable FMRP in peripheral blood. His mother had a normal pregnancy, and J. P. was delivered by cesarean section; his birth weight was 9 pounds, 5½ ounces.

J. P. was mildly delayed in development. He sat at 7 months, crawled at 11 months, walked at 21 months, and began speaking in phrases between 2 and 3 years. He had significant reflux in the newborn period and was a very colicky baby. His parents noticed that his behavior was unusual even in the first year. J. P. would frequently arch his back and focus on ceiling fans; he displayed hand flapping and poor eye contact, as well as tactile defensiveness. Concerned about J. P.'s behaviors, his parents had him evaluated at an autism clinic. J. P. was diagnosed as autistic, which qualified him to receive appropriate special education preschool services, as well as speech/language and occupational therapy. It was not until J. P. was 3½ years old that the diagnosis of FXS was made.

J. P. is hyperactive with a very short attention span; he has tantrums, but these are not aggressive episodes. He has difficulty with transitions and anxiety on a daily basis. Although some of his autistic behavior has improved with therapy, J. P. continues to seek self-stimulatory input and perseverates in spinning and twirling objects. On the Vineland Adaptive Behavior Scales, his Adaptive Behavior Composite score is 54, with an age equivalent of 24 months of age. His other scores are as follows: Communication, 65; Daily Living Skills, 54; Socialization, 65; and Motor Skills, 51.

As noted above, J. P. is already receiving special education and various therapies. He also spends part of the school day integrated into a regular kindergarten, where he is assisted by an aide. Mainstreaming J. P. into the normal classroom is beneficial for him, because he can learn from and imitate other children who are performing at a normal level. J. P. has outgrown some of his autistic tendencies, and his interest in others and socialization skills have improved over time. However, he continues to be easily overwhelmed and overstimulated, and he utilizes approach–withdrawal behavior in many interactions.

J. P.'s medical history includes a history of sinusitis and recurrent otitis media infections, with more than 20 infections beginning at 6 months of age. He has not had hernias or joint dislocations, and his only surgery was for PE tubes because of the recurrent otitis media infections. Upon physical examination, his height is at the 50th percentile, his weight is at the 75th percentile, and his head circumference is at the 98th percentile for his age. His forehead and ears are prominent, but his face is not long. J. P. has a high-arched palate, hyperextensible joints, and flat feet, but does not have double-jointed thumbs, a single palmar crease, or hand calluses. Cardiac exam shows a normal rhythm, without murmur or click. His testicular volume is 3 ml bilaterally, which is normal for his age.

MOLECULAR–CLINICAL CORRELATIONS AND ADULT OUTCOME

As described earlier, the majority of males with FXS present with mental retardation, although approximately 13% do not have a retarded IQ at presentation (Hagerman et al., 1994a). This number may increase when younger children are examined. Freund, Peebles, Aylward, and Reiss (1995) found that approximately 50% of preschool boys with FXS had intellectual functioning in the normal or borderline range. Children with FXS may present with normal or near-normal expressive vocabulary abilities, and they also do well on visual matching tasks, so their initial IQ may look fairly good. However, IQ usually declines with age as more demands are made in reasoning (Lachiewicz, Gullion, Spiridigliozzi, & Aylsworth, 1987; Hagerman et al., 1989; Hodapp et al., 1990). Significant IQ decline may occur in approximately 30% of individuals with the full mutation (Wright-Talamante et al., 1996).

A few males are able to maintain an IQ in the normal or borderline range in adolescence and adulthood. These individuals usually have variant DNA patterns and are producing a significant level of FMRP. For high-functioning males, a typical pattern is a full mutation that is completely or almost completely unmethylated (Hagerman et al., 1994a; Merenstein et al., 1994; Merenstein et al., 1996; Tassone et al., 1999; Hagerman, 1999). In addition, individuals with a mosaic pattern (i.e., some cells with the premutation and other cells with the full mutation) may also be high-functioning, particularly if a high percentage of cells demonstrates the premutation (Tassone et al., 1999). The higher the FMRP level, the more likely the patient is to maintain an IQ in the borderline or normal range. Studies have shown that the average IQ in adulthood for a male with the full mutation that is fully methylated is 41;

the average IQ for a mosaic male is 60; and the average IQ for patients with a lack of methylation, or at least 50% of the mutation unmethylated, is 88 (Merenstein et al., 1996). Therefore, it appears that the level of FMRP produced by the gene correlates with an improved prognosis in adulthood (Tassone et al., 1999).

Case 3

D. C. is a 12-year-old boy who was diagnosed as carrying the premutation at 8 years of age, when DNA testing demonstrated a CGG repeat number of 79. D. C.'s mother had a normal pregnancy; she delivered at full term; and the birth weight was 6 pounds, 4½ ounces. D. C. did well in the newborn period and exhibited normal developmental milestones, including sitting at 6 months, walking at 11 months, riding a tricycle at 3½ years of age, and riding a bicycle by 7 years of age. His coordination has been quite good, and he has played soccer and other sports, but he has had mild difficulty with handwriting and drawing. In the language area, D. C. said words in the first year and sentences by 2 years of age. However, he was noted to be hyperactive as a toddler, and this persisted into his school years; his significant attentional problems and impulsivity led to a diagnosis of ADHD. He had both recurrent otitis media infections and sinusitis infections in earlier childhood. His mother is a premutation carrier, and his father had a history of a high energy level at least in adulthood.

As treatment for his ADHD, he was started on dextroamphetamine (Dexedrine, 5-mg spansules) when he was 8 years old, and he did well on this medication. His dose was gradually increased, and at 12 years of age he is using 15-mg spansules of Dexedrine each morning, with normal growth parameters.

D. C.'s behavior has not included hand flapping or hand biting, but he had approximately one tantrum per week in middle childhood, and he has shown more significant problems with aggressive behavior both at home and at school within the last year. His mother has remarried during the last year, and D. C. dislikes his stepfather. A more detailed psychological evaluation was recently carried out because of his history of aggression. His emotional assessment demonstrated severe problems with anger, mood instability, and dysthymia. It also revealed obsessive thinking focused on violent ideation. His aggressive ideation toward his stepfather was severe, and intensive counseling was initiated, in addition to a positive behavioral program in school.

Cognitive testing at age 8 years, 10 months with the K-ABC yielded an overall Mental Processing Composite score of 100, with a Sequential Processing score of 108 and a Simultaneous Processing score of 95. Cognitive testing at 12 years of age with the third edition of the Wechsler Intelligence Scale for Children yielded a Full Scale IQ of 103, a Verbal IQ of 99, and a Performance IQ of 107.

Because D. C.'s recent evaluation revealed not only severe ADHD but aggression and violent ideation, clonidine was added to his Dexedrine after a baseline normal electrocardiogram (EKG). He improved on clonidine with a gradual increase to 0.1 mg three times a day, but his obsessive and violent thinking persisted, and so fluvoxamine (Luvox) was initiated at a dose of 50 mg at bedtime; this has proved helpful for his obsessive symptoms.

Recent DNA testing for D. C. demonstrated the presence of a premutation at 66 repeats, and this was completely unmethylated in 83.6% of his cells. However, in addition, a light smear in the full-mutation range was seen at 230 repeats, and this was present in 16.3% of his cells and was methylated. Subsequent FMRP levels were obtained, and only 70% of his lymphocytes demonstrated FMRP (Tassone et al., 1999). D. C. is therefore a mosaic male with FXS; his cognitive abilities are in the normal range, but he has significant emotional and behavioral problems, including ADHD, violent ideation, and depression.

MILD INVOLVEMENT IN SOME INDIVIDUALS

Individuals with the premutation do not have cognitive deficits but may be mildly affected in a variety of ways. Women with the premutation are more likely to have prominent ears and other physical features of FXS than control patients are (Hull & Hagerman, 1993; Riddle et al., 1998). In addition, women with the full mutation have approximately a 25% risk of premature menopause and have three times the twinning rate seen in normal populations (Schwartz et al., 1994; Turner, Laing, Robinson, Wake, & Wright, 1995). Moreover, Franke et al. (1996) demonstrated a higher incidence of anxiety disorders, mood lability, and depression in women with the premutation than in controls, who included women with autistic children who did not carry the FMR1 mutation. It was previously thought that emotional problems only occurred in women with the premutation because they were raising difficult children with FXS. However, there does appear to be a biological predisposition for anxiety disorders and worrying in women with the premutation. When these problems are severe enough to interfere with sleep and daily life, they typically respond well to a selective serotonin reuptake inhibitor (SSRI), such as fluoxetine (Prozac) or sertraline (Zoloft).

Some women with the full mutation may be only mildly affected by FXS, and DNA testing of normal mothers occasionally demonstrates the full mutation instead of a premutation. Women with a high AR (see above) are less affected than women with a low AR. This is because of the increased protein expression due to the higher percentage of cells with the normal X chromosome as the active X chromosome (Tassone et al., 1999).

Case 4

L. H. is an 11-year-old girl who has a full mutation with an AR of 0.5. L. H. was born after a normal pregnancy and weighed 7 pounds, 12 ounces. She walked at 13 months and was speaking in phrases by 3 years of age. She has a long face and a high-arched palate. She had mild attentional problems without hyperactivity in school, so she was treated with Dexedrine (5-mg spansules). L. H. is a shy girl with poor eye contact, and significant anxiety developed in middle childhood. L. H. was tested with the K-ABC at 11 years of age, and she obtained a Mental Processing Composite score of 64, a Sequential Processing score of 69, and a Simultaneous Processing score of 65.

On examination at 11 years, L. H. hyperventilated throughout; according to her mother, this occurs regularly in anxiety-provoking circumstances. She has been treated with Prozac (10 mg/day), which has been helpful for her anxiety and her social interactions. She has also done well with individualized special education support for math and language therapy, in addition to group counseling in school to develop social skills.

ASSESSMENT ISSUES: WHO REQUIRES TESTING?

Children and adults with FXS may often present with other diagnoses. These may include a pervasive developmental disorder (PDD), such as autism or Asperger syndrome; schizotypal personality disorder; or other diagnoses with specific etiologies, such as Tourette syndrome, Pierre Robin sequence, Soto syndrome, or even Prader–Willi syndrome. Tics are seen in approximately 20% of patients with FXS, and abrupt mood swings and ADHD are common in FXS, as they are in Tourette syndrome. Children with Tourette syndrome do not usually demonstrate the cognitive deficits that are present in FXS, however. The large head circumference in childhood frequently causes FXS to be confused with Soto syndrome or cerebral gigantism. Approximately 5% of patients with FXS can have a cleft palate, which can be confused with other clefting syndromes, including Pierre Robin sequence. As previously discussed, autism also overlaps with FXS. Obsessive–compulsive behavior is often seen in FXS, and occasionally the obsessive behavior may focus on eating, which can lead to obesity and a phenotype similar to Prader–Willi syndrome. However, patients with FXS typically have large testicles by adolescence, instead of small testicles or hypogonadism, which is seen in Prader–Willi syndrome.

It is important to consider fragile X testing in all individuals who have mental retardation, or Autism or another PDD, when etiology is unknown. In addition, if there is a family history of mental retardation, the chance that this could be due to FXS increases dramatically. As noted earlier, FXS causes 30% of X-linked mental retardation, and in general FXS is the most common inherited form of mental retardation known.

Not all children with hyperactivity should be tested for FXS. However, if a hyperactive child has cognitive deficits or typical physical features associated with FXS, or exhibits autistic-like features such as hand flapping, hand biting, or poor eye contact, then the diagnosis of FXS should be strongly considered and DNA testing should be carried out. Similarly, not all learning-disabled children need to be tested for FXS. However, if a learning disability involves math deficits (particularly in a female), and it is combined with shyness, social anxiety, or physical features related to FXS and/or with a family history of mental retardation, then this child should be tested for FXS. In addition, patients who have selective mutism or schizotypal personality disorder and other features consistent with FXS should be tested.

The diagnosis of FXS is important from two perspectives. First, it allows genetic counseling to be given to multiple family members who may be carriers of or affected by FXS. In addition, the diagnosis of FXS helps in the development of treatment programs, including the various interventions described below.

TREATMENT

There is no cure for FXS, but a variety of interventions and treatments are helpful for affected children and adults. The treatment team should include multiple professionals, including a special education teacher, a speech and language pathologist, an occupational therapist, a physician, and a psychologist (Hagerman, 1996b; Scharfenaker et al., 1996a; Sobesky 1996).

Medical Follow-Up and Psychopharmacology

The medical treatment of FXS includes vigorous intervention for recurrent otitis media infections, which can further exacerbate the language delays in FXS (Hagerman et al., 1989). In addition, approximately 20% of patients have seizures; these can further interfere with normal development and academic progress, and they require treatment (Hagerman, 1996b; Hagerman, 1999). Other medical problems associated with loose connective tissue include rare hernias, rare joint dislocations, mitral valve prolapse, sinus infections, and gastroesophageal reflux (Hagerman, 1996b).

Medical intervention can be most helpful for the behavior problems that are usually present in FXS. For the preschool child, tantrums and hyperarousal are common difficulties, in addition to a short attention span. Stimulant medications (see below) may benefit some preschool children but may exacerbate behavioral problems in others (Hagerman, Murphy, & Wittenberger, 1988). Clonidine may be tried to calm behavior and improve attention and organization. Clonidine is an antihypertensive that comes in both a pill and a patch form. The most common side effect is sedation, but in approximately 70% of individuals with FXS it can be helpful for improving ADHD symptoms and decreasing outburst behavior (Hagerman, 1996b). Folic acid has also been reported to be helpful, although there are multiple arguments both for and against its use in FXS (see review by Turk, 1992). In our clinical experience, this treatment is helpful for approximately 50% of young children with FXS; however, it appears to work similarly to a weak stimulant medication, and other interventions described here are often more powerful than folic acid therapy alone (Hagerman, 1996b).

Stimulant medications are helpful in approximately 60% of school-age children for improving attention and concentration, and for decreasing impulsivity and aggression (Hagerman et al., 1988). Stimulants include methylphenidate (Ritalin), dextroamphetamine (Dexedrine and Adderall), and pemoline (Cylert). Stimulant treatment should start with a low dose, since higher doses may cause an increase in irritability even in a school-age child. Additional side effects of stimulants include cardiovascular stimulation, decrease in appetite, and difficulty in falling asleep at night. It is important for children who are treated with stimulants to be followed regularly by their physicians to document their response and their growth, as well as to review the side effects. Patients who become more irritable on Ritalin or Dexedrine often respond well to Cylert, but Cylert has a risk of significant liver dysfunction, and thus its use requires regular liver function studies. A recent Food and Drug Administration report stated that 13 cases of liver failure related to Cylert have occurred in the last 20 years of its use (Hagerman, 1999). This report should stimulate caution in prescribing, and careful follow-up of treatment with Cylert. In general, Cylert causes less cardiovascular stimulation and perhaps less appetite suppression than to the other stimulants. A newer medication, a mixture of four dextro- and levoamphetamine salts (Adderall) appears to be efficacious; however, controlled studies are still underway.

If severe mood lability or aggression occurs, the anticonvulsants carbamazepine (Tegretol) or valproic acid (Depakote) can be helpful to stabilize mood and decrease aggression (Hagerman, 1996b). They are also utilized to treat seizures in FXS. These medications have significant side effects, however, and they require careful monitoring of blood count, platelet count, electrolytes, and liver function.

For the treatment of moodiness, aggression, anxiety and obsessive–compulsive behavior, the SSRIs have been remarkably helpful in FXS (Hagerman et al., 1994a; Hagerman, 1996b). The SSRIs include fluoxetine (Prozac), sertraline (Zoloft), paroxetine (Paxil), citalopram (Celexa), and fluvoxamine (Luvox). They are relatively safe and easy to monitor because they do not require regular blood work or EKGs. The side effects include diarrhea, agitation, hyperactivity, sleep disturbances, abdominal pain, and the rare occurrence of mania. They are commonly used in adolescence and adulthood, and limited experience is available regarding their use in childhood. Controlled studies are needed to document their efficacy, specifically in FXS.

Speech/Language and Occupational Therapy

All children who are significantly affected by FXS can benefit from speech/language therapy and occupational therapy (Scharfenaker et al., 1996a; Schopmeyer & Lowe, 1992). Speech and language deficits in FXS include auditory processing problems, cluttering, mumbling, poor pragmatics, motor dyspraxia, and difficulties with abstract reasoning. Speech and language therapy can focus on each of these deficits. Even in a nonretarded child, deficits in higher linguistic skills and pragmatics may exist. Strengths in the language area include memory and imitation skills, a fine sense of humor, and empathy in social interactions. The memory strengths and the imitation skills can be well utilized in a therapy intervention program (Scharfenaker et al., 1996a).

Sensory integration and occupational therapy can also be helpful for children with FXS. Physical calming techniques such as brushing of the arms and legs, joint compression, and deep back rubs can be helpful in decreasing hyperarousal behavior or aggression. In addition to sensory integration therapy, a focus on fine and gross motor coordination and on motor planning is helpful in therapy. Hypotonia also improves with time and with intervention.

Additional techniques can be used to improve oral strength and verbalization. For jaw and mouth strength, several approaches are helpful. For instance, introducing a variety of textured foods can help decrease oral sensitivity. Bagels, fruit leather, and chewy candy are excellent at improving oral function. Simple games, such as playing tug of war with a wet washcloth during bathtime, can promote increased jaw strength (Scharfenaker et al., 1996a). Other methods can be used for stimulating verbal expression, including the use of rhythm, movement, dancing, and singing. The combination of speech and language therapy with occupational therapy can be helpful, particularly for less verbal children with FXS (Scharfenaker et al., 1996a). Therapies can be even more effective when they are implemented at home as well as in school.

The use of augmentative and alternative communication (AAC) can be successful for children with FXS who are nonverbal. Many different methods of communication can be used to "augment" a child's speech production or provide an "alternative" to speech (Beukelman & Mireuda, 1992), and an AAC evaluation can determine which of these may be useful. For instance, some children may use signs and gestures to communicate with others. Pointing to pictures can also be a useful form of communication and choice making. Parents and teachers can create picture books or cards to help a child communicate his or her needs (e.g., the child can point to a picture of a glass of water when he or she is thirsty). For choice making, the child can choose between pictures of two things or activities (e.g., pictures of going outside or of playing in the house). More complicated picture boards can also be successful in generating expressive language. For instance, the child can select pictures that represent the words "I," "want," and "hug," to generate the sentence "I want [a] hug." Finally, speech output devices may be used to help a child communicate his or her needs through synthesized or digitized speech (Hagerman, 1999). An AAC evaluation can be very beneficial to the child and to parents and educators if the child is still not talking or is having difficulty communicating with others (Beukelman & Mireuda, 1992).

Computer-Based Interventions

Computer technology is a useful adjunct to the educational experience for children with FXS. They usually enjoy working on computers, and they show talent in this area. Computers can be utilized to enhance attention and build vocabulary skills, in addition to improving written language output. Adaptive peripherals, such as an expanded keyboard or IntelliKeys, can be useful in helping children with FXS to use the computer (IntelliTools, Inc., 1996). Another adjustment that can make a computer user-friendly to a child with

FXS is a "track ball." A track ball is a type of inverted mouse with a stationary base that makes it easier for many children to use.

The use of both visual and auditory feedback computer technology is most beneficial for children with FXS. Computers can help sustain attention in some children with FXS who are otherwise easily distracted in standard learning environments. There is such a wide variety of software available in different topics of learning that it is important to evaluate a child's cognitive level and visual–spatial, memory, motor, and language skills, in order to match a beneficial program to the child (Scharfenaker et al., 1996a). Some helpful programs include IntelliTalk from IntelliTools, which is a talking word processor that can speak letters, words, sentences, and a combination of all three (IntelliTools, Inc., 1996; Scharfenaker et al., 1996b), and Co-Writer from Don Johnston, Inc., which is a combination of a dictionary and software that uses artificial intelligence to predict what a person wants to say (Scharfenaker et al., 1996b; D. Johnston, Inc., 1997). Programs such as Co-Writer were initially established to aid people with physical limitations, but children with learning and mental disabilities have also benefited tremendously from these programs. A list of computer centers for children with FXS in each state can be found in Scharfenaker et al. (1996b).

Behavioral and Educational Interventions

The use of behavioral intervention techniques, including structure and positive behavioral reinforcement, is most beneficial for children with FXS. Brown, Braden, and Sobesky (1991) describe behavioral intervention techniques in detail. Topics of high interest to a particular child can be utilized in behavioral interventions and academic programs. For instance, a young man who was extremely interested in fish was given fish stickers on a regular basis throughout the school day when he completed academic tasks. Such themes can be tied into academic presentations; for instance, writing words within an outline of a fish in paper can help improve the attention of a child who is interested in fish.

Children with FXS can be often educated in an inclusion setting in the regular classroom (Spiridigliozzi et al., 1994). If cognitive deficits or behavioral problems are significant, then an aide or paraprofessional can be utilized in the classroom to modify assignments or to give extra explanation to the child with FXS (and perhaps others who need it). An inclusion setting helps to improve social skills, since the child imitates the normal and appropriate behavior of the other children. Education in a segregated program exclusively with children who have special needs can be problematic, particularly if all of the other children are lower-functioning, since the child with FXS will imitate the behaviors and language of the lower-functioning children. Therefore, an inclusion setting is recommended for a child with FXS whenever possible, so that the other children in the class can model appropriate behavior for the child with FXS.

The treatment of children with FXS always necessitates creativity on the part of the therapist and the treatment team. Often nontraditional approaches can be most helpful, particularly when one considers the behavioral phenotype of FXS.

Conclusions

The broad spectrum of involvement in FXS requires a variety of interventions specific to each individual. Although there are similar physical, cognitive, and behavioral characteristics among children with FXS, there is no set curriculum that will be effective for every child. For instance, some children who are carriers of FXS may not require medical or educational intervention, while others may benefit from medication to help with anxiety or tutoring to help with school difficulties. Children who are affected by FXS usually benefit from special education support, speech/language and occupational therapy, and medication; however, there is no set formula as to the extent of therapy and the specific medications that will be most helpful for each individual child. For this reason, it is essential for children with FXS to be seen by a physician and a team of professionals who are familiar with FXS and can create an appropriate program for the child.

Once a family knows of the FXS diagnosis, it is helpful for the family to contact the National Fragile X Foundation, which has a network of parent support groups and resource centers around the country and internationally. The phone number of the National Fragile X Foundation is (800) 688-8765 or (303) 333-6155. The National Fragile X Foundation can also provide educational information in papers, books, videos, and conferences for both parents and professionals.

ACKNOWLEDGMENTS

This work was partially supported by a grant from Maternal Child Health (No. MCJ -089413), a grant from the National Institute of Child Health and Human Development (No. HD36071), the Denver Foundation, and the Kenneth Kendall King Foundation. We also thank Annette Taylor and Flora Tassone from Kimball Genetics, and Louise Staley-Gane from the Fragile X Treatment and Research Center, Children's Hospital, for their research and support. We would also like to thank Rebecca O'Connor, Sarah Scharfenaker, Mela Barrios, Barbara Wheeler, and Beverly Rogers of the Child Development Unit, Children's Hospital, for their expertise and support.

REFERENCES

Abbeduto, L., & Hagerman, R. J. (1997). Language and communication in fragile X syndrome. *Mental Retardation and Developmental Disabilities Research Reviews, 3*, 313–322.

Abrams, M. T., & Reiss, A. L. (1995). The neurobiology of fragile X syndrome. *Mental Retardation and Developmental Disabilities Research Reviews, 1*, 269–275.

Abrams, M. T., Reiss, A. L., Freund, L. S., Baumgardner, T. L., Chase, G. A., & Denckla, M. B. (1994). Molecular–neurobehavioral associations in females with the fragile X full mutation. *American Journal of Medical Genetics, 51*, 317–327.

Baumgardner, T., Reiss, A. L., Freund, L. S., & Abrams, M. T. (1995). Specifications of the neurobehavioral associations in males with fragile X syndrome. *Pediatrics, 95*, 744–752.

Bell, M. V., Hirst, M. C., Nakahori, Y., MacKinon, R. N., Roche, H., Flint, T. J., Jacobs, P. A., Tommerup, N., Tranebjaerg, L., Froster-Iskenius, U., Kerr, B., Turner, G., Lindenbaum, R. H., Winter, R., Pembrey, M., Thibodeau, S., & Davies, K. E. (1991). Physical mapping across the fragile X: Hypermethylation and clinical expression of the fragile X syndrome. *Cell, 64*, 861–866.

Belser, R. C., & Sudhalter, V. (1995). Arousal difficulties in males with fragile X syndrome: A preliminary report. *Developmental Brain Dysfunction, 8*, 252–269.

Beukelman, D. R., & Mireuda, P. (1992). *Augmentative and alternative communication: Management of severe communication disorders in children and adults.* Baltimore: Paul H. Brookes.

Brown, J., Braden, M., & Sobesky, W. (1991). The treatment of behavioral and emotional problems. In R. J. Hagerman & C. Silverman (Eds.), *Fragile X syndrome: Diagnosis, treatment, and research* (pp. 311–326). Baltimore: Johns Hopkins University Press.

Brown, W. T. (1996). The molecular biology of the fragile X mutation. In R. J. Hagerman & A. C. Cronister (Eds). *Fragile X syndrome: Diagnosis, treatment, and research* (2nd ed., pp. 88–113). Baltimore: Johns Hopkins University Press.

Brown, W. T., Jenkins, E. C., Cohen, I. L., Fisch, G. S., Wolf-Schein, E. G., Gross, A., Waterhouse, L., Fein, D., Mason-Brothers, A., Ritvo, E., Rittenberg, B. A., Bentley, W., & Castells, S. (1986). Fragile X and autism: A multicenter survey. *American Journal of Medical Genetics, 23,* 341–352.

Butler, M. G., Allen, M. G., Haynes, J. L., Singh, D. N., Watson, M. S., & Breg, W. R. (1991). Anthropometric comparison of mentally retarded males with and without the fragile X syndrome. *American Journal of Medical Genetics, 38,* 260–268.

Cohen, I. L. (1995). Behavioral profiles of autistic and nonautistic fragile X males. *Developmental Brain Dysfunction, 8,* 252–269.

Cohen, I. L., Brown, W. T., Jenkins, E. C., French, J. C., Raguthu, S., Wolf-Schein, E. G., Sudhalter, V., Fisch, G., & Wisniewski, K. (1989). Fragile X syndrome in females with autism [Letter to the editor]. *American Journal of Medical Genetics, 34,* 302–303.

Cohen, I. L., Sudhalter, V., Pfadt, A., Jenkins, E. C., Brown, W. T., & Vielze, P. M. (1991). Why are autism and the fragile X syndrome associated?: Conceptual and methodological issues. *American Journal of Human Genetics, 48,* 195–202.

Cronister, A. C. (1996). Genetic counseling. In R. J. Hagerman & A. C. Cronister (Eds.), *Fragile X syndrome: Diagnosis, treatment, and research* (2nd ed., pp. 251–282).Baltimore: Johns Hopkins University Press.

deVries, B. B. A., Fryns, J.-P., Butler, M. G., Canziani, F., Wesby-van Swaay, E., vanHemel, J. O., Oostra, B. A., Halley, D. J. J., & Niermeyer, M. F. (1993). Clinical and molecular studies in fragile X patients with a Prader–Willi-like phenotype. *Journal of Medical Genetics, 30,* 761–766.

deVries, B. B. A., Robinson, H., Stolte-Dijkstra, I., Gi, C. V. T. P., Dijkstra, D. F., vanDoorn, J., Halley, D. J. J., Oostra, B. A., Turner, G., & Niermeijer, M. F. (1995). General overgrowth in the fragile X syndrome: Variability in the phenotype expression of the FMR1 gene mutation. *Journal of Medical Genetics, 32,* 764–769.

deVries, B. B. A., Wiegers, A. M., Smits, A. P. T., Mohkamsing, S., Duivenvoorden, H. J., Fryns, J.-P., Curfs, L. M. G., Halley, D. J. J., Oostra, B. A., van den Ouweland, A. M. W., & Niermeijer, M. F. (1996). Mental status of females with an FMR1 gene full mutation. *American Journal of Human Genetics, 58,* 1025–1032.

Eichler, E. E., & Nelson, D. L. (1996). Genetic variation and evolutionary stability of the FMR1 CGG repeat in six closed human populations. *American Journal of Medical Genetics, 64,* 220–225.

Franke, P., Maier, W., Iwers, B., Hautzinger, M., & Froster, U. G. (1996). Fragile X carrier females: Evidence for a distinct psychopathological phenotype? *American Journal of Medical Genetics, 64,* 334–339.

Freund, L. S., Peebles, C. D., Aylward, E., & Reiss, A. L. (1995). Preliminary report on cognitive and adaptive behaviors of preschool aged males with fragile X. *Developmental Brain Dysfunction, 8,* 242–251.

Freund, L. S., & Reiss, A. L., (1991). Cognitive profiles associated with fragile X syndrome in males and females. *American Journal Medical Genetics, 38,* 542–547.

Freund, L. S., Reiss, A. L., & Abrams, M. (1993). Psychiatric disorders associated with fragile X in the young female. *Pediatrics, 91,* 321–329.

Hagerman, R. J. (1996a). Physical and behavioral phenotype. In R. J. Hagerman & A. C. Cronister (Eds.), *Fragile X syndrome: Diagnosis, treatment, and research* (2nd ed., pp. 3–87). Baltimore: Johns Hopkins University Press.

Hagerman, R. J. (1996b). Medical follow-up and psychopharmacology. In R. J. Hagerman & A. C. Cronister (Eds.), *Fragile X syndrome: Diagnosis, treatment, and research* (2nd ed., pp. 283–331). Baltimore: Johns Hopkins University Press.

Hagerman, R. J. (1999). Fragile X syndrome. In *Neurodevelopmental disorders: Diagnosis and treatment.* New York: Oxford University Press.

Hagerman, R. J., Hull, C. E., Safanda, J. F., Carpenter, I., Staley, L. W., O'Connor, R. O., Seydel, C., Mazzocco, M. M., Snow, K., Thibodeau, S., Kuhl, D., Nelson, D. L., Caskey, C. T., & Taylor,

A. (1994a). High functioning fragile X males: Demonstration of an unmethylated, fully expanded FMR-1 mutation associated with protein expression. *American Journal of Medical Genetics, 51,* 298–308.

Hagerman, R. J., Murphy, M. A., & Wittenberger, M. (1988). A controlled trial of stimulant medication in children with fragile X syndrome. *American Journal of Medical Genetics, 30,* 377–392.

Hagerman, R. J., Schreiner, R., Kemper, M., Wittenberg, M., Zahn, B., & Habitcht, K. (1989). Longitudinal IQ changes in fragile X males. *American Journal of Medical Genetics, 33,* 513–518.

Hagerman, R. J., Wilson, P., Staley, L. W., Lang, K. A., Fan, T., Uhlhorn, C., Jewell-Smart, S., Hull, C., Flom, K., & Taylor, A. K. (1994b). Evaluation of school children at high risk for fragile X syndrome utilizing buccal cell FMR-1 testing. *American Journal of Medical Genetics, 51,* 474–479.

Hodapp, R. M., Dykens, E. M., Hagerman, R. J., Schreiner, R., Lachiewicz, A. M., & Leckman, J. F. (1990). Developmental implications of changing trajectories of IQ in males with fragile X syndrome. *Journal of the American Academy of Child and Adolescent Psychology, 29,* 214–219.

Hull, C., & Hagerman, R. J. (1993). A study of the physical, behavioral, and medical phenotype, including anthropometric measures of females with fragile X syndrome. *American Journal of Diseases of Children, 147,* 1236–1241.

Imbert, G., Feng, Y., Nelson, D. L., Warren, S. T., & Mandel, J. L. (1998). FMRI and mutations in fragile X syndrome: Molecular biology, biochemistry, and genetics. In R. D. Wells & S. T. Warien (Eds.), *Genetic instabilities and hereditary neurological diseases* (pp. 27–53). New York: Academic Press.

IntelliTools, Inc. (1996). *IntelliTools: Access to learning through technology.* Novato, CA: Author.

Johnston, D. Inc. (1997). *Solutions for struggling students.* Wauconda, IL: Author.

Lachiewicz, A. M., & Dawson, D. V. (1994). Do young boys with fragile X syndrome have macroorchidism? *Pediatrics, 93,* 992–995.

Lachiewicz, A. M., Gullion, C., Spiridigliozzi, G., & Aylsworth, A. (1987). Declining IQs of young males with the fragile X syndrome. *American Journal of Mental Retardation, 92,* 272–278.

Loesch, D. Z., Huggins, R. M., & Hoang, N. H. (1995). Growth in stature in fragile X families: A mixed longitidinal study. *American Journal of Medical Genetics, 58,* 249–256.

Mazzocco, M., Pennington, B., & Hagerman, R. (1993). The neurocognitive phenotype of female carriers of fragile X: Further evidence for specificity. *Journal of Developmental and Behavioral Pediatrics, 14,* 328–335.

Merenstein, S. A., Shyu, V., Sobesky, W. E., Staley, L., Taylor, A., & Hagerman, R. J. (1994). Fragile X syndrome in a normal IQ male with learning and emotional problems. *Journal of the American Academy of Child and Adolescent Psychiatry, 33,* 1316–1321.

Merenstein, S. A., Sobesky, W. E., Taylor, A. K., Riddle, J. E., Tran, H. X., & Hagerman, R. J. (1996). Molecular-clinical correlations in males with an expanded FMRI mutation. *American Journal of Medical Genetics, 64,* 388–394.

Oberlé, I., Rousseau, F., Heitz, D., Kretz, C., Devys, D., Hanauer, A., Boue, J., Bertheas, M. F., & Mandel, J. L. (1991). Instability of a 550-base pair DNA segment and abnormal methylation in fragile X syndrome. *Science, 52,* 1097–1102.

Oostra, B. A. (1996). FMR1 protein studies and animal model for fragile X syndrome. In R. J. Hagerman, & A. C. Cronister (Eds.), *Fragile X syndrome: Diagnosis, treatment, and research* (2nd ed., pp. 193–209). Baltimore: Johns Hopkins University Press.

Opitz, J. M., Westphal, J. M., & Daniel, A. (1984). Discovery of a connective tissue dysplasia in the Martin–Bell syndrome. *American Journal of Medical Genetics, 17,* 101–109.

Pieretti, M., Zhang, F., Fu, Y.-H., Warren, S. T., Oostra, B. A., Caskey, C. T., & Nelson, D. L. (1991). Absence of expression of the FMR-1 gene in fragile X syndrome. *Cell, 66,* 817–822.

Reiss, A., Abrams, M., Greenlaw, R., Freund, L., & Denckla, M. (1995). Neurodevelopmental effects of the FMR-1 full mutation in humans. *Nature Medicine, 1,* 159–167.

Reiss, A. L., Aylward, E., Freund, L. S., Joshi, P. K., & Bryan, R. N. (1991a). Neuroanatomy of the fragile X syndrome: The posterior fossa. *Annals of Neurology, 29,* 26–32.

Reiss, A. L., & Freund, L. (1990). Fragile X syndrome, DSM-III-R, and autism. *Journal of the American Academy of Child and Adolescent Psychiatry, 29*, 885–891.

Reiss, A. L., & Freund, L. (1991). Behavioral phenotype of fragile X syndrome: DSM-III-R autistic behavior in male children. *American Journal of Medical Genetics, 43*, 35–46.

Reiss, A. L., Freund, L., Abrams, M. T., Boehm, C., & Kazazian, H. (1993). Neurobehavioral effects of the fragile X premutation in adult women: A controlled study. *American Journal of Human Genetics, 52*, 884–894.

Reiss, A. L., Freund, L., Tseng, J. E., & Joshi, P. K. (1991b). Neuroanatomy in fragile X females: The posterior fossa. *American Journal of Human Genetics, 49*, 279–288.

Reiss, A. L., Lee, J., & Freund, L. (1994). Neuroanatomy of fragile X syndrome: the temporal lobe. *Neurology, 44*, 1317–1324.

Reiss, A. L., Patel, S., Kumar, A. J., & Freund, L. (1988). Preliminary communication: neuroanatomical variations of the posterior fossa in men with the fragile X (Martin–Bell) syndrome. *American Journal of Medical Genetics, 31*, 407–414.

Reyniers, E., Vits, L., De Boulle, K., Van Roy, B., Van Velzen, D., de Graaff, E., Verkerk, A. J. M. H., Jorens, H. Z. J., Darby, J. K., Oostra, B., & Willems, P. (1993). The full mutation in the FMR-1 gene of male fragile X patients is absent in their sperm. *Nature Genetics, 4*, 143–146.

Riddle, J. E., Cheema, A., Sobesky, W. E., Gardner, S. C., Taylor, A. K., Pennington, P. F., & Hagerman, R. J. (1998). Phenotype in females with the FMRI gene mutation. *American Journal of Mental Retardation, 102*, 590–601.

Rousseau, F., Heitz, D., Oberlé, I., & Mandel, J.-L. (1991). Selection in blood cells from female carriers responsible for variable phenotypic expression of the fragile X syndrome: Inverse correlation between age and proportion of active X-carrying the full mutation. *Journal of Medical Genetics, 28*, 830–836.

Rousseau, F., Morel, M.-L., Rouillard, P., Khandjian, E. W., & Morgan, K. (1996). Surprisingly low prevalence of FMR1 premutation among males from the general population. *American Journal of Human Genetics, 59*(Suppl.), 1069.

Rousseau, F., Rouillard, P., Morel, M.-L., Khandjian, E. W., & Morgan, K. (1995). Prevalence of carriers of premutation-sized alleles of the FMR1 gene—and implications for the population genetics of the fragile X syndrome. *American Journal of Human Genetics, 57*, 1006–1018.

Scharfenaker, S., O'Connor, R., Stackhouse, T., Braden, M., Hickman, L., & Gray, K. (1996a). An integrated approach to intervention. In R. J. Hagerman & A. C. Cronister (Eds.), *Fragile X syndrome: Diagnosis, treatment, and research* (2nd ed., pp.349–411). Baltimore: Johns Hopkins University Press.

Scharfenaker, S., O'Connor, R., Stackhouse, T., Braden, M., Hickman, L., & Gray, K. (1996b). Computer software information. In R. J. Hagerman & A. C. Cronister (Eds.), *Fragile X syndrome: Diagnosis, treatment, and research* (2nd ed., pp. 453–462). Baltimore: Johns Hopkins University Press.

Schwartz, C., Dean, J., Howard-Peebles, P., Bugge, M., Mikkelsen, M., Tomerup, N., Hull, C., Hagerman, R., Holden, J., & Stevenson, R. E. (1994). Obstetrical and gynecological complications in fragile X carriers: A multicenter study. *American Journal of Medical Genetics, 51*, 400–402.

Shapiro, M. B., Murphy, D. G. M., Hagerman, R. J., Azari, N. P., Alexander, G. E., Meizejeski, C. M., Hinton, V. J., Horwitz, B., Haxby, J. V., Kumar, A., White, B., & Brady, C. L. (1995). Adult fragile X syndrome: Neuropsychology, brain anatomy and metabolism. *American Journal of Medical Genetics, 60*, 480–493.

Sherman, S. (1996). Epidemiology. In R. J. Hagerman & A. C. Cronister (Eds.), *Fragile X syndrome: Diagnosis, treatment, and research* (2nd ed., pp. 165–192). Baltimore: Johns Hopkins University Press.

Shopmeyer, B., & Lowe, F. (1992). *The fragile X child*. San Diego: Singular.

Slaney, S. F., Wilkie, A. O. M., Hirst, M. C., Charlton, R., McKinley, M., Pointon, J., Christodoulou, Z., Huson, S. M., & Davies, K. E. (1995). DNA testing for fragile X syndrome in schools for learning difficulties. *Archives of Disease in Childhood, 72*, 33–37.

Sobesky, W. E. (1996). The treatment of emotional and behavioral problems. In R. J. Hagerman & A. C. Cronister (Eds.), *Fragile X syndrome: Diagnosis, treatment, and research* (2nd ed., pp. 332–348). Baltimore: Johns Hopkins University Press.

Sobesky, W. E., Pennington, B. F., Porter, D., Hull, C. E., & Hagerman, R. J. (1994). Emotional and neurocognitive deficits in fragile X. *American Journal of Medical Genetics, 51,* 378–384.

Sobesky, W. E., Porter, D., Pennington, B. F., & Hagerman, R. J. (1995). Dimensions of shyness in fragile X females. *Developmental Brain Dysfunction, 8,* 280–292.

Sobesky, W. E., Taylor, A. K., Pennington, B. F., Riddle, J. E., & Hagerman, R. J. (1996). Molecular/clinical correlations in females with fragile X. *American Journal of Medical Genetics, 64,* 340–345.

Spiridigliozzi, G., Lachiewicz, A., MacMurdo, C., Vizoso, A., O'Donnell, C., McConkie-Rosell, A., & Burgess, D. (1994). *Educating boys with fragile X syndrome: A guide for parents and professionals.* Durham, NC: Duke University Medical Center.

Sutherland, G. R. (1977). Fragile sites on human chromosomes: Demonstration of their dependence on the type of tissue culture medium. *Science, 197,* 265–266.

Tassone, F., Dyer, P. D., Lampe, M., Willemsen, R., Oostra, B., Hagerman, R. J., & Taylor, A. K. (1999). FMRP expression as a potential prognostic indicator in fragile X syndrome. *American Journal of Medical Genetics, 84,* 250–261.

Taylor, A., Safanda, J. F., Fall, M. Z., Quince, C., Lang, K. A., Hull, C. E., Carpenter, I., Staley, L.W., & Hagerman, R. J. (1994). Molecular predictors of involvement in fragile X females. *Journal of American Medical Association, 271,* 507–514.

Turk, J. (1992). Fragile X syndrome and folic acid. In R. J. Hagerman & P. McKenzie (Eds.), *1992 International Fragile X Conference Proceedings* (pp. 195–200). Dillon, CO: National Fragile X Foundation/Spectra.

Turner, G., Laing, S., Robinson, H., Wake, S., & Wright, F. (1995, August). *The prevalence of the fragile X syndrome in NSW prior to counseling of females at risk.* Paper presented at the 7th International Workshop on the Fragile X and X-Linked Mental Retardation, Tromsø, Norway.

Turner, G., Robinson, H., Laing, S., & Purvis-Smith, S. (1986). Preventive screening for the fragile X syndrome. *New England Journal of Medicine, 315,* 607–609.

Turner, G., Webb, T., Wake, S., & Robinson, H. (1996). Prevalence of the fragile X syndrome. *American Journal of Medical Genetics, 64,* 196–197.

Verkerk, A. J., Pieretti, M., Sutcliffe, J. S., Fu, Y.-H., Kuhl, D. P., Pizzuti, A., Reiner, O., Richards, S., Victoria, M. F., Zhang, F., Eussen, B.E., van Ommen, G. J., Blonden, L. A. J., Riggins, G. J., Chastain, J. L., Kunst, C. B., Galjaard, H., Caskey, C. T., Nelson, D. L., Oostra, B. A., & Warren, S. T. (1991). Identification of a gene (FMR-1) containing a CGG repeat coincident with a breakpoint cluster region exhibiting length variation in fragile X syndrome. *Cell, 54,* 905–914.

Wahlstrom, J., Gillberg, C., Gustavson, K., & Holmgren, G. (1986). Infantile autism and the fragile X: A Swedish multicenter study. *American Journal of Medical Genetics, 23,* 403–408.

Warren, S. T., & Ashley, C. T. (1995). Triplet repeat expansion mutations: The example of fragile X syndrome. *Annual Review of Neuroscience, 18,* 77–99.

Webb, T. P., Bundey, S., Thake, A., & Todd, J. (1986). The frequency of the fragile X chromosome among school children in Coventry. *Journal of Medical Genetics, 23,* 396–399.

Wright-Talamante, C., Cheema, A., Riddle, J. E., Luckey, D. W., Taylor, A. K., & Hagerman, R. J. (1996). A controlled study of longitudinal IQ changes in females and males with fragile X syndrome. *American Journal of Medical Genetics, 64,* 350–355.

Yu, S., Pritchard, M., Kremer, E., Lynch, M., Nancarrow, J., Baker, E., Holman, K., Mulley, J. C., Warren, S. T., Schlessinger, D., Sutherland, G. R., & Richards, R. I. (1991). Fragile X genotype characterized by an unstable region of DNA. *Science, 252,* 1179–1181.

Zhong, N., Kajanoja, E., Smits, B., Pietrofesa, J., Curley, D., Wang, D., Ju, W., Nolin, S., Dobkin, C., Ryynnan, M., & Brown, W.T. (1996). Fragile X founder effects and new mutations. *American Journal of Medical Genetics, 64,* 226–233.

13

THE MUCOPOLYSACCHARIDOSES

MICHAEL B. BROWN

The mucopolysaccharidoses (MPS disorders) are a group of genetic abnormalities of muco-polysaccharide metabolism characterized by varying degrees of physical, sensory, cognitive, and behavioral impairments (Cervantes & Lifshitz, 1990; Levine, 1991). Mucopolysac-charides are complex compounds that are present in bone, skin, connective tissues, and major organs, and are commonly broken down or metabolized by a series of enzymes. Enzyme mutations result in an excess of incompletely metabolized mucopolysaccharides accumulating in bone and connective tissues, resulting in the patterns of features and com-plications that characterize these disorders. There are six types of MPS disorders, several of which have a number of subtypes (see Table 13.1).

The MPSs are relatively rare, and accurate epidemiological data are difficult to obtain. The prevalence of Hurler syndrome has been estimated at 1 in 100,000 live births. Scheie syndrome is believed to occur in 1 in 600,000 live births (Neufeld & Muenzer, 1995). Few reports exist of patients with Hurler–Scheie syndrome (Matalan, 1996); therefore, prevalence figures are not available. Hunter syndrome is estimated to occur in approximately 1 in 130,000 to 150,000 male births (Sinclair, 1979; Young & Harper, 1982), with a much higher preva-lence of 1 in 36,000 births in Israel (Schaap & Bach, 1980). Sanfilippo syndrome has been reported in 1 in 25,000 births in the United Kingdom (Cleary & Wraith, 1993). Morquio syndrome has a prevalence of 3 per 1,000,000 persons (Goldberg, 1996). Maroteaux–Lamy syndrome occurs in 1 in 216,000 births (Lowry, Applegarth, Toone, MacDonald, & Thunem, 1990). Very few cases of Sly syndrome have been reported (Neufeld & Muenzer, 1995).

ETIOLOGY, FEATURES, AND COURSE

Pathophysiology

The mucopolysaccharidoses are lysosomal storage disorders (Pennock, 1994). Lysosomes are intracellular particles containing enzymes that can break down or digest complex molecules. The complex molecules are brought into the lysosomes for degradation in the course of normal physiological processes. In the MPS disorders, there is a failure of spe-

TABLE 13.1. Classification of the MPS Disorders

MPS IH	Hurler syndrome
MPS IS	Scheie syndrome
MPS IHS	Hurler–Scheie syndrome
MPS II	Hunter syndrome
MPS IIIA	Sanfilippo syndrome, Type A
MPS IIIB	Sanfilippo syndrome, Type B
MPS IIIC	Sanfilippo syndrome, Type C
MPS IIID	Sanfilippo syndrome, Type D
MPS IVA	Morquio syndrome, Type A
MPS IVB	Morquio syndrome, Type B
MPS IVC	Morquio syndrome, Type C
MPS VI	Maroteaux–Lamy syndrome
MPS VII	Sly syndrome

cific genes to produce adequate levels of active enzymes necessary to break down the mucopolysaccharides, which are components of connective tissue and bone. As a result, large quantities of the incompletely metabolized material accumulate in the lysosomes. The abnormal accumulation produces the symptoms and complications of these disorders. There are several enzymes required for the degradation of mucopolysaccharides, and each of the MPS disorders has a specific enzyme defect that is responsible for the disorder (Christodoulou & McInnes, 1998; see Table 13.2).

Genetics

All of the MPS disorders, with the exception of Hunter syndrome, are autosomal recessive disorders. In an autosomal recessive disorder each parent must be a carrier of the abnormal gene for a child to develop the disorder (Pennock, 1994). Both males and females can be affected by these MPS disorders. There are several alleles (genetic sites) believed to be responsible for correct enzyme production. This accounts for the variations in severity of clinical manifestations of the disorders in different individuals (Menkes, 1990).

Hunter syndrome is a recessive, sex-linked disorder, with the affected gene site located on the X chromosome. Females carry the recessive gene for the disorder. The disorder there-

TABLE 13.2. Enzyme Deficiencies in MPS Disorders

Type of disorder		Enzyme deficiency
MPS IH	Hurler syndrome	Alpha-L-iduronidase
MPS IS	Scheie syndrome	Alpha-L-iduronidase
MPS IHS	Hurler–Scheie syndrome	Alpha-L-iduronidase
MPS II	Hunter syndrome	Iduronate sulfatases
MPS IIIA	Sanfilippo syndrome, Type A	Heparan-N-sulfatase
MPS IIIB	Sanfilippo syndrome, Type B	Alpha-N-acetylglucosaminidase
MPS IIIC	Sanfilippo syndrome, Type C	Acetyl CoA-alpha-glucosaminide-acetyltransferase
MPS IIID	Sanfilippo syndrome, Type D	N-Acetylglucosamine-6-sulfatase
MPS IVA	Morquio syndrome, Type A	Galactosamine-6-sulfate sulfatase
MPS IVB	Morquio syndrome, Type B	Beta-galactosidase
MPS VI	Maroteaux–Lamy syndrome	N-Acetylgalactosamine-4-sulfatase
MPS VII	Sly syndrome	Beta-glucuronidase

fore occurs almost exclusively in males, as they receive only one X chromosome and there is no other X chromosome to provide a dominant (normal) version of the gene to override the effect of the recessive (impaired) gene. Females can be affected if there has been an inactivation of the normal X chromosome or a balanced translocation of part of the X chromosome (Roberts, Upadhyaya, Sarfarazi, & Harper, 1989). The disorder is seen primarily in persons of European descent, and only rarely in members of other racial/ethnic groups (Pennock, 1994). There is a report that Hunter syndrome occurs more frequently in persons of Jewish ancestry (Schaap & Bach, 1980). Like the other MPS disorders, it is genetically heterogeneous, in that mutations in different allelic sites are responsible for the variation in expression of the disorder.

Major Features

The most striking features of the MPS disorders are their skeletal effects. The complete range of skeletal features occurs in Hurler syndrome; these features occur to varying degrees in each of the other MPS disorders. The abnormal accumulation of incompletely metabolized mucopolysaccharides also affects other organ systems, most notably the cardiovascular, respiratory, and nervous systems. Neurological involvement results in progressive dementia in many of the MPS disorders.

MPS I (Hurler Syndrome, Scheie Syndrome, and Hurler–Scheie Syndrome)

Children with Hurler syndrome have characteristic skeletal effects known as "dysostosis multiplex" (Neufeld & Muenzer, 1995; Goldberg, 1996). Specific features include (1) widened collarbone and ribs; (2) progressive curvature of the lower spine (lumbar kyphoscoliosis); (3) significant shortening of stature; (4) shortened neck; (5) stubby, claw-like hands; (6) contractions of the joints; (7) enlarged head; (8) flattening of the bridge of the nose, wide nostrils, thick lips, and large and protruding tongue with open mouth; and (9) thick hair and excessive body hair. Hurler syndrome is the most severe of the three syndromes; Scheie and Hurler–Scheie syndromes have less severe skeletal expressions. Rapidly progressing cognitive impairment is the rule in Hurler syndrome, while cognitive functioning is spared in Scheie and Hurler–Sheie syndromes.

MPS II (Hunter Syndrome)

The features of Hunter syndrome include (1) a depressed nasal bridge and distortion of facial bones; (2) enlarged head; (3) a distinctive posture of hunched shoulders, with the joints of the limbs held in partial flexion; (4) joint stiffness and a claw-like hand deformity; (5) very short stature or dwarfism; (6) a thickening and overgrowth of hair on the body (hypertrichosis); and (7) raised, thickened skin nodules over the shoulder blades (Finlayson, 1990; Pennock, 1994; Christodoulou & McInnes, 1998; Young, Harper, Newcombe, & Archer, 1982b).

MPS III (Sanfilippo Syndrome)

The presentation of Sanfilippo syndrome is dominated by severe neurodegenerative disturbance (Cleary & Wraith, 1993). Progressive mental retardation occurs rapidly, along with serious behavior problems (Nidiffer & Kelly, 1983). Children exhibit hyperactive behavior, physical aggression, noncompliance, and self-stimulatory behaviors. There is usually only mild somatic involvement of the sort typical of the other MPS disorders at least until late in the course of the disorder (Matalan, 1996). Stature is near normal, and the coarsened facial features common to the other MPS disorders are usually not present. Joint stiffness is mild and rarely causes mobility problems.

MPS IV (Morquio Syndrome)

The primary features of Morquio Syndrome are severe skeletal deformities, with secondary effects on the nervous and cardiovascular systems (Watts & Gibbs, 1986). Persons with the disorder have normal or near-normal intelligence (Cervantes & Lifschitz, 1990). The characteristic features include (1) shortened trunk, neck, legs, and arms; (2) short stature or dwarfism, depending on the severity of the disorder; (3) unstable knee joints; (4) enlarged elbows and wrists; (5) flattened vertebrae, with underdevelopment of a portion of the cervical vertebrae; (6) expanded thoracic rib cage, with marked inward curvature of the lumbar spine (kyphoscoliosis); (7) waddling gait and inward-turned knees; (8) finger and joint stiffness, and early arthritis in hips and knees; (9) depressed nasal bridge and protruding lower jaw; (10) broad mouth, with the appearance of a permanent grin; and (11) dental abnormalities, including thin and pitted enamel, widely spaced conical teeth, and excessive tooth wear (Cervantes & Lifshitz, 1990; Goldberg, 1996; Nelson & Kinirons, 1988; Watts & Gibbs, 1986).

MPS VI (Maroteaux–Lamy Syndrome)

Children with Maroteaux–Lamy syndrome have dysostosis multiplex, the same characteristic skeletal effects as in Hurler syndrome (see above). Unlike children with Hurler syndrome, however, those with Maroteaux–Lamy sundrome may exhibit variations in the severity of the skeletal manifestations. Moreover, intellectual functioning remains in the normal range (Pennock, 1994).

MPS VII (Sly Syndrome)

Sly syndrome is characterized by skeletal manifestations similar to those of Hurler syndrome (Matalan, 1996). Unusual facial appearance, hepatosplenomegaly, and short stature are common. However, mild and severe forms of the disorder have been reported, along with a form of the disorder that is present at birth (Neufeld & Muenzer, 1995).

Developmental Course

The features of the MPS disorders generally become apparent in early childhood, though some of these disorders may first be diagnosed as late as adolescence. Although there may be individual variations, each of the disorders has a typical developmental course that includes the age of onset of symptoms and the progression of impairment.

MPS I (Hurler, Scheie, and Hurler–Scheie Syndromes)

Children with Hurler syndrome appear normal at birth and grow rapidly during their first year (Nelson & Crocker, 1992). A deceleration of growth occurs at some point between 6 and 18 months of age (Neufeld & Muenzer, 1995). Motor skills are usually limited, and language development is severely affected. Learning peaks in the second or third year of life, and afterward developmental regression occurs, with a loss of previously learned skills. Progressive mental retardation results. The ability to walk is gradually lost, as is language facility. Most children remain incontinent (Bax & Coville, 1995). Many have difficulty feeding themselves because of poor coordination and swallowing difficulties. The children also become less interested in the environment. Maximum functional age is usually between 2 and 4 years. Death frequently occurs by age 10 (Neufeld & Muenzer, 1995), typically as a result of cardiovascular disorders, respiratory problems, or complications of neurological damage (Nelson & Crocker, 1992).

The symptoms of Hurler–Scheie syndrome usually begin between 3 and 8 years of age (Neufeld & Muenzer, 1995). Children develop mild facial deformities, corneal clouding, and shortness of stature (Matalan, 1996). Joints are stiffened and contracted. Hepatosplenomegaly and hernia are frequent complications. Visual losses may occur due to corneal clouding or glaucoma. Intellectual development is typically normal or only mildly impaired. Hydrocephaly is common. Deafness and heart valve disorders are typical. Persons with this syndrome usually survive into adulthood.

Scheie syndrome is at the milder end of the clinical spectrum of these disorders (Goldberg, 1996). This disorder is characterized by joint stiffness, corneal clouding, and no mental retardation. The stature is usually normal, and children with the disorder develop an excess of body hair. The face may be coarsened in appearance, and the tongue is large (Pennock, 1994). Glaucoma may be present. The diagnosis is usually made in the teens, and life expectancy is not affected.

MPS II (Hunter Syndrome)

Two forms of Hunter syndrome, mild and severe, have been identified based on onset, complications, and course of the disorder (Pennock, 1994; Menkes, 1990; Young, Harper, Newcombe, & Archer, 1982a, 1982b). Within each form, however, considerable individual variation can exist (Tsuzaki, Matsuo, Nagai, Osano, & Orii, 1987). The mild or late-onset form has an average age of onset of 4.3 years and an average age at death of 21.7 years (Young & Harper, 1982). Development is typically normal at first, with the abnormal facial configuration and growth defects becoming evident by early childhood (Avery & First, 1994). Mental retardation is typically absent, with relatively normal intellectual performance. Survival is possible into the fourth decade and beyond, and persons with the disorder may continue their education, marry, and have children. Death is usually caused by cardiac or pulmonary complications (Young & Harper, 1982).

The severe or early-onset form of Hunter syndrome has an average age of onset of 2.5 years, with an average age at death of 11.8 years (Young & Harper, 1983). This form of the disorder is marked by progressive neurological involvement, which results in a plateau of learning and developmental skills at some point between ages 2 and 6. The plateau is followed by a regression in cognitive skills and behavior. Mental retardation has an insidious onset and becomes profound. Seizure disorder is common, especially past age 10. The children become emaciated, and there is significant wasting of body mass (neurodevelopmental cachexia). Ninety percent of those affected are bedridden by age 10. Death usually results from pulmonary complications of the cachexic state (Young & Harper, 1983).

MPS III (Sanfilippo Syndrome)

Children with Sanfilippo syndrome are typically first diagnosed at about age 5 (Cleary & Wraith, 1993; Neufeld & Muenzer, 1995; Nidiffer & Kelly, 1983). The features of the disorder begin to appear between 2 and 6 years of age. The rate of achievement of developmental milestones is normal up to this time, although delay or loss of language and memory may be the most notable early symptoms. The presenting symptoms include hyperactivity, developmental delay, hirsutism, and poor sleep. There may also be increasingly severe temper tantrums, as well as aggressive behavior that may result in destructiveness. Some children have panic-like symptoms in unfamiliar places. Cognitive decline continues with progressive dementia. The skeletal features common to the MPS disorders are usually less severe in Sanfilippo syndrome and tend to become obvious only in the later stages of the disorder. Some children develop episodes of intractable diarrhea.

After age 10 the behavioral symptoms are less severe. Typical problems include falls caused by lack of coordination, and difficulty with feeding as a result of impaired swallowing. Joint stiffness and spasticity interfere with mobility and may necessitate the use of a wheelchair. Claw-like deformities of the hand may be present. Seizures are not uncommon. Most individuals with Sanfilippo syndrome survive into their teens, although some more mildly impaired persons live into their second or third decade.

There are four forms of Sanfilippo syndrome(MPS III), designated as IIIA, IIIB, IIIC, and IIID, each associated with a different enzyme abnormality. The clinical presentation of each type appears similar. Not every child will fit the profile described above (Ozand et al., 1994); there are reports of persons whose behavior was not problematic until their late teens (Kim, Berger, Bunner, & Carey, 1996), and others who were still mobile into their 20s (Cleary & Wraith, 1993).

MPS IV (Morquio Syndrome)

Individuals with Morquio syndrome (MPS IV) appear normal at birth, and the characteristics of the disorder develop during infancy or childhood. Almost all of the children in a sample of children in the United Kingdom were fluent speakers (Bax & Coville, 1995). There have traditionally been two widely recognized forms of this disorder, designated as MPS IVA and MPS IVB, which differ in the severity of symptoms and the age at detection (Neufeld & Muenzer, 1996). Persons with MPS IVA, the severe form of the disorder, have all the classic features enumerated above. They appear normal at birth, and shortened stature appears by about 1 year of age. Final height is usually less than 50 inches. Younger children have difficulty with continence, although most children over 10 are continent (Bax & Coville, 1995). The diagnosis of the severe form of the disorder is usually made between 1 and 3 years of age. Individuals with the severe variant of the disorder usually live until their third or fourth decade. Death is typically a result of cardiopulmonary complications (Matalan, 1996).

Children with MPS IVB, the intermediate form of the disorder, have the classic characteristics in a less severe form. They have a final height greater than 50 inches. They usually have normal-appearing dentition. The diagnosis of this form is usually made during the childhood years. A recent typology (Goldberg, 1996) proposes a third variant of Morquio syndrome, MPS IVC. This mild variant of the disorder results in much less severe clinical manifestations. Stature is nearly normal, with only mild skeletal abnormalities. This form is usually first diagnosed in adolescence.

MPS VI (Maroteaux–Lamy Syndrome)

The severe form of Maroteaux–Lamy syndrome includes pronounced skeletal deformities with intact intellectual functioning (Matalan, 1996; National MPS Society, n.d.; Neufeld & Muenzer, 1995). The head is usually large, with a short neck, broad flat nose, and wide nostrils. The skin and hair are thick and course. Liver enlargement is common, and the abdomen may protrude. The spine may be curved, and joint mobility may be limited. Stature is significantly shortened and is noticable by age 2. Growth usually stops at about age 7 (Pennock, 1994). There is wide variation in the presentation of the disorder, including a mild version of the disorder that results in less severe skeletal involvement.

MPS VII (Sly Syndrome)

Individuals with Sly syndrome may vary in the expression of the symptoms of the disorder (Neufeld & Muenzer, 1995). The more severe, early-onset type of this disorder begins by age 3. Skeletal abnormalities are moderately severe and result in shortened stature. Mental retardation is frequently moderate, but not progressive. The later-onset form of the disorder occurs after age 4. Skeletal involvement may be mild or severe. Intelligence is usually normal. A severe neonatal form of the disorder can be present and has caused infant death.

MEDICAL, PSYCHOLOGICAL, AND SOCIAL COMPLICATIONS

Medical Complications

Complications of MPS disorders occur in many organ systems (Avery & First, 1994; Goldberg, 1996; Neufeld & Muenzer, 1996). Enlargement of the liver and spleen (hepatosplenomegaly) results in a protuberant abdomen. Hernia frequently occurs. Chronic, intractable diarrhea is frequently found in Hunter and Sanfilippo syndromes. Carpal tunnel syndrome (entrapment of nerves in the wrist) can result in further impairment in the use of the hands and arms.

Cardiovascular problems, especially valvular disorders, are usually evident in older children and adolescents with MPS disorders. Respiratory disorders are common, including increased incidence of respiratory infections, airway obstruction, and pulmonary hypertension. Sleep apnea may result from obstructions in the respiratory system.

Ear infections frequently occur. Deafness, due to both progressive thickening of the skull (conduction loss) and sensory impairment, is likely in the severest forms of the disorders (Pennock, 1994; Tachdjian, 1990). Glaucoma and retinitis pigmentosa can occur, which, along with corneal clouding, can affect vision.

Dentition is frequently affected in the MPS disorders, especially in Morquio and Maroteaux–Lamy syndromes (Nelson & Kinirons, 1988; Smith, Hallett, Hall, Wardrop, & Firth, 1995). Delayed eruption and abnormalities of tooth morphology can occur, along with weaknesses in enamel. The teeth may be widely spaced and have a sharp, conical shape. Excessive wear on the tooth surface may result.

The abnormal formation of the cervical vertebrae, especially in Morquio syndrome, may lead to misalignment of these vertebrae (atlantoaxial subluxation). This can cause spinal cord compression, leading to disability and death (Ashraf, Crockard, Ransford, & Stevens, 1991; Neufeld & Muenzer, 1995). Spinal misalignment and narrowing of the airway also create potentially serious problems with establishing an airway and providing anesthesia if surgery is needed.

Neuropsychological Complications

Hydrocephaly (an accumulation of cerebrospinal fluid surrounding the brain) is likely to occur, especially in Hurler and Hunter syndromes. Children with Sanfilippo syndrome and the severe form of Hunter syndrome commonly have seizures (Cleary & Wraith, 1993; Young et al., 1982b). Neurological symptoms may also be caused by spinal cord compression due to a buildup of extradural soft tissue (Goldberg, 1996). The presence of these complications makes the determination of the primary neuropsychological effects of the disease more difficult.

There is little specific knowledge about the neuropsychological aspects of the MPS disorders (Shapiro & Klein, 1994), because there has been little neuropsychological study of children with these disorders. Children with the MPS disorders have rarely been referred for neuropsychological assessment; reasons have included the lack of treatment available for the disorders, as well as the advanced stage of the disorders by the time diagnoses are usually made. The excessive storage of mucopolysaccharides in the tissues does affect both the gray and white matter of the brain. The primary neuropsychological complication of the MPS disorders is progressive dementia. Dementia differs from mental retardation in that mental retardation is a slowing in the attainment of developmental milestones, whereas dementia is a reduction in the previously attained level of functioning. In those MPS disorders that result in dementia, there is an initial slowing of development, followed by a plateau in level of functioning. Skills that have been developed are subsequently lost. Language delays occur in the severe form of Hunter syndrome and in Sanfilippo syndrome (Shapiro, Lockman, Balthazar, & Krivit, 1995). All patients with Hurler syndrome, in one study, who had been treated with bone marrow transplantation have had residual learning problems, although none had severe mental retardation (Guffon, Souillet, Maire, Straczek, & Guibaud, 1998).

Behavioral Complications

Children with MPS disorders have been found to have a high incidence of certain behavior problems (Bax & Colville, 1995). Parents of children with Hurler syndrome describe their children as anxious or fearful. Many are considered to be restless, with little aggressive behavior. Sleep problems are seen in some children, but these are reflections of their medical problems rather than of a behavior problem. In children with Hunter syndrome overactivity is common up to age 10. There is a high incidence of aggressive/destructive behavior in children under 5. Excessive fearfulness occurs in most and is especially likely in younger children. Problems with sleep, such as difficulty settling and going to sleep, are very common. Behavior problems (overactivity, aggression, and defiance) tend to occur early in the course of the disorder in children with the severe form of the disorder. In the mild form of Hunter syndrome, behavioral problems are more likely to occur in adolescence, presumably because of the adjustment problems posed by the patients' unusual appearance and their knowledge of the prognosis for early death (Young et al., 1982b).

Sanfilippo syndrome causes the most dramatic behavioral symptoms of all the MPS disorders (Bax & Coville, 1995; Nidiffer & Kelly, 1983). Restlessness is a common feature in children with MPS III. They commonly wander around home and school, and they mouth clothing and other objects. Parents often describe their children as unpredictable, with frequent aggressive and destructive behaviors, including hitting others. These behaviors seem unprovoked and do not appear to be accompanied by anger on a child's part. Difficult behavior at night is also common, including staying up during the nighttime hours, wandering, and restlessness. Many families have had to use secure sleeping arrangements or resort to having a child sleep in a parent's room so as to provide nighttime supervision.

Children with Morquio syndrome have a relatively low level of behavioral problems, compared to those with the other MPS disorders. Sleep problems are present, especially in the 5- to 9-year-old group. Many children between ages 10 and 14 are described by their parents as fearful (Bax & Colville, 1995).

Social Complications

Family stress often occurs because of the multiple demands of the MPS disorders (Bax & Coville, 1995; Nidiffer & Kelly, 1983). Parents are unlikely to have regular outside help in managing the day-to-day care of a child with such a disorder. They often feel uncomfortable leaving their child with other caregivers, sometimes because of the fear that the child may die while the parents are gone. In addition, parents often face increased pressures caused by repeated medical procedures, associated behavior problems, and the financial demands of having a child with a major chronic disorder. Relatively few families receive any type of assistance from a mental health care provider.

Parents feel a great deal of distress when their child becomes so impaired that they are unable to communicate with him or her (Bax & Coville, 1995). They are also concerned about the effect of the MPS child on siblings (Nidiffer & Kelly, 1983). Sibling relationships may be affected by jealousy because of the extra parental attention to the needs of the child with MPS, or the burden of providing extra care for an ill sibling. Siblings may also be concerned that their own acceptance by their peers will be affected by the presence of a sibling with such significant problems.

Parents are very concerned and frequently worried about their child's prognosis. Many are frustrated by the lack of information available to parents and professionals at the local level. There is often a lack of adequate community support and assistance. Parents frequently feel helpless (Nidiffer & Kelly, 1983) and isolated (Bax & Coville, 1995).

IDENTIFICATION, TREATMENT, AND INTERVENTION

Because the MPS disorders are rare, parents, school personnel, and local health care providers are likely to have little firsthand experience with them. Definitive diagnosis is available, however, as is the ability to screen parents for these disorders. Early identification is important to allow for early treatment and intervention. Multiple interventions are commonly required.

No research has addressed interventions for the specific educational and psychosocial problems posed by the MPS disorders. Adaptation of methods and technologies currently used for children with multiple handicaps may be helpful. A variety of medical, educational, and allied health care specialists are required for optimal care, especially for those children with more severe forms of the disorders (see Table 13.3). Close communication and collaboration among parents, educators, and health care providers are vital to create an atmosphere of trust and support, which is necessary in dealing with these disorders.

Diagnosis

Children with MPS disorders are usually brought for diagnosis as a result of developmental delay or the development of characteristic skeletal features. Diagnosis is possible through several means (Goldberg, 1996). Because excess mucopolysaccharide metabolites accumulate in the urine, urine mucopolysaccharide levels can be measured to provide initial diag-

TABLE 13.3. Treatment Providers Involved in Comprehensive Care for MPS Disorders

Physicians	Educational specialists
Anesthesiologist	Early intervention specialist
Cardiologist	Special education teacher
Child psychiatrist	Instructional aide
Neurologist	School psychologist
Neurosurgeon	
Ophthalmologist	
Orthopedic surgeon	
Pulmonary specialist	
Health care providers	
Pediatric dentist	
Occupational therapist	
Physical therapist	
Psychologist	
Rehabilitation counselor	
Speech/language clinician	

nosis, although urinary screening is sometimes inaccurate. Definitive diagnosis requires an enzyme assay of cultured fibroblasts or leukocytes (white blood cells). In this procedure, cell samples are taken from the child and grown in a culture medium. The cells are then subjected to a chemical test for the presence of the enzyme in question.

Prenatal diagnosis is possible and is routinely conducted when there is a known risk that the fetus will be affected by one of the disorders (Gahl, 1999; Neufeld & Muenzer, 1995). Fetal fibroblasts circulating in the amniotic fluid can be obtained through amniocentesis from the 13th to the 16th week of gestation. These cells can then be cultured and assayed for the pertinent enzyme activity. Chorionic villus sampling obtains small pieces of the placenta through needle biopsy from the sixth to the eighth week of gestation. These cells are then analyzed for enzyme activity, although this test may not be accurate for Hurler, Scheie, and Hurler–Scheie syndromes.

The differential diagnosis for MPS disorders includes those diseases that produce dysostosis multiplex and physical appearance similar to that often seen in the MPSs (Matalan, 1996; see Table 13.4). The differential diagnosis of these disorders is based on laboratory findings. The hyperactivity and tantrum behaviors present in Sanfilippo syndrome may be misdiagnosed as attention-deficit/hyperactivity disorder. This underscores the importance of a medical workup on all children with developmental difficulties as part of an evaluation of behavioral problems.

TABLE 13.4. Genetic Diseases Considered in the Differential Diagnosis of the MPS Disorders

GM_1 gangliosidosis	Mucolipidosis III
Mannosidosis	Mucolipidosis IV
Fucosidosis	Multiple sulfatase deficiency
Aspartylglucosaminuria	Kneist syndrome
Mucolipidosis I	Spondyloepiphyseal dysplasias
Mucolipidosis II (I-cell disease)	

Carrier Identification and Genetic Counseling

The identification of genetic risk is an important factor in the management of MPS disorders. Carrier detection tests are used to identify the carriers of genetic diseases before they have affected children. Widespread population screening for the MPS disorders does not occur at this time (Gahl, 1999). Screening of the mother's family is warranted for known cases of Hunter syndrome, which is an X-linked disorder. Attention to future pregnancies is prudent for the other MPS disorders, which are autosomal recessive disorders; testing will permit the identification of risk for future children who may be born with an MPS disorder. A significant problem, however, for parents of children with Sanfilippo syndrome is that this diagnosis is usually made relatively late, making effective genetic counseling more difficult. It is not uncommon for parents to have additional children with Sanfilippo syndrome prior to having a diagnosis made on their first child (Nidiffer & Kelly, 1983).

Genetic counseling services can be useful for families with a history of an MPS disorder. The geneticist or genetic counselor will take a detailed history of the family to help determine the risk of the specific disorder in future children (Batshaw & Rose, 1997). The geneticist can also discuss the risks and benefits of prenatal diagnostic tests after pregnancy occurs. The genetic counselor can assist the parents in considering their reproductive options (such as artificial insemination with donor sperm or eggs) if the parents are found to be carriers of the affected genes.

Key Issues Regarding Psychoeducational Assessment

The child with an MPS disorder should receive careful evaluation of adjustment, cognitive functioning, and behavior. Psychological testing can serve several functions (Shapiro & Klein, 1994). Tests can document deterioration of function over time, allowing the clinician to determine the progression of the disease. Improvement in functioning can be determined by psychological testing as a means of providing outcome data for treatment. This may be useful for those children who have been treated with bone marrow transplantation (BMT; see below).

Psychoeducational assessment may be useful in determining the appropriate curriculum and school placement for children with MPS disorders. Documentation of deterioration may help teachers adjust their expectations and strategies for those children who have progressive dementia. The documentation of normal intellectual functioning may also help teachers and parents have appropriately high academic and vocational expectations for children with MPS disorders that result in alterations of physical appearance without intellectual impairment.

Shapiro and Klein (1994) have described several issues that are relevant to the assessment of individuals with the MPS disorders, particularly the more severe variants of these disorders. Sensory deficits, including hearing loss and vision impairment (due to corneal clouding and cataracts), complicate the assessment of cognitive abilities. The behavioral problems that are characteristic of Sanfilippo syndrome, including restlessness, hyperactivity, limited attention span, disruptive behavior, and tantrums, pose serious obstacles to testing. Attention deficits, distractibility, and hyperactivity are noted in children with Hurler syndrome in early childhood. Hearing loss, vision impairment, and movement difficulties also affect the selection of psychoeducational tests. Strategies for selecting and administering tests for children with handicaps are available elsewhere (McLean, Bailey & Wolery, 1996; Sattler, 1992; Shapiro & Klein, 1994; Teeter & Semrud-Clikeman, 1997; Vess & Douglas, 1996).

Medical Issues and Interventions

There has historically been no successful direct treatment for the MPS disorders, and supportive treatment has been the most commonly provided intervention (Gahl, 1999). Supportive treatment focuses on the alleviation of the manifestations and complications of the disorders (Neufeld & Muenzer, 1995). Children commonly need intervention for cardiovascular complications and respiratory difficulties. Upper-airway obstruction and sleep apnea may require surgical intervention (Adachi & Chole, 1990). Respiratory infections and middle-ear infections need prompt and aggressive treatment (Nelson & Crocker, 1992). Because of the difficulties of maintaining an airway, persons with MPS disorders who need general anesthesia must be cared for in a setting that has experience in providing anesthesia services for this group (Neufeld & Muenzer, 1995).

Interventions for hearing loss are frequently necessary (Alpern, 1992). Children should receive regular evaluation for sensory and conductive hearing loss. Hearing aids can be helpful for many children with MPS disorders who also have hearing loss. Auditory training, such as instruction in making use of residual hearing and lip reading, may be useful for some children. Alternative communication skills may be necessary for higher-functioning children and adults who have tracheotomies because of airway obstruction, or who have total hearing loss.

Regular dental examination is important in dealing with the potential dental problems. Surgical treatment of impacted teeth may be necessary. Prophylactic treatment is indicated to prevent the occurrence of infective endocarditis secondary to dental procedures. The possibility of endocarditis is increased by the presence of cardiovalvular disease, which is commonly present in the MPS disorders.

Skeletal and mobility difficulties are common problems for children with severe forms of these disorders. Both surgical and nonsurgical interventions are used in the management of the orthopedic problems of the MPS disorders (Loder, 1996). Nonsurgical treatments have included gentle physical therapy to minimize joint contractures, and bracing as a preoperative procedure to prevent the need for surgical correction of joint contractures and as a postoperative tool to maintain surgical correction. Surgical intervention may be necessary to correct spinal deformity and to stabilize cervical instability in those situations where the instability may lead to neurological impairment. Surgical treatment is also indicated to reduce median nerve compression in those MPS disorders that lead to carpal tunnel syndrome. Some children will need a wheelchair or buggy to assist in mobility (Penso, 1992).

A number of definitive biological efforts to correct the basic defects that cause the MPS disorders or to provide adequate levels of enzymes in the body have been made. Plasma and lymphocyte transfusions have been used in hope of providing the missing enzymes. Neither method of enzyme replacement has proven successful in ameliorating or reversing the disorders (Bach, 1986), although some success has been reported with animal models (Crawley et al., 1996). This lack of success is probably due to the inability of such techniques to provide high enough levels of the enzymes for normal functioning.

Ideally, replacing the defective gene with a normal gene would thereby prevent or reverse the damage caused by the disorders (Trent, 1997). The identification of the location and functions of specific genes involved in the MPSs has paved the way for this method of treatment, usually called "gene therapy." In gene therapy, a normal copy of the relevant gene is spliced into the genetic material of a retrovirus. The retrovirus is used to transfer the normal gene into a culture of cells of the affected person (in the case of MPS disorders, it could be bone marrow cells). The virus implants itself and the normal gene into the cell, which can then be transplanted into the person and begin production of the missing enzyme. Gene therapy is presently being studied in animal research and human trials and remains a prospect for future treatment (Bergstrom, Quinn, Greenstein, & Ascensao, 1994; Goldberg, 1996; Maria, Medina, Hoang, & Phillips, 1997).

BMT is a form of treatment that replaces abnormal cells or supplements the production of the genetic product (Haskins et al., 1991). BMT has been attempted for many of the MPS disorders. The use of sibling donor marrow has the greatest likelihood of success (Shapiro & Klein, 1994). The evaluation of the success of BMT has been hindered in earlier research because of diagnostic uncertainties, lack of standardized longitudinal study of neuropsychological status, and the failure of researchers to document the characteristics of enzymatic activity (Krivit & Shapiro, 1991).

Krivit and Shapiro (1991) provide a comprehensive summary of the use of BMT for the MPS disorders. In general, once engraftment is established for 1 year, the correction of the metabolic defect persists. The visceral aspects of the MPS disorders improve after long-term engraftment. There is also some improvement in facial features. In most children, developmental and intellectual functioning stabilize, but many continue to have significant mental impairments.

Some studies have documented a decrease of hydrocephaly after BMT. The musculoskeletal effects of the disorders have not been ameliorated by transplantation in most subjects, probably because of poor penetration of the enzyme into the musculoskeletal tissues (Field, Buchanan, Copplemans, & Aichroth, 1994). Cardiac damage and the reduction of hepatosplenolomegaly have also been reported, along with improved vision due to a reduction of corneal clouding. Hearing also improves (Penso, 1992).

In their study of neuropsychological outcomes of BMT for the MPSs, Shapiro et al. (1995) found that BMT prior to age 2 resulted in stabilization of intellectual functioning for those children with Hurler syndrome who had an IQ above 70 prior to the procedure. BMT did not alter the progressive course in any children with Sanfilippo syndrome. No children with Hunter syndrome were transplanted prior to the age of 2, and all but one of the children failed to show an alteration in the course of the disease. There are reports of successful BMT for children with Hurler syndrome (Whitley et al., 1993) for a child with the mild variant of Hunter syndrome (Bergstrom et al., 1994), and a child with Sly syndrome (Yamada et al., 1997). This may demonstrate that the severity of the disease and the age at onset are important factors in successful outcomes of BMT. BMT, like any organ transplantation, remains an expensive procedure with significant mortality and morbidity rates (Batshaw, 1997), and further research will be required to develop more effective and safer procedures.

Psychosocial Issues and Interventions

Unfortunately, psychological services are rarely provided in the ongoing management of children with these disorders, despite the very common presence of significant behavioral complications (Bax & Colville, 1995). The typical approach to dealing with the difficult behavior of children with developmental delays and multiple handicaps has been the use of operant conditioning paradigms, with the assumption that behavior problems are caused by the antecedents and consequences of the behaviors (Parrish, 1997). Clinical experience has found that the difficult behaviors of children with MPS disorders (such as the aggressive outbursts of children with Sanfilippo syndrome) frequently do not respond well to behavioral intervention strategies (Nidiffer & Kelly, 1983). Behavioral interventions have been successful in decreasing sleep problems of children with Sanfilippo syndrome (Coville, Watters, Yule, & Bax, 1996). Discomfort, changes in routine, and level of environmental stimulation may exacerbate difficult behavior, and a thorough assessment of behavioral problems should include an assessment of antecedents and consequences of the behavior as well as an evaluation of the child (Jacob-Timm & Daniels, 1998).

Few studies have been conducted of psychopharmacological intervention for behavioral difficulties of children with MPS disorders. The response to psychopharmacological intervention has been variable (Cleary & Wraith, 1993). Methylphenidate has not been useful in reducing the hyperactivity of children with Sanfilippo syndrome (Jacob-Timm & Daniels, 1998). Thioridazine and haldol do reduce the hyperactivity, although these drugs also had potential side effects (Wraith, 1995). Wraith also found that benzodiazepines and chloral hydrate were both effective sleep medications for children with Sanfilippo syndrome. Carbamazepine has been successfully used to reduce overactivity, aggressive outbursts and labile mood in an adolescent with Sanfilippo syndrome (Kim et al., 1996).

Parents have many stressors that result from having a child with a progressive genetic disorder. Empathy and emotional support are very helpful responses from treatment providers. Training parents in behavior management techniques, or providing referrals for parent counseling and/or psychopharmacological interventions, may help parents cope with their child's behavior problems. Parents may also need assistance in accessing the necessary medical care for the complications of this disorder. Providing information and helping parents locate support groups (see Table 13.5) can be of great benefit to parents overwhelmed by the enormous challenges of a child with an MPS disorder.

In the case of Hurler syndrome or Hunter syndrome, where the disorder is likely to cause death during childhood, the family members may also benefit from support and counseling to help them deal with issues of grief and loss. Deterioration in the child's con-

---

TABLE 13.5. Information and Support Resources for Parents and Professionals

---

Alliance of Genetic Support Groups
35 Wisconsin Circle
Suite 440
Chevy Chase, MD 20815
(800) 336–4363
http://medhlp.org/www/agsg.htm

  Information on support groups in the local community.

The Canadian Society for Mucopolysaccharide and Related Disease, Inc.
P.O. Box 64714
Unionville, ON L3R 0M9
(905) 479–8701
http://neuro-www2.mgh.harvard.edu/MPS/mpsmain.html

  An information and advocacy organization for persons with MPSs.

National MPS Society, Inc.
17 Kraemer Street
Hicksville, NY 11801
(516) 931–6338
http://members.aol.com/mpssociety/index.html

  A support and advocacy organization for MPS disorders. Information, names of specialists who treat these disorders, and ways to contact other families who have children with these disorders are available.

---

dition is likely to cause a renewal of the feelings of loss, grief, and helplessness that arose when the initial diagnosis was made. Referral to resources that can assist with grief support and in-home care in the later stages of the disorder (such as a hospice) may be useful.

Educational Issues and Interventions

Most children with MPS disorders are likely to need assistance in school through special education services, and usually can be served under the current "other health-impaired" category. Difficulties with behavior management, socialization, and medical/health care will need to be addressed. There are several specific issues to consider in providing services for children with these disorders.

Early Intervention

Infants and very young children with Hurler syndrome (Nelson & Crocker, 1992), and children with the other MPS disorders, may obtain substantial benefit from an early intervention and stimulation program in which maximum intellectual gain can be encouraged (prior to the inevitable deterioration of cognitive skills in several of these disorders). The resulting gains in cognitive, language, self-help, and motor skills will be especially important as early plateaus in learning occur. Therefore, enrolling a child in a preschool early intervention program as soon as a diagnosis is made is warranted. Coordination of educational and support services during the transition from the infant/toddler program to the school setting is an essential area for professional attention.

Individualized Education Planning

Because of the rather rapid regression in skills and behavior experienced in the severe forms of the MPS disorders frequent monitoring is required so that changes in the individualized education plan (IEP) can quickly be made to support the child whose skills are deteriorating. Educational strategies should encourage appropriate participation, new learning, or the preservation of established skills. Alterations in the learning environment and in methods of instruction are frequently necessary to adapt to a child's cognitive, mobility, or behavior problems.

The IEP should include rapidly increasing support and assistance as regression in behavior and cognitive skills occurs. Planning and goal development may be difficult for personnel who do not have experience with children whose disorders are progressive, since the traditional focus is on improvement in skills and lessened support as improvement occurs. Plans should be based on short-term goals. Teachers frequently need additional support to accept a child's limited skills and deteriorating course.

Academic and Career Expectations

Children with Scheie syndrome, Hurler–Scheie syndrome, Morquio syndrome, Maroteaux–Lamy syndrome, and the less severe variant of Hunter syndrome are likely to have normal or only mildly delayed intellectual development, along with a longer life expectancy. Teachers and parents should not assume from the outward skeletal manifestations of the disorders that there is significant retardation of intellectual development. Appropriately high expectations of academic achievement will foster realistic self-appraisal and enhanced academic achievement.

Vocational maturity in adolescents with chronic health concerns is largely contingent on the attitudes and efforts of parents, teachers, and counselors (Brolin, 1980). Academic and vocational programming should foster independence and autonomy. Vocational goals should be set realistically high. Planning for transition from school to postsecondary education or the world of work should focus on helping students pursue vocations in a manner similar to that of their peers (Davis, Anderson, Linkowski, Berger, & Feinstein, 1991).

Teacher Education and Support

Teachers and peers should be educated about the condition, abilities, and special needs of a child with an MPS disorder. Teachers may be unsure of their ability to teach children with these disorders. Their competence should be supported, as they will find that many of the skills they use in teaching nonimpaired children are the skills that will enable them to work well with children who have these syndromes. Teachers and peers will need support in dealing with their feelings of loss in a case where the child's condition worsens and the child dies.

Medical Care Needs

Specific medical and health care needs are likely to require intervention by specialized health care personnel. Mobility problems, respiratory difficulties, and cardiovascular problems are commonly encountered in the school setting. Sleep apnea may be noticed by school personnel as daytime sleepiness. Special attention is required to identify and monitor hearing loss and to improve communication. A more detailed framework for assessment, intervention, and program planning for children with hearing loss can be found elsewhere (Vess & Douglas, 1996).

Problems with Behavior

It is important to treat the behavior difficulties as complications of the medical condition and not as misbehavior per se. Alterations to the learning environment and methods of instruction may be helpful in decreasing some behavior problems. Teachers and administrators may need additional assistance in managing the behavior problems that may occur in children with these syndromes. This includes training and consultation in interventions for overactivity, restlessness, and fearfulness. Behavior support and behavior management principles should be used to improve behavior, with an emphasis on use of reinforcements. Appropriate psychopharmacological intervention may be necessary as an adjunct to behavioral and educational interventions.

Socialization

School attendance and socialization is to be encouraged and fostered through classroom integration and specific social skills interventions. Independence should be supported. Teachers can do much to improve the acceptance of a child through instructional activities, such as cooperative learning and encouraging support for all children in the classroom. Additional support and education is necessary during adolescence, especially for adolescents with Morquio, Maroteaux–Lamy, Scheie, and Hurler–Scheie syndromes and the mild form of Hunter syndrome, when sexuality and physical appearance become especially important.

SUMMARY

The MPS disorders are a group of rare disorders resulting from genetic mutations affecting the metabolism of mucopolysaccharides, which are constituents of bone and connective tissue. These defects result in the deposition of incompletely metabolized mucopolysaccharides in the connective tissues, bone, and major organs. The disorders are all characterized by varying degrees of physical, sensory, cognitive, and behavioral impairments.

Children with certain of the MPS disorders have been found to have a higher incidence of behavior problems, including overactivity, aggressiveness, restlessness, and fearfulness. They are likely to need assistance in school through special education services, where difficulties with behavior management, socialization, and medical/health care will need to be addressed. Because of the multiple demands of these chronic disorders, family stress levels are often high.

There has historically been no successful direct treatment for the MPS disorders, and supportive treatment has been most commonly provided. Supportive treatment focuses on alleviating the manifestations and complications of the disorders. BMT has proven successful for some of the disorders, and gene therapy offers hope for a more effective intervention in the future. A multidisciplinary approach to assessment and intervention will be necessary for most children. Local providers are unlikely to have experience with these disorders, and information and evaluation from regional or national specialists may be required. Close communication and collaboration among parents, educators, and health care providers are essential in dealing with these disorders.

REFERENCES

Adachi, K., & Chole, R. A. (1990). Management of tracheal lesions in Hurler's syndrome. *Archives of Otolaryngology—Head and Neck Surgery, 116,* 1205–1207.

Alpern, C. S. (1992). Hunter's syndrome and its management in a public school setting. *Language, Speech, and Hearing Services in Schools, 23,* 102–106.

Ashraf, J., Crockard, H. A., Ransford, A. O., & Stevens, J. M. (1991). Transoral decompression and posterior stabilisation in Morquio's disease. *Archives of Diseases in Childhood, 66,* 1318–1321.

Avery, M. E., & First, L. R. (1994). *Pediatric medicine.* Baltimore: Williams and Wilkins.

Bach, G. (1986). Disorders of mucopolysaccharide metabolism. In A. Milunsky (Ed.), *Genetic disorders and the fetus.* New York: Plenum Press.

Batshaw, M. L. (1997). PKU and other inborn errors of metabolism. In M. L. Batshaw (Ed.), *Children with disabilities.* Baltimore: Paul H. Brookes.

Batshaw, M. L., & Rose, M. C. (1997). Birth defects, prenatal diagnosis, and fetal therapy. In M. L. Batshaw (Ed.), *Children with disabilities.* Baltimore: Paul H. Brookes.

Bax, M. C., & Colville, G. A. (1995). Behaviour in mucopolysaccharide disorders. *Archives of Disease in Childhood, 73,* 77–81.

Bergstrom, S. K., Quinn, J. J., Greenstein, R., & Ascensao, J. (1994). Long-term follow-up of a patient transplanted for Hunter's disease type IIB: A case report and literature review. *Bone Marrow Transplantation, 14,* 653–658.

Brolin, D. E. (1980). *Vocational preparation of persons with handicaps.* Columbus, OH: Merrill.

Cervantes, C. D., & Lifshitz, F. (1990). Skeletal dysplasias with primary abnormalities in carbohydrate, lipid, and amino acid metabolism. In S. Castells & L. Finberg (Eds.), *Metabolic bone disease in children.* New York: Marcel Dekker.

Christodoulou, J., & McInnes, R. R. (1998). A clinical approach to inborn errors of metabolism. In A. M. Rudolph & R. K. Kamei (Eds.), *Rudolph's fundamentals of pediatrics.* Stamford, CT: Appleton & Lange.

Cleary, M. A., & Wraith, J. E. (1993). Mangement of mucopolysaccharidosis type III. *Archives of Disease in Childhood, 69,* 403–406.

Coville, G. A., Watters, J. P., Yule, W., & Bax, M. (1996). Sleep problems in children with Sanfilippo syndrome. *Developmental Medicine and Child Neurology, 38,* 538–544.

Crawley, A. D., Brooks, D. A., Muller, V. J., Petersen, B. A., Isaac, E. Ol, Bielicki, J., King, B. M., Boulter, C. D., Moore, A. J., Fazzalari, N. L., Anson, D. S., Byers, S., & Hopwood, J. (1996). Enzyme replacement therapy in a feline model of Maroteaux–Lamy syndrome. *Journal of Clinical Investigation, 97,* 1864–1873.

Davis, S. E., Anderson, C., Linkowski, D. C., Berger, K., & Feinstein, C. F. (1991). Developmental tasks and transitions of adolescents with chronic illnesses and disabilities. In R. P. Marinelli & A. E. Dell Orto (Eds.), *The psychological and social impact of disability.* New York: Springer.

Field, R. E., Buchanan, J. A. F., Copplemans, M. G. J., & Aichroth, R. M. (1994). Bone-marrow transplantation in Hurler's syndrome. *Journal of Bone and Joint Surgery, 76-B,* 975-981.

Finlayson, L. A. (1990). Hunter syndrome (mucopolysaccharidosis II). *Pediatric Dermatology, 7,* 150–152.

Gahl, W. A. (1999). Lysosomal storage diseases. In F. D. Burg, J. R. Ingelfinger, E. R. Wald, & R. A. Polin (Eds.), *Gellis and Kagan's current pediatric therapy.* Philadelphia: W. B. Saunders.

Goldberg, M. J. (1996). Syndromes of orthopaedic importance. In R. T. Morrissy & S. L. Weinstein (Eds.), *Lovell and Winter's pediatric orthopaedics.* Philadelphia: Lippincott-Raven.

Guffon, N., Souillet, G., Maire, I., Straczek, J., & Guibaud, P. (1998). Follow-up of nine patients with Hurler syndrome after bone marrow transplantation. *Journal of Pediatrics, 133,* 119–125.

Haskins, M., Baker, H. J., Birkenmeier, E., Hoogerbrugge, P. M., Poorthuis, B., Sakiyama, T., Shull, R. M., Taylor, R. M., Thrall, M. A., & Walkley, S. U. (1991). Transplantation in animal models. In R. J. Desnick (Ed.), *Treatment of genetic diseases.* New York: Churchill Livingstone.

Jacob-Timm, S., & Daniels, J. A. (1998). Sanfilippo syndrome. In L. Phelps (Ed.), *Health related disorders in children and adolescents.* Washington, DC: American Psychological Association.

Kim, W. J., Berger, P., Bunner, S., & Carey, M. P. (1996). Behavioral manifestations of genetic disorder. *Journal of the American Academy of Child and Adolescent Psychiatry, 35,* 976–977.

Krivet, W., & Shapiro, E. (1991). Bone marrow transplantation for storage diseases. In R. Desnick (Ed.), *Treatment of genetic diseases.* Edinburgh: Churchill Livingstone.

Levine, M. I. (1991). *Jolly's diseases of children.* Oxford: Blackwell Scientific.

Loder, R. T. (1996, October). *Orthopaedic considerations in the muopolysaccharidoses.* Paper presented at the annual conference of the National MPS Society, Hartford, CT.

Lowry, R. B., Applegarth, D. A., Toone, J. R., MacDonald, E., & Thunem, N. Y. (1990). An update on the frequency of mucopolysaccharide syndromes in British Columbia. *Human Genetics, 85*(3), 389–390.

Maria, B. L., Medina, C. D., Hoang, K. B., & Phillips, M. I. (1997). Gene therapy for neurologic disease: Benchtop discoveries to bedside applications. *Journal of Child Neurology, 12,* 77–84.

Matalan, R. K. (1996). Disorders of mucopolysaccharide metabolism. In R. E. Behrman, R. M. Kliegman, W. E. Nelson, & V. C. Vaughan (Eds.), *Nelson textbook of pediatrics.* Philadelphia: Saunders.

McLean, M., Bailey, D. B., & Wolery, M. (1996). *Assessing infants and preschoolers with special needs.* Englewood Cliffs, NJ: Prentice-Hall.

Menkes, J. H. (1990). *Textbook of child neurology.* Malvern, PA: Lea & Febiger.

National MPS Society. (n.d.). *Maroteaux–Lamy syndrome.* Hicksville, NY: Author.

Nelson, J., & Kinirons, M. (1988). Clinical findings in 12 patients with MPS IV A (Morquio's disease). Further evidence for heterogeneity. Part II: Dental findings. *Clinical Genetics, 33,* 121–125.

Nelson, R. P., & Crocker, A. C. (1992). The child with multiple disabilities. In M. R. Levine, W. B. Carey, & A. C. Crocker (Eds.), *Developmental–behavioral pediatrics*. Philadelphia: Saunders.

Neufeld, E. F., & Muenzer, J. (1995). The mucopolysaccharidoses. In C. R. Scriver, A. L. Beaudet, W. S. Sly, & D. Valle (Eds.), *The metabolic and molecular bases of inherited disease*. New York: McGraw–Hill.

Nidiffer, F. D., & Kelly, T. E. (1983). Developmental and degenerative patterns associated with cognitive, behavioural and motor difficulties in the Sanfilippo syndrome: An epidemiological study. *Journal of Mental Deficiency Research*, 27, 185–203.

Ozand, P. T., Thompson, J. N., Gascon, G. G., Sarvepalli, S. B., Rahbeeni, Z., Nester, M. J., & Brismar, J. (1994). Sanfilippo type D presenting with acquired language disorder but without features of mucopolysaccharidosis. *Journal of Child Neurology*, 9, 408–411.

Parrish, J. M. (1997). Behavior management: Promoting adaptive behavior. In M. L. Batshaw (Ed.), *Children with disabilities*. Baltimore: Paul H. Brookes.

Pennock, C. A. (1994). Lysosomal storage disorders. In J. B. Holton (Ed.), *The inherited metabolic diseases*. New York: Churchill Livingstone.

Penso, D. E. (1992). The mucopolysaccharidoses: Classification, symptoms, and the role of the occupational therapist. *British Journal of Occupational Therapy*, 55, 44–48.

Roberts, S. H., Upadhyaya, M., Sarfarazi, M., & Harper, P. S. (1989). Further evidence localizing the gene for Hunter's syndrome to the distal region of the X chromosome long arm. *Journal of Medical Genetics*, 26, 309–313.

Sattler, J. M. (1992). (3rd ed.). *Assessment of children*. San Diego, CA: Jerome M. Sattler, Publisher.

Schaap, T., & Bach, G. (1980). Incidence of mucopolysaccharidoses in Israel: Is Hunter disease a Jewish disease? *Human Genetics*, 56, 221–226.

Shapiro, E. G., & Klein, K. A. (1994). Childhood dementia: neuropsychological assessment with application to the natural history and treatment of degenerative storage diseases. In M. Tramontano & S. Hooper (Eds.), *Advances in child neuropsychology* (Vol. 2). New York: Springer-Verlag.

Shapiro, E. G., Lockman, L. A., Balthazar, M., & Krivit, W. (1995). Neuropsychological outcomes of several storage diseases with and without bone marrow transplantation. *Journal of Inherited Metabolic Diseases*, 18, 413–429.

Sinclair, L. (1979). *Metabolic disease in childhood*. Oxford: Blackwell Scientific.

Smith, K. S., Hallett, K. B., Hall, R. K., Wardrop, R. W., & Firth, N. (1995). Mucopolysacchariosis: MPS VI and associated delayed tooth eruption. *International Journal of Oral and Maxillofacial Surgery*, 24, 176–180.

Tachdjian, M. O. (1990). *Pediatric orthopedics*. Philadelphia: W. B. Saunders.

Teeter, P. A., & Semrud-Clikeman, M. (1997). *Child neuropsychology: Assessment and interventions for neurodevelopmental disorders*. Needham Heights, MA: Allyn & Bacon.

Trent, R. J. (1997). *Molecular medicine*. New York: Churchill Livingstone.

Tsuzaki, S, Matsuo, N., Nagai, T., Osano, M., & Orii, T. (1987). An unusually mild variant of Hunter's syndrome in a 14-year-old boy. *Acta Paediatrica Scandinavica*, 76, 844–846.

Vess, S., & Douglas, L. (1996). Best practices in program planning for children who are deaf or severely hard of hearing. In A. Thomas & J. Grimes (Eds.), *Best practices in school psychology*. Washington, DC: National Association of School Psychologists.

Watts, W. E., & Gibbs, D. A. (1986). *Lysosomal storage diseases: Biochemical and clinical aspects*. London: Taylor & Francis.

Whitley, C. B., Belani, K. G., Chang, P., Summers, C. G., Blazar, B. R., Tsai, M. Y., Latchaw, R. E., Ramsay, N. K. C., & Kersey, J. H. (1993). Long-term outcome of Hurler syndrome following bone marrow transplantation. *American Journal of Medical Genetics*, 46, 209–218.

Wraith, J. E. (1995). Behavior management, mobility, and medication. *The Canadian Connection*, pp. 32–37.

Yamada, Y., Kato, K., Sukegawa, K., Tomatsu, S., Fukuda, S., Emura, S., Kojima, S., Matsuyama, T., Sly, W. S., Kondo, N., & Orii, T. (1997). Treatment of MPS VII (Sly disease) by allogenieic BMT in a female with homozygous A619V mutation. *Bone Marrow Transplantation*, 21, 629–634.

Young, I. D., & Harper, P. S. (1982). Mild form of Hunter's syndrome: Clinical delineation based on 31 cases. *Archives of Disease in Childhood, 57,* 828–836.

Young, I. D., & Harper, P. S. (1983). The natural history of the severe form of Hunter's syndrome: A study based on 52 cases. *Developmental Medicine and Child Neurology, 25,* 481-489.

Young, I. D., Harper, P. S., Newcombe, R. G., & Archer, I. M. (1982a). A clinical and genetic study of Hunter's syndrome: I. Heterogeneity. *Journal of Medical Genetics, 19,* 401–407.

Young, I. D., Harper, P. S., Newcombe, R. G., & Archer, I. M. (1982b). A clinical and genetic study of Hunter's syndrome: II. Differences between mild and severe forms. *Journal of Medical Genetics, 19,* 408–411.

14

NOONAN SYNDROME

PHYLLIS ANNE TEETER

Biogenetic disorders of childhood are of interest to neuropsychologists because they frequently interfere with children's neuropsychological, cognitive, psychosocial, and academic development. Medical complications accompany many biogenetic disorders, and place added stress on family members. These interrelated variables have been systematically investigated for more common syndromes (e.g., Tourette syndrome), but other genetic disorders are less well understood. However, clinicians have long been interested in how genetic disorders affect children's development, interfere with their neuropsychological and cognitive functioning, and affect their overall psychological adjustment across environments—home, school, and community. In order to provide ecologically valid assessment and intervention planning, neuropsychologists should consider the impact of biogenetic disorders on these various dimensions, and should provide meaningful interventions to address these needs. Noonan syndrome (NS) is discussed in this chapter, with a focus on clinical presentation, common characteristics and associated medical and neuropsychological complications, assessment issues, and intervention planning.

NS is accompanied by multiple congenital anomalies with variable expressivity across individuals, and may be hard to detect in mildly affected individuals (Johannes, Garcia, De Vaan, & Weening, 1995). It is characterized by craniofacial anomalies, including ptosis, hypertelorism and epicanthus, an anti-mongoloid slant of palpebral fissures, low-set, posteriorly angulated ears, a deeply grooved philtrum with high wide peaks of the vermillion border of the upper lip, a high arched palate, and micrognathia. In addition to these features the syndrome is often accompanied by congenital heart disease (pulmonary valve stenosis), skeletal abnormalities (short stature, webbed neck and thorax abnormalities), genital malformations, and mental retardation. (Johannes et al., 1995, p. 571)

In 1883, Kobylinski reported a case of a 20-year-old male who presented with unusual features (for a review of this and other early studies, see Noonan, 1994). The patient's characteristics included small stature, low-set ears, webbed neck, micrognathia (i.e., unusual smallness of the jaw), and other symptoms overlapping with those of several present-day syndromes, including NS (Noonan, 1994). In 1930, Ullrich published case studies of children with physical anomalies resembling those of Kobylinski's patient (e.g., webbed neck and short stature) and sexual infantilism (i.e., small testes). In 1938 Turner described female children who had similar physical characteristics (e.g., webbed neck, short stature, and sexual infantilism) and whose underlying disorder was later identified as a sex chromosome abnormality. "Ullrich–Turner syndrome" (UTS) or "Turner syndrome," as this disorder came to be called, thus was defined as a complete or partial absence of, or other anomaly in, the X chromosome in some or all body cells (Wiederman, Kunze, & Dibbem, 1992).

Ullrich expanded his interests in rat research conducted by Bonnevie, who produced mice with webbed necks and swollen limbs through genetic mutations (Noonan, 1994). Europeans adopted the term "Ullrich–Bonnevie syndrome" to describe children who are now considered to have NS. Noonan and Ehmke (1963) published reports of nine patients (six males and three females) who were believed to represent a distinct syndrome. These children had small stature and various facial abnormalities, including hypertelorism (i.e., abnormally large distance between eyes), ptosis (i.e., drooping of the eyelid), and low-set ears. Some of the males had undescended testes. Other abnormalities included chest deformities, and all the patients had vascular pulmonary stenosis (Noonan, 1994). Opitz and Weaver (1985) confirmed that this indeed was a separate syndrome, and suggested the name "Noonan syndrome." Although the term "Turner phenotype" remained in use for a number of years, NS became more prevalent in the literature in about 1968; it was also soon dissociated from sex-linked abnormalities, as it was found in both males and females (Noonan, 1994). "Soon it was realized that some female patients with normal chromosomes previously diagnosed as having the UTS were in fact females with the 'male Turner syndrome,' i.e., the same syndrome described by Noonan" (Mendez & Opitz, 1985, p. 494). (Incidentally, the term "UTS" is now considered in U.S. medical usage to refer to NS rather than to Turner syndrome; *Dorland's Illustrated Medical Dictionary*, 1994.)

Because of the relative newness of NS in the literature, "many pediatricians have only a limited knowledge of this condition" (Noonan, 1994, p. 548). Although not sex-linked, NS is considered to be an autosomal dominant inherited condition that typically involves the cardiovascular system (50%), with other associated physical characteristics (e.g., short stature, chest deformity) (Noonan, 1994).

PREVALENCE RATES

Estimates of prevalence rates vary from 1 per 1,000 births to 1 per 2,500 (Nora, Nora, & Sinka, 1974) in some studies. Others suggest higher rates, ranging from 1 per 1,000 for severe symptoms (Mendez & Opitz, 1985) to 1 per 100 for milder expression (Noonan, 1994). Males and females are equally affected (Fakouri & Fakouri, 1998). There appear to be no racial differences in its occurrence, and the syndrome has been found in countries all over the world. NS is the most common genetic disorder in children with congenital heart disease (it is found in 1.4% of children with cardiac defects), and its rate of occurrence is even higher for children undergoing surgery for pulmonary stenosis (17%; Noonan, 1994).

GENETIC FACTORS, FAMILIAL TRANSMISSION, AND PATHOGENESIS

Although the symptoms of NS have a superficial resemblance to the symptoms of Turner syndrome (which involves an absent or defective chromosome), a sex-linked inheritance has not been verified, in that NS occurs in both males and females. A number of NS patients also have von Recklinghausen neurofibromatosis (NFvR), so speculations that chromosome 17 (which is abnormal in NFvR patients) was involved in NS were also investigated, without positive findings (Sharland, Taylor, Patton, & Jeffrey, 1992). At this time, the exact genetic anomaly for NS has not been found (Noonan, 1994). However, close relatives of individuals with NS are likely to have some features of the syndrome (Ghaziuddin, Bolyard, & Alessi, 1994).

In some cases NS can be sporadically transmitted (i.e., only one family member is affected), but recent research suggests that parent-to-child transmission is more common than originally noted (Graham, 1996). Mother-to-child inheritance seems likely, as many males have cryptorchidism (i.e., undescended testes) and are sometimes infertile (Noonan, 1994). Approximately 30–75% of cases result from parent-to-child transmission (Graham, 1996).

The variable expressivity of NS makes detection of mild cases difficult, so individuals may carry the gene but may not be aware of it. The phenotypic changes over the lifespan from birth to adulthood may be misleading, because a parent may not look like a child, but infant pictures of the parent will show similarities. Consequently, Noonan (1994) suggests that a careful review of family pictures at various ages on both maternal and paternal sides of the family may reveal whether a particular case is sporadic or familial in nature. The risk that subsequent offspring will have NS is reduced if it is a sporadic case; however, if it is familial, Noonan (1994) believes there is a 50% risk that an offspring will also have the disorder.

Despite the presumed genetic link, the exact etiology of NS is unknown, but it may be similar to that hypothesized for Turner syndrome (Grandy, 1993). It has been hypothesized that NS patients have a genetic defect that alters prenatal development of the lymphatic vessels (lymphangiectasia), and that disrupts tissue migration and organ placement during a critical period (Grandy, 1993). The manner in which the genetic defect causes the anomalies associated with NS is not well known, however. Fetal lymphedema (swelling due to lymph flow obstruction) may cause some of the associated characteristics (Govaert et al., 1992; Mendez & Opitz, 1985). An alternative explanation is that the fetal branchial arch field is developmentally altered. There may be more than one way in which this set of physical findings occurs (Graham, 1996).

DEVELOPMENTAL CONSIDERATIONS

Prenatal Period and Early Infancy

Individuals with NS generally have an unremarkable prenatal history. About one-third of NS pregnancies do have complications caused by polyhydramnios (excess of amniotic fluid). Fetal edema has also been found with ultrasound technology, and excessive weight loss in the first week of life has been reported as well (Noonan, 1994).

Feeding problems are relatively common; 39% of babies with NS have moderate difficulties, and 24% show severe problems that require tube feeding (Sharland, Burch, McKenna, & Patton, 1992). Projectile vomiting may also be present (Gilbert, 1996). Failure to thrive has been reported in up to 40% of NS infants (Graham, 1996), and lethargy, poor feeding, and vomiting may lead to hospitalization, according to Noonan (1994). The feeding difficulties do resolve themselves in later infancy, although repeated concerns about failure to thrive may be part of the early developmental picture. Hypotonia may also be observed (Noonan, 1994), and motor delays are also commonly found (Graham, 1996).

Childhood and Early Adolescence

Both physical and cognitive/intellectual delays have been found in a relatively large number of children diagnosed with NS. Short stature is found in the majority of children (80%), and a 2-year gap between bone age and chronological age is common (Gilbert, 1996). Treatment with growth hormone (GH) has been tried, but the results have not been well studied (Gilbert, 1996). Delayed puberty has also been reported in the literature; undescended testes are frequently observed, as noted earlier, with small size and infertility reported in later stages (Gilbert, 1996; Mendez & Opitz, 1985).

Thomas and Stanhope (1993) suggest that patients who are below the 3rd percentile for height before puberty should be considered as candidates for GH treatment. These authors have found that patients' height increases once they are treated, although growth velocity may decrease with age. Ahmed et al. (1991) likewise reported initial increases in height in five children treated with GH. However, Thomas and Stanhope (1993) caution that GH treatment needs further study, and that it may not be beneficial in changing the final stature of individuals with NS because it reduces the duration of puberty, which is already a problem.

Adulthood

Although weight and length are within normal limits at birth, the mean height of adults with NS is two standard deviations below the norm (Noonan, 1994). Ultimate adult height is affected by parental size, and wide variations have been found, but most females reach 5 feet and males reach 5 feet, 5 inches. In a cross-sectional study of 100 patients with NS, Allanson, Hall, Hughes, Preus, and Witt (1985) documented "marked change of phenotype with age from the newborn period, infancy, childhood, and adolescence to adulthood. . . . Our study, while not ruling out casual heterogeneity, suggests that the change of phenotype with age may have been falsely perceived as clinical heterogeneity" (p. 507).

PSYCHOSOCIAL COMPROMISE

The psychosocial features of NS are not well documented, but social interactions may be compromised as a result of other complications. First, children with NS often have poor muscle tone, which tends to affect their athletic ability (Gilbert, 1996). Children with NS are thus frequently poor at sports, and this fact may reduce their natural opportunities for play and socialization. Because they also tend to mature late, they often prefer to play with younger children (Gilbert, 1996). The social consequences of chronic medical complications (e.g., cardiac, orthopedic, etc.) need further study in patients with NS. However, it is important to note that there is no evidence of consistent psychiatric or behavioral disorders in patients with NS (Graham, 1996).

NEUROLOGICAL COMPROMISE

Various neurological problems in patients with NS have been described. Sharland, Burch, et al. (1992) reported that recurrent seizures are a problem for 13% of NS patients. Infrequent peripheral neuropathy has also been reported. For example, Noonan (1994) found mild myelomeningocele (protrusion of the cord and meninges from a defect in the vertebral column) in a patient with recurring tethered cord. "Other neurologic complications have included spina bifida occulta, subarachnoid hemorrhage from aneurysm, and syringomyelia," as well as optic glioma and medulloblastoma (Noonan, 1994, p. 552). Malignant schwannoma was reported by Kaplan, Opitz, and Gosset (1968), while Noonan (1994) also found a number of benign schwannomas.

As noted earlier, Noonan (1994) indicates that hypertonia is common, and it can be associated with poor coordination. The interaction of hypertonia with visual problems may account for the coordination difficulties.

MEDICAL RISKS

Congenital Heart Disease

A number of congenital heart diseases are associated with NS and are identifiable at birth (Gilbert, 1996). Pulmonary stenosis, in which the valve in the pulmonary artery is misshapen (narrowed) or not adequately formed, is the most common (50%); atrial septal defect, in which the wall dividing the right and left upper heart chambers is improperly formed, is not uncommon (10%); ventricular septal hypertrophy, where there is an increase in the wall separating the right and left lower heart chambers, is also found (10%); and ventricular septal defects, where there is a hole between the right and left lower chambers, are found in approximately 5% of NS patients (Allanson, 1996; Noonan, 1994). Noonan (1994) indicates that virtually every type of cardiac defect has been found in individuals with NS. Hypertrophic cardiomyopathy, including both the obstructive and the nonobstructive types, occurs in 20–30% of patients. Cardiomyopathy frequently involves both the right and the left ventricles, is noticeable at birth or develops in later infancy or childhood, and involves muscle disarray and thick walls in the coronary arteries. Other cardiac problems include dysplastic pulmonary valve and mitral valve prolapse.

Various congenital defects may require surgery or medications, while others may not need further treatment (Gilbert, 1996). Electrocardiograms are used to identify abnormal defects (e.g., left-axis deviation or dominant S wave over the precordium) and sometimes can be helpful or confirmatory in the diagnosis of NS (Noonan, 1994). Noonan (1994) suggests that all patients with NS should undergo cardiac evaluations as soon after birth as possible, as well as frequent, periodic checkups, because not all cardiac problems present at birth.

Thrombocytopenia

In some patients with NS, decreased numbers of blood platelets have been found (Mendez & Opitz, 1985). Various bleeding abnormalities have been reported, including factor IX deficiency and von Willebrand disease (Grandy, 1993; Mendez & Opitz, 1985). Flick, Sing, Kizer, and Lazarchick (1991) estimate that as many as 20% of patients with NS have clinically significant coagulation abnormalities. In a case study, Flick et al. (1991) found that a 23-year-old patient with chronic idiopathic thrombocytopenic purpura also had cyclooxygenase deficiency, which was thought to be the primary mechanism for the patient's platelet defect.

Lymphatic System Difficulties

Although it is not pathognomonic for NS, lymphatic involvement has been found in NS patients (Mendez & Opitz, 1985). Lymphatic dysplasia (abnormal or obstructed drainage of the lymphatic system) has produced various complications, including edema and protein-losing enteropathy. Lymphatic conditions can also create complications after surgery.

Leukemia

Johannes et al. (1995) found two cases of acute lymphocytic leukemia (ALL) in children with NS. These authors hypothesize a possible linkage between chromosome 22 and NS; because a linkage with this chromosome has also been reported in ALL, this "can lead to speculation that there may be a connection between the two related abnormalities [NS and ALL] on the chromosome" (Johannes et al., 1995). Previous reports of leukemia in NS patients found that one patient also had malignant schwannoma (Kaplan et al., 1968), while another had acute promyelocytic leukemia and congenital hypoplastic anemia (Krishan, Wegner, & Garg, 1978).

Genitourinary Problems

The fact that the majority of males with NS have undescended testes (cryptorchidism), often bilaterally, may result in deficient spermatogenesis and infertility (Grandy, 1993). Male puberty may be delayed for as much as 2 years; this appears related to bone age (Noonan, 1994). Moreover, secondary sexual characteristics may not be adequately developed (Grandy, 1993). Females are not typically infertile, and they may have either normal or delayed puberty (Grandy, 1993). Maternal transmission of NS is three times greater than paternal transmission; this appears likely to be due to male infertility resulting from cryptorchidism. Noonan (1994) also reports that patients with NS may have renal abnormalities (10%), but that most of these have little serious medical impact on the affected individuals.

Orthopedic Problems

A number of different orthopedic problems have been found in individuals with NS, with as many as 90% of patients showing chest deformity (i.e., prominent-pectus cariatum or hallowed-pectus excavatum; Graham, 1996). Other orthopedic problems have been reported, including scoliosis (10–15%), talipes equinovarus (a deformity of the foot in which the heel is turned inward and is plantar-flexed—typical clubfoot; 10–15%), radioulnar synostosis, cervical spine fusion, or contractures of the joints (Noonan, 1994). The hypotonia that is common may improve with age. Other anomalies include abnormal angle of the elbow, curved fifth finger, blunt and squared fingertips, shield-like chest, and widely spaced nipples (Noonan, 1994).

NEUROPSYCHOLOGICAL IMPAIRMENTS

Most of the research on NS to date has been directed at documenting the physical characteristics of NS, with limited information about the central nervous system or neuropsychological features (intellectual, speech, or hearing problems) of the disorder (Hopkins-Acos & Bunker, 1979). A few isolated studies or single-subject designs have investigated specific neuropsychological deficits, but these investigations should be considered preliminary. Noonan (1994) reported that hypotonia is common and poor coordination is also reported (Fakouri & Fakouri, 1998).

Attention and Concentration

There are no documented studies investigating attention and concentration difficulties in patients with NS.

Intellectual and Academic Development

The intellectual functioning of individuals with NS can range from mild mental deficiency (Noonan, 1994) to superior abilities (Finnegan & Hughes, 1988; Money & Kalus, 1979). Mendez and Opitz (1985) reviewed 63 papers reporting the intellectual functioning of individuals with NS and found that 24% of these individuals were mentally retarded. Others have reported higher rates of mental deficiencies, with 70% close to the deficient range of ability (cited in Graham, 1996). In a study of 100 students with NS, 5% attended schools for the physically disabled, 11% were in programs for slow learners, and 84% attended regular education classrooms and had good school performance (Sharland, Burch et al., 1992).

A Full Scale IQ (e.g., on the third edition of the Wechsler Intelligence Scale for Children) may mask specific abilities when there are significant Verbal–Performance discrepancies. In a small-scale study of children with NS, profile analysis showed that individuals varied in their pattern of verbal and nonverbal strengths. In one case, a patient did show a specific deficit in verbal reasoning skills; however, in four cases, praxic or nonverbal abilities were compromised (Money & Kalus, 1979). Specifically, the latter cases showed difficulty with the visual constructional aspects of the Wechsler scales. These authors hypothesized that the visual constructional disabilities found in NS patients "as well as Turner's syndrome, despite the disparity of the two syndromes cytogenetically, puts constraints on what importance may be attributed to the missing chromosome of 45,X Turner's syndrome in formulating theories regarding the X and Y chromosome as determinants of sex difference in hemispheric dominance and verbal–praxic disparity in 'normal girls' and boys" (Money & Kalus, 1979, p. 850). Further study is needed to confirm this hypothesis and to delineate more clearly any differences between verbal and nonverbal abilities in patients with NS.

Sensory, Motor, and Visual Perceptual Skills

There is ample evidence to suggest that motor, visual perceptual, and sensory deficits are associated with NS (Grandy, 1993; Hopkins-Acos & Bunker, 1979; Noonan, 1994). Motor difficulties that may be secondary to hypertonia and poor muscle tone appear early in life (e.g., poor sucking in infancy) and often continue into early childhood (Gilbert, 1996). Children with NS are often described as clumsy, are frequently poor in sports, and have a tendency to "knock into objects" (Gilbert, 1996, p. 216). Visual perceptual difficulties have also been reported, and squinting and myopia (nearsightedness) may be problems as well (Gilbert, 1996).

Language Skills

Delays in language acquisition are quite common (25%) in children with NS, with a majority of children showing articulation problems (Allanson, 1996). Speech and hearing deficits were reported in a case study of a 3½-year-old boy with NS (Hopkins-Acos & Bunker, 1979). In this young child, "slightly depressed pure-tone thresholds" were reported with a "slight downward shift for both ears on the typanograms," which were consistent with a "mild conductive loss" (Hopkins-Acos & Bunker, 1979, p. 497). Further speech/ language evaluation showed that the child was functioning significantly below expected age levels on measures of language comprehension, with more pronounced difficulties on verbal expressive skills. A functional assessment of his communication intentions and behaviors, via systematic, structured observations of the child in his home interacting with his mother, his brother, and the clinician, also yielded signs of significant delays.

Hopkins-Acos and Bunker (1979) suggested a relationship among the child's congenital heart problems, reduced sensory–motor exploration experiences, and speech/language delays. The child did show improvement with an early intervention program designed to treat speech/language delays. When he was later placed in a normal kindergarten classroom, he made improvements in language comprehension, including three-part commands, same–different, and other verbal concepts; reading through visual recognition of letters; writing his name; social interactions; and independent and group activities. He continued to show below-average abilities in the perceptual–motor area and had difficulty catching and throwing a ball, balancing on one foot, and working with pencils or crayons. Delays were most significant in visual perceptual, motor, and phonological development (Hopkins-Acos & Bunker, 1979). Remediation efforts focused on increasing functional skills to facilitate communication by combining nonverbal signs with appropriate verbalizations that encouraged the "reciprocal nature of social-linguistic behavior" (Hopkins-Acos & Bunker, 1979, p. 503).

The extent to which other children with NS evidence speech/language delays warrants further investigation. Consideration of the effects of early cardiac problems and restriction of sensory–motor experiences is also of interest. The extent to which children respond to early intervention is of primary concern. In addition, Graham (1996) suggests that the possibility of hearing problems should be investigated early.

Organization, Sequencing, Learning, Memory, and Executive Functions

An extensive review of MEDLINE and Psyclit indicated that no research to date has explored problems with organization, sequencing, learning, memory, or executive functions in individuals with NS. Gilbert (1996) does indicate that children with NS may have specific difficulties in learning to speak and may be slow to mature. The extent to which individuals with NF have compromised intellectual abilities may predict difficulties in these areas as well, but research and clinical case reports are needed to verify this hypothesis.

In conclusion, as Hopkins-Acos and Bunker (1979) commented, most research to date has focused on the physical characteristics associated with NS, with less emphasis on neuropsychological abilities. Thus it is difficult to predict which individuals will display select deficits, apart from generalized difficulties associated with low intellectual functioning.

ASSESSMENT AND DIAGNOSTIC ISSUES

Clinical Findings That Aid in Diagnosis

The diagnosis of NS is made from clinical findings (Noonan, 1994). Typically the facial features are helpful for making a diagnosis, although these are difficult to discern in newborns. Noonan (1994) indicates that the following features are typically present: (1) sloping forehead; (2) thick ears, which may be posteriorly positioned; (3) hypertelorism, with downslanting of the palpebral fissures (folds protecting eyes), a deep-set philtrum (groove of the upper lip), and sometimes retrognathia (jaw positioned in the back of the frontal plane); (4) marked edema of the neck, with excess nuchal skin (skin on the back of the neck); (5) relatively enlarged head from infancy through age 2 years; (6) flat cheekbones with prominent, round eyes; (7) depressed nasal bridge; (8) stocky body, with chest deformities that become more prominent with age; and (9) short neck. These features do change in childhood, and the face becomes more coarse, triangular, and sharper in adolescence and adulthood. A low hairline in back may obscure web-like features on the neck. Adults tend to have obvious nasolabial folds, with a high hairline in front, and transparent, wrinkled skin (Noonan, 1994).

Although a scoring system for clinicians was devised by Duncan, Fowler, & Farkas (1981), the diagnosis of NS is still subjective (Noonan, 1994). However, it is important to determine the maternal use of alcohol or other teratogens (e.g., anticonvulsants) and to identify other chromosomal abnormalities, to rule out competing diagnoses.

Several cases of individuals with NS showed fetal edema (Bowle & Black, 1986) and cystic hygroma (i.e., watery tumor on the neck; Donnefeld, Nazir, Sindoni, & Libviggi, 1991) *in utero*. Graham (1996) suggests that diagnosis for mildly affected individuals can be made after a careful cardiac evaluation and consideration of the adult expression of the disorder.

Key Issues in Regard to Differential Diagnosis

A number of other syndromes should be excluded when one is making a diagnosis of NS, including Turner syndrome, NFvR, and Aarskog syndrome. These syndromes are briefly reviewed in order to highlight the major features and characteristics that distinguish NS.

Turner Syndrome

As noted earlier, Turner syndrome occurs when there is a partial or complete absence of, or other abnormality in, the X chromosome (Wiederman et al., 1992). This syndrome (see Powell & Schulte, Chapter 11, for a full discussion occurs only in females and is characterized by the following: short stature, webbed neck, redundant skin folds or edema of the neck, lymphedema of the feet and hands, ptosis of the eyelids, micrognathia, renal anomalies, cardiac defects (i.e., coarctation of the aorta), poor development of secondary sexual characteristics, and primary amenorrhea. A child with Turner syndrome may not be diagnosed at birth. Despite physical features (i.e., webbed neck, ptosis, short stature) and medical problems (e.g., cardiac defects) similar to those of NS, Turner syndrome can be reliably differentiated through genetic tests.

von Recklinghausen Neurofibromatosis

NFvR (also known as NF1) is characterized by multiple *café au lait* spots and skin tumors, with skeletal (i.e., club foot, dislocation of the hips) and neurological signs (Wiederman et al., 1992; see Nilsson & Bradford, Chapter 15, this volume, for a full discussion). NFvR is thought to be an autosomal dominant disorder with variable expressivity, and chromosome 17 has been implicated. Children may show classic signs of NFvR with NS, and are generally diagnosed as having "neurofibromatosis–Noonan syndrome" (NFNS; Wiederman et al., 1992). In some cases the NS signs may be subtle but nonetheless clinically evident (Opitz & Weaver, 1985). Opitz and Weaver (1985) suggest that NFNS is nosologically discrete, not an unusual form of either syndrome; that it is as common as NFvR; and that it has an unknown pathogenesis, although males have different manifestations of the syndrome (fusiform swelling of nerve strands) compared to females (classic cutaneous neurofibromas and a propensity to develop retroperitoneal/visceral neurofibromas. Allanson, Hall, and Van Allen (1985) have also reported patients with NFNS, and likewise suggest that this is a single disorder distinct from the separate syndromes.

Aarskog Syndrome

Although Aarskog syndrome is considered an X-linked recessively inherited syndrome, there is some evidence that it can be partially manifested in females (i.e., short stature with facial and hand features), so there may be an autosomal recessive inheritance linkage as well (Wiederman et al., 1992). Features of Aarskog syndrome that resemble those of NS include short stature, unusual facial features (hypertelorism, antimongoloid slant of the palpebral fissures, ptosis). Aarskog syndrome and NS can be differentiated, however, as NS "does not include the penoscrotal anomaly, but includes pulmonary stenosis, pterygium, [and] mental retardation" (Wiederman et al., 1992, p. 194).

TREATMENT AND INTERVENTION PLANNING

Medical Treatment

Cardiac surgery may or may not be warranted, depending upon the severity and symptoms of the heart disease (Noonan, 1994). Although balloon valvoplasty has been used to treat pulmonary stenosis, difficulties have been noted when the valve is dysplastic (i.e., abnormal in size or shape; Marantz et al., 1988). In these instances, if balloon valvoplasty is not successful, then surgery is an alternative. Noonan (1994) also notes that in some cases the valve may need to be resected to relieve obstructions. Other surgical procedures may be needed to treat the various cardiac problems associated with NS. In rare cases, NS children with cardiomyopathy have undergone heart transplants, but the general course and prognosis for cardiomyopathy are not well known.

Bleeding problems and easy bruising may also need attention; in such cases, platelet counts should be tracked, and aspirin products should be avoided (Noonan, 1994). As noted earlier, cases of ALL have been reported in children with NS, although it is not known whether NS places a child at higher risk for other malignancies. Obviously, medical screening and follow-up treatment are important in these cases.

Although GH deficiency is not considered to be a typical correlate of Noonan's, GH treatment has been used to increase height, as described earlier (Gilbert, 1996). There have been reports of improved growth velocity in prepubertal and pubertal children with NS; however, there is not sufficient longitudinal evidence of change in overall adult stature (Ahmed et al., 1991). Ahmed, Allen, Sharma, MacFarlane, and Dunger (1993) recommend that a community-wide growth screening for height be used in conjunction with a health surveillance program.

Gilbert (1996) suggests that in some cases, surgery may be warranted to treat unde-scended testes. Surgical intervention prior to school age may increase fertility and may decrease other malignant complications.

Psychosocial, Educational, and Emotional Interventions

Although specific treatment plans have not been investigated, techniques for addressing cognitive, visual perceptual, and academic difficulties may prove helpful. Access to special education services may be appropriate under the special education category of "other health-impaired." It is apparent that some children with NS may require psychological support for other issues associated with coping with a chronic medical disease. Further long-term follow-up is needed to determine whether children with NS have a predictable develop-mental course, particularly when cognitive diffiulties are present, or whether the syndrome is so heterogeneous that its progression remains highly individual. Vocational training or preparation for the work force may be particularly challenging for individuals with asso-ciated cognitive difficulties or more serious medical problems.

Parents may benefit from counseling and realistic planning for a child's future. Fam-ily education and support are also recommended, as families may not be well informed about the disorder. Further research is needed to more clearly establish effective practices for children and adolescents with NS and their families.

CONCLUSIONS

A multidisciplinary approach is recommended for an individual with NS, so that medical follow-up, psychoeducational interventions, vocational training, and parental support can be coordinated. These interventions should be monitored regularly so that the child will have the best possible adult outcome. For children with NS, a neuropsychologist needs to move beyond being a diagnostician into playing the role of advocate and counselor. The Individu-als with Disabilities Education Act of 1990 empowers disabled children, adolescents, and adults to gain the vocational and educational training needed for life success. The extent to which we can foster this kind of ecologically valid intervention may optimize the potential for individuals with NS to become self-reliant, self-sufficient, and/or completely independent.

ACKNOWLEDGMENT

I would like to extend my thanks to Jane Walczak, the librarian at Children's Hospital in Milwau-kee, Wisconsin, for her assistance in accessing many of the references for my research on NS.

REFERENCES

Ahmed, M. L., Allen, A. D., Sharma, A., MacFarlane, J. A., & Dunger, D. B. (1993). Evaluation of a distrinct growth screening programme: The Oxford Growth Study. *Archives of Disease in Childhood, 69*, 361–365.
Ahmed, M. L., Foot, A. B. M., Edge, J. A., Lamkin, V. A., Savage, M. O., & Dunger, D.B. (1991). Noonan's syndrome: Abnormalities of the growth hormone/IGF-I axis and the response to treat-ment with human biosynthetic growth hormone. *Acta Paediatrica Scandinavica, 80*, 446–450.

Allanson, J. E. (1996). *The Noonan syndrome factsheet* [On-line]. Available: http://www.paston. co.uk/users/maygurney/tnssg4. html.

Allanson, J. E., Hall, J. G., Hughes, H. E., Preus, M., & Witt, R. D. (1985). Noonan syndrome: The changing phenotype. *American Journal of Medical Genetics, 21,* 507–514.

Allanson, J. E., Hall, J.G., & Van Allen, M. I. (1985). Noonan phenotype associated with neuro-fibromatosis. *American Journal of Medical Genetics, 21,* 457–462.

Bowle, E. V., & Black, V. (1986). Non-immune hydrops fetalis in Noonan's syndrome. *American Journal of Diseases of Children, 140,* 758–760.

Donnefeld, A. E., Nazir, M. A., Sindoni, F., & Libviggi, R. J. (1991). Prenatal sonographic documentation of cystic hygroma regression to Noonan syndrome. *American Journal of Medical Genetics, 39,* 461–465.

Dorland's illustrated medical dictionary (28th ed.). (1994). Philadelphia: W. B. Saunders.

Duncan, W. J., Fowler, R. S., & Farkas, L. G., (1981). A comprehensive scoring system for evaluating Noonan syndrome. *American Journal of Medical Genetics, 10,* 37–50.

Fakouri, C., & Fakouri, E. (1998). Noonan syndrome. In L. Phelps (Ed.), *A guidebook for understanding and educating health-related disorders in children and adolescents* (pp. 474–479). Washington, DC: American Psychological Association.

Finnegan, J. A., & Hughes, H. E. (1988). Very superior intelligence in a child with Noonan syndrome. *American Journal of Medical Genetics, 31,* 385–389.

Flick, J. T., Sing, A. K., Kizer, J., & Lazarchick, J. (1991). Platelet dysfunction in Noonan's syndrome: A case with a platelet cyclooxygenase-like deficiency and chronic idiopathic thrombocytopenic purpura. *American Journal of Clinical Pathology, 95,* 739–742.

Ghaziuddin, M., Bolyard, B., & Alessi, A. (1994). Autistic disorder in Noonan syndrome. *Journal of Intellectual Disability Research, 38,* 67–72.

Gilbert, P. (1996). *The A–Z reference book of syndromes and inherited disorders.* San Diego, CA: Singular.

Govaert, P., Leroy, J. G., Pauwels, R., Vanhaesebrouck, P., De Praeter, C. Van Kets, H., & Goeteyn, M. (1992). Perinatal manifestations of maternal yellow nail syndrome. *Pediatrics, 89,* 1016–1018.

Graham, J. M. (1996). *Aspects of Noonan syndrome* [On-line]. Available: http://www.paston.co.uk/ users/maygurney/tnssg4. html.

Grandy, A. (1993). *Noonan syndrome* [On-line]. Available: http://www.ciondata.com/health/ pedbase/files/noonansy.htm.

Hopkins-Acos, P., & Bunker, K. (1979). A child with Noonan syndrome. *Journal of Speech and Hearing Disorders, 44,* 494–503.

Johannes, J. M., Garcia, E. R., De Vaan, G. A. M., & Weening, R. S. (1995). Noonan's syndrome in association with acute leukemia. *Pediatric Hematology and Oncology, 12,* 571–575.

Kaplan, M. S., Opitz, J. M., & Gosset, F. R. (1968). Noonan's syndrome: A case with elevated serum alkaline phosphatase levels and malignant schwannoma of the left forearm. *American Journal of Diseases of Children, 116,* 359–366.

Krishan, E. U., Wegner, K., & Garg, S. K. (1978). Congenital hypoplastic anemia terminating in acute promyelitic leukemia. *Pediatrics, 61,* 898–901.

Marantz, P. M., Huta, J. C., Mullins, C. E. (1988). Results of balloon valvoplasty in typical and dysplastic pulmonary valve stenosis: Doppler echocardiographic follow-up. *Journal of the American College of Cardiology, 12,* 476–479.

Mendez, H. M. M., & Opitz, J. M. (1985). Noonan syndrome: A review. *American Journal of Medical Genetics, 21,* 493–506.

Money, J., & Kalus, M. (1979). Noonan's syndrome: IQ and specific disabilities. *American Journal of Diseases of Children, 133,* 846–850.

Noonan, J. A. (1994, September). Noonan syndrome: An update and review for the primary physician. *Clinical Pediatrics,* 548–555.

Noonan, J. A., & Ehmke, D. A. (1963). Associated noncardiac malformations in children with congenital heart disease. *Journal of Pediatrics, 63,* 468–469.

Nora, J. J., Nora, A. H., Sinka, A. K., (1974). The Ullrich–Noonan syndrome. *American Journal of Diseases of Children, 127*, 48–55.

Opitz, J. M., & Weaver, D. D. (1985). Editorial comments: The neurofibromatosis–Noonan syndrome. *American Journal of Medical Genetics, 21*, 477–490.

Sharland, M., Burch, M., McKenna, W. M., & Patton, M. A. (1992). A clinical study of Noonan syndrome. *Archives of Disease in Childhood, 67*, 178–183.

Sharland, M., Taylor, R., Patton, M. A., & Jeffrey, S. (1992). Absence of linkage of Noonan syndrome to the neurofibromatosis type I locus. *Journal of Medical Genetics, 29*, 188–190.

Thomas, B. C., & Stanhope, R. (1993). Long-term treatment with growth hormone in Noonan's syndrome. *Acta Paediatrica, 82*, 853–855.

Wiederman, H. R., Kunze, J., & Dibbem, H. (1992). *Atlas of clinical syndromes: A visual aid to diagnosis for clinicians and practicing physicians.* St. Louis, MO: Mosby/Year Book.

15

NEUROFIBROMATOSIS

DAVID E. NILSSON
LYNNE W. BRADFORD

Neurofibromatosis (NF) is a relatively common autosomal dominant genetic disorder resulting in development of both benign and malignant tumors at an increased frequency within the central nervous system (CNS) and the peripheral nervous system (Riccardi & Eichner, 1992; Riccardi, 1991; Huson & Hughes, 1994). Although John Merrick, the renowned "Elephant Man," brought considerable attention to NF, current opinion is that he was misdiagnosed; a more likely diagnosis for Merrick would have been Proteus syndrome, a rare somatic cell genetic disease. NF occurs in both sexes and in all races and ethnic groups. Since a German pathologist, Friedrich von Recklinghausen, first noted in 1882 that the tumors propagated from nerve cells, knowledge of NF has progressively increased. Two distinct forms of the disorder are currently identified, NF1 and NF2, although other forms may exist. Given the greater prevalence of NF1 and the relatively larger body of research literature available addressing its neurocognitive and neurobehavioral characteristics and outcomes, NF1 is the primary focus of this chapter. NF2 is discussed whenever there are relevant comparable data available. In spite of the growing body of research literature, our knowledge of the specific neurodevelopmental consequences of NF remains limited.

CLINICAL PRESENTATION

NF1 is a disorder of abnormal peripheral nerve cell growth with an unusually heterogeneous clinical presentation. Although it is generally considered to be a peripheral neuropathy, brain tumors and other lesions within the brain are often present. It has a prevalence of 1 in 4,000 live births. Despite medical and genetic advances in the understanding of NF1, a diagnosis is still made on the basis of clinical criteria. Symptoms of NF1 are usually present in childhood, but as a result of the progressive nature of the disease, symptoms may become more pronounced during puberty, pregnancy, or hormonal changes.

Specific diagnostic criteria, as originally identified by the National Institutes of Health (NIH) Consensus Development Conference (1988), consist of two or more of the following: (1) six or more *café au lait* (CAL) spots more than 5 mm in diameter prior to puberty or more than 15 mm in diameter after puberty; (2) two or more neurofibromas of any type, or one plexiform neurofibroma (subcutaneous cluster of nerve and skin fiber); (3) freckling in the axillary or inguinal regions (Crowe's [1964] sign); (4) an optic pathway tumor (i.e., optic glioma); (5) two or more Lisch nodules (benign iris hamartomas—i.e., clumps of pigment in the iris); (6) bowing of bone structure (commonly seen in shin bowing or in the spine as scoliosis; and/or (7) a first-degree relative with NF1 based on the preceding criteria.

Diagnostic criteria for NF1 are usually met by age 10 (Korf, 1992). The most common manifestations of NF1 are CAL spots, neurofibromas, Lisch nodules, and auxiliary or inguinal (i.e., skin fold) freckling (Gutmann et al., 1997). Pain or other physical discomfort may be present, particularly in more severe clinical manifestations of the disease. The severity of symptoms and rate of progression vary across patients. The severity of NF is directly related to the location and type of neurofibromas, and in some cases to the size of the tumors. Although some centers use a four-level grading scale for the severity of NF1, such a clinical grading system is of limited value, given the variability of clinical presentation and the lack of correlation between disease severity and underlying genetic mutation in NF1.

Neuromas, one of the most common types of tumors, may develop anywhere in the body where there are nerve cells, but most characteristically develop in the peripheral nervous system. Although NF1 can affect almost any organ, many patients experience relatively few symptoms. Skin lesions may be apparent as CAL spots, named for their color (which resembles the color of coffee with milk). These may be present at birth or may appear later. CAL spots may also appear in the general population, but are usually smaller and fewer in number. The frequency of axillary or inguinal freckling is reported to be 81% by 6 years of age (Obringer, Meadows, & Zackai, 1989) and 89% by the fourth decade of life (Huson, Harper, & Compston, 1988). Most visible neurofibromas may be seen as small bumps on the surface of the skin, approximately the size of a mosquito bite. Neurofibromas can produce disfiguring plexiform growths in multiple areas of the body, but such growths are relatively rare. Unlike cutaneous neurofibromas, plexiform neurofibromas can undergo malignant transformation, with increased incidence of sarcomas and leukemias. NF increases the risk of malignant cancer by an estimated 5% over that of the general population. Evolving pain or rapid growth in neurofibromas is a prompt for immediate medical follow-up.

Tumors of the optic pathway (i.e., optic gliomas) are more common than plexiform neurofibromas, and are sometimes found as a thickening of the optic nerve with no symptoms present. They infrequently progress to visual loss (Listernick, Darling, Greenwald, Strauss, & Charrow, 1995). Tumors may compromise vision, create hydrocephalus, and often require neurosurgical intervention through resection or debulking. Such tumors are typically low-grade and do not require additional treatment or chemotherapy. Accelerated head growth (i.e., macrocephaly) is often present, but is not always associated with neurological manifestations (Obringer et al., 1989). The deformity of bone structure is relatively rare, occurring predominantly in facial bones. Such deformity does not typically develop later in life (Korf, 1994); it almost always presents initially in infancy. Scoliosis may not become apparent until a child is of school age, however. Bowing of the shin bones may also be observed. Other complications include headaches, hypertension, seizures, short stature, weakness, and precocious puberty.

From 30% to 60% of individuals with NF1 will present with nonenhancing hyperintensities (often referred to as "unidentified bright objects" or UBOs) evident on magnetic resonance imaging (MRI); these are most commonly found in the cerebellum, basal ganglia, thalamus, and brain stem regions (Gutmann et al., 1997.) Neurodevelopmental disruption—including developmental delay in roughly 20% of NF1 children and learning disabilities (LDs) in an estimated 50% (Riccardi and Eichner, 1992)—occurs, although these estimates are considered by many to be low and poorly conceptualized. It has been suggested that LDs probably represent the most common problem in childhood NF (Hofman, Harris, Bryan, & Denckla, 1994). Intuitively, a disease that is so intimately associated mechanically, structurally, and probably neurochemically with the nervous system should have the potential for negative influence on neurocognitive and neurobehavioral functioning. Equally intuitively, the disruption in the neurodevelopmental progression of the individual should be dependent upon the specific idiosyncratic presentation of the disease, the individual's characteristics, and his or her age at disruption.

NF2 is much less prevalent than NF1 (1 in 40,000) and is manifested most commonly in acoustic or central neuromas. Cataract formation and hearing loss are often associated with NF2. Some of the manifestations are progressive and result in considerable morbidity or mortality. Diagnosis of NF2, like that of NF1, is based on clinical criteria. As outlined by Gutmann et al. (1997), the original NIH Consensus Development Conference criteria for NF2 included (1) bilateral vestibular schwannomas on MRI or (2) a first-degree relative with NF2 and either unilateral eighth-nerve masses or two of the following: neurofibroma, meningioma, glioma, schwannoma, or juvenile posterior subcapsular ventricular opacity (Mulvihill et al., 1990). The new criteria for confirmed or definite NF2 (Gutmann et al., 1997) differ only slightly, including (1) bilateral vestibular schwannomas on MRI or (2) a parent, sibling, or child with NF2 plus (a) unilateral vestibular schwannoma detected before the age of 30 years or (b) any two of the following: angioma, glioma, schwannoma, or juvenile posterior subcapsular ventricular opacity. Cerebral calcifications have been suggested as an additional diagnostic feature of NF2, although there are no convincing data to justify their inclusion, as they appear to represent relatively nonspecific findings. In only 10% of cases do individuals with NF2 become symptomatic before 10 years of age. The clinical management of an individual with NF2 includes an annual neurological evaluation with cranial MRI and follow-up ophthalmological evaluations. In the case of NF2, unlike that of NF1, there are sufficient data to support the existence of severe and mild forms, suggesting the potential benefit of a clinical grading system.

GENETIC RESEARCH

Evolving technology has allowed a progressively greater understanding of the genetics of NF. Cell differentiation, regulation of cell growth, and interactions between cells of various structures are directly affected by the NF1 gene. NF1 is known to be precipitated by deletions on chromosome 17, although there has been a wide diversity of genetic mutation in NF1, including deletions, insertions, duplications, point mutations, and chromosome rearrangements. Although 50% of new cases diagnosed are results of direct genetic transmission, the other 50% are new-mutation original cases (NIH Consensus Development Conference, 1988). In 1990, an NF1 gene was cloned and its protein product, neurofibromin, was identified (Cawthon et al., 1990; Viskochil et al., 1990; Wallace et al., 1990). Deletions or insertions, as well as other mutations of this gene, may affect cell growth differentially during the developmental period for CNS networks, which continues in some form until at least the onset of puberty and possibly beyond. Lazaro et al. (1996) found sex differences in the mutation rate and mutational mechanism in NF1, with the paternal transmission more likely to be a point mutation and the maternal transmission more likely to be a deletion. Lazaro et al. (1996) also suggest that it is likely that the male germ has a higher rate of mutation. Patients with deletions characteristically have more severe manifestations (Wu, Austin, Schneider, Boles, & Korf, 1995), including severe developmental delay, minor and major physical anomalies (e.g., bilateral iris colobomas), multiple cutaneous fibromas, and plexiform neurofibromas present before age 5.

Giordano, Mahadeo, He, Geist, and Gutmann (1996) found that neurofibromin functions as a tumor suppressor and is elevated in response to cerebral ischemia, suggesting involvement in growth regulatory pathways associated with cellular remodeling responses to injury. Supplementary to this activity of NF1 is the finding of Gutmann et al. (1996, 1997) that neurofibromin expression is increased in astrocytic tumors in response to feedback regulation provided by increasing levels of activated p21-ras. Other genetic differences—not only in neurodevelopment but in tumor growth (Giordano et al., 1996) and other characteristics of the disease (Norton, Mahadeo, Geist, & Gutmann, 1996; Pollock, Shultz, & Mulvihill, 1996; Lazaro et al., 1996)—are manifested with apparent sex differences. Norton et al. (1996) report that NF1 expression occurs late in cell growth arrest and may contribute to the maintenance of the differential state of the cell. Consistent with these findings, Pollack et al. (1996) found that the biological behavior of brain stem lesions in patients with NF1 differed significantly from that of the lesions in patients without NF1. Histological differences also exist between NF1 children with and without learning disabilities (LDs) (Castillo et al., 1995). Castillo et al. (1995) found that N-acetyl-aspartate–creatine ratios were 1.83 (± 0.14) in NF1 with LDs, as opposed to 1.63 (± 0.2) in NF1 without LDs. The significance of this finding is not understood.

The NF2 gene has been linked to chromosome 22q. In 1993, an NF2 gene was cloned and its protein product, merlin or schwannomin, was identified (Rouleau et al., 1993; Trofatter et al., 1993). Merlin or schwannomin has been identified as a tumor suppressor protein.

For individuals who desire prenatal diagnosis, genetic testing and counseling can be provided. Unfortunately, NF1 exhibits considerable clinical variability within families, and these tests will tell only *whether* an individual at risk is affected, not *how severely* he or she will be affected. Future research may facilitate improved DNA or biochemical diagnostic testing (Gutmann et al., 1997). In most families with more than one affected individual, linkage analysis for NF2 still remains the test of choice, as this will indicate the presence of NF2 with greater than 99% certainty (Gutmann et al., 1997).

NEURORADIOLOGICAL MANIFESTATIONS AND OUTCOME CORRELATIONS

The progression of technology for neuroimaging has greatly facilitated our understanding of the nervous system over the past 20 years. Although by current standards computed tomography (CT) is relatively punitive, introduction of the CT scan allowed the first glimpses of the structure of the brain within a living being. Progression of MRI greatly expanded the structural neurodiagnostic capabilities. The rapid evolution of the computer and its application to neuroimaging technology (in single-photon emission computed tomography [SPECT] and other new imagining methods, PET, MRA, fMRI, MEG) have not only enhanced the detail of the visible structure, but have begun to expand our *functional* understanding of the CNS. Although evolving neuroradiology has contributed significantly to our evolving understanding of NF, just as there is considerable heterogeneity in the clinical presentation of symptoms, there is also impressive diversity in neuroradiological manifestations. The complete mechanism of the neurodevelopmental progression of the CNS neuromas and the hyperintensities (i.e., UBOs) identified on MRI is unknown. There is limited understanding of the logic of presentation of lesions, their developmental progression, and particularly their significance for outcome. Even less is known about the functional consequences of the occurrence of lesions.

Although preliminary, several studies across a variety of populations have contributed somewhat to our understanding of the significance of MRI lesions identified in NF1 patients. Menor and colleagues (Menor, Marti-Bonmati, Mulas, Cortina, & Olague, 1991; Menor & Marti-Bonmati, 1992) reported the results of a study of NF1 patients that utilized both CT and MRI. Out of 41 children (24 males, 17 females) aged 2 to 13 (mean age = 8 years), T2-weighted hyperintensities were found in the globus pallidus in 22 cases (54%), in the internal capsule in 6 cases (15%), in the corpus callosum in 2 cases (5%), in the anterior commissure in 1 case (2%), and in the semioval center in 2 cases (5%). Less clearly defined intensities were found in cerebellar white matter in 21 cases (51%) and the brain stem in 21 cases (51%). None of the cases displayed enhancement with gadolinium-DPTA. Predictably, MRI was found to distinguish the presence of the abnormalities more clearly than CT.

Ferner, Hughes, and Weinman (1996) and DiMario, Ramsby, Greenstein, Langshur, and Dunham (1993) found similar hyperintensities. Ferner et al. studied a group including both children and adults (mean age = 25 years). Half of the 16 children in the study presented with hyperintensities in the basal ganglia, cerebellum, or brain stem. DiMario et al. found the highest percentage of hyperintensities in the globus pallidus and in the cerebellar white matter. Ferner et al. (1996) failed to detect any significant correlation between the presence of hyperintensities and measures of intelligence; this is not surprising, given the relative insensitivity of IQ measures to neurocognitive change. Other researchers, such as Denckla et al (1996) and Moore, Slopis, Schomer, Jackson, and Levy (1996), have reported a correlation between the hyperintensities and intellectual functioning. Denckla et al. (1996) demonstrated a correlation between lower IQ and the *distribution* of UBOs, not just their *presence*. The percentage of volume of brain tissue found in the UBOs did not reflect a correlation with IQ, supporting a study by Castillo et al. (1995) with SPECT, which asserted that hyperintensities are similar to normal brain tissue. Moore et al. (1996) failed to find a statistically significant relationship between the presence or absence of hyperintensities and neuropsychological scores, but they did find that IQ scores, as well as scores on measures of memory, motor function, distractibility, and attention, were significantly lower for children with hyperintensities in the thalamus. Hofman et al. (1994), found a significant correlation between the lowering of Full Scale IQ scores and Judgment of Line Orientation scores in children with NF1 and the *number* of locations in which T2–weighted intensities were found. They also found that NF1 children had significant LDs for written language and reading, in addition to deficits in neuromotor function, when they were compared to unaffected siblings.

North et al. (1994) found a relation between NF1 patients with hyperintensities and a correlating shift in Full Scale IQ, although mean scores were not out of the "normal" range. NF1 children without the hyperintensities (UBOs) did not significantly differ from published norms for any measure of ability or performance. North et al. suggested that the pathology underlying the hyperintensities changes over time; they proposed that "Mutations of the NF1 gene may result in abnormal cell differentiation in the brains of a subgroup of patients with NF1. Areas of dysplastic gliosis and aberrant myelination disrupt important neuronal circuits involving higher cognitive processing and in turn these appear as increased T2 signal intensity in MRI" (1994, p. 882). The majority of lesions were found in the basal ganglia and in the subcortical white matter, which is consistent with the findings of other researchers. The presence of T2 UBOs correlated with lower mean IQ scores, lower language scores, impaired visual–motor integration, and coordination deficits. However, coordination deficits were found to improve after age 17. Although differences were found in the presence of UBOs, there was no correlation between the number of hyperintensities and any measure of performance. Given the diversity of presentation (combining NF with non-NF individual genetic manifestations, such correlations would be difficult with the relatively small n's of the studies.

The observations of North et al. (1994) were somewhat supported by sequential, prospective, and retrospective MRI studies of 44 children and adults ranging in age from 1 to 37 years (Terada, Barkovich, Edwards, & Circillo, 1996). When grouped according to age, 28 of 30 subjects (93%) younger than 15 had hyperintensities, 4 of 7 subjects (57%) between 16 and 30 had them, and only 2 of 7 (29%) over 31 had them. Somewhat more interesting was the finding that a group of children with a mean age of 3.7 years displayed lesions found to increase in size. For a group with a mean age of 6.2 years, the lesions remained unchanged. For a group with a mean age of 11.4 years, the lesions were found to have decreased or disappeared. In older patients, the lesions were small and unilateral; in younger patients, lesions were large and bilateral. Lesions in the cerebellum appeared to disappear sooner than those in the basal ganglia structures and the brain stem. Although deep gray and white matter lesions were found in families of 86% of the children, only 17% of the parents had them. Since some of these data may reflect the development of sporadic cases, additional longitudinal studies are needed to improve our understanding of the natural history and developmental progression of lesions—not only across groups, but for individual patients.

Moore, Ater, Needle, Slopis, and Copeland (1994) compared children with brain tumors, children with NF1, and children with both conditions, finding that those with only brain tumors scored highest, the NF1-only group was next, and the group with both conditions scored lowest. Unfortunately, Moore et al. did not compare groups for nontumor intensities. Leguis, et al. (1995) failed to find a significant relationship between T2 hyperintensities and intelligence among children with NF1, but noted lower mean Full Scale IQ scores for the group that displayed other neurological symptoms; this finding is not surprising, given the additional mechanisms for disruption of CNS function. Proton MRI spectroscopy, completed by Castillo et al. (1995) with NF1 patients, showed spots of increased signal that were different from gliomas and more similar to normal brain tissue. These were termed "hamartomas." Boardman, Anslow, and Renowden (1996), in a discussion of neuronal migration, postulated that hamartomas may not be as transient as Itoh et al. (1994) suggested a majority of T2 hyperintensities to be. Es, North, McHugh, and Silva (1996) studied hyperintensities of both T1 and T2 and found no association with neurological deficits or the occurrence of macrocephaly; intellectual functioning was not analyzed. A spontaneous decrease in the size of lesions was supported in the study, consistent with the findings of others (North et al. 1994). Terada et al. (1996) have theorized that the hyperintensities represent a reparative process of myelin and maturation abnormality in cells. Prolonged T2 relaxation in the basal ganglia approximates the T2 prolongation in the white matter of the posterior fossa. Short T1 relaxation is characteristic of only the basal ganglia, not the posterior fossa or the white matter hyperintensities, but does not appear to regress over periods as long as 90 months.

NEUROPSYCHOLOGICAL IMPAIRMENTS

Given the rather intimate association of NF with the CNS, there is, not surprisingly, a growing body of research literature reflecting neurocognitive and neurobehavioral consequences of NF1. Children with NF have been found to have an increased incidence and surprising diversity of LDs, and to be at significant risk for academic difficulties (Hofman et al., 1994; Denckla et al., 1996). It has been suggested by Denckla and others that LDs are the most common problems associated with NF. However, the pattern of neurocognitive deficits or LDs is less than clearly understood or predictable—a situation not unlike that in research on other neurological conditions (e.g., traumatic brain injury, seizures, brain tumors). Our understanding of neuroanatomy as it relates to neurofunction is incomplete at best; our understanding of individual neurodevelopment subsequent to neurological compromise for almost all populations is even more limited. Neurobehavioral developmental progression (e.g., progression in affective disorders, moods, temperament) is possibly the least understood area, although a body of research literature is evolving.

As in many neuropsychological outcome studies, the apparent basic assumption in the NF1 outcome research literature has been that patients are more similar than dissimilar as a clinical group. However, not only is the individual clinical manifestation of NF1 extremely varied, but additional individual patient characteristics are also extremely diverse across a variety of factors (e.g., levels of intellectual ability, genetic predisposition to LDs, comorbidity with other genetic disorders, comorbidity with emotional/behavioral disorders). Perhaps the single most complicating factor is individual variance. Although it is substantial for school-age populations in general, it is even greater for populations with neurological and neurodevelopmental difficulties, given the interaction of genetic predisposition with specific neurological characteristics of individual children. A patient can be mentally retarded or gifted, independent of NF disease manifestations. A patient can be language-disordered generally or more specifically dyslexic, with or without NF. It has been suggested that there may be a selective pairing factor, a process of some self-selection in marriage for the NF population. The 50% new-mutation figure would seem to decrease that contribution, however. As such, it is not surprising that global scores have reflected substantial variability and hence inconsistent findings. Combining the individual variability into global scores becomes predictably misleading and ambiguous. With the magnitude of variability present, an overwhelming effect would need to be present for consistent, specific findings. There are no reported efforts to partial out the variance attributable to familial characteristics, genetic predisposition to LDs, or factors of potential comorbidity. Similarly, there is limited understanding for the neurodevelopmental progression of NF. Given the early occurrence of the disease, it would seem likely that the progression of the neurodevelopmental acquisition of skills would dictate not only outcome, but the manifestation of symptoms through developmental stages on into adulthood. If, as has been suggested, neurological injury or neurodevelopmental disruption compromises ongoing neurodevelopment, later-developing functions will be disrupted, but this will perhaps not be apparent earlier in development. It appears that when neurodevelopmental disorder (e.g., NF) interacts with additional neurological injury, the effects are magnified (Moore et al., 1994).

In addition to idiosyncratic individual characteristics, another obstacle to conceptualizing LDs in NF1 is that of the "either–or" approach to LDs. When a deviation quotient is used, specific LDs are identified, primarily those associated with academic skills. However, other neurodevelopmental disabilities, such as nonverbal LDs (NLDs) or deficits in executive function, are not identified—let alone recognized or accommodated. Further compounding the problem is the use of such terms as "within normal limits" or "average" to refer to the relative level of test performance. What would a child's test profile have been like *without* NF1 contribution? Many studies use very limited measures, relying heavily upon global scores (e.g., the third edition of the Wechsler Intelligence Scale for Children [WISC-III]). Other measures have obvious potential ceiling effects (e.g., a continuous-performance test). There is considerable diversity reported across studies in the breadth (and depth) of neuropsychological measures used.

Group studies have not been specific or consistent in their demonstration of a specific profile of neurocognitive and neurobehavioral characteristics for NF patients. Again, this is a common problem in the neuroscience literature on other neurological patient populations. Given the number of subjects in most studies and the seemingly unmanageable array of individual characteristics and variables, it is virtually impossible to study NF children with current applications of research design. For example, a child's age of the child at the time of assessment is a critical variable, given what we know about the neurodevelopment of cognition. Specific measures become more critical relative to their sensitivity for a given age group. Individual level of intellectual ability is another important factor. A bright child is more likely to adapt to the structural demands of testing more productively, and this may mask some of his or her deficits. Genetic predisposition to cognitive difficulties (e.g., language difficulties, LDs, attention-deficit/hyperactivity disorder [ADHD]) and emotional/behavioral problems (e.g., depression, anxiety) also contribute to cloud the NF group profile. The presence of other contributing neurological conditions (e.g., seizures, brain tumors, hydrocephalus, vascular anomalies) further confounds the comparison.

Although the neuropsychological deficits found in NF children have been demonstrated to be both language-based and visual–spatial/perceptual–motor, the latter have been more consistently reported in the research literature. Such a pattern of "nonverbal learning disability" (NLD) has been researched extensively in a general population of children with LDs by Rourke (1989, 1995) and colleagues. Rourke (1995) and Harnadek and Rourke (1994) have proposed a diagnostic profile for NLDs that includes the following: bilateral tactual perceptual deficit (usually more marked for the left side); bilateral psychomotor coordination deficits (more marked for the left side); deficiencies in visual–spatial/organization ability; deficits in higher levels of language and verbal problem solving; hypothesis testing in understanding cause-and-effect relationships; deficits in computational arithmetic skills, relative to well-developed rote verbal memory and word recognition; deficits in adapting to novel or complex situations; and deficits in social perception and judgment. Many of these deficits lead to disturbances in cognition that affect ongoing development and learning. Continuing research has demonstrated similar profiles of NLDs in a variety of populations, but most notably in patient populations with neurological injury, disease, or neurodevelopmental disorder. Rourke has proposed a model of white matter disease, although it would appear that there are potentially multiple etiologies. Later-developing skills, such as visual–spatial/perceptual–motor functions or higher-order intellectual abilities and executive functions, seem to take the biggest "hit." Intellectual ability is often "average," and it has often been assumed that there is no cognitive disruption as a result. As is commonly the case, a patient can be of "average" or "above-average" intellectual ability, but can exhibit *substantial* neurocognitive deficits, given the disruptions to higher-order intellectual abilities, executive functions, and visual–spatial functions. More recent research also suggests disruption of language-based academic skills (e.g., reading, spelling), as reported in North et al. (1997). It would thus appear likely that a more mixed neurodevelopmental model is in operation. Visual–spatial deficits are not independent of language-based academic skills (Hofman et al., 1994; North et al., 1997).

Various other studies have suggested cognitive and behavioral phenotypes for NF1. There are several discrepancies, but many similarities. Again, characteristics of NLDs tend to predominate in many NF1 patients, although a variety of LD combinations have been reported. There is some evidence suggesting that severity of developmental disabilities is directly related to the presence of UBOs and other neuroradiological findings (e.g., tumors). As noted above, however, many factors make it difficult to interpret previous and future studies addressing LDs in NF1 and other neurological/neurodevelopmental disorders. In support of the overall profile of NLDs, Dilts et al. (1996) found a significant number of mild deficits in NF1 children compared to same-sex siblings. That study proposed a model for a cognitive phenotype consistent with NLDs, including difficulty with visual–spatial/ perceptual–motor functions, dysfunction of higher-order language abilities, problems with attention, sensory–motor deficits, problems with visual–motor integration functions (e.g., writing, copying, drawing), and psychosocial difficulties (including lack of peer support and probable social perception deficits).

Yet another problem area relative to research has to do with the issue of behavior or "psychopathology." The assumption is that, similar to the health care industry, the brain is divided into "major medical" and "emotional/behavioral" compartments. In reality, the brain regulates everything. With neuropathy, certain neurobehavioral characteristics are generated; these are often described as irritability, emotional volatility, impulsivity, anxiety, depression, and others. Often the most disruptive influences are specific to such problems of self-regulation. Many such patients will exhibit difficulty maintaining and sustaining attention. Some researchers suggest that the neuropathy may exaggerate underlying genetic predisposition. Although they are difficult to distinguish, the neurological bases of behavior and behavior change must be factored into the equation. It would be logical to assume that the development of personality would be similarly disrupted by any neurological injury or neurodevelopmental influence (e.g., NF, Tourette syndrome). Cognition also contributes significantly to the development of what we refer to as behavior or personality.

An improved understanding of the neurocognitive and neurobehavioral outcomes for NF should lead not only to a better understanding of the disease, but also to improved neurodevelopmental support, treatment interventions, and educational support to enhance quality of life and productive outcome. Since age has long been recognized as an apparent critical neurodevelopmental variable in neurological compromise, it would seem to be of importance for NF1 as well. The heterogeneity of individual manifestation of the disease makes a clear understanding difficult. It seems logical that the disruption to neurodevelopmental progression, interacting with individual characteristics, would explain individual manifestations; this would make the interaction of age and natural history of the disease important considerations. It is this understanding that should drive the assessment process and subsequent intervention.

NEUROPSYCHOLOGICAL TESTING APPLICATIONS

The research literature is nonspecific in regard to neuropsychological strategies for assessing children with NF. There is relatively little consistency in comparable test measures across studies, as noted earlier. General functional categories are assessed, but the different measures used contribute significantly to the overall variability in scores. The lack of a demonstrably consistent neurocognitive phenotype for NF is not surprising, given the diversity of measures used, the relative lack of control of multiple variables (e.g., disease severity, idiosyncratic presentation), and the multitude of individual characteristics of patients (e.g., individual levels of performance, genetic predisposition) NF is also not the only genetic variant in operation for any given patient. A patient may exhibit manifestations of genetic dispositions toward LDs, ADHD, mental retardation, affective disorders, or other such characteristics, and independent of NF. Again, it is likely that bright NF patients are able to adapt and compensate better, thus masking cognitive deficits in traditional standardized testing. Such factors are difficult to quantify or qualify. As for many neurological disorders and injuries, the neuropathy probably tends to intensify or exacerbate (and perhaps to be exacerbated by) comorbid functional deficits, although little quantification is available (Moore et al., 1994). The brain appears to make specific accommodations neurobiologically, neurofunctionally, and neurochemically, although the models for such are clearly inadequate to explain the process. Surprisingly little research is available addressing changes over time.

Several basic principles should drive all neuropsychological assessment, including children with NF. The value of neuropsychological assessment is in identifying specific intervention strategies for specific patients. This is particularly critical for children in a managed health care environment. The major disruption of NF, as for any neurological compromise or disorder, is a disruption of ongoing neurodevelopment. Measurable functional deficits at age 6 will present very differently at age 16. Neuropathy is more likely to compromise later-developing functions, given "sparing models" (Satz, Strauss, Hunter, & Wada, 1994). A broad-based functional assessment is critical to understanding neurodevelopmental progression and functional capacity. No single measure provides an adequate assessment of functional ability.

A critical part of the assessment should cover the higher-order cognitive functions developing later in neurodevelopmental progression. Assessment should carefully consider such functions as attention/concentration, psychomotor speed (e.g., speed of processing), regulation of moods and emotion, conceptual organization, and speed and efficiency of language use. Global scores are not likely to be as sensitive to the needs of the individual patient as scores on more specialized tests. As described earlier, higher-order reasoning/ problem solving, attention/concentration, mental organization, planning, and other self-regulation functions are most likely to be disrupted, and this will have an adverse impact on continuing neurodevelopment, psychosocial development, and academic performance. However, as children progress in school, the greater demands for independence, self-regulation, and speed of processing begin to take a toll, both academically and relative to stress and anxiety, even though traditional LDs are not identified.

The model of LDs currently based upon skill production (i.e., reading, writing), rather than functional abilities or processing skills, is particularly limiting from the perspective of neurodevelopmental intervention. A disruption of neurodevelopmental progression creates changes in a child's abilities to self-regulate, organize, plan, or completely integrate information. In particular, patients with NLDs struggle in this manner. Although this is especially evident on visual–spatial/perceptual–motor tasks (right hemisphere), the lesion is probably more global than is currently understood, as has been observed for hydrocephalus. NF1 is likely to be characterized by the same pattern, consistent with the test data, although other factors (e.g., specific lesions, genetic predisposition, age) may alter its manifestations.

Given these basic principles, we present the following suggestions for generating a functionally valuable assessment of the individual patient—his or her specific idiosyncratic risk factors, the most productive means of adaptation and compensation, and possible specific neurodevelopmental interventions. It is critical to include in an assessment anecdotal observations, teacher reports, and parent reports. A well-done history is probably one of the most sensitive measures that we have of neurodevelopmental disorder.

Understanding Familial/Genetic Predisposition

A critical part of the evaluation is determining the genetic history of the nuclear and extended family. School records of siblings (e.g., achievement tests) may be helpful in achieving a better understanding of familial characteristics. A family history LDs (e.g., language disorders, reading disorders, poor school performance), affective disorders (e.g., anxiety, depression), or ADHD is of potential value in predicting the developmental course of the individual patient. It also helps in understanding the specific risk factors for the patient in addition to NF. Like neurologial injury and other neurodevelopmental disorders, NF potentially exacerbates other genetic predispositions. For example, a child with a reading disorder is potentially even more impaired for reading globally as a consequence of NF. Similarly, a child with a predisposition to anxiety is likely to exhibit even greater levels of anxiety.

Understanding Family Characteristics

Various characteristics of the family will have an impact on specific treatment and developmental interventions, and these should be carefully considered. The parents' level of education and financial circumstances will affect their ability to understand and implement recommendations, to follow up with the school, or to follow up with medical specialists. A parent who also has NF may either overreact or underreact to his or her child's symptoms, depending upon the parent's own clinical experience. The number of children in the family and their specific needs will also affect the parents' ability to respond to the patient's needs. Sometimes older children in the family can be a resource for providing developmental and school support to the patient.

Understanding the Patient's Previous Neurodevelopmental Progression

A thorough neurodevelopmental history is critical to an understanding of the developmental context for any given patient. Whether this is obtained through a well-rehearsed, structured clinical interview or an interview in combination with a parent history form, an understanding of the patient from birth to the present—especially of additional risk factors (e.g., traumatic brain injury, diabetes, seizures) potentially contributing to neurodevelopmental status—is critical. Previous school records for the patient are also important, not only for an initial assessment, but also as part of the patient file so that ongoing developmental and academic progression can be monitored. Previous individual and group testing is particularly helpful in better understanding individual neurodevelopment.

Monitoring Changes in Development over Time

Just as it is not appropriate to administer a neuropsychological test battery every year, it is inappropriate to complete only one neuropsychological test battery, as if this single "snapshot" of the child could illuminate all of his or her neurodevelopmental complexities, past, present, and future. In today's managed health care environment, and with characteristic underfunding for children's health care in particular, some creativity and adaptability must be applied. Collaboration with the school system, using a combination of routine school testing (e.g., the WISC–III, the Woodcock–Johnson Psycho-Educational Battery—Revised, the Wechsler Individual Achievement Test, etc.) with neuropsychological testing support, not only is cost-efficient but facilitates a team effort by community and health care providers. Some school systems exhibit impressive sophistication in evaluation; others are less fortunate. A collaborative effort serves not only to provide support to the individual child, but to educate health care providers and educators—to the benefit of other children with similar neurodevelopmental disruptions.

Assessing Emotional/Behavioral Characteristics in Relation to Neurobehavioral Status

Another critical part of any assessment is understanding the emotional/behavioral characteristics of the child as they relate to his or her neurobehavioral status. The answer to the question "Is this behavior a result of genetic predisposition, NF [i.e., neurobehavioral status], or environment?" is always "Yes!" The relative contributions for any given child are different. For some, genetic predisposition to anxiety tempers all interventions and reactions. For others, the neurological disruption is greater. For still others, factors of fear, pain, and social context of the disease are paramount. An anxious child is likely to respond with greater sensitivity than a less anxious child to certain aspects of NF.

Conducting a Broad-Based Neuropsychological Assessment

Although there are numerous neuropsychological measures available and more are being published monthly, the specific list of test measures is less significant than a thorough, broad-based functional assessment strategy addressing multiple areas of functioning (e.g., attention/concentration, language functions, visual–spatial reasoning, executive function, sensory–motor function). As emphasized throughout this discussion, it is particularly critical to monitor a child's ongoing neurodevelopment in relation to higher-order cognitive skills. For example, many children with NF, in addition to exhibiting characteristics of NLDs, exhibit many subtle neurodevelopmental consequences. As these children grow and develop, higher-order intellectual functions (e.g., reasoning, judgment, problem solving) and executive functions (i.e., self-regulation) tend to be compromised. As such, they begin after a period of time to have difficulty keeping up, and their performance begins to trail off. For others, problems are apparent from the outset.

Understanding NF

A final important part of the assessment of a child with NF is the neuropsychologist's understanding of the disease, the risk factors of the disease, and the contributing symptom constellations as they relate to that child. It is equally critical to assess the family's understanding of the disease. Often there are others in the immediate family who have the disease, and the family is well educated and experienced. Given the number of new mutations that occur, however, this may not be the case. It is particularly critical as part of a competent neuropsychological evaluation to know the specific characteristics of the disease, to evaluate the parents' understanding of risk factors and treatment resources, and to determine whether or not they are receiving services from a multidisciplinary team in the region. Although many such families are, it is surprising, if not disheartening, how often a family has never recognized or understood the need to be monitored regularly for the disease. It is important that the neuropsychologist be able to identify local resources and refer the patient to a team, either through the family physician or directly. In completing a neuropsychological assessment, it is critical to consider the multidisciplinary needs of the patient as the foundation for recommending or planning intervention strategies.

NEURODEVELOPMENTAL INTERVENTION

This chapter advocates a neurodevelopmental approach to interventions for children with NF, particularly in *anticipating* specific neurodevelopmental interruption and intervening accordingly. This is more consistent with the prevention model of medicine, as opposed to the management-by-crisis model practiced in the past. Rather than anticipating difficulty, professionals would wait for the illness to develop and provide intervention at that time. Much of special education has operated on a form of this model, waiting until a child's level of educational achievement is 2 years or 40% below projected intellectual ability. Many children with NF, if allowed to fall 2 years behind, will never catch up. The preceding section has addressed assessing the individual needs of the patient; in this section, the focus is on application of the information obtained through a thorough neuropsychological/neurodevelopmental assessment of the child.

Another premise of this approach is the need to provide multidisciplinary support, using public, private, and family resources. It is critical for the neuropsychologist to recognize potential "resource people" and collaborate with them. The first critical level of intervention is with the parents, other family members, and the child himself or herself (if old enough), helping them to understand the child's developmental needs and how they can best support that development. The second is maximizing school support, given the amount of the child's life spent in that environment. The third is identifying private and public programs available and necessary for support.

Parent and Child Education

It is critical that parents understand the developmental and behavioral "logic" of their child and anticipate his or her needs, as well as their own role in maintaining the child's development. This allows the parents to intervene at home, as well as to advocate for the child at school. Unless parents understand the need to advocate and have the specific skills to advocate, advocacy is not likely to occur. This is not to downplay the neuropsychologist's role in educating the school directly. The one ongoing, continuous relationship in the child's life is the one with his or her parent(s), and given the mobility of much of our society, a parent has a critical role in that process.

Similarly, a school-age child must understand his or her own learning characteristics in order to implement strategies that permit maximum adaptation and compensation. This will maximize the child's developmental potential into adulthood. The long-term goals are total self-sufficiency and self-advocacy. Many patients experience a "healthy" denial in response to the uncertainty of the NF1 disease. It is essential for the clinician to understand the complexities and subtleties of the individual child's neurodevelopment, the child's understanding of the disease, and his or her fears about the disease (in order to separate uninformed fears from well-informed fears). The particular role of the neuropsychologist is to educate both parent and child about the neurodevelopmental complications and risk factors, and to intervene as necessary. The written evaluation is critical as an educational tool, as is the specific feedback to the parents. Each parent is unique not only in his or her ability to understand, but also in his or her reaction to the child's specific emotional/behavioral and medical needs.

Education and Support of School Personnel

Since children are required to be in school, the most time- and cost-efficient use of treatment and neurodevelopmental intervention within the school setting must be made. If school personnel understand the logic behind interventions, they are typically very willing to provide not only educational, but also psychosocial and other support. Traditionally, school intervention is remedial in nature (e.g., teaching a student to read). By contrast, many of the intervention needs for NF patients tend to be adaptive and compensatory in nature; that is, they involve the development of more productive, less frustrating means of learning. Rourke's 1995 book *Syndrome of Nonverbal Learning Disabilities* contains an appendix addressing specific learning characteristics and intervention strategies, which are particularly applicable to school settings. NF patients should be considered as at-risk patients, and intervention and monitoring should be initiated early to facilitate optimal school support for each individual patient. Given the high prevalence of NLD characteristics, stimulating development of mental organization and conceptual integration early is critical, in terms of both teaching the student specifically to formulate concepts and helping him or her to develop adaptive and compensatory strategies.

Not all NF1 children will require specific special education placement. Some districts will allow such a placement, or accommodations within a regular classroom setting, on the basis of "other health-impaired" or "traumatic brain injury" (liberally interpreted). For many NF children, the accommodations are often related to pace and volume of work. Untimed or more structured (e.g., oral) testing formats are often of benefit. Use of a calculator can be helpful for children with motor disabilities.

Cognitive Rehabilitation

In many respects, there is no "rehabilitation" necessary, as nothing has been lost; "habilitation" may be a better concept, given that many of NF children's skills are merely not developed. Cognitive rehabilitation strategies, particularly those developed for rehabilitation of right-hemisphere lesions, are of particular benefit. It has been suggested that many of the skills that most of us learn by just growing up and living day to day, are not learned automatically by children with neurological compromise or neurodevelopmental disorders such as NF. It thus becomes critical to teach such a child to conceptually integrate and organize information, as well as to facilitate reasoning, judgment, problem solving, and related skills. Again, it is particularly important that the child recognize and understand the specific characteristics of his or her learning. Such basic skills are the foundation to learning and developmental progression; they allow the child to process larger quantities of information much more rapidly and efficiently as he or she grows older. Failure to develop such skills disrupts ongoing development considerably, contributing to considerable levels of stress. This failure appears to be the basis of the dropping IQ scores observed over time for some patients.

There is probably a limit to how much can be developed, and thus adaptation and compensation become critical elements. Teaching productive use of a day planner is critical to organizational functions. Using outlines, "skeletons," "brain mapping," and related devices is also suggested. In addition, having the child "think aloud" or verbalize his or her thinking and reasoning both provides a direct means of understanding the child's conceptual processes and can be a way of coaching the child specifically in thinking, judgment, reasoning, and problem solving. It is critical to explain in greater detail the specifics of an interaction or event to increase the child's understanding. Through such verbalization, either by parents or aloud to themselves, patients are more likely to acquire the skills. Finally, it is critical for patients to ask for additional information when they are uncertain or do not understand.

Behavior Management Strategies

Using behavior management strategies at home and at school can provide important neurodevelopmental support to children with neurodevelopmental disorders such as NF. Various characteristics of a good behavior program will greatly facilitate the process of development for the individual child. The process of writing goals or identifying target behaviors increases both the patient's and the parent's or educator's level of awareness. Perhaps more importantly, a good, well-applied behavior management program provides additional levels of structure through setting specific goals and identifying particular target behaviors. It also allows for specific, immediate feedback, which not only greatly facilitates the child's learning, but improves his or her understanding of cause-and-effect relationships. Finally, self-esteem can be enhanced through the patient's success in achieving goals, as well as the focus on levels of reinforcement.

Social Skill Development

To varying degrees, many children with NF require help in developing basic social skills. Given the prevalence of NLD characteristics to varying degrees, a child with NF often appears to have difficulty in reading nonverbal social cues and using them to understand cause-and-effect relationships within social interactions. Many children are at risk for relative social isolation, given the disease, but often the underlying etiology is as much cognitive as behavioral. Tending to be shy, they struggle with understanding social relationships and anticipating consequences of social interaction. As such, they need to learn consciously what comes very naturally to most people. In other words, they must learn "manually."

Medication Strategies

With current neuropharmacology, the primary goals are to facilitate regulation of mood and emotion; to reduce irritability, reactivity, and emotional volatility; and to improve attention and concentration. Although such medications are not a cure, they reduce neurodevelopmental consequences and complications. For example, children who tend to be very anxious, easily stressed, and overwhelmed tend to avoid social interaction and are less likely to follow through with specific intervention and support strategies. In many cases, a trial-and-error approach is necessary to identify optimal medication strategies.

SUMMARY

NF is a relatively common, autosomal dominant genetic disorder resulting in development of benign and malignant tumors at an increased frequency within the CNS and the peripheral nervous system. Children with NF demonstrate myriad cognitive, emotional, and behavioral sequelae. Often this population of children demonstrates a pattern of NLDs that, unless understood, is often difficult to diagnose and treat. Given the potentially debilitating long-term impact of NF on children's developing lives and ultimate adult outcome, an anticipatory model of assessment and intervention is suggested, in which risk factors are identified early and children are provided with supportive and preventive, rather than reactive, treatment for their particular neurodevelopmental problems.

REFERENCES

Boardman, P., Anslow, P., & Renowden, S. (1996). Pictorial review: MR imaging of neuronal migration anomalies. *Clinical Radiology, 4*(51), 3–13.

Castillo, M., Green, C., Kwock, L., Smith, K., Wilson, D., Schiro, S., & Greenwood, R. (1995). Proton MR spectroscopy in patients with neurofibromatosis type 1: Evaluation of hamartomas and clinical correlation. *American Journal of Neuroradiology, 16,* 141–147.

Cawthon, R. M., Weiss, R., Xu, G. F., Viskochil, D., Culver, M., Stevens, J., Robertson, M., Dunn, D., Gesteland, R., O'Connell, P. et al. (1990). A major segment of the neurofibromatosis type 1 gene: cDNA sequence, genomic structure, and point mutations. *Cell, 62,* 193–201.

Crowe, F.W. (1964). Axillary freckling as a diagnostic aid in neurofibromatosis. *Annals of Internal Medicine, 61,* 1142–1143.

Denckla, M., Hoffman, K., Mazzocco, M., Melhem, E., Reiss, A., Bryan, R., Harris, E., Lee, J., Cox, C., & Schuerlolz, L. (1996). Relationship between T2-weighted hyperintensities (unidentified bright objects) and lower IQS in children with neurofibromatosis-1. *American Journal of Medical Genetics (Neuropsychiatric Genetics), 67,* 98–102.

Dilts, C., Carey, J., Kircher, J., Hoffman, R., Creel, D., Ward, K., Clark, E., & Leonard, C. (1996). Children and adolescents with neurofibromatosis 1: A behavioral phenotype. *Journal of Developmental and Behavioral Pediatrics, 17*(4), 229–241.

DiMario, F., Ramsby, G., Greenstein, R., Langshur, S., & Dunham, B. (1993). Neurofibromatosis type 1: Magnetic resonance imaging findings. *Journal of Child Neurology, 8,* 32–39.

Es, S., North, K., McHugh, K., & de Silva, M. (1996). MRI findings in children with neurofibromatosis type 1: A prospective study. *Pediatric Radiology, 26,* 478–487.

Ferner, R., Hughes, R., & Weinman, J. (1996). Intellectual impairment in neurofibromatosis 1. *Journal of the Neurological Sciences, 138,* 125–133.

Giordano, M., Mahadeo, D., He, Y., Geist, R., & Gutmann, D. (1996). Increased expression of the neurofibromatosis 1 (NF1) gene product, neurofibromin, in astrocytes in response to cerebral ischemia. *Journal of Neuroscience Research, 43,* 246–253.

Gutmann, D. H., Aylsworth, A., Carey, J. C., Korf, B., Marks, J., Pyeritz, R. E., Rubenstein, A., & Viskochil, D. (1997). Diagnostic evaluation and multidisciplinary manangement of neurofibromatosis 1 and neurofibromatosis 2. *Journal of the American Medical Association, 278*(1), 51–57.

Gutmann, D., Giordano, M., Mahadeo, K., Lau, N., Silbergeld, D., & Guha, A. (1996). Increased neurofibromatosis 1 gene expression in astrocytic tumors: Positive regulation by p21-ras. *Oncogene, 12,* 2121–2127.

Harnadek, M., & Rourke, B. (1994). Principal identifying features of the syndrome of nonverbal learning disabilities in children. *Journal of Learning Disabilities, 27*(3), 144–154.

Hofman, K. J., Harris, E. L., Bryan, N., & Denckla, M. (1994). Neurofibromatosis type 1: The cognitive phenotype. *Journal of Pediatrics, 124*(4), S1–S8.

Huson, S. M., Harper, P. S., & Compston, D. A. S. (1988). von Recklinghausen neurofibromatosis: A clinical and population study in South East Wales. *Brain, 111,* 1355–1381.

Huson, S. M., & Hughes, R. A. C. (1994). *The neurofibromatoses: A pathogenetic and clinical overview.* London: Chapman & Hall.

Itoh, T., Magnaldi, S., White, R., Denckla, M., Hofman, K., Naidu, S., & Bryan, R. (1994). Neurofibromatosis type 1: Type evolution of deep gray and white matter MR abnormalities. *American Journal of Neuroradiology, 15,* 1513–1519.

Korf, B. R. (1992). Diagnostic outcome in children with multiple café au lait spots. *Pediatrics, 90,* 924–927.

Korf, B. R. (1994). *Neurofibromatosis type one: A guide for educators.* New York: National Neurofibromatosis Foundation.

Lazaro, C., Gaona, A., Ainsworth, P., Tenconi, R., Viduad, D., Kruyer, H., Ars, E., Volpini, V., & Estivill, X. (1996). Sex differences in mutational rate and mutational mechanism in the NF1 gene in neurofibromatosis type 1 patients. *Human Genetics, 98,* 696–699.

Leguis, E., Descheemacker, M., Steyaert, J., Spaepen, A., Vlietinck, R., Casaer, P., Demaerel, P., & Fryns, J. (1995). Neurofibromatosis type 1 in childhood: Correlation of MRI findings with intelligence. *Journal of Neurology, Neurosurgery and Psychiatry, 59,* 638–640.

Listernick, R., Darling, C., Greenwald, M., Strauss, L., & Charrow, J. (1995). Optic pathway tumors in children: The effect of neurofibromatosis 1 on clinical manifestations and natural history. *Journal of Pediatrics, 127,* 718–722.

Menor, F., & Marti-Bonmati, L. (1992). CT detection of basal ganglion lesions in neurofibromatosis type 1: Correlation with MRI. *Neuroradiology, 34*(4), 305–307.

Menor, F., Marti-Bonmati, L., Mulas, F., Cortina, H., & Olague, R. (1991). Imaging considerations of central nervous system manifestations in pediatric patients with neurofibromatosis type 1. *Pediatric Radiology, 21,* 389–394.

Moore, B., Ater, J., Needle, M., Slopis, J., & Copeland, D. (1994). Neuropsychological profile of children with neurofibromatosis, brain tumor, or both. *Journal of Child Neurology, 9,* 368–377.

Moore, B., Slopis, J., Schomer, D., Jackson, E., & Levy, B. (1996). Neuropsychological significance of areas of high signal intensity on brain MRIs of children with neurofibromatosis. *Neurology, 46,* 1660–1668.

Mulvihill, J. J., Parry, D. M., Sherman, J. L., Pikus, A., Kaiser-Kupfer, M. I., & Eldridge, R. (1990). Neurofibromatosis 1 (Recklinghausen disease) and neurofibromatosis 2 (bilateral acoustic neurofibromatosis): An update. *Annals of Internal Medicine, 113,* 39–52.

National Institutes of Health (NIH) Consensus Development Conference. (1988). Neurofibromatosis: Conference statement. *Archives of Neurology, 45,* 575–578.

North, K. N., Joy, P., Yuille, D., Cocks, N., Mobbs, E., Hutchings, P., McHugh, K., & de Silva, M. (1994). Specific learning disability in children with neurofibromatosis type 1: Significance of MRI abnormalities. *Neurology, 44,* 878–883.

North, K. N., Riccardi, V., Samango-Sprouse, C., Ferner, R., Moore, B., Legius, E., Ratner, N., & Denckla, M.B. (1997). Cognitive function and academic performance in neurofibromatosis 1: Consensus statatement from the NF1 Cognitive Disorders Task Force. *Neurology, 48,* 1121–1127.

Norton, K., Mahadeo, K., Geist, R., & Gutmann, D. (1996). Expression of the neurofibromatosis 1 (NF1) gene during growth arrest. *Neuroreport, 7,* 601–604.

Obringer, A. C., Meadows, A. T., & Zackai, E. H. (1989). The diagnosis of neurofibromatosis 1 in the child under the age of 6 years. *American Journal of Diseases of Children, 143,* 717–719.

Pollack, I., Shultz, B., & Mulvihill, J. (1996). The management of brainstem gliomas in patients with neurofibromatosis 1. *Neurology, 46,* 1652–1660.

Riccardi, V. M. (1991). Neurofibromatosis: Past, present, and future. *New England Journal of Medicine, 324,* 1283–1285.

Riccardi, V. M., & Eichner, J. E. (1992). *Neurofibromatosis: Phenotype, natural history, and pathogenesis* (2nd ed.). Baltimore: Johns Hopkins University Press.

Rouleau, G. A., Merel, P., Lutchman, M., Sanson, M., Zucman, J., Marineau, C., Hoang-Xuan, K., Dernczuk, S., Desmaze C., Plougastel, B. et al. (1993). Alteration in a new gene encoding a putative membrane-organizing protein causes neurofibromatosis type 2. *Nature, 363*, 515–521.

Rourke, B. P. (1989). *Nonverbal learning disabilities: The syndrome and the model.* New York: Guilford Press.

Rourke, B. P. (Ed.). (1995). *Syndrome of nonverbal learning disabilities: Neurodevelopmental manifestations.* New York: Guilford Press.

Satz, P., Strauss, E., Hunter, M., & Wada, J. (1994). Re-examination of the crowding hypothesis: Effects of age of onset. *Neuropsychology, 8*(2), 255–262.

Terada, H., Barkovich, A., Edwards, M., & Circillo, S. (1996). Evolution of high-intensity basal ganglia lesions on T1-weighted MR in neurofibromatosis type 1. *American Journal of Neuroradiology, 17*, 755–760.

Trofatter, J. A., MacCollin, M. M., Rutter, J. L., Murrell, J. R., Duyao, M. P., Parry, D. M., Eldridge, R., Kley, N., Menon, A. G., Pulaski, K. et al. (1993). A novel moesin-, ezrin-, radixin-like gene is a candidate for the neurofibromatosis 2 tumor suppressor. *Cell, 72*, 1–20.

Viskochil, D., Buchberg, A. M., Xu, G., Cawthon, R. M., Stevens, J., Wolff, R. K., Culver, M., Carey, J. C., Copeland, N. G., Jenkins, N. A. et al. (1990) Deletions and a translocation interrupt a cloned gene at the neurofibromatosis type 1 locus. *Cell, 62*, 187–192.

Wallace, M. R., Marchuk, D. A., Andersen, L. B., Letcher, R., Odeh, H. M., Saulino, A. M., Fountain, J. W., Brereton, A., Nicholson, J., Mitchell, A. L. et al. (1990). Type 1 neurofibromatosis gene: Identification of a large transcript disrupted in three NF1 patients. *Science, 249*, 181–186.

Wu, B., Austin, M., Schneider, G., Boles, R., & Korf, B. (1995). Deletion of the entire NF1 gene detected by the FISH: Four deletion patients associated with severe manifestations. *American Journal of Medical Genetics, 59*, 528–535.

16

SICKLE CELL DISEASE

JULIEN T. SMITH

The term "sickle cell disease" (SCD) refers to a broad category of chronic hematological disorders. It is an autosomal recessive genetic pathology of the hemoglobin (the oxygen-binding molecules of the blood), which affects approximately 50,000 people of African and Mediterranean descent in North America alone (Wasserman, Williams, Fairclough, Mulhern, & Wang, 1991). One infant in every 600 live births will have the disease (Des-Forges, Milner, Wethers, & Whitten, 1978). "Sickle cell anemia" (SCA) refers to the pathological variant of hemoglobin (HbS) present in the red blood cells. The HbS contains two normal and two abnormal amino acid chains.

The inherited homozygous condition, HbSS, leads to SCD. The inheritance of a single allele leads to the heterozygous condition, HbAS, and the individual will be a carrier of the sickle cell trait but will not exhibit the full disease state. The symptoms of SCD are not evident at birth; they usually begin to present during the first year. By the preschool years, delayed growth and development are apparent, and many children experience delayed puberty (Pearson, 1987).

PHYSIOPATHOLOGY

Oxygen bonds to a healthy erythrocyte (red blood cell) in order to be carried to peripheral tissues. As blood vessels decrease in diameter, the erythrocytes can bend, flex, and contort through the tight spaces while retaining the oxygen, releasing and delivering it appropriately to critical areas and returning to the lungs for reoxygenation. HbS allows crystal formation on the erythrocytes after releasing oxygen, leaving them less stable, unable to bond oxygen properly, unmalleable, and with a shorter lifespan. During the deoxygenation process in the vasculature, the presence of abundant HbS molecules causes the collapse and "sickling" of the red blood cell. Because sickled cells are rigid, they are unable to pass through the vasculature properly, and interfere with the blood flow or may become lodged in the vessel. Accumulations of sickled cells lead to slowed movement of blood, referred to as "sludging," as the healthy, oxygenated blood cells cannot pass around the rigid cells that collect in increasing numbers. The collection of many of these trapped sickled cells can cause vaso-occlusion, not only blocking blood flow, but preventing the oxygenation of cells in the immediate and ensuing surrounding tissue. Low oxygenation creates low tissue oxygen; this increases acidosis and ischemic necrosis, which can then lead to further sickling of unstable erythrocytes.

For years, infarct was thought to be the main mechanism of neurologic impairment in SCD; with improved radiological studies, however, the process of injury is better understood. Using magnetic resonance imaging (MRI), computerized tomography (CT), and angiograms, researchers have found that bleeding can occur in minute veins and arterioles, where occlusion and low oxygenation cause seepage (hypoperfusion) from the vessel into surrounding tissue (Adams, et al., 1992; Adams, et al., 1988; Armstrong et al., 1996; Ris et al., 1996; National Institutes of Health, 1986; Pavlakis et al., 1988; Wiznitzer et al., 1990). Arterial border zones ("watershed regions") are most susceptible to cerebral hypoperfusion. Smaller vessels naturally have less flow and increased pressure, and are further at risk in SCD due to involvement of the larger vessels. Reduced pressure from large-vessel disease causes slower flow rates of blood between vessels in watershed regions. Reduced flow pressure and reduced erythrocyte oxygen content then lead to hypoperfusion. The chronic anemia and hemodynamic insufficiency of SCD lead to vulnerability and "inadequate perfusion in border zone regions present[ing] a mechanism for cerebral infarction" (Pavlakis et al., 1988, p.128). The large vessels most commonly affected by SCD tend to be the distal internal carotid artery, the proximal middle cerebral artery, and the proximal anterior cerebral artery. The most common sites of cerebrovascular accident (CVA) or stroke are the internal carotid artery, the anterior an middle cerebral arteries, and their boundary zones (Craft, Schatz, Glauser, Lee, & DeBaun, 1993). Infarct is usually first suspected from symptoms of hemiplegia, visual disturbance, loss of consciousness, seizure, or focal neurological abnormalities (Mercuri et al., 1995). "Silent" strokes may also occur without obvious clinical symptoms. Children are more likely to evidence pure motor involvement following central nervous system (CNS) stroke, due to better collateral blood flow (Pavlakis et al., 1988). Neurological sequelae can affect intellectual, academic, and social functioning (Wasserman et al., 1991; see below).

Many other specific crises can occur in SCD, including splenic sequestration, sepsis, aplastic crises, and hyperhemolytic crises. Vaso-occlusive crises and splenic sequestration commonly result in negative cognitive outcome (Swift et al., 1989). Vaso-occlusive crises can occur anywhere in the low-oxygen-tension areas of the body, but are most common in the bones, joints, and CNS. Repeated or severe occlusion often leads to secondary organ damage, infarction or stroke, and subsequent neurological compromise. Sequestration is most common in children aged 8 months to 5 years and occurs acutely when large amounts of blood are trapped in the abdominal organs. Shock is an immediate threat, and death can occur within hours (Pearson, 1987). Thrombus formation is most likely in the spleen, retina, placenta, kidneys, and CNS. Sepsis and stroke from thrombus formation are the leading causes of death in SCD (Partington, Aronyk, & Byrd, 1994). Severe bacterial infections result from splenic dysfunction and developmental humoral immunity (Pearson, 1987). Finally, the lifespan of an erythrocyte is only 10–20 days in a patient with SCD, whereas it is 120 days in a healthy person; the bone marrow compensates for this by increasing the erythrocyte production rate. Aplastic crises occur when the compensatory erythrocyte production rate falls off, reducing the ratio of healthy to sickled erythrocytes and leading to increased respiration, heart rate, and fatigue.

MEDICAL RISK FACTORS IN SICKLE CELL TRAIT

It is estimated that 8% of African Americans are carriers of the sickle cell trait (HbAS) (DesForges et al., 1978). Sickle cell trait is considered to be a relatively innocuous condition, except under rare low-oxygen situations (e.g., hypoxia, sepsis, general anesthesia, dehydration, and postoperative periods) (Kramer, Rooks, & Pearson, 1978; McCormack et al., 1975; Partington, et al., 1994). The hemoglobin is abnormal, but does not lead to as frequent sickling or short a lifespan in erythrocytes as in SCD. Under low-oxygen conditions sickling can occur, leading to medical complications that include organ and CNS infarction/stroke, hematuria, renal papillary necrosis/failure, retroperitoneal fibrosis, renal arterial occlusion, and increased risk for low-birth-weight offspring. Increasing reports of neurological compromise and postmortem CNS findings are found in the literature, suggesting that even trait carriers can exhibit neurological compromise. Precautionary measures such as avoidance of very-low-oxygen situations (e.g., air travel, diving) and genetic counseling are warranted, but other interventions are seldom necessary.

Sickle cell trait is not benign in regard to physical growth and development, and carriers may be susceptible to pathophysiological symptoms of SCD (McCormack et al., 1975). Clearly there are cognitive risks related to neurological events in SCD, but the risks to trait carriers are not definitively known. Risk factors for developmental compromise in pediatric trait carriers have been documented, such as hypoxic episodes, developmental impairment, stroke, and ischemic cerebral infarction (Greenberg & Massey, 1985; Katz, Lubin, & Armstrong, 1974; Kramer et al., 1978; McCormack et al., 1975; Partington et al., 1994; Riggs, Ketonen, Wang, & Valanne, 1995). No neuropsychological data have been collected from these case reports to help clarify developmental issues resulting from neurological injury. The risk of stroke complications in trait carriers has not been clearly determined, but may be similar to risk factors in SCD patients.

Outside of high-risk conditions, might a trait carrier also be at risk for other pathological effects of the disease? McCormack et al. (1975) found no significant difference in intellectual functioning between adolescent trait carriers and normal peers, but did find the trait carriers to have reduced physical growth and development. Because the groups were not matched, it is difficult to determine the true cause of the findings. Kramer et al. (1978) matched subjects at birth for gender, postnatal medical factors, and socioeconomic status. Results indicated no significant differences between trait carriers and normal hemoglobin matches, suggesting that trait carriers were not at increased risk for cognitive deficits. Wasserman et al. (1991) matched trait carriers with sibling controls (HbAS or HbAA) on intellectual, academic, and neuropsychological status. Siblings with sickle cell trait performed no differently from normal-hemoglobin siblings, supporting the findings of previous researchers, and suggesting that neuropsychological impairment is more likely with pathological effects of the trait than with the trait alone.

DEVELOPMENTAL CONSIDERATIONS

Effects of Strokes and Other Symptoms on Brain Development

The earliest presentation of the symptoms of SCD, including anemia and vaso-occlusive crises, occurs between 6 and 24 months of age (Cohen, Branch, McKie, & Adams, 1994; Listianingsih, Harriman, Griffith, Hurtig, & Keehn, 1991; Swift et al., 1989; Wasserman et al., 1991). Children with SCD have an increased risk of major cerebral events such as CVAs, which occur with more frequency than in adults (Fowler, Whitt, Lallinger, Nash, Atkinson, Wells, & McMillan, 1988; Swift et al., 1989).

Strokes occur in 6–10% of all patients with SCD, 80% of whom are under 15, with the average age at onset being 6 years (Cohen et al., 1994; Listianingsih et al., 1991; Wasserman et al., 1991). Sixty-seven percent of children who have one stroke have another stroke, 80% of which occur within 36 months. Seventy-five percent of the children who experience CVA have cerebral infarction, while 20% have intracerebral hemorrhage. For uncertain reasons, children are more likely to experience infarct, whereas adults are more likely to experience hemorrhage (Pavlakis, Prohovnik, Piomelli, & Devivo, 1989). Some investigators hypothesize that changes in cerebral blood flow, which is age-dependent, may relate to this difference. The majority of spontaneous brain function recovery occurs within 3 to 6 months of the stroke (Listianingsih et al., 1991), but the long-term complications are quite variable. For this reason, physical and cognitive rehabilitation are crucial in the immediate period following stroke, especially for children who are on a critical developmental curve.

The first 2 years of life are a critical period of brain development, during which glial proliferation, myelinization, dendritic branching, and development of synaptic connections are abundant, and vulnerability to neurological compromise is profound. Neurological insult during this period may have long-term cognitive and behavioral consequences, because optimal brain activity is interrupted during an imperative growth period. This debilitation is often overlooked by medical and educational professionals, as compensatory strategies develop with physical recovery and time, and these can obscure underlying deficits temporarily or in specific situations. Neurological injury is often viewed as an acute illness that ends at about the time of discharge from the hospital, and long-term sequelae are not linked to the original injury. Early injury, however can lead to a globally compromised CNS that has been forced to reconstruct the interactive neuronal network. Theories of neurological maturation suggest that the developing brain is "plastic," or malleable to alterations in functional area. Plasticity implies that the functions of a damaged area of the brain can be "reassigned" to another, undamaged area. Although this is immediately effective in enabling an individual to regain a certain level of skill, it can lead to longer-term problems when the area of the brain that has taken over a specific ability is called upon to perform its original function. According to Teuber's "crowding principle" (Woods & Teuber, 1973), recovery by reassignment occurs at the expense of other abilities. When functions are shifted in an attempt to compensate, areas become congested and less efficient. Early injury therefore jeopardizes long-term developmental progress, although this may not be immediately evident.

Further clarification of the impact of SCD on brain development is provided by research in early nutritional issues. Multiple or severe hypoglycemic episodes, or severe malnutrition in early development, can compromise brain growth (Swift et al., 1989). Iron deficiency anemia in the critical CNS growth period can clearly compromise long-term cognitive development; the effects include reduced attention, fatigue, behavioral problems, and poor academic achievement. Iron deficiency anemia can also lead to neurological "soft signs," such as poor coordination and balance. Presumably, neurodevelopmental compromise is highly likely.

Painful Crises and Psychological Development

The effects of recurrent pain on psychological development are not well understood, but they can be assumed to have an impact. A child undergoing repeated painful experiences, many of which result in extended hospitalizations, is likely to have his or her development affected. The effects of pain at different levels of psychosexual, psychosocial, and moral development vary, as children's perceptions of themselves change with cognitive and emotional development. The bonding process may be disrupted in infancy as a result of recurrent hospitalizations and feelings of fear and helplessness in the parents. The egocentric toddler may feel that his or her pain is a consequence for perceived misbehavior. The school-age child may exaggerate reports of pain to avoid school, where he or she is teased or ridiculed. The adolescent may become depressed, withdrawn, rebellious, or angry as a result of years of being either coddled or ignored. Teenagers who are struggling with identity have an added burden in developing a sense of self, as they must become increasingly independent in self-care and self-esteem in the face of a chronic illness that isolates and differentiates them from their peers. As the next section disccuses in more detail, such periods of poor coping are likely to have a negative impact or academic as well as social and interpersonal development if they are not properly perceived and addressed.

It is important to discuss with SCD patients the relationship between stress and illness. Many patients resist such discussions, as they feel accused of exaggerating or feigning painful crises. As with any chronic illness (e.g, asthma, diabetes, cystic fibrosis), stress plays an important role in the expression and intensity of the symptoms. Although some patients may malinger, the vast majority of patients frequently exaggerating pain are probably individuals with poor coping skills whose bodies are reactive to emotional and psychological tension. It may be beneficial to help children with frequent pain crises and their parents explore environmental patterns, predisposing factors, and possible coping skills for reducing the invasive nature of pain crises. A healthy psychological state in a patient with SCD may be a combination of knowledge, acceptance, self-esteem, motivation, and hope that develops throughout the lifespan.

PSYCHOSOCIAL COMPROMISE AND ITS EFFECTS ON COGNITIVE COMPROMISE

It is not clearly known whether the cognitive impairment in SCD is due to an encephalopathy inherent in the disease or solely to the physiological deficits caused by complications. Except in very extreme cases, cognitive impairment is not associated with age of onset, frequency of crises, or number and length of hospitalizations, suggesting that something about SCD other than crises and anemia alone is related to the cognitive impairment (Swift et al., 1989).

The psychosocial factors that accompany SCD—including the stress of living with a chronic illness, recurrent painful crises, ongoing uncertainty, school absence, and financial and other burdens on the family—appear to increase the possibility of academic and developmental risk factors, and most certainly contribute to the extensive impact of SCD. Living with a potentially painful illness that can strike unpredictably can overwhelm any family, and can specifically interfere with interpersonal relationships between parents and siblings (Burlew, Evans, & Oler, 1989). Although preventative measures are helpful (e.g., avoiding extreme temperatures, dehydration, and overexertion), they cannot consistently avert a crisis. Families whose members are more educated about the illness and have greater social support networks tend to cope better (Burlew et al., 1989) as a result of better daily management and less emotional turmoil. In addition, the financial strain of a chronic illness places a family at increased risk for stress. Finances are strapped by frequent medical appointments, hospitalizations, and/or the profound financial burden of a medical crisis or long-term care. Although theories are abundant, it is unclear why a disproportionate number of families are living with SCD in depressed socioeconomic situations. The environmental impact of poverty in relation to the overall stressors of this particular illness needs to be more clearly elucidated.

As suggested above, adolescents appear to have an increased risk of poor coping with SCD, compared to children and adults (Hurtig & Park, 1987; Hurtig & White, 1986). This vulnerability to poor coping is related to the common course of adolescence in all North

America, but is also linked to the additional burdens created by the unique manifestations of the illness (e.g., delayed development, school absences, social/activity restrictions, etc.). For adolescents, delayed growth, sexual development, and physical development have a profound impact on their identity and social adjustment. When a teenager is struggling with issues of identity, independence, self-image, and role in the cohort, these differences of appearance can be quite devastating. Adolescent boys tend to have more behavioral problems (somaticizing, immaturity, and hyperactivity), while adolescent girls tend to have less coping competency in families with increased levels of conflict (Hurtig & White, 1986).

There is an increased existence of reported behavioral problems in children with SCD. Physiological interpretations suggest that "silent" strokes and abnormal blood glucose metabolism in the frontal lobes create an increased risk of deficits in executive functioning, which in turn affect social interaction and self-management. Psychosocial explanations focus on the developmental impact of chronic illness and the physical differences that isolate these children. Again, a disproportionate number of children with SCD also live in depressed socioeconomic situations, suggesting that poverty and destitute environments may relate to behavioral challenges.

SCD places children at greater risk for academic difficulty, although why this occurs has not been well defined. Children with SCD tend to experience repeated school absences because of medical appointments and painful crises. Their illness creates the need for attentive care within school, such as adapted physical education, appropriate hydration, and adult awareness of emergent care. The academic issues are probably not solely related to the CNS impairments, as not all SCD patients have CNS disease. The progressive functional impairments in children with SCD are also affected by genetic variables, physical factors (small stature, fatigue, crises, etc.), and neuropsychological variables, which function either together or independently. In addition, the psychosocial factors associated with SCD (low socioeconomic status, effects of a chronic illness, frequent hospitalizations, family stress, etc.) contribute to overall cognitive performance (Chapar, 1988). Cognitive deficits are best understood through identifying the broad presentation of organic mechanisms and psychosocial factors.

Given these discussions and studies about poor coping in patients with SCD, one might conclude that the vast majority have moderate to severe psychosocial impairment as a result of the disease. In actuality, most patients with SCD fare well in coping with the illness. Unfortunately, research bias tends to lead to writing primarily about the problem cases rather than the successes. According to Williams, Earles, and Pack (1983), only 35% of patients have repeated hospitalizations, with only 5% having more than three hospitalizations within a single year. The majority of research on patients with SCD and coping has probably been performed on a very small percentage of the total population presenting to hospitals for treatment, and should not be overinterpreted as representative of the majority of patients with SCD or their families.

ASSESSING NEUROLOGICAL AND NEUROPSYCHOLOGICAL COMPROMISE

Determining the Nature of CNS Damage

The process of CNS injury in SCD has only recently begun to be physiologically understood. It was originally hypothesized that CNS damage came solely from ischemic and aneurysmal injury in the smaller vessels, which would be evident on most imaging studies. Therefore, if there were no indications of stroke on MRI or CT scan, no damage would be diagnosed. With the understanding of the effects of sickling in arterial border zones and hypoperfusion, it became more apparent that SCD places children at far greater risk of subtle CNS compromise, which may not appear in imaging studies. Large-vessel disease and multiple infarcts clearly increase the risk of global neurological and developmental compromise. Secondary cognitive compromise can also result from other specific crises, including splenic sequestration, aplastic crises, hyperhemolytic crises, thrombus formation, and severe bacterial infections.

Any blood vessel in the body is susceptible to the effects of vaso-occlusion. Many SCD-related strokes are so small that they are not easily recognized. Ongoing, subtle neurological deficits caused by minute vaso-occlusions (called "silent" strokes), ischemia, and hypoxia are not characteristically apparent on a standard neurological exam (Fowler et al., 1988; Mercuri et al., 1995; Swift et al., 1989). Neurological "soft signs" are minor motor impairments indicative of subtle neurological damage that are not always part of a standard neurological exam, but that may indicate the presence of a silent stroke. Subtle cerebral impairment may be evident only as sensory deficits, soft signs, or higher-order cognitive deficits. Neuroimaging studies can have false-negative occurrences and may not identify silent strokes. Others are apparently "abnormal" but inconclusive and do not necessarily isolate the cause of the abnormal findings.

Silent strokes may lead to developmental compromise in long-term intellectual, academic, and social functioning (Fowler et al., 1988). Although the subtle deficits caused by these strokes may not be apparent on routine neurological exam or more sophisticated tests such as MRI, they are likely to appear on specific neuropsychological assessment, which can isolate the functional deficit. Identifying the compromised function through neuropsychological evaluation, which is not usually a part of a neurological evaluation in SCD, may be more cost-efficient and increase the probability of locating the specific area of neurological damage (Fowler et al., 1988). Subtle neurological compromise is not easily detectable by routine standardized testing, but requires the specialized and focused assessment of a neuropsychologist. Even so, neuropsychological evaluations can only estimate location of impact by function, which is certainly less accurate than imaging techniques. Given this limitation, the purpose of neuropsychological assessment should be not only to estimate area of lesion, but, more importantly, to determine the pattern of functional impairment and suggest specific interventions for each deficit identified through detailed therapeutic and academic recommendations.

There is an ongoing debate in available literature about whether or not SCD in and of itself places children at increased risk of academic and intellectual compromise. Clearly, children who have experienced obvious physiological complications are at increased risk; however, children who are experiencing silent strokes are also likely to be at risk for complications affecting neurocognitive functioning.

Physical Findings and Their Relation to Neuropsychological Findings

When the functional outcomes of patients by lesion site are compared, a clearer picture of specificity of injury can be observed. No current physiological study is without a margin of error, and many false-negative studies are completed, as noted earlier. There have been a variety of efforts to find the single most accurate method of locating injury. Although all are valid, none is perfect.

Pavlakis et al. (1988) found most MRI abnormalities in the arterial border zones (watershed regions), which are most susceptible to cerebral hypoperfusion. This occurs because of reduced pressure between vessel flow areas, which leads to seepage between these areas.

Large-vessel disease (lesions of the intima in major arteries), reduced flow pressure, and reduced red blood cell oxygen content lead to hypoperfusion in these more vulnerable areas. The patient's increased risk of cerebral infarction is the result of unstable hemodynamics and inadequate perfusion in border zone regions.

Transcranial Doppler ultrasonography (TDU) is a noninvasive measure of blood flow velocity that can detect high levels associated with severe stenosis. Adams et al. (1992) used TDU to potentially identify asymptomatic SCD children at increased risk for stroke, with encouraging results. Although they acknowledged that further research in the study design and use of TDU is necessary, their early data suggested that it may identify patients at increased risk, providing the opportunity to enlist preventative treatments such as transfusion therapy.

Intra-arterial angiography can identify and localize arterial lesions, but is invasive, requires contrast medium (which can increase sickling), and can damage the vasculature. The noninvasive magnetic resonance angiography (MRA) can isolate the vasculature from surrounding tissue, providing a view of stenosis, occlusion, or vascular malformation that may suggest increased risk for stroke, or identifying a minute area of injury. Wiznitzer et al. (1990) utilized MRA to detect abnormalities in the internal carotid artery and circle of Willis that placed children with SCD at increased risk for stroke. Results suggested that MRA may be advantageous because it is noninvasive, brief, and lacking in contrast, and can also be connected to MRI studies. However, false-positive results can occur when rapidly alternating vessel direction creates flow turbulence that is misidentified as narrowing or occlusion (Wiznitzer et al., 1990).

Neuroimagery studies cannot always definitively isolate vascular involvement, and the false negative rates can be 20–30%, even with documented clinical symptoms. Other studies are clearly required to minimize false-negative rates. Positron emission tomography (PET) scans were found to detect changes in blood glucose metabolism that resulted from the clotting of abnormal cells (National Institutes of Health, 1986). Researchers found significantly higher levels of abnormal glucose metabolism in the frontal lobes of sickle cell patients, consistent with the intellectual and behavioral changes so frequently reported. Studies are needed to link metabolic testing to neuropsychological measures so that children at risk for CNS dysfunction can perhaps be identified prior to showing overt neurological signs; longitudinal studies are also needed to monitor subtle CNS dysfunction over time (Fowler et al., 1988). The correlation between neuropsychological findings and PET scan hypothesized by Rodgers, et al. (1988) may suggest a return to utilizing neuropsychological measures diagnostically to determine brain abnormalities, in order to save expense and broaden application (Wasserman et al., 1991).

Efforts to pinpoint factors that place children at increased risk for stroke have resulted in mixed findings. Some researchers have suggested increased CNS infection, cardiomegaly, lower hemoglobin, higher reticulocyte levels, abnormal liver function, and sepsis to be linked to higher stroke rates, although no study was definitive (Pavlakis et al., 1989). Children with SCD who have a sibling with cerebrovascular involvement have been found to be three times more likely to have a stroke themselves (Pavlakis et al., 1989).

Although multiple studies such as these suggest that early detection of risk factors may provide the opportunity to offer preventative therapy, known treatment mechanisms come with their own sets of risk factors. Chronic transfusion therapy places patients at increased risk of such complications as infection, anaphylaxis, alloimmunization, high blood iron levels, and undetected blood-borne diseases. Discontinuation of chronic transfusion also presents increased risk of CVA. Bone marrow transplant has been proposed as a possible treatment, but comes with excessively high risk factors, such as immunocompromise, graft-versus-host disease, and long-term neuropsychological compromise due to radiation of the brain and high dose chemotherapy.

Few studies to date have combined neuropsychological and neuroimaging evaluations. Comparing MRI findings and neuropsychological assessment, Armstrong et al. (1996) found that SCD children with a history of stroke had significantly lower neuropsychological scores than children with silent strokes or children without MRI abnormality. Children with silent strokes also had significantly lower scores than children without MRI abnormality. Craft et al. (1993) looked at neuropsychological functioning according to site of lesion on MRI. In all spatial measures, children with diffuse lesions had significantly lower scores than sibling controls. Those with anterior lesions had significantly more intrusions (inappropriate addition of visual information) than a sibling group. On spatial measures, children with silent, diffuse strokes had significant impairment compared to those with anterior lesions and siblings.

There is a need to use a broad battery of neuropsychological measures to detect patterns of deficits according to area of lesion. Both clinically obvious and silent strokes can produce lesion-specific neuropsychological deficits. Cognitive abnormalities may not be evident with standard psychometric testing, particularly in children with anterior lesions, even though subtle neuropsychological deficits may be present. Anterior deficits may be so selective that they do not show up on global function tests as these are currently constructed and standardized. "For some patients neuropsychological testing may be more sensitive in detecting the presence of stroke than neurologic history, neurologic examination, or both" (Craft et al., 1993, p. 716).

SPECIFIC NEUROPSYCHOLOGICAL IMPAIRMENTS

Attention and Concentration

Multiple studies have documented the commonly reported problems in attention and concentration skills in pediatric SCD patients. Fowler et al. (1988) found that children with SCD had more impaired attention/distractibility than their sibling control group, and significantly more impairment than the mean for their ages. Craft et al. (1993) found that on tests of visual perception, children with SCD performed faster but made significantly more errors than their matched siblings, suggesting increased impulsivity and reduced self-regulation. Those with anterior lesions had significantly more intrusive errors than the sibling group. The authors questioned whether this finding was related to findings of increased anterior and diffuse infarcts found in the SCD group, which may have led to symptoms resembling those of attention-deficit/hyperactivity disorder (ADHD). Patients with increased frontal lobe involvement may be more likely to evidence attentional impairments. However, even studies that have not examined physiological findings have found more attentional and behavioral problems in SCD children (Burlew et al., 1989; Hurtig & Park, 1987; Hurtig & White, 1986). Obviously, some physiological aspect of the disease or its psychosocial impact has negative consequences in the areas of attention and concentration. Multiple dimensions of the illness, including the socioeconomic, psychosocial, and neuropsychological areas, are likely to contribute to impaired attentional function.

The process of human attention involves multiple interconnected abilities. The sensory system is the initial contact with the tangible world. Attention begins with the arousal of the neurological system. With adequate arousal follows the ability to scan the environment with the senses and to use the sensory register to screen relevant from irrelevant environmental input. Following a generalized screening is the next step of increasing focus on the part of the environment that is deemed crucial and decreasing focus on the part that is not. Focused attention to the crucial element is increased and maintained for a relevant period of time. During this time, mental flexibility, sequential skills, shifting, and continued environmental monitoring are required to manage ongoing environmental input and maintain the focus on the selected stimulus. Next, focused attention must be closed off and return to the scanning stage for transition to a new stimulus. This process of scanning, screening, focusing, maintaining, and concluding attention can be disrupted at any stage, although any such disruption will always be labeled merely "poor attention." Many SCD children are inappropriately diagnosed with ADHD because the diagnosing professional does not clearly understand the complicated labyrinth of attentional skills and its relationships to neurological dysfunction. Because of the diffuse nature of stroke in SCD children, any one level or multiple levels of attentional skill can be compromised. Neuropsychologists must take the time and effort to evaluate and dissect skill levels and to identify specific deficits, as the interventions for children and the education of adults working with them will vary according to the particular weaknesses found.

Intellectual and Academic Development

Early studies compared the intellectual status of SCD patients and healthy peers, finding discrepancies that were clearly confounded by racial, economic, and cohort issues. For this reason, research began to turn toward comparing SCD patients with healthy siblings to control for these threats to internal validity. Even with such controls, subsequent studies have found lower overall scores in intellectual development in SCD children who have experienced stroke (Fowler et al., 1988; Kramer et al., 1978; Listianingsih et al., 1991; McCormack et al., 1975).

Early concerns that the pathological hemoglobin of sickle cell might be related in and of itself to lower intellectual status have not been supported through research findings, although the specific nature of deficits in children who have not experienced a documented stroke has yet to be determined. Wasserman et al. (1991) matched SCD patients with sibling controls on intellectual, academic, and neuropsychological measures. As noted earlier, siblings with sickle cell trait (HbAS) performed no differently from normal-hemoglobin subjects (HbAA); this supported the findings of previous researchers (Kramer et al., 1978; McCormack et al., 1975), who had hypothesized that the abnormal hemoglobin found in SCD and sickle cell trait is not the primary factor in lower intellectual and academic performance.

Clearly, children with SCD and some trait carriers are at increased risk for learning problems, given their significantly lower academic abilities, a larger discrepancy between IQ and academic achievement, higher rates of retention in grade, and greater use of special services than matched siblings (Fowler et al., 1988). Something related to the presence of SCD or sickle cell trait is associated with increased risk for intellectual and academic difficulty. Remember that, as previously discussed, the pathological effects of the abnormal hemoglobin are not always readily observable via neurological exam or imaging techniques, and patients with SCD as well as trait carriers are at risk for hypoxia, stroke, and ischemic injury. "Silent injury" in this population may be occurring to elevate the probability of subtly compromised intellectual and academic development. Not only lower IQ, but reduced language functions and a trend toward lower total adjustment, have been found (Listianingsih et al., 1991). As noted earlier, it is likely that subtle physiological consequences of the illness, in conjunction with the psychosocial impact (living with a chronic illness, painful crises, school absence, financial burdens, etc.), are at the foundation of compromised development.

Armstrong et al. (1996) found that SCD children with a history of stroke had significantly lower neuropsychological scores than children with silent strokes or children without MRI abnormality. Children with silent strokes had significantly lower scores than children without MRI abnormality in arithmetic, vocabulary, visual–motor speed, and coordination. Even with documented physical impairment and subtle neuropsychological deficits, the effects of focal silent strokes may not appear on generalized cognitive or academic assessments. Comprehensive neuropsychological measures are essential in detecting patterns of subtle deficit according to area of lesion.

Sensory, Motor, Visual–Spatial, and Visual Perceptual Skills

An increased presence of fine motor, tactile, visual perceptual, and visual–motor integration impairments has been found in children with SCD. Although some areas of lesion are clear, many children may have subtle deficits that negatively affect their abilities to attend to, organize, and sequence visual information, and to understand relationships, directionality, dimensionality, and orientation.

Cohen et al. (1994) compared patients with documented hemispheric lesions and found increased constructional dyspraxia and significantly weaker perceptual organization in the SCD group than in sibling controls or in an age-referenced normative group. Patients with a history of right cerebral infarct clearly had nonverbal deficits affecting visual–motor integration, visual–spatial construction, and arithmetic skills. Interestingly, some of these deficits were also common in children with a history of left cerebral infarct (LCI): LCI subjects had impairments in visual–spatial construction. (These subjects, however, had a broader pattern of impairments in other areas; see below.)

Spatial organization and processing deficits have been found to be more likely in SCD children with a history of diffuse injury. Craft et al. (1993) found that children with silent diffuse stroke showed significantly more impairment on spatial measures than did either children with anterior lesions or healthy siblings. As noted earlier, the subjects with anterior lesions had more impairment on attentional tasks, which subsequently reduced visual discrimination, scanning, sequencing, and organization. This pattern can also be found in other types of diffuse neurological injury, such as hypoxia, traumatic brain injury, or infectious processes. Such deficits increase proportionally with the size of the neurological injury, regardless of the specific location.

Language Skills

As is well known, language impairments are related to left-hemisphere compromise. Cohen et al. (1994) found that their LCI patients had a global impairment in verbal abilities (expressive language, verbal and auditory memory, oral reading) consistent with aphasia. Although this and other studies have found impaired language function in children with SCD, not all are specifically related to left cerebral injury. There are clearly reductions in Full Scale IQ, reading, spelling, and written language, which suggest an underlying language weakness. Cohen et al. (1994) found significantly lower verbal function in the SCD group than in either their sibling control group or the age-referenced normative group. Listianingsih et al. (1991) found reduced language functions in children with SCD who did not have a documented history of stroke, suggesting the possibility of either inherent neuropathology or the occurrence of silent stroke. Wasserman et al. (1991) also found language difficulties on the Luria–Nebraska, but did not find supportive evidence of language compromise on the Wechsler Intelligence Scale for Children, third edition (WISC-III). Interestingly a recent parental survey of a population of SCD infants and preschoolers indicated more concern regarding physical development than language development (Gentry, Hall, & Dancer, 1997). However, the awareness of language developmental milestones at younger ages may not be generally understood by nonprofessionals, and, therefore, is under reported. More subtle language-based impairments may not be apparent until later years, when academic and social demands increase.

Organization, Sequencing, Learning, and Memory

The evidence of weaker attention in children with diffuse and anterior stroke suggests that the process of acknowledging, acquiring, organizing, retaining, and recalling information is likely to be compromised. The process of learning and accessing knowledge requires a sequence of attending, organizing, planning, and storing information in an efficient and accessibe style. If a child cannot attend efficiently, then impairments in learning and memory are likely to result, but these may or may not reflect a specific memory deficit. In addition, weak organization and sequencing can subsequently interfere with efficient learning and memory. Memory impairments are often diagnosed when the actual underlying deficit occurs in a related neuropsychological function. True memory deficits should be isolated from impairments that lead to reduced memory, as the interventions are likely to be different.

Cohen et al. (1994) found significantly reduced attention and memory (including visual–spatial memory) in the SCD group compared with their sibling control group and the age-referenced normative group. Short-term visual memory was more impaired in SCD adolescents than in their matched peers (Chapar, Doctors, Radel, & Coupey, 1986). It is likely that with the previously discussed impairments in attention, visual organization, self-monitoring, perceptual skills, and language skills, learning and memory will be affected.

Executive Functions

Higher levels of deficits in executive functions are consistently found in poststroke SCD patients (Cohen et al., 1994). "Executive functions" are those operations that direct and control thought and behavior, including obvious social pragmatics and behavior, as well as subtle cognitive processes. Young children are not expected to have adequate self-regulation, as their managerial monitors are under development. Inappropriate executive skills are often viewed as immaturity, ADHD, or delayed social development, and children with such problems are expected to "catch up" with time. Children who have experienced early CNS injury often recover acutely and appear to perform adequately or have only subtle deficits in preschool and primary grades. Families and medical personnel often label these "miracle children" and unintentionally downplay subtle impairments in comparison to the original trauma. Some children are seen as awkward or different, but not "impaired," and consequently do not receive interventions during a critical period of development. It is not until later grades, when the executive functions are socially demanded, that the impairments become more obvious and less tolerable to peers, parents, and teachers. Increasing social, behavioral, and academic problems, unregulated by an impaired executive system, pose greater threats to ongoing development. Many parents or professionals do not believe that these problems could have anything to do with the original injury—a belief that is reinforced by the "dramatic" recovery seen acutely. Often referred to as "developmental regression," the failure to progress at the same rate as peers is in fact what creates the increasing difficulty. Standardized test scores may decrease over time, but these do not necessarily indicate a loss of abilities or neurological regression. Often a failure to sustain developmental gains will appear as losses because the child is continually compared to normally developing peers in normative samples on standardized tests. Such late effects of CNS injury can be frightening and devastating, and need to be clearly understood, explained, and anticipated by the professional intervening with families (Riva & Cazzaniga, 1986).

Lateralized Deficits and Poststroke Functioning

Early in the development of neuropsychological theories, it was proposed that cerebral lateralization occurs as a consequence of the development process. With the advent of better imaging techniques (especially functional MRI), and the improved understanding of anatomy, physiology, and neurobehavior, there is growing evidence of specific functional specialization in infancy and even during prenatal development (Hynd & Willis, 1988). The idea of specialization was once so extreme that specific areas were posited to have circumscribed functions. Therefore, it was thought that if damage to a structure occurred, that area's function was destroyed. Better understanding of the recovery of neurologically impaired patients now makes it clear that even a demarcated lesion affects multiple functional behaviors. Although brain areas can be delineated by primary function, there is also evidence that each functional ability is regulated by the interconnection of many cerebral areas. It is this interconnection that has yet to be well understood.

Clarifying specificity can be assisted by comparing functional outcomes of patients according to lesion site. Nass, Koch, Janowsky, and Stiles-Davis (1985) found that patients with left-hemisphere lesions had a higher Full Scale IQ on the WISC-R, with significant verbal sparing. No significant differences between these patients and patients with right-hemisphere lesions were found on Performance IQ. These results provide support for Teuber's "crowding principle" (Woods & Teuber, 1973)—that is, the principle that the brain can compensate for early damage, at a cost to efficiency. The undamaged hemisphere is adept at moderating the cognitive functions after a unilateral lesion, which leads to adequate generic functioning. This recovery process comes at a price to generalized functioning, however, as remaining CNS functions become overwhelmed with the additional burden of conducting their original function while also taking over the functions of the damaged area. Crowding then interferes with such neuropsychological abilities as attention, cognitive flexibility, acquisition, and organization. Nass et al. (1985) found more evidence of crowding with early (infancy) left-hemisphere lesions. The more "plastic" right hemisphere is less traumatized by injury and associated with better recovery and less long-term general compromise; this has been supported by neuropsychological data (Cohen et al., 1994; Craft et al., 1993; Nass et al., 1985; Woods, 1980).

General neuropsychological deficits seem to be associated with the CNS injuries caused by abnormal hemoglobin in SCD (e.g., ischemia, stroke, infarct, etc). Children with SCD on transfusion therapy have been found to exhibit significant declines in intellectual functioning, falling in the borderline to mildly mentally handicapped range (Listianingsih et al., 1991). Most children are prescribed transfusion therapy following a neurological injury, or following the indication of increased risk (e.g., abnormal imaging studies). Swift et al. (1989) found poststroke sickle cell patients to have intelligence scores significantly below those of their sibling controls. Poststroke patients appear to have increased higher cortical impairments, as well as significantly lower IQs, than patients without clinical stroke (Cohen et al., 1994; Listianingsih et al., 1991).

Neuropsychological deficits increase proportionally with the size of the lesion, regardless of location. Craft et al. (1993) suggested that stroke patterns influence specific neuropsychological profiles; as described above, they found children with diffuse stroke to be more impaired on spatial tasks, and those with anterior lesions to be more impaired on attentional tasks. Cohen et al. (1994) found that children with LCI tended to have more global impairment, including problems with visual–spatial construction and memory, expressive language, verbal/auditory memory, academic skills, and attention. Children with right cerebral infarct tended to have more specific nonverbal deficits affecting visual–motor integration, visual–spatial construction and memory, and arithmetic skills.

Neurocognitive abnormalities occurring in children after stroke may not be evident with standard psychometric testing. Executive functioning deficits are more common in poststroke populations (Cohen et al., 1994), but are more difficult to identify with standardized tests. Anterior deficits may be difficult to isolate on global function tests, because the skills associated with such areas are less well defined on standard measures. Both clinically identifiable and silent strokes in children with SCD are associated with specific neuropsychological deficits. Neuropsychological testing may discriminate the presence of stroke more readily than neurological history or neurological examination may, because of its ability to discriminate neurological operations by function.

FUTURE DIRECTIONS IN NEUROPSYCHOLOGICAL RESEARCH

For many years, it was believed that children with SCD who showed no evidence of CVA had no neuropsychological impairment (Craft et. al., 1993). Until 1996, no studies had combined neuroradiographic with clinical findings in an attempt to identify silent strokes and their neuropsychological correlates. Using MRI to classify patients with overt stroke, silent stroke, and normal findings, Armstrong et al. (1996) compared these findings to neuropsychological findings; as described earlier, they found that children with silent strokes were more likely to have neuropsychological impairments than children without MRI abnormality. With the increasing evidence that silent strokes contribute to developmental compromise, future directions are examining the predictability of risk. Many studies examining neuropsychological functioning have excluded patients with a history of CVA, but have not identified those who may have had a silent stroke. With a mean age for stroke of 6, many subjects are eliminated from studies early. However, because silent strokes and subtle effects may be present, covert disease may lead to poorer performance in the younger age groups.

The impact of early CVA and silent stroke has not been well examined. Older children may have learned to compensate for deficits over time, suggesting that very early developmental injury can be accommodated. As noted above, however, the risk for developmental regression in patients with early neurological injury is quite high, and acute recovery does not predict long-term outcome. Does early injury heal with time and intervention or with time alone? In particular, because transient ischemic episodes occur more frequently in younger children, can these be "outgrown" with appropriate intervention or merely with time? (Wasserman et al., 1991). With the improvement of neuropsychological evaluation and neuroimaging studies, children who are at increased risk might be identified, and preventative measures taken prior to the injury. However, prevention may also come at a financial or physiological cost. At this time, chronic transfusion is the treatment of choice for preventing sickle crises and CVA, but it can be costly, demanding, and risky. It is also currently unclear whether subtle early findings on neuroimaging, TDU, and neuropsychological tests contribute reliably to predictability of future strokes (Adams et al., 1992; Wasserman et al., 1991); this question needs to be more rigorously examined.

In addition, more attention is needed to psychosocial components of neuropsychological findings, which (as discussed earlier) can affect neurodevelopment and test performance. Almost all research to date has focused on the small percentage of the total SCD population attending clinics and treatment centers, and this focus may overrepresent poor coping and impairment in this disease.

Increased exploration into the risk–benefit ratio of noninvasive techniques and neuropsychological evaluations is needed as well. Further comparisons of the results of brain recording techniques (e.g., TDU, functional MRI, etc) with neuropsycholgical and functional performance will help to elucidate true risk factors and consequences of the disease. What is needed is a comprehensive effort to use neuropsychological and physiological imaging to clarify the pathophysiology and neurodevelopmental variability of neurological injury in SCD (Bigler, 1991; Tzika et al., 1993).

A final caveat is that the sensitivity of neuropsychological measures to the complex neurobehavioral sequelae of neurological injury, especially frontal lobe deficits, is not well known. Given the findings of increased behavioral and attentional problems in children with anterior lesions, neuropsychological measures should be structured to be more sensitive to these functions. There may also be better ways to represent neuropsychological findings than merely giving standard scores; these may include performance patterns, variability, and suggestive signs of pathological processes. Neurodevelopmental studies need to represent more clearly how specific and global neurological processes become cognitively and behaviorally apparent over time.

The most critical aspect of future directions will be in the increased awareness of potential neurocognitive concerns and ongoing assessment for early identification of neuropsychological concerns. Including neuropsychological evaluation as part of medical protocols (American Academy of Pediatrics, 1996) will allow more comprehensive treatment of the SCD patient.

REFERENCES

Adams, R. J., McKie, V., Nichols, F., Carl, E., Zhang, D., McKie, K., Figueroa, R., Litaker, M., Thompson, W., & Hess, D. (1992). The use of transcranial ultrasonography to predict stroke in sickle cell disease. *New England Journal of Medicine, 326*(9), 605–610.

Adams, R. J., Nichols, F. T., McKie, V., McKie, K., Milner, P., & Gammel, G. T. (1988). Cerebral infarction in sickle cell anemia: Mechanisms based on CT and MRI. *Neurology, 38,* 1012–1017.

American Academy of Pediatrics (1996). Health supervision for children with sickle cell diseases and their families. *Pediatrics, 98*(3), 467–472.

Armstrong, F., Thompson, R., Wang, W., Zimmerman, R., Pegelow, C., Miller, S., Moser, F, Bello, J., Hurtig, A., & Vass, K. (1996). Cognitive functioning and brain magnetic resonance imaging in children with sickle cell disease. *Neuropsychology, 97*(6), 864–870.

Bigler, E. D. (1991). Neuropsychological assessment, neuroimaging, and clinical neuropsychology: A synthesis. *Archives of Clinical Neuropsychology, 6,* 113–132.

Burlew, A. K., Evans, R., & Oler, C. (1989). The impact of a child with sickle cell disease on family dynamics. *Annals of the New York Academy of Sciences, 565,* 161–171.

Chapar, G. N. (1988). Chronic disease of children and neuropsychological dysfunction. *Journal of Developmental and Behavioral Pediatrics, 9*(4), 221.

Chapar, G. N., Doctors, S. R., Radel, E., & Coupey, S. M. (1986). Minimal neurological deficits in adolescents with sickle cell disease. *Journal of Developmental and Behavioral Pediatrics, 7*, 205.

Cohen, M. J., Branch, W. B., McKie, V. C., & Adams, R. J. (1994). Neuropsychological impairment in children with sickle cell anemia and cerebrovascular accidents. *Clinical Pediatrics, 33*(9), 517–524.

Craft, S., Schatz, J., Glauser, T. A., Lee, B., & DeBaun, M. R. (1993). Neuropsychological effects of stroke in children with sickle cell anemia. *Journal of Pediatrics, 123*(5), 712–717.

DesForges, J. F., Milner, P., Wethers, D. L., & Whitten, C. F. (1978). Sickle cell disease: Tell the facts, quell the fables. *Patient Care, 12*(11), 1–28.

Fowler, M. G., Whitt, J. K., Redding-Lallinger, A. R., Nash, K. B., Atkinson, S. S., Wells, R. J., & McMillan, C. (1988). Neuropsychologic and academic functioning of children with sickle cell anemia. *Journal of Developmental and Behavioral Pediatrics, 9*, 213–220.

Gentry, B., Hall, L., Danier, J. (1997). A parental survey of speech, language and physical development of infants and toddlers with sickle cell disease. *Perceptual and Motor Skills, 83*(3), 1105–1106.

Greenberg, J., & Massey, E. W. (1985). Cerebral infarction in sickle cell trait. *Annals of Neurology, 18*, 354–355.

Hurtig, A. L., & Park, K. B. (1987). Adjustment and coping in adolescents with sickle cell disease. *Annals of the New York Academy of Sciences*, 172–181.

Hurtig, A. L., & White, L. S. (1986). Psychosocial adjustment in children and adolescents with sickle cell disease. *Journal of Pediatric Psychology, 11*(3), 411–427.

Hynd, G. W., & Willis, W. G. (1988). *Pediatric neuropsychology*. Boston: Allyn & Bacon.

Katz, S., Lubin, B., & Armstrong, D. (1974). Growth of adolescents with sickle cell trait. *Lancet, 1*, 814–815.

Kramer, M. S., Rooks, Y., & Pearson, H. A. (1978). Growth and development in children with sickle cell trait. *New England Journal of Medicine, 299*, 686–489.

Listianingsih, M. F., Hariman, M. D., Griffith, E. R., Hurtig, A. L., & Keehn, M. T. (1991). Functional outcomes of children with sickle-cell disease affected by stroke. *Archives of Physical Medicine and Rehabilitation, 72*, 498–502.

McCormack, M. K., Scarr-Salapatek, S., Polesky, H., Thompson, W., Katz, S. H., & Barker, W. B. (1975). A comparison of the physical and intellectual development of black children with and without sickle-cell trait. *Pediatrics, 56*, 1021–1025.

Mercuri, E., Faundez, J., Roberts, I., Flora, S., Bouza, H., Cowan, F., Pennock, J., Bydder, G., & Dubowitz, L. (1995). Neurological 'soft' signs may identify children with sickle cell disease who are at risk for stroke. *European Journal of Pediatrics, 154*, 150–156.

Nass, R. D., Koch, D. A., Janowsky, J., & Stiles-Davis, J. (1985). Differential effects on intelligence of early left versus right brain injury. *Annals of Neurology, 18*, 393.

National Institutes of Health. (1986). PET Scans pinpoint brain metabolism changes in sickle cell disease. *Journal of American Medical Assocation, 256*(13), 1692.

Partington, M. D., Aronyk, K. E., & Byrd, S. E. (1994). Sickle cell trait and stroke in children. *Pediatric Neurosurgery, 20*(2), 148–51.

Pavlakis S. G., Bello, J., Prohovnik, I., Sutton, M., Ince, C., Mohr, J. P., Piomelli, S., Hilal, S., & Devivo, D. C. (1988). Brain infarction in sickle cell anemia: Magnetic resonance imagery correlates. *Annals of Neurology, 23*(2), 125–130.

Pavlakis, S. G., Prohovnik, I., Piomelli, S., & Devivo, D. C. (1989). Neurologic complications of sickle cell disease. *Advances in Pediatrics, 36*, 247–276.

Pearson, H. A. (1987). Sickle cell diseases: Diagnosis and management in infancy and childhood. *Pediatric Review, 9*, 121–130.

Riggs, J. E., Ketonen, L. M., Wang, D. D., & Valanne, L. K. (1995). Cerebral infarction in a child with sickle cell trait. *Journal of Child Neurology, 10*(3), 253–254.

Ris, M. D., Kalinyak, K. A., Ball, W. S., Noll, R. B., Wells, R. J., & Rucknagel, D. (1996). Pre- and post-stroke MRI and neuropsychological studies in sickle cell disease: A case study. *Archives of Clinical Neurology, 11*(6), 481–490.

Riva, D., & Cazzaniga, L. (1986). Late effects of unilateral brain lesions sustained before and after age one. *Neuropsychologia, 24,* 423–428.

Rodgers, G., Clark, C., Larson, S., Rapport, S., Nienhuis, A., & Schechter, A. (1988). Brain glucose metabolism in neurologically normal patients with sickle cell disease. *Archives of Neurology, 45,* 78–82.

Swift, A. V., Cohen, M. J., Hynd, G. W., Wisenbaker, J. M., McKie, K. M., Makari, G., & McKie, V. C. (1989). Neuropsychological impairment in children with sickle cell anemia. *Pediatrics, 84*(6), 1077–1085.

Tzika, A. A., Massoth, R. J., Ball, W. S., Majumdar, S., Dunn, R. S., & Kirks, D. R. (1993). Dynamic contrast enhanced T2-weighted MR images: Detection of cerebral perfusion in children. *Radiology, 187,* 449–458.

Wasserman, A. L., Williams, J. A., Fairclough, D. L., Mulhern, R. K., & Wang, W. (1991). Subtle neuropsychological deficits in children with sickle cell disease. *American Journal of Pediatric Hematology–Oncology, 13,* 14–20.

Williams, I., Earles, A. N., & Pack, B. (1983). Psychological considerations in sickle cell disease. *Nursing Clinics of North America, 18*(1), 215–229.

Wiznitzer, M., Ruggeri, P. M., Masaryk, T. J., Ross, J. S., Modic, M. T., & Berman, B. (1990). Diagnosis of cerebrovascular disease in sickle cell anemia by magnetic resonance angiography. *Journal of Pediatrics, 117*(4), 551–555.

Woods, B. T. (1980). The restricted effects of right-hemisphere lesions after age one: Wechsler test data. *Neuropsychologia, 16,* 65–70.

Woods, B. T., & Teuber, H. L. (1973). Early onset of complimentary specialization of cerebral hemispheres in man. *Transactions of the American Neurological Association, 98,* 113–117.

17

DOWN SYNDROME

HEATHER CODY
RANDY W. KAMPHAUS

Down syndrome was named after the physician John Langdon Down, who in 1866 published a description of patients he identified as "Mongolian." In addition to delineating the physical features of this syndrome, Down noted that these individuals were responsive to training and could benefit from intervention (Carr, 1995). In the United States, the prevalence rate of Down syndrome is reported to be approximately 1 per 600 live births, and an estimated 7,000 babies are born each year with it (Wishart, 1988). This estimate is lower than earlier ones, due to efforts to screen pregnant women over the age of 35, who are felt to be at greater risk for giving birth to a child with Down syndrome. However, because approximately 70% of babies born with Down syndrome are born to younger mothers and because some women may refuse screening (Carr, 1995; Sadovnick & Baird, 1992), this figure is still high. Gender differences are evident, in that males commonly outnumber females (the sex ratio is 1.3:1); this may be due to a higher mortality rate in females during infancy (Carr, 1995).

GENETIC AND FAMILIAL ISSUES RELATED TO ETIOLOGY

Down syndrome is classified as one of the chromosomal disorders, meaning that the syndrome has been traced to malformations in the genes of individuals who display the syndrome. There are actually several different types of Down syndrome, with the most prevalent being trisomy 21 (94%), where there is actually a third chromosome 21 in addition to the usual two (Prescott, 1988). Trisomy occurs in approximately 4% of all pregnancies, making it the most common chromosomal abnormality in humans (Hassold, Sherman, & Hunt, 1995). Genetic anomalies have also been found on chromosome 21, in particular band q22. Specific regions of chromosome 21 have been mapped and are associated with the various features of Down syndrome. Currently, approximately 25–40 genes have been mapped to chromosome 21 through techniques such as gene linkage. This is one reason for the wide range of individual variation found within the Down syndrome population (Korenberg,

Pulst, & Gerwehr, 1992). Other types of Down syndrome consist of translocation 21, mosaicism, and partial trisomy 21 (Coleman, 1988; Pueschel, 1992b). Translocation 21 results when one part of chromosome 21 has been transferred to a different location. Mosaicism occurs when not all of the cells display the chromosomal trisomy, although a majority do display trisomy 21. Some research indicates that individuals with this condition have higher mean cognitive scores than those with trisomy 21.

Relative risk for giving birth to a child with Down syndrome is approximately 1%, plus the amount of risk associated with the mother's age during pregnancy. The risk for having a child with Down syndrome increases exponentially with maternal age. For example, a 20-year-old mother has a 1 in 1,923 chance of giving birth to an infant with Down syndrome, while the chance for a 49-year-old mother is 1 in 12 (Prescott, 1988). Procedures such as amniocentesis and chorionic villi sampling can be used to screen for Down syndrome. The etiology behind the maternal age effect has not yet been determined, although it appears to be related to an increase in trisomy at conception rather than a decrease in the ability to abort a trisomic fetus naturally (Hassold et al., 1995).

MEDICAL CONCERNS AND COMORBID DISORDERS

Although Down syndrome is primarily known as one of the chief causes of mental retardation, it also includes distinctive physical characteristics, as Down noted in his 1866 report. These may include brachycephaly (broad head), a delay in the closure of the fontanels, hypoplasia of the midfacial bones, obliquely placed palpebral fissures, epicanthal folds, depressed nasal bridge, hyper- or hypotelorism, Brushfield spots (white spots on the periphery of the iris), an overlapping or folding of the helix of the ear, thickened lips, tongue protrusion and/or fissured tongue with increasing age, short and broad neck, umbilical hernias, broad and stubby hands and feet, a single palmar transverse crease, partial or complete syndactyly, and a wide space between the first and second toes (Pueschel, 1992b). Certain features have been found to change over time. For example, the epicanthal folds and large neck may become less noticeable over time, while other features (e.g., a fissured tongue and dental problems) become more problematic with increasing age (Pueschel, 1992b). The mental retardation evident with Down syndrome may range from mild to profound (according to the American Association on Mental Retardation classification), which adds to the heterogeneity of this population.

Ophthalmological Concerns

Ophthalmological problems can be major disabilities for individuals with Down syndrome. The most common causes of loss of vision are cataracts and acute keratoconus. Functionally, individuals may suffer from strabismus, blepharitis, and high refractive errors, which if untreated may be debilitating (Catalano, 1992; Niva, 1988). Fortunately, medical intervention is available for all of these conditions; therefore, parents, teachers, and health professionals should be aware of these potential difficulties and seek medical evaluation for them.

Oral Problems

Since the maxilla and mandible are smaller in persons with Down syndrome than in most individuals, the tongue may appear to be larger than normal. As a result of the smaller oral cavity and relatively larger tongue, oral hygiene may be difficult. In addition, individuals with Down syndrome may have a furrowed tongue or cleft palate, which may further complicate oral health. The tongue protrusion also contributes to the split, inflamed lips that are commonly seen in these individuals. Other common problems include malocclusions, anomalies in the dentition (e.g., congenitally missing teeth, delayed eruption of teeth, delayed shedding of primary teeth), and periodontal disease (e.g., gingivitis is seen in almost all persons with Down syndrome) (Vigild, 1992).

Cardiac Problems

The incidence of congenital heart malformations in persons with Down syndrome has been reported to be as high as 50% (for trisomy 21), and cardiac anomalies remain the main cause of death, especially in the first few years of life (Marino, 1992). The most common types of anomalies found in these children are defects in the atrioventricular canal. These anomalies produce an increased risk of congestive heart failure. Certain types of cardiac defects result in decreased pulmonary blood flow, which may contribute to pulmonary artery hypertension and pulmonary vascular obstructive disease (Howenstein, 1992). Early diagnosis and corrective surgery may improve survival rates to 80–90% of children who may otherwise fail to reach their 15th year (Marino, 1992). A survival rate as high as 87.8% was reported for individuals with Down syndrome who had surgery for cardiovascular lesions. In contrast, a survival rate of 41.4% was reported for those who did not undergo surgery (Hijii, Fukushige, Igarashi, Takahashi, & Ueda, 1997).

Respiratory Concerns

Respiratory problems may result from the physical abnormalities observed in children with Down syndrome. For example, the small oral cavity and hypoplasia of the midfacial region create problems with airways. In addition, lungs in individuals with Down syndrome have been found to be smaller than average (Howenstein, 1992). Pneumonia continues to be one of the major causes of death, and there is an overall predisposition for contracting infectious diseases in the lower respiratory tract. Lower respiratory tract infections have also been linked to the increased mortality rates in this population. These conditions are related to the many structural and functional disorders associated with Down syndrome (Howenstein, 1992). Sinus infections and chronic rhinitis are common, and cases of bacterial pneumonia and viral infections are typically more severe in these individuals. Sleep apnea, which is characterized by snoring, restless sleep, interrupted breathing while asleep, mouth breathing, and daytime somnolence, has also been reported.

Gastrointestinal Anomalies

A number of gastrointestinal anomalies are associated with Down syndrome, but among the most common are esophageal atresia, tracheoesophageal fistula, duodenal atresia or stenosis, and Hirschsprung disease (Levy, 1992). The etiology of these conditions can be traced to malformation during embryonic development. A child with esophageal atresia may have difficulty breathing, due to the increased production of oropharyngeal secretions. Children may also exhibit a balky cough as a result of tracheoesophageal fistula. Both of these conditions are complicated by gastroesophageal reflux. Corrective surgery is available for these anomalies, and therefore early detection and intervention should prevail. Beasley, Allen, and Myers (1997) reported that despite treatment, individuals with Down syndrome who have oesophageal atresia have a high mortality, perhaps due to the other physical anomalies associated with Down syndrome. Claims that children with Down syndrome have difficulty with absorption of some foods (e.g., protein, fat, and vitamins) have not been supported conclusively.

Dermatological Conditions

Although there is no dermatological condition that is characteristic of Down syndrome, several conditions are seen frequently (>50%) in this population. These maladies include dry skin, atopic dermatitis, fungal infections of the feet and nails, and mucosal anomalies (e.g., inflammation of the lip, scrotal tongue) (Benson & Scherbenske, 1992). With proper treatment, these conditions should not become disabling.

Other Physical Difficulties

In infancy and early childhood, ear infections are a significant problem for individuals with Down syndrome. This is an important medical concern, since frequent ear infections are known to contribute to developmental delays in language skills. The cause for the increased number of ear infections may be related to the abnormalities of the ear that are associated with Down syndrome. For this reason, hearing should be closely monitored and screened semiannually through age 8 (Downs & Balkany, 1988).

Disorders of the liver, such as hepatitis, have been linked to Down syndrome. Individuals with Down syndrome who are institutionalized are at particular risk for contracting hepatitis B. Proper hygiene and immunization may provide protection against hepatitis B. In addition, persons with Down syndrome seem to be susceptible to leukemia (Scola, 1992).

The genitourinary system may also be affected in persons with Down syndrome. Research has identified smaller-than-normal kidneys, obstructive lesions along the urinary tract, and difficulty with uric acid and creatinine clearance (Ariel & Shvil, 1992). Additional characteristics involve the genitalia. One commonly observed characteristic has been hypogenitalism, particularly with males. In addition, trisomy 21 has been found to be concomitant with other sex-related syndromes, such as Klinefelter, XYY, XXX, and Turner syndromes. At one time it was hypothesized that hypospadias and cryptorchidism were also linked to Down syndrome, but more recent findings have disproven such reports (Ariel & Shvil, 1992). In females, there may be the occurrence of hypermenorrhea or menorrhagia with the onset of puberty (Elkins, 1992). This problem may be due to a number of factors, such as hypothyroidism and/or obesity, both of which are associated with Down syndrome.

Neuromuscular abnormalities are commonly reported in cases of Down syndrome, and often these contribute to the increased mortality rates within this population. Among the problems reported, subluxation and dislocation of the cervical spine, hip, and patella are the most life-threatening (Pueschel & Solga, 1992). Each of these conditions may impede physical activity by causing severe discomfort, which in turn contributes to decreased mobility and physical activity. Other orthopedic difficulties may arise from cervical spine instability in the atlanto-occipital and atlantoaxial regions. Persons with Down syndrome may suffer from severe scoliosis and typically have problems with collapsing flat feet and bunion deformity (Pueschel & Solga, 1992). Additional difficulties result from hypotonia, or low muscle tone, which is considered to be a major universal characteristic and is related to delays found in gross motor development.

Neurological and Psychiatric Conditions

Down syndrome has been found to interfere with the fetal development of the central nervous system and to result in brain abnormalities. These anomalies include a reduction in the total number of neurons throughout several cortical areas, abnormalities within the neurons themselves, and abnormalities in the ability of the neurons to communicate with each other (Florez, 1992). Although brain weight at birth is close to normal, brain weight estimates for children with Down syndrome tend to fall in the below-average range over time. This condition may be related to a reduction in the neuronal density in cortical areas and decreased dendritic arborization (Florez, 1992). However, the most affected area of the brain in persons with Down syndrome is the cerebral cortex, where the reduction in the number of neurons, existence of dendritic spines, and poor synaptic connections contribute to difficulties in cognitive and learning processes (e.g., attention, information processing, integration, short- and long-term memory, and language skills) (Florez, 1992).

Other neurological problems that some children with Down syndrome face are seizure disorders. Increased rates of seizure disorders have been associated with Down syndrome, with prevalence rates reported as high as 33% in some studies (Pueschel, 1992b). Most seizures will begin before age 1 (40%) or after individuals reach their 30s (40%).

Early accounts of Down syndrome portrayed a general decline in IQ over the lifespan. However, Carr (1995) summarized this research and found that there is actually little evidence that IQ, memory, or practical skills deteriorate significantly before the age of 50. In addition, fewer than 50% of individuals with Down syndrome show clear signs of dementia. Individuals with Down syndrome who live to be over age 40 have been found to show the characteristic features of Alzheimer disease in the central nervous system; these consist of cortical atrophy, neurofibrillary tangles, and neuritic plaques (Lai, 1992; Mufson, Benzing, & Kordower, 1995). Visser, Aldenkamp, van Huffelen, and Kuilman (1997) found an increasing prevalence rate for dementia in a group with Down syndrome. After age 40, prevalance rates fell at 11% between ages 40–49 and increased up to 77% between ages 60–69. Efforts to find a genetic link between Down syndrome and Alzheimer disease have had mixed results, with some indication that a gene for Alzheimer disease may be located on the long arm of chromosome 21. The dementia resulting from Alzheimer disease is difficult to establish in persons with mental retardation, especially in severe cases, and therefore clinical studies attempting to establish the presence of dementia in Down syndrome populations are difficult to carry out. Moreover, hypothyroidism, poor nutrition, and depression may all masquerade as dementia and are also common problems for persons with Down syndrome. This scenario makes differential diagnosis hard to accomplish. The clinical dementia associated with Alzheimer disease does, however, become evident in persons with Down syndrome who live to be 50. The symptomatic presentation is essentially the same as that for groups without Down syndrome, but it may appear to be somewhat exaggerated, due to the physical and cognitive features already associated with Down syndrome (Lai, 1992). New research using magnetic brain imaging (MRI) to examine the brains of adults with Down syndrome and dementia indicated smaller total brain, left hippocampus, and left amygdala volumes when compared to the nondemented subjects with Down syndrome (Pearlson et al., 1998). Additionally, the adults with Down syndrome and dementia showed more generalized atrophy than their peers.

Myers (1992) reviewed the literature on other psychiatric conditions that are comorbid with Down syndrome. She found that in children under the age of 20, externalizing problems such as attention-deficit/hyperactivity disorder, oppositional defiant disorder, conduct disorder, and aggressive behavior account for most of the disturbances. In persons over age 20, aggressive behavior, major depressive disorder, and stereotypic behavior are reported most frequently. Myers also stated that although children and adolescents with Down syndrome show lower risk for developing a psychiatric disorder than other individuals with mental retardation, they are still at greater risk than the general population. Individuals with Down syndrome are at increased risk for depression, and therefore symptoms of depression should be investigated seriously.

Systemic Problems

Persons with Down syndrome have a higher susceptibility to bacterial infections, malignancies, and autoimmunine disturbances, as a result of a mild immune deficiency (Ugazio, Maccario, & Burgio, 1992). Further complications result from several hematological abnormalities that are unique to Down syndrome. These irregularities include transient myelodysplasia in infancy (the presentation of which resembles congenital leukemia), red cell macrocytosis, and increased susceptibility to leukemia (Lubin, Cahn, & Scott, 1992). At one time, Down syndrome was felt to be caused by generalized endocrine failure; however, the majority of persons with Down syndrome do not suffer from endocrine dysfunction (Pueschel & Bier, 1992). On the other hand, the prevalence rate for endocrine disturbances is greater for those with Down syndrome than for the general population. Among the most common findings are problems related to thyroid functioning, specifically hypothyroidism (Pueschel & Bier, 1992). This condition may predispose individuals with Down syndrome to become overweight.

Mortality

The greatest likelihood of death resulting from medical complications such as congenital anomalies, circulatory problems, and respiratory illness occurs during the first year of life, with ages 1–9 being the largest age group at risk for early death (Sadovnick & Baird, 1992). With advances in medical treatment and early intervention for such difficulties as cardiac and gastrointestinal defects, survival rates should improve in the future.

When he originally characterized Down syndrome, Down (1866) commented on the shorter life expectancy for these individuals. This phenomenon held true until the 1940s, when average life expectancy figures rose from approximately 9 years to 12 years of age. Current trends indicates that nearly half (44%) of the children born between 1952 and 1981 will live to be at least 60 years old (Carr, 1995; Sadovnick & Baird, 1992). Although the shorter life expectancy had at one time been accounted for by the congenital heart defects that often accompany Down syndrome, this hypothesis has not been substantiated in studies comparing individuals with Down syndrome who did not have heart defects to a matched group with mental retardation but not Down syndrome (Sadovnick & Baird, 1992). A more recent study (1986–1991) looking at the mortality rates of a large sample of individuals with Down syndrome found that up to age 35, mortality rates were comparable to a sample with mental retardation. However, after age 35, the mortality rates for the group with Down syndrome increased at a greater rate than for the group with mental retardation (Strauss & Eyman, 1996).

DEVELOPMENTAL COURSE

Although the majority of children with Down syndrome display delayed motor function, cognitive development, and language acquisition, there are individual variations in rate and level of achievement. Children with Down syndrome experience a period of rapid growth and development during their first 3 years of life, much as other children do. Their special needs may require some environmental supports in order for them to achieve their developmental milestones, however. Developmental stages generally mimic those found in normal children in the domains of sensorimotor functioning, conservation, and mastery of space, time, and moral judgment, although these skills are acquired at a slower rate (Hodapp & Zigler, 1990). This finding is supported by the work of Tingey, Mortensen, Matheson, and Doret (1991), who found that infants and young children with Down syndrome were more similar to normal children on the Personal, Social, and Adaptive domains of the Battelle Developmental Inventory, and less similar in the Communication and Cognitive domains. This discrepancy was found to widen as the children's age approached 36 months.

Temperament

Biological studies have found that children with Down syndrome may be less reactive to novelty, and thus may appear more passive or less generally reactive, than other children of similar age (Ganiban, Wagner, & Cicchetti, 1990). In many other regards, however, children with Down syndrome display the same temperamental variability as any other children. Zickler, Morrow, and Bull (1998) found infants with Down syndrome were rated as more active, less intense, more distractible, and tended to demonstrate more approach behaviors when compared to normally developing infants. When maternal ratings of temperamental qualities for children with Down syndrome are compared to those for non-handicapped children, the developmental stages of temperament appear to be the same. However, mothers of a Down syndrome group have reported lower adaptability and a greater need for stimulation for their children (Vaughn, Contreras, & Seiter, 1994). A study of older children and adolescents with Down syndrome, using maternal and teacher ratings of temperamental characteristics, found that mothers perceived their children as less active, more predictable, more positive in mood, less persistent, and more distractible (Gunn & Cuskelly, 1991). Mothers and teachers agreed on which children were viewed as easy or difficult overall, but the reports of individual characteristics constituting these categories varied for the two sets of raters.

Cognitive Development

Given that most children with Down syndrome suffer from some degree of mental retardation (mild, moderate, severe, or profound), the degree of cognitive development that may be evident is dependent on how severe the cognitive deficits may be. The difficulty of using standardized tests to evaluate a child with mental retardation, and the problems with obtaining longitudinal data, make research in this area difficult to generalize to a population that is known for its heterogeneity. Although standardized intelligence tests have been found to be useful in classifying an individual as either mentally retarded or not, they are of more limited utility in discriminating between the various levels of mental retardation (Kamphaus, 1993).

Perhaps the most consistent finding regarding cognitive development in children with Down syndrome is that there is a general decline in their developmental rate as the children get older (Carr, 1885). Children with mosaicism have been found to score 10–30 points higher on IQ measures than those with trisomy 21, and have demonstrated normal skills of visual-perceptual skills as well (Fishler & Koch, 1991). However, Wishart (1995) cautions that, generally speaking, there is no fixed "ceiling" of cognitive development for individuals with Down syndrome, and that research findings show learning to continue well beyond adolescence for this population.

Language Development

Language is closely linked to cognitive ability, in that the rate and degree of language attainment will depend heavily on the amount of cognitive deficit that exists. However, in comparison to the development of nonretarded children, language skills are acquired more slowly in children with Down syndrome than are other motor or cognitive skills. In addition, language development fails to proceed at a consistent pace but rather in spurts, with a great deal of development occurring before the age of 7 (Fowler, 1988). This discrepancy can first be seen in infancy and grows larger as children become older. For example, although the rate of vocabulary learning in children with Down syndrome is typically consistent with their developmental age, it does not progress at a rate that is consistent with their other cognitive skills (Miller, 1995). Children with Down syndrome may communicate more effectively through the use of gestures rather than verbal expression (Weitzner-Lin, 1997). Language production appears more deficient than language comprehension. Within expressive language, the grammatical/syntactical components of language rather than the lexical or nonverbal aspects seem to show the greatest impairments (Fowler, 1988; Miller, 1995). Children with Down syndrome are found to have a specific language impairment characterized by fewer total words used in an utterance, fewer number of different words used, and less than average length of their utterance (Chapman, Seung, Schwartz, & Bird, 1998). When adaptive behaviors were assessed with the Vineland Adaptive Behavior Scales in a group of children with Down syndrome aged from 1 to 11½ years, a relative weakness in communication compared with daily living and socialization skills was found (Dykens, Hodapp, & Evans, 1994). Within the communication domain, there was more deficiency with expressive language than with receptive language. This finding is supported by Miller's work.

Some factors that lead to the delays in language acquisition are related to the physical characteristics associated with Down syndrome. Problems with otitis media, cognitive dysfunction (e.g., memory, attention, arousal), and visual disturbances may impede a child's ability to gather auditory and visual cues concerning language.

Social Development

Because of the motor, perceptual, cognitive, and language delays that children with Down syndrome exhibit, their ability to gain social competence may also be diminished. For this reason, they may seek out developmentally matched rather than age-matched children for peer interactions. Play development has been reported to follow developmental trajectories as well (Beeghly, Perry, & Cicchetti, 1989). Earlier hypotheses that children with Down syndrome are more sociable than other retarded children and that this is a defining quality of the whole group have not been definitively supported by research, although some sex differences in sociability have been described. Ruskin, Kasari, Mundy, and Sigman (1994) found that young children with Down syndrome paid more attention to people during a social interaction paradigm than did mental-age-matched controls, demonstrating a greater focus of attention to the social cues provided. However, when presented with ambiguous stimuli paired with either positive or negative facial expressions from their parents, toddlers with Down syndrome were found to display significantly less appropriate responses (e.g., they responded with positive affect to negative expression) than did mental-age-matched controls (Knieps, Walden, & Baxter, 1994). Therefore, although children with Down syndrome may be as socially responsive as other children, they fail to learn socially referenced cues. Landry, Miller-Loncar, and Swank (1998) found that children with Down syndrome have a more difficult time transferring goal-directed play skills used with their mothers in a joint-play session to independent play situations than control children. In other words, children with Down syndrome benefit from structured (directed) play but have trouble using these skills on their own and may continue to need structured play time.

Growth and Motor Development

Individual factors (e.g., cardiac and skeletal problems, hypotonia, obesity, vision and hearing disturbances, and perceptual problems) may have an impact on the growth and motor development of any child with Down syndrome. Aspects of significance are height and weight. Prenatally, fetuses with Down syndrome have been found to be smaller than when compared to normals. The largest deficit appears between birth and 36 months of age, where statistical differences have been found between children with Down syndrome (both males and females) and normal controls, with children with Down syndrome being smaller than average. Potential factors affecting growth in infancy may include prematurity, cardiac disease, and genetics. During middle childhood, growth rates become closer to normal, although adolescents experience smaller pubertal growth spurts as well as delayed onset of menses for females (i.e., later than the typical onset of 10–14 years) (Elkins, 1992). They will, however, have normal development of secondary sex characteristics. By adulthood, individuals with Down syndrome are typically two standard deviations below normal in height (Cronk & Anneren, 1992). Individuals with Down syndrome are commonly found to be overweight because of excessive weight gain during infancy and childhood (Cronk & Anneren, 1992; Rubin, Rimmer, Chicoine, Braddock, & McGuire, 1998). The etiology of this weight gain has not yet been determined conclusively, although there are some indications that it may be a factor of hypothyroidism and/or hypotonia (deficient muscle tone). Although their metabolic rates do not differ from normal, individuals with Down syndrome have less body mass and slower growth, and therefore require fewer calories (Pipes, 1992).

Generally, motor development is delayed in children with Down syndrome, with the most frequently cited causal factors being the hypotonia and hyperflexia seen in almost all of these children. However, individual variations are seen in both the qualitative and quantitative motor skills exhibited. Dunst (1990) concluded that sensorimotor development in children with Down syndrome, despite its slower pace, was more like that of nonretarded children. In a cross-sectional study of 6- to 16-year olds with Down syndrome, using a range of manual tasks, Thombs and Sugden (1991) found evidence of an increased use in precision grips among older children. The older children were also found to be faster on the speeded tasks. The authors concluded that on measures of speed, strategies, and types of grip, there are general developmental advances across age groups. Children with Down syndrome may display difficulty with gross and fine motor skills, balance, posture, strength, and flexibility. In a small study using neuropsychological tests, children with Down syndrome were found to have below average tactual perception (Brandt, 1996). However, one longitudinal study tracking motor development in school-age children with Down syndrome found that there was a wide range of skill levels and rates of progress between groups and among individuals (Jobling, 1998). Therefore, intervention should be tailored to individual children, based on their medical and health conditions. An excellent review of the literature on motor development in children with Down syndrome has been provided by Block (1991).

COGNITIVE, EMOTIONAL, AND BEHAVIORAL PRESENTATION

Cognitive Presentation

As noted earlier, a wide range of cognitive abilities can be observed in individuals with Down syndrome, creating a heterogeneous population. Interestingly, females have been found to have higher average scores than males in both childhood and adulthood (Carr, 1995). Many arguments have been made regarding this finding, but to date there are no established conclusions about any gender differences. When compared to other groups of disabled children, those with Down syndrome may not appear that different in the classroom. One study comparing the cognitive skills of adolescents with Down syndrome to those of children with cerebral palsy or nonspecific mental retardation found no significant differences between any of the groups (Smith & Phillips, 1992). The Down syndrome group did fail to show progress in language acquisition on a second assessment, but they also displayed some gains in cognition and copying skills, compared to the group with nonspecific mental retardation. Other cognitive deficits noted in children with Down syndrome include limited memory functioning (particularly for spatial stimuli), reduced task persistence and distractibility, slowed reaction time and information-processing speed, and difficulty with reasoning and judgment (Gibson, 1991).

Children with Down syndrome have been found to have delayed acquisition of language skills that is not commensurate with their mental age. This deficit may be due to the presence of central auditory processing abnormalities. For example, dichotic listening studies have found that individuals with Down syndrome have reversed hemispheric dominance (right- rather than left-hemisphere dominance) for processing speech (Dahle & Baldwin, 1992). Almost all of the literature on Down syndrome discusses language difficulties, particularly within expressive language, as constituting a hallmark of this disorder. New research using volumetric magnetic resonance imaging (MRI) measures have found that individuals with Down syndrome have a smaller planum temporale volume than controls (Frangou et al., 1997). This region has been associated with language functioning. The implications of a smaller planum in individuals with Down syndrome is still unclear, as the authors were unable to find a direct relationship between size and performance on their language testing.

Due to their neurological abnormalities, individuals with Down syndrome will display reduced short-term memory and will have greater difficulty recalling auditory than visual information (Florez, 1992). Difficulties in language development involve (1) an asynchrony in language production relative to language understanding and other cognitive skills; (2) an onset of productive deficits that coincides with vocabulary growth; (3) a slowness in the development of syntactic skills; and (4) heterogeneous language development for the population (Florez, 1992). In addition, difficulties with articulation may be exacerbated by hypotonia of facial muscles and related congenital abnormalities.

Emotional Presentation

Emotionally, individuals with mental retardation demonstrate greater susceptibility to stressors than the general population. The developmental delay and language impairments associated with mental retardation may contribute to the finding that individuals with Down syndrome are at slightly greater risk for autism than the general population (Myers, 1992). Children with Down syndrome may display impairment in school, occupational, or social functioning as a result of an adjustment disorder. These lags may be manifested in mood disturbances (anxiety or depression), physical complaints, social withdrawal, or work inhibition (Myers, 1992). Although depression in children with Down syndrome has not been well documented in the literature, adults have been found to exhibit depression, as noted earlier. The prevalence of major affective disorders in adults with mental retardation has been estimated to be 1–3.5% (Myers, 1992).

Behavioral Presentation

Cuskelly and Dadds (1992) performed a study of mother, father, and teacher ratings of behavior problems in children with Down syndrome compared to their siblings. On the Revised Behavior Problem Checklist, all raters reported that the group with Down syndrome exhibited significantly more total behavior problems and significantly more attention/immaturity problems than their siblings. There were also significant gender differences as viewed by the raters. Mothers reported the same level of problem behaviors for each gender, whereas fathers reported that the girls displayed more problems, and teachers experienced greater problems with boys. In an interesting follow-up study, Cuskelly and Gunn (1993) found that mothers of children with Down syndrome reported significantly more conduct problems in the female siblings than mothers who did not have a child with Down syndrome reported in their daughters. This finding may indicate that mothers of children with disabilities may have some misperceptions regarding "typical" behavior. It may also show that siblings of children with Down syndrome, especially girls, could experience greater adjustment problems and should be considered to be at risk for developing an adjustment disorder.

KEY ASSESSMENT ISSUES AND TOOLS

Diagnosis of Down syndrome is typically made at birth (35%) or within the first 2 years of life (46%), although there are some cases where a diagnosis has been made after the third year (Quine & Rutter, 1994). For this reason, most children enter preschool with a diagnosis. However, as Quine and Rutter (1994) found, parents are often not provided with detailed explanations of their children's impairments and its associated features. Psychologists should be aware that they may frequently need to educate parents and families.

Often parental reports constitute a chief source of assessment information regarding the developmental status of children with disabilities such as Down syndrome. When rating scales and interview data are being employed, estimates of a child's functioning must sometimes rely on the judgment of the parent who fills out the form. In a study comparing maternal and professional estimates of developmental status among children with handicaps, it was concluded that mothers provided higher estimates of ability across all developmental domains (Sexton, Thompson, Perez, & Rheams, 1990). Additional findings showed that maternal and professional ratings were highly correlated, with children's intellectual functioning being the most significant variable contributing to this correlation. In other words, mothers and professionals tended to agree more closely when children's intellectual functioning was closer to average.

Cognitive Assessment

Children with Down syndrome were found to exhibit a general deficit in the Sequential Processing domain of the Kaufman Assessment Battery for Children, as were children with fragile X syndrome and children with nonspecific mental retardation (Hodapp et al., 1992). Gestalt Closure appeared to be the most difficult subtest for all three groups, with Hand Movements being a significant strength for males with Down syndrome. A concurrent validity study between two editions of the Stanford–Binet (L-M and the fourth edition) with mentally retarded children found a strong relationship between these two tests, but also concluded that the fourth edition of the Stanford–Binet may be better suited for young children in this population (Bower & Hayes, 1995). Assessment of this group may be difficult for a variety of reasons, one being the instability of test performance. Variability has been found within a population of young children with Down syndrome (Wishart & Duffy, 1990). Failure to engage in the task and a variability in responding were factors that added to the instability of their evaluations.

Behavioral Assessment

There are no characteristic behaviors associated with Down syndrome. Rather, the full range of behaviors seen in nondisabled children may be exhibited by children with Down syndrome. Obstinance, aggression, withdrawal, and self-injurious behaviors are among the most frequently seen behaviors, and they are also the ones that elicit the most frustration from parents and educators. Behavior management techniques such as positive and negative reinforcement have been shown to be effective in decreasing problem behaviors and increasing target behaviors. In a study using descriptive analysis to ascertain the function of problem behaviors in a small sample of children with mental retardation, contingent reinforcement and teaching functionally equivalent behaviors were found to be effective in reducing problem behaviors for these children (Lalli, Browder, Mace, & Brown, 1993). In addition, because the students were required to communicate their requests, they concurrently improved their verbal skills.

Medical Assessment and Intervention

In 1991, the National Down Syndrome Society (NDSS) sponsored a conference on health care in Down syndrome, where suggestions were made for important medical interventions (Lott & McCoy, 1992). It was recommended that during the neonatal period and early infancy there should be an attempt to establish chromosomal karyotype, communicate the diagnosis to parents, and refer parents to available support groups. In addition, several types of screenings were recommended, based on the known health concerns for children with Down syndrome. These included screening for cataracts, blockage in the gastrointestinal tract, congenital heart disease, thyroid dysfunction, and hearing problems. It was advised that these exams should continue annually into early adulthood. The NDSS also advocated enrolling these children in early intervention programs.

During the preschool and school years, early efforts should focus on remediating common orthopedic problems (e.g., bunions, severe flat feet, dislocated hips) and dental problems, as well as on providing additional vaccinations (e.g., against influenza, pneumococcal infections, and hepatitis B) for at-risk children. Special behavioral programs may be beneficial to improve self-help skills, communication, and nutrition, as well as problems related to aggression, self-injurious behavior, and school adjustment. For example, some children with Down syndrome display food behavior problems, such as throwing or hoarding food (Pipes, 1992). Psychoeducational evaluation and remediation should also take place as early as possible, with follow-up provided throughout children's academic careers.

Over the years, numerous treatments have been sought to help "cure" various dysfunctions caused by Down syndrome. Whereas some of these treatments have sought to improve intellectual functioning and others have attempted to alleviate physical conditions, they are considered unconventional, and practitioners may wish to familiarize themselves with these in order to discuss them competently with parents who show an interest in these therapies. Some of the more popular of these are as follows: (1) pituitary extract, given to improve intellectual and social development; (2) glutamic acid; (3) thyroid hormone, given to improve intellectual functioning; (4) 5-hydroxytryptophan, given to improve behavioral and motoric functioning; (5) dimethyl sulfoxide, given to improve behavior and learning; (6) sicca cells (fetal cell therapy), given to increase intellectual functioning and growth; (7) vitamins, minerals, enzymes, and hormones, administered to treat mental retardation; and (8) facial plastic surgery, intended to improve characteristic features (for a detailed review, see Pueschel, 1992a). Parents may be willing to try these alternative therapies, despite evidence that demonstrates their lack of efficacy. Often they are influenced by positive expectations of improvement and may attribute any change to the therapy. However, at all times, the health and best interest of a child should remain the primary focus.

OPTIONS FOR TREATMENT OF PSYCHOSOCIAL, EDUCATIONAL, AND EMOTIONAL PROBLEMS

Infants with Down syndrome commonly display delays in gross and fine motor, cognitive, personal, social, emotional, and language development (Dmitriev, 1988). These areas may be improved with training, and certain characteristics of children with Down syndrome facilitate such education. These factors include the following: (1) Infants with Down syndrome are more like normal infants than not and will respond to social gestures; (2) they will respond positively to physical assistance (e.g., shaping) while learning; (3) they are reinforced by their own successes; and (4) they have higher receptive than expressive language skills and good visual discrimination (Dmitriev, 1988). Interventions should also include a child's family, since there are some indications that maternal responsiveness to a preschooler with Down syndrome may be improved by the existence of available maternal supports (Lojkasek, Goldbert, Marcovitch, & MacGregor, 1990). The effectiveness of early intervention programs for children with disabilities has not gone without debate, since available research is often plagued by methodological flaws. Shonkoff, Hauser-Cram,

Krauss, and Upshur (1992) reviewed the existing literature on the effects of early intervention services, and concluded that most programs for infants and toddlers with disabilities are only moderately effective in producing short-term benefits as measured by traditional cognitive or developmental measures. However, other studies suggest that longer, more intense interventions may be more effective in the age range from birth to 5 years. Not only has functioning been found to be closer to normal development with early infancy training programs, but there are indications that early entry into intervention programs is more cost-effective than later entry into such programs (Warfield, 1994). In other words, the earlier that treatment for developmental skills is available for infants, the better.

Dmitriev (1988) has advocated an interdisciplinary training model for effectively teaching children with Down syndrome—a model in which medical, educational, and parental participation is essential. The educational program should also include parent training in behavior management and developmental concerns. Developing a sequence of tasks and skills to be obtained will provide parents with a hierarchy of skills required for their child to master certain developmental goals. In one study, Wishart (1991) found that, compared to nonhandicapped infants, those with Down syndrome made inefficient use of the cognitive abilities that they did have and would often remain passive even when a task was within their ability level. The implications are that the delayed developmental rate seen in children with Down syndrome may be due to an interaction between inadequate motivation levels and deficient learning. Fewell and Oelwein (1991) examined the effectiveness of the Model Preschool Program, which focused on children with Down syndrome and developmental delay. They found that of the six skill areas emphasized (gross motor skills, fine motor skills, cognition, receptive communication, expressive communication, and social/self-help skills), the children with Down syndrome made gains in all areas with the exception of gross motor skills on the Classroom Assessment of Development Skills. However, on the Battelle Developmental Inventory, expressive language in addition to fine and gross motor skills failed to show developmental improvements. Nonetheless, the project presented evidence that early intervention could be successful in some areas of development.

Behavioral interventions designed to incorporate functional communication training have been shown to be effective (Arndorfer, Miltenberger, Woster, Rortvedt, & Gaffaney, 1994). Although the number of families involved in this study was limited, the researchers utilized behavioral interviews, direct observation, and experimental analysis to determine the functions of the children's problem behaviors. The researchers then used functional communication training as an intervention. This procedure involved teaching a child a response that resulted in the same desired consequence as a problem behavior. Others have endorsed the use of naturalistic teaching to gain acquisition of targeted skills (Fox & Hanline, 1993). A methodology of this nature would involve using the natural environment, natural consequences, and child initiation to teach new tasks. However, both approaches need to be researched empirically in order to determine whether these methods are truly successful. In another experiment designed to increase vocal responsiveness in preschoolers with Down syndrome, positive reinforcement was found to be successful (Drash, Raver, Murrin, & Tudor, 1989). Children were trained using positive reinforcement (PR) alone, PR combined with dimming of lights, and PR combined with visual screening. All conditions were successful in increasing vocal responsiveness, with the two methods combining PR with other techniques producing the most improvement. It should be noted that a commonly used reinforcer (food) was not employed, in an effort to create a more socially valid paradigm. The results indicate that behavioral management techniques may be employed successfully to teach language skills.

Skills that preschool programs should concentrate on in order to increase independence include separation from parents, eating and drinking, handwashing, toileting, gross and fine motor skills, social skills, and language acquisition (see Love, 1988, and Oelwein, 1988, for model instructional plans). Cuskully, Zhang, and Gilmore (1998) advocate training self-regulation skills, such as the ability to delay gratification and mastery motivation, early in development to help foster greater independence later in adulthood. Principles of applied behavior analysis are often successful when instructors are attempting to teach such tasks as feeding, toileting, cessation of habitual tongue protrusion, and gross and fine motor skills. Since the developmental age of children with Down syndrome often lags behind their chronological age, it is necessary to maintain an awareness of which activities a child is ready to perform successfully.

Placement in a regular classroom may also improve academic attainment in children with Down syndrome. One study of academic attainment in children with Down syndrome aged 6–14 years found that although cognitive ability level had the greatest impact on achievement, type of school attended was the next largest contributing factor (Sloper, Cunningham, Turner, & Knussen, 1990). Additional factors influencing academic attainment were gender (female), paternal locus-of-control ratings, and chronological age. In a naturalistic classroom setting, 3-year-olds with Down syndrome were compared to normal 2- and 3-year-olds, as well as to another group with mild to moderate mental retardation, on some classroom behaviors (Bronson, Hauser-Cram, & Warfield, 1995). Both groups of children with developmental disabilities were found to perform lower on task mastery behaviors than either the typical 2-year-olds or 3-year-olds. The developmentally disabled groups completed only half as many tasks successfully as the typical children. In addition, both groups had higher rates of interaction with the teacher (i.e., more frequent demands for assistance). Compared to the other children with mental retardation, the children with Down syndrome actually made fewer requests of the teacher and peers, but their requests were more successful. These findings indicate that children with Down syndrome may benefit from working within a buddy system, given that they experience lower task mastery but relatively advanced social interaction skills. Some research has indicated that developmental gains in children with Down syndrome are not associated with time spent in an integrated classroom, and in fact that slightly higher gains in expressive language are made in nonintegrated settings (Fewell & Oelwein, 1990).

The use of computers to teach language skills has been advocated as another teaching tool (Meyers, 1988). In this forum, the computer provides structure and scaffolding for the acquisition of spoken and written language skills such as vocabulary, spelling, comprehension, and sentence construction. Language intervention, as advocated by Miller (1995), should be family-based. Parents and siblings should encourage communication about daily activities and events, and should be responsive to a child's interests and initiation of communication.

Beginning in adolescence, the child's emotional health should be carefully monitored for symptoms of depression. Individuals with Down syndrome are at increased risk for developing major depression and have also been noted to develop learned helplessness (Harris, 1988). Activities to build self-esteem and self-concept, as well as to provide training in vocational matters, should be initiated during middle or high school.

Parents and families of children with Down syndrome may be in need of support services as well. These children, as a result of their cognitive and physical limitations, may require a great amount of parental care. Barnett and Boyce (1995) found that parents of children with Down syndrome devoted more time to child care and spent less time in social activities than parents without a disabled child. Both mothers and fathers made accommodations in the amount of time they spent doing daily household activities. Single parents, who were not sampled in this study, may therefore have even greater difficulty responding to the needs of children with Down syndrome. As mentioned earlier, the siblings of children with Down syndrome may be at risk for developing behavior problems and adjustment disorders. Another study that examined ratings of parental stress found that parents of a child with Down syndrome reported more stress than comparison families (Cuskelly, Chant, & Hayes, 1998). For these reasons, it is important to provide these families with such resources as parent and sibling support groups.

ADOLESCENCE AND ADULTHOOD OUTCOMES

As a child with Down syndrome enters young adulthood, concerns regarding vocation and independent living emerge. Prior to the implementation of Public Law 94-142, the Education for All Handicapped Children Act of 1975, vocational training was not considered to be an integral part of service for adolescents with disabilities. Individuals should be prepared to function as independently as possible in society, and therefore should receive training in vocational and independent living skills. A greater range of opportunities currently exists for adolescents with Down syndrome as they approach completion of their educational careers. Sheltered workshops and other less restricted job sites are common places of eventual employment. On-the-job training may be provided through vocational schools, job coaches, community colleges, or sheltered workshops (Renzaglia & Hutchins, 1988).

Additional counseling should focus on further development of social skills, on sexuality, and on separation from parents. Brown (1996) advocates training adaptive work and social behaviors early in development to help prepare individuals for independent living later in life. Reproductive counseling for females is especially important, given the risk of producing a child with Down syndrome or congenital anomalies (Elkins, 1992). Most importantly, individuals with Down syndrome should be viewed as people first, with the same desires as nondisabled individuals for developing relationships and becoming productive adults. Assistance should focus on the development of well-rounded persons who can live in the least restrictive environment possible, whether that means independently in the community, in supervised semi-independent settings, or within group homes.

REFERENCES

Ariel, I., & Shvil, Y. (1992). Genitourinary system. In S. M. Pueschel & J. K. Pueschel (Eds.), *Biomedical concerns in persons with Down syndrome*. Baltimore: Paul H. Brookes.

Arndorfer, R. E., Miltenberger, R. G., Woster, S. H., Rortvedt, A. K., & Gaffaney, T. (1994). Home-based descriptive and experimental analysis of problem behaviors in children. *Topics in Early Childhood Special Education, 14*, 64–87.

Barnett, W. S., & Boyce, G. C. (1995). Effects of children with Down syndrome on parents' activities. *American Journal on Mental Retardation, 100*, 115–127.

Beasley, S. W., Allen, M., & Myers, N. (1997). The effects of Down syndrome and other chromosomal abnormalities on survival and management in oesophageal atresia. *Pediatric Surgery International, 12*, 550–551.

Beeghly, M., Perry, B. W., & Cicchetti, D. (1989). Structural and affective dimensions of play development in young children with Down syndrome. *International Journal of Behavioral Development, 12*, 257–277.

Benson, P. M., & Scherbenske, J. M. (1992). In S. M. Pueschel & J. K. Pueschel (Eds.), *Biomedical concerns in persons with Down syndrome*. Baltimore: Paul H. Brookes.

Block, M. E. (1991). Motor development in children with Down syndrome: A review of the literature. *Adapted Physical Activity Quarterly, 8,* 179–209.

Bower, A., & Hayes, A. (1995). Relations of scores on the Stanford Binet fourth edition and Form L-M: Concurrent validation study with children who have mental retardation. *American Journal on Mental Retardation, 99,* 555–563.

Brandt, B. R. (1996). Impaired tactual perception in children with Down's syndrome. *Scandinavian Journal of Psychology, 37,* 312–316.

Bronson, M. B., Hauser-Cram, P., & Warfield, M. E. (1995). Classroom behaviors of preschool children with and without developmental disabilities. *Journal of Applied Developmental Psychology, 16,* 371–390.

Brown, R. I. (1996). Partnership and marriage in Down syndrome. *Down Syndrome: Research and Practice, 4,* 96–99.

Carr, J. (1995). *Down's syndrome: Children growing up.* Cambridge, England: Cambridge University Press.

Catalano, R. A. (1992). Ophthalmologic concerns. In S. M. Pueschel & J. K. Pueschel (Eds.), *Biomedical concerns in persons with Down syndrome*. Baltimore: Paul H. Brookes.

Chapman, R. S., Seung, H., Schwartz, S. E., & Bird, E. K. (1998). Language skills of children and adolescents with Down syndrome: II. Production deficits. *Journal of Speech Language and Hearing Research, 41,* 861–873.

Coleman, M. (1988). Medical care of children and adults with Down syndrome. In V. Dmitriev & P. L. Oelwein (Eds.), *Advances in Down syndrome*. Seattle, WA: Special Child.

Cronk, C. E., & Anneren, G. (1992). Growth. In S. M. Pueschel & J. K. Pueschel (Eds.), *Biomedical concerns in persons with Down syndrome*. Baltimore: Paul H. Brookes.

Cuskelly, M., Chant, D., & Hayes, A. (1998). Behaviour problems in the siblings of children with Down syndrome: Associations with family responsibilities and parental stress. *International Journal of Disability, Development and Education, 45,* 295–311.

Cuskelly, M., & Dadds, M. (1992). Behavioral problems in children with Down's syndrome and their siblings. *Journal of Child Psychology and Psychiatry, 33,* 749–761.

Cuskelly, M., & Gunn, P. (1993). Maternal reports of behavior of siblings of children with Down syndrome. *American Journal on Mental Retardation, 97,* 521–529.

Cuskelly, M., Zhang, A., & Gilmore, L. (1998). The importance of self-regulation in young children with Down syndrome. *International Journal of Disability, Development and Education, 45,* 331–341.

Dahle, A. J., & Baldwin, R. L. (1992). Audiologic and otolaryngologic concerns. In S. M. Pueschel & J. K. Pueschel (Eds.), *Biomedical concerns in persons with Down syndrome*. Baltimore: Paul H. Brookes.

Dmitriev, V. (1988). Programs for children with Down syndrome and other developmental delays: Development of an educational model. In V. Dmitriev & P. L. Oelwein (Eds.), *Advances in Down syndrome*. Seattle, WA: Special Child.

Downs, M. P., & Balkany, T. J. (1988). Otologic problems and hearing impairment in Down syndrome. In V. Dmitriev & P. L. Oelwein (Eds.), *Advances in Down syndrome*. Seattle, WA: Special Child.

Drash, P. W., Raver, S. A., Murrin, M. R., & Tudor, R. M. (1989). Three procedures for increasing vocal response to therapist prompt in infants and children with Down syndrome. *American Journal on Mental Retardation, 94,* 64–73.

Dunst, C. J. (1990). Sensorimotor development of infants with Down syndrome. In V. Dmitriev & P. L. Oelwein (Eds.), *Advances in Down syndrome*. Seattle, WA: Special Child.

Dykens, E. M., Hodapp, R. M., & Evans, D. W. (1994). Profiles and development of adaptive behavior in children with Down syndrome. *American Journal on Mental Retardation, 98,* 580–587.

Elkins, T. E. (1992). Gynecologic care. In S. M. Pueschel & J. K. Pueschel (Eds.), *Biomedical concerns in persons with Down syndrome*. Baltimore: Paul H. Brookes.

402

Fewell, R. R., & Oelwein, P. L. (1990). The relationship between time in integrated environments and developmental gains in young children with special needs. *Topics in Early Childhood Special Education, 10,* 104–116.

Fewell, R. R., & Oelwein, P. L. (1991). Effective early intervention: Results from the Model Preschool Program for children with Down syndrome and other developmental delays. *Topics in Early Childhood Special Education, 11,* 56–68.

Fishler, K., & Koch, R. (1991). Mental development in Down syndrome mosaicism. *American Journal on Mental Retardation, 96,* 345–351.

Florez, J. (1992). Neurologic abnormalities. In S. M. Pueschel & J. K. Pueschel (Eds.), *Biomedical concerns in persons with Down syndrome.* Baltimore: Paul H. Brookes.

Fowler, A. E. (1988). Language abilities in children with Down syndrome: Evidence for a specific syntactic delay. In V. Dmitriev & P. L. Oelwein (Eds.), *Advances in Down syndrome.* Seattle, WA: Special Child.

Fox, L., & Hanline, M. F. (1993). A preliminary evaluation of learning within developmentally appropriate early childhood settings. *Topics in Early Childhood Special Education, 13,* 308–327.

Frangou, S., Aylward, E., Warren, A., Sharma, T., Barta, P., & Pearlson, G. (1997). Small planum temporale volume in Down's syndrome: A volumetric MRI study. *American Journal of Psychiatry, 154,* 1424–1429.

Ganiban, J., Wagner, S., & Cicchetti, D. (1990). Temperament and Down syndrome. In D. Cicchetti & M. Beeghly (Eds.), *Children with Down syndrome: A developmental perspective.* New York: Cambridge University Press.

Gibson, D. (1991). Searching for a life-span psychobiology of Down syndrome: Advancing educational and behavioral management strategies. *International Journal of Disability, Development and Education, 38,* 71–89.

Gunn, P., & Cuskelly, M. (1991). Down syndrome temperament: The stereotype at middle childhood and adolescence. *International Journal of Disability, Development and Education, 38,* 59–70.

Harris, J. C. (1988). Psychological adaptation and psychiatric disorders in adolescents and young adults with Down syndrome. In S. M. Pueschel (Ed.), *The young person with Down syndrome: Transition from adolescence to adulthood.* Baltimore: Paul H. Brookes.

Hassold, T., Sherman, S., & Hunt, P. A. (1995). The origin of trisomy in humans. In C. J. Epstein, T. Hassold, I. T. Lott, L. Nadel, & D. Patterson (Eds.), *Etiology and pathogenesis of Down syndrome.* New York: Wiley-Liss.

Hijii, T., Fukushige, J., Igarashi, H., Takahashi, N., & Ueda, K. (1997). Life expectancy and social adaptation in individuals with Down syndrome with and without surgery for congenital heart disease. *Clinical Pediatrics, 36,* 327–332.

Hodapp, R. M., Leckman, J. F., Dykens, E. M., Sparrow, S. S., Zelinsky, D. G., & Ort, S. I. (1992). K-ABC profiles in children with fragile X syndrome, Down syndrome, and nonspecific mental retardation. *American Journal on Mental Retardation, 97,* 39–46.

Hodapp, R. M., & Zigler, E. (1990). Applying the developmental perspective to individuals with Down syndrome. In D. Cicchetti & M. Beeghly (Eds.), *Children with Down syndrome: A developmental perspective.* New York: Cambridge University Press.

Howenstein, M. S. (1992). Pulmonary concerns. In I. T. Lott & E. E. McCoy (Eds.), *Down syndrome: Advances in medical care.* New York: Wiley-Liss.

Jobling, A. (1998). Motor development in school-aged children with Down syndrome: A longitudinal perspective. *International Journal of Disability, Development and Education, 45,* 283–293.

Kamphaus, R. W. (1993). *Clinical assessment of children's intelligence.* Needham Heights, MA: Allyn & Bacon.

Kneips, L. J., Walden, T. A., & Baxter, A. (1994). Affective expressions of toddlers with and without Down syndrome in a social referencing context. *American Journal on Mental Retardation, 99,* 301–312.

Korenberg, J. R., Pulst, S. M., & Gerwehr, S. (1992). Advances in the understanding of chromosone 21 and Down syndrome. In I. T. Lott & E. E. McCoy (Eds.), *Down syndrome: Advances in medical care.* New York: Wiley-Liss.

Lai, F. (1992). Alzheimer disease. In S. M. Pueschel & J. K. Pueschel (Eds.), *Biomedical concerns in persons with Down syndrome.* Baltimore: Paul H. Brookes.

Lalli, J. S., Browder, D. M., Mace, F. C., & Brown, D. K. (1993). Teacher use of descriptive analysis data to implement interventions to decrease students' problem behaviors. *Journal of Applied Behavior Analysis, 26,* 227–238.

Landry, S. H., Miller-Loncar, C. L., & Swank, P. R. (1998). Goal-directed behavior in children with Down syndrome: The role of joint play situations. *Early Education and Development, 9,* 375–392.

Levy, J. (1992). Gastrointestinal concerns. In S. M. Pueschel & J. K. Pueschel (Eds.), *Biomedical concerns in persons with Down syndrome.* Baltimore: Paul H. Brookes.

Lojkasek, M., Goldberg, S., Marcovitch, S., & MacGregor, D. (1990). Influences on maternal responsiveness to developmentally delayed preschoolers. *Journal of Early Intervention, 14,* 260–273.

Lott, I. T., & McCoy, E. E. (Eds.). (1992). *Down syndrome: Advances in medical care.* New York: Wiley-Liss.

Love, P. L. (1988). The early preschool program: The bridge between infancy and childhood. In V. Dmitriev & P. L. Oelwein (Eds.), *Advances in Down syndrome.* Seattle, WA: Special Child.

Lubin, B. H., Cahn, S., & Scott, M. (1992). Hematologic manifestations. In S. M. Pueschel & J. K. Pueschel (Eds.), *Biomedical concerns in persons with Down syndrome.* Baltimore: Paul H. Brookes.

Marino, B. (1992). Cardiac aspects. In S. M. Pueschel & J. K. Pueschel (Eds.), *Biomedical concerns in persons with Down syndrome.* Baltimore: Paul H. Brookes.

Meyers, L. F. (1988). Using computers to teach children with Down syndrome spoken and written language skills. In L. Nadel (Ed.), *The psychobiology of Down syndrome.* Cambridge, MA: MIT Press.

Miller, J. F. (1995). Individual differences in vocabulary acquisition in children with Down syndrome. In C. J. Epstein, T. Hassold, I. T. Lott, L. Nadel, & D. Patterson (Eds.), *Etiology and pathogenesis of Down syndrome.* New York: Wiley-Less.

Mufson, E. J., Benzing, W. C., & Kordower, J. H. (1995). Dissociation of galaninergic and neruotrophic plasticity in Down syndrome and Alzheimer disease. In C. J. Epstein, T. Hassold, I. T. Lott, L. Nadel, & D. Patterson (Eds.), *Etiology and pathogenesis of Down syndrome.* New York: Wiley-Liss.

Myers, B. A. (1992). Psychiatric disorders. In S. M. Pueschel & J. K. Pueschel (Eds.), *Biomedical concerns in persons with Down syndrome.* Baltimore: Paul H. Brookes.

Niva, R. A. (1988). Eye abnormalities and their treatment. In V. Dmitriev & P. L. Oelwein (Eds.), *Advances in Down syndrome.* Seattle, WA: Special Child.

Oelwein, P. L. (1988). Preschool and kindergarten programs: Strategies for meeting objectives. In V. Dmitriev & P. L. Oelwein (Eds.), *Advances in Down syndrome.* Seattle, WA: Special Child.

Pearlson, G. D., Breiter, S. N., Aylward, E. H., Warren, A. C., Grygorcewizc, M., Frangou, S., Barta, P. E., & Pulsifer, M. B. (1998). MRI brain changes in subjects with Down syndrome with and without dementia. *Developmental Medicine and Child Neurology, 40,* 326–334.

Pipes, P. L. (1992). Nutritional aspects. In S. M. Pueschel & J. K. Pueschel (Eds.), *Biomedical concerns in persons with Down syndrome.* Baltimore: Paul H. Brookes.

Prescott, G. H. (1988). Genetic counseling for families about Down syndrome. In V. Dmitriev & P. L. Oelwein (Eds.), *Advances in Down syndrome.* Seattle, WA: Special Child.

Pueschel, S. M. (1992a). General health care and therapeutic approaches. In S. M. Pueschel & J. K. Pueschel (Eds.), *Biomedical concerns in persons with Down syndrome.* Baltimore: Paul H. Brookes.

Pueschel, S. M. (1992b). Phenotypic characteristics. In S. M. Pueschel & J. K. Pueschel (Eds.), *Biomedical concerns in persons with Down syndrome.* Baltimore: Paul H. Brookes.

Pueschel, S. M. (1995). *Babies with Down syndrome: A new parents' guide* (2nd ed.). Bethesda, MD: Woodbine House.

Pueschel, S. M., & Bier, J. B. (1992). Endrocrinologic aspects. In S. M. Pueschel & J. K. Pueschel (Eds.), *Biomedical concerns in persons with Down syndrome.* Baltimore: Paul H. Brookes.

Pueschel, S. M., & Solga, P. M. (1992). Musculoskeletal disorders. In S. M. Pueschel & J. K. Pueschel (Eds.), *Biomedical concerns in persons with Down syndrome.* Baltimore: Paul H. Brookes.

Quine, L., & Rutter, D. R. (1994). First diagnosis of severe mental and physical disability: A study of doctor–parent communication. *Journal of Child Psychology and Psychiatry, 35,* 1273–1287.

Renzaglia, A., & Hutchins, M. P. (1988). Establishing vocational training programs for school-age students with moderate and severe handicaps. In S. M. Pueschel (Ed.), *The young person with Down syndrome: Transition from adolescence to adulthood.* Baltimore: Paul H. Brookes.

Rubin, S. S., Rimmer, J. H., Chicoine, B., Braddock, D., & McGuire, D. E. (1998). Overweight prevalence in persons with Down syndrome. *Mental Retardation, 36,* 175–181.

Ruskin, E. M., Kasari, C., Mundy, P., & Sigman, M. (1994). Attention to people and toys during social and object mastery in children with Down syndrome. *American Journal on Mental Retardation, 99,* 103–111.

Sadovnick, A. D., & Baird, P. A. (1992). Life expectancy. In S. M. Pueschel & J. K. Pueschel (Eds.), *Biomedical concerns in persons with Down syndrome.* Baltimore: Paul H. Brookes.

Scola, P. S. (1992). Disorders of the liver. In S. M. Pueschel & J. K. Pueschel (Eds.), *Biomedical concerns in persons with Down syndrome.* Baltimore: Paul H. Brookes.

Sexton, D., Thompson, B., Perez, J., & Rheams, T. (1990). Maternal versus professional estimates of developmental status for young children with handicaps: An ecological approach. *Topics in Early Childhood Special Education, 10,* 80–95.

Shonkoff, J. P., Hauser-Cram, P., Krauss, M. W., & Upshur, C. C. (1992). Development of infants with disabilities and their families: Implications for theory and services delivery. *Monographs of the Society for Research in Child Development, 57*(6, Serial No. 230), 1–17.

Sloper, P., Cunningham, C., Turner, S., & Knussen, C. (1990). Factors related to the academic attainments of children with Down's syndrome. *British Journal of Educational Psychology, 60,* 284–298.

Smith, B., & Phillips, C. J. (1992). Attainments of severely mentally retarded adolescents by aetiology. *Journal of Child Psychology and Psychiatry, 33,* 1039–1058.

Strauss, D., & Eyman, R. K. (1996). Mortality of people with mental retardation in California with and without Down syndrome, 1986–1991. *American Journal of Mental Retardation, 100,* 643–653.

Thombs, B., & Sugden, D. (1991). Manual skills in Down syndrome children ages 6 to 16 years. *Adapted Physical Activity Quarterly, 8,* 242–254.

Tingey, C., Mortensen, L., Matheson, P., & Doret, W. (1991). Developmental attainment of infants and young children with Down syndrome. *International Journal of Disability, Development and Education, 38,* 15–26.

Ugazio, A. G., Maccario, R., & Burgio, G. R. (1992). Immunologic features. In S. M. Pueschel & J. K. Pueschel (Eds.), *Biomedical concerns in persons with Down syndrome.* Baltimore: Paul H. Brookes.

Vaughn, B. E., Contreras, J., & Seifer, R. (1994). Short-term longitudinal study of maternal ratings of temperament in samples of children with Down syndrome and children who are developing normally. *American Journal on Mental Retardation, 98,* 607–618.

Vigild, M. (1992). Oral health conditions. In S. M. Pueschel & J. K. Pueschel (Eds.), *Biomedical concerns in persons with Down syndrome.* Baltimore: Paul H. Brookes.

Visser, F. E., Aldenkamp, A. P., van Huffelen, A. C., & Kuilman, M. (1997). Prospective study of the prevalence of Alzheimer-type dementia in institutionalized individuals with Down syndrome. *American Journal on Mental Retardation, 101,* 400–412.

Warfield, M. E. (1994). A cost-effectiveness analysis of early intervention services in Massachusetts: Implications for policy. *Educational Evaluation and Policy Analysis, 16,* 87–99.

Weitzner-Lin, B. (1997). A comparison of international communication in children who have Down syndrome with typical children matched for developmental and chronological age. *Infant-Toddler Intervention, 7,* 123–132.

Wishart, J. G. (1991). Taking the initiative in learning: A developmental investigation of infants with Down syndrome. *International Journal of Disability, Development and Education, 38,* 27–44.

Wishart, J. G. (1995). Cognitive abilities in children with Down syndrome: Developmental instability and motivational deficits. In C. J. Epstein, T. Hassold, I. T. Lott, L. Nadel, & D. Patterson (Eds.), *Etiology and pathogenesis of Down syndrome.* New York: Wiley-Liss.

Wishart, J. G., & Duffy, L. (1990). Instability of performance on cognitive tests in infants and young children with Down's syndrome. *British Journal of Educational Psychology, 60,* 10–22.

Zickler, C. F., Morrow, J. D., & Bull, M. J. (1998). Infants with Down syndrome: A look at temperament. *Journal of Pediatric Health Care, 12,* 111–117.

18

KLINEFELTER SYNDROME

HEATHER CODY
GEORGE HYND

Klinefelter syndrome (KS) is a disorder seen in males resulting from an abnormality found at the chromosomal level. It was first described in 1942 by Klinefelter, Reifenstein, and Albright, who used the term to describe a small group of infertile men. More than a decade later, the discovery of an extra X chromosome was used to further distinguish the syndrome. Consequently, KS is considered a sex chromosome disorder. Normally, males are born with 46 chromosomes, with their gender being defined by a pairing of an X and a Y sex chromosome. Males born with KS, however, typically show an XXY pattern. There are some other variations, such as XXXY or XXXXY, and also cases considered to reflect mosaicism, which is characterized as a combination of normal and abnormal cells. The prevalence of KS has been estimated at between 1 in 700 and 1 in 900 live-born males (Drugan, Isada, Johnson, & Evans, 1996b; Rovet, Netley, Keenan, Bailey, & Stewart, 1996). Estimates conducted in Denmark of all males born during a 13-year period reported the incidence rate to be as high as 1 in 426 (Nielsen & Wohlert, 1991).

Earlier studies of males with KS found an increased risk for psychiatric disorders, criminality, and mental retardation (Forssman, 1970; Schroder, Chapelle, Hokola, & Virkkunen, 1981). These studies, however, had serious methodological problems, as they were generally conducted with institutionalized or imprisoned populations (Cohen & Durham, 1985). Unfortunately, even some fairly recent literature tends to rely on these early findings to describe individuals with KS as having high rates of incarceration and mental problems (Gilbert, 1993).

More recent research indicates that although some individuals with KS experience significant cognitive, psychiatric, and/or behavioral problems, outcomes are not as grim as the earlier conceptualizations indicated. Several longitudinal studies have contributed to our understanding of developmental outcomes in KS. For example, large prospective studies conducted during the late 1960s and early 1970s compiled outcome data for children born with sex chromosome abnormalities. Bender and Berch (1991) outlined the most important findings from this research. First, children with sex chromosome disorders appear to display increased risk for developmental, language, learning, and behavioral problems, compared to nondisabled children; however, their profiles appear relatively "normal" when contrasted with earlier stereotypes, thus supporting the notion that earlier studies examined biased samples. Second, there is a great deal of variability in the phenotype of children with the same syndrome, and family influences may mediate the amount of dysfunction displayed. Because of the significant variability associated with KS, our description of KS in this chapter addresses the most recent and well-accepted findings regarding these children and their neuropsychological functioning.

GENETIC AND FAMILIAL ISSUES RELATED TO ETIOLOGY

There are several different types of genetic disorders. These include autosomal dominant disorders (e.g., Huntington chorea), autosomal recessive disorders (e.g., phenylketonuria), X-linked disorders (e.g., Lesch–Nyhan syndrome), and those that involve chromosome abnormalities. KS falls into this last category, since it is caused by a sex chromosome abnormality. The phenomenon that results in the abnormality is referred to as "nondisjunction." This occurs when a pair of chromosomes fail to separate during either the first or second division of meiosis. When nondisjunction occurs, it results in "aneuploidy" (the addition or absence of a single chromosome). Aneuploidy is the most common type of chromosome anomaly found in live births or spontaneous abortions, occurring in approximately 3% of all confirmed pregnancies (Evans, Drugan, Pryde, & Johnson, 1996). Rather than the normal XY genotype that signifies the male gender, these boys will typically display a trisomy or XXY pattern of sex chromosomes. Roughly 50% of KS cases are caused by maternal meiotic errors, with three-fourths of these reported to show significant effects of maternal age (Gardner & Sutherland, 1996). Some have reported maternal age to be a contributing factor in approximately 60% of a sample of males with KS (Drugan et al., 1996b), while others have found rates of paternal nondisjunction to occur in slightly over half (57%) of the cases, with the exception of those directly linked to advanced maternal age (Evans et al., 1996). Approximately 10% of individuals with KS exhibit mosaicism, meaning that not all cells examined display trisomy of the sex chromosomes; instead, some show a normal XY pattern (Pierce, 1990).

KS is one of the most frequently occurring sex chromosome abnormalities seen in males. In general, the sex chromosome abnormalities produce less significant impairments than do abnormalities in autosomes (e.g., Down syndrome, Edwards syndrome). Hynd and Willis (1988) noted two hypotheses for this distinction. First, the Y sex chromosome appears to carry only information necessary for gender determination; second, any number of X chromosomes greater than the normal one appears to become relatively inactive in early fetal development.

A diagnosis of KS is made through karyotyping of the chromosome. This may be done either prenatally or postnatally through amniocentesis or chorionic villus sampling (Pierce, 1990). There are no familial indicators that would suggest a higher risk for producing a child with KS, although females with trisomy XXX have been reported to be at greater risk for producing offspring with KS or XXX, and, in fewer cases, offspring with trisomy 21 and monosomy XO (Drugan et al., 1996b). Maternal age is a risk factor for any pregnancy, and in these cases a prenatal diagnosis of KS may be possible. Characteristic physical features may or may not be present at birth, and therefore the existence of an extra X chromosome may not be discovered until puberty or during testing for infertility (Drugan, Isada, Johnson, & Evans, 1996a). In most cases, the physical characteristics (e.g., small testes, abnormal leg length) are not visible at birth, and there is no obvious reason for genetic testing to be conducted. In an overview of genetic disorders and their onset, Weatherall (1991) placed the average age for first appearance of KS-related impairments at age 5. These are most likely to be the abnormal growth rate and elongated leg length. Abramsky and Chapple (1998) conducted a four-year study on the diagnosis of boys with KS and determined that the most common indicator leading to karotyping (and diagnosis) was hypogonadism and/or infertility. They noted that otherwise these children would have been undiagnosed.

MEDICAL CONCERNS AND COMORBID DISORDERS

As noted above, the sex chromosome disorders generally have less of an impact on the phenotype than do autosomal disorders. With autosomal trisomies, for example, there may be multiple affected systems and greater physical anomalies. The sex chromosome trisomies cause less global impairment. However, the development and function of the sex organs, hormonal production, and reproduction are all negatively affected by sex chromosome trisomies (Evans et al., 1996).

Genital Anomalies

In a review of the literature on the physical characteristics of KS, Theilgaard (1984) found several classic attributes common among these individuals. Among the chief features of this syndrome are endocrinological disturbances, which impair normal genital and sexual development. According to Schwartz and Root (1991), KS is the most common cause of hypogonadism in males. This becomes problematic during puberty, as secondary sex characteristics may be diminished by restricted levels of testosterone. At puberty, hyalinization and atrophy of the seminiferous tubules are also common. Normally, the seminiferous tuberules make up 85% of the volume in the testes, but in males with KS the testes are often noted by midchildhood to be abnormally small in size (Bender & Berch, 1991; Schwartz & Root, 1991). Typically, although testes size is smaller than average (3–5 ml volume), penis size is normal (Ratcliffe, Bancroft, Axworthy, & McLaren, 1982a). Infertility is caused by azoospermia and is one of the primary disabling features of KS because it is not treatable.

Hormonal Disturbances

Increased levels of gonadotropin produced by the pituitary have been reported in males with KS, as well as decreased androgen production in the testes. In addition, males display lower levels of testosterone and higher concentrations of luteinizing hormone (LH) and follicle-stimulating hormone (FSH) upon entering adolescence (Robinson et al., 1986). LH stimulates testosterone secretion, while FSH stimulates the development of sperm during puberty. Therefore, although males with KS will enter puberty at a normal age, inadequate testosterone secretion prevents normal puberty (Styne, 1991). There have been some mixed accounts of thyroid conditions (particularly hypothyroidism) in these children, with some studies indicating an increased incidence for congenital hypothyroidism and others showing no significant findings (Schwartz & Root, 1991). There have also been accounts of acne conglobata associated with KS, which was linked to elevated LH and FSH (Wollenberg et al., 1997).

Neurological Findings

Some literature indicates that abnormal electroencephalograms and seizure activity are seen more frequently in males with KS than in the general population. Whether or not there is an increased incidence of epilepsy in these males has not been determined conclusively. Neuromuscular findings show that when compared to controls, boys with KS have lower scores on tasks involving fine and gross motor skills, coordination, speed and dexterity, and strength (Robinson et al., 1986).

Other Physical Features

Older case descriptions associate cryptorchidism and hypospadias with KS, but these are not common problems. Boys with KS are typically taller than average because of elongated legs, and this feature can be seen prior to puberty. They appear to be at an increased risk for osteoporosis as a result of their androgen deficiency, which causes a decrease in bone mineral content (Schwartz & Root, 1991). A clinical study of 24 adult males with KS found a higher-than-average occurrence of tall stature, obesity, diabetes mellitus, hyperlipemia, hypercholesterolemia, gall bladder disease, chronic pulmonary infection, and peptic ulcer (Zuppinger, Engel, Forbes, Mantooth, & Claffey, 1967). Interestingly, this investigation found that a family history of diabetes mellitus was present in a majority of these cases, leading to the hypothesis that a genetic predisposition for diabetes may exist in some individuals with KS. Later work has found that patients with KS do have a higher incidence of diabetes mellitus, and when compared to normal controls, they are found to display insulin resistance (Pei, Sheu, Jeng, Liao, & Fuh, 1998). Another description by Evans et al. (1996) included increased occurrence of elbow dysplasia, elongated limbs, chronic bronchitis, and poor fine motor coordination. They found diabetes to occur in 8% of their total population of individuals with KS. Some variants of KS (e.g., XXXY and XXXXY) have been associated with short stature or radioulnar synostosis (Schwartz & Root, 1991).

Reports of comorbidity for renal, cardiac, or lymphatic conditions have not been confirmed in this population (Evans et al., 1996). Other nonspecific features include increased occurrence of fatigue, venous stasis ulcers, or essential tremor (Schwartz & Root, 1991). Leg ulceration has also been associated with KS, resulting from elevations in plasminogen activator inhibitor-1 (PAI-1) (Zollner et al., 1997). At times, patients with leg ulcerations may be found to have KS, as discovered in a 47-year-old man suffering from recurrent leg ulcers who was noted to be hypogonadal (Tyler, Kungl, & Green, 1998). Of the few accounts of cardiac defects associated with KS, these appear to occur more frequently in the rarer cases of polysomy (e.g., XXXXY) than in cases of the typical XXY presentation (Elias & Yanangi, 1981). The number and severity of these cardiac defects may also be correlated with the degree of polysomy. A large study of cancer incidence in a group of 696 men (Hasle, Mellemgaard, Nielsen, & Hansen, 1995) found increased risk of cancer (mediastinal germ cell) in the 15–30 year age group. Bebb, Grannis, Paz, Slovak, and Chilcote (1998) reported on a case of a child treated for a mediastinal mass. They state that among patients with KS, germ cell tumors are 50 times more common than in the general population, present at an early age, and are seldom testicular in location. Others (Hultborn et al., 1997) report that males with KS have a prevalance rate of 7.5 percent for breast cancer, putting them at greater risk than the normal male population. Low grade B-cell non-Hodgkin lymphoma has also been reported in KS, but at a lesser rate (Humphreys, Lavery, Morris, & Nevin, 1997).

DEVELOPMENTAL COURSE

Schwartz and Root (1991) outlined common clinical presentations at the various developmental stages. During infancy, KS may be discovered during routine evaluations of hypospadias, microphallus, or cryptorchidism. School-age children may present with learning or behavioral problems. During adolescence, clinical presentations may result from gynecomastia, delayed onset of puberty, abnormally tall stature, small testes, or eunuchoid habitus. Adults may be discovered during evaluations for malignancies and/or tumors, and also during investigations of infertility.

Physical Development and Puberty

Generally, physical development in KS follows normal patterns until the child reaches adolescence, when specific disturbances in puberty result. Motor developmental milestones are not significantly different from normal. Height is usually greater than normal, due to abnormally long legs (Pierce, 1990). Bender and Berch (1991) noted that these males typically display reduced sensory–motor integration and motor strength. These children may also appear to be slower and less coordinated than their siblings.

For the purposes of comparison, normal pubertal development is briefly reviewed. Normal secondary sexual development in males involves genital development and pubic hair growth. Features of puberty related to the external genitalia may begin to develop at any time from age 11 to 15 years (Wheeler, 1991); this process involves the growth of the testes, maturation of the scrotum, and growth of the penis. In males with KS, the size of the penis is within normal limits, but the testes begin to be distinguished by diminished size and maturation. Androgens control pubic hair growth, and (as mentioned above) males with KS have decreased androgen production, which results in diminished or absent hair growth. Normally, pubic hair growth as well as axillary and facial hair growth follow on the heels of genital development. In KS, this growth may be delayed, diminished, or absent. During puberty, the voice normally deepens and the bulbourethral glands enlarge. Both processes may be abnormal in KS. In addition, while some breast enlargement is typical in normal adolescence, in KS there may be significant gynecomastia (Wheeler, 1991). Other major features characteristic of normal pubertal development in males include alterations in lean body mass and fat distribution, and rapid skeletal growth. In males with KS, fat distribution may mimic that of females (e.g., hip and thigh) (Wheeler, 1991). Figure 18.1 is a photograph of a typical individual with KS.

Therefore, physical features at puberty may involve absent or diminished growth of facial, chest, and pubic hair. Gynecomastia, eunuchoidism, and feminine fat distribution may also be present in these males, although varying degrees of these conditions have been reported (Pierce, 1990). Schwartz and Root (1991) estimate that from 30% to 60% or more of all children with KS will exhibit gynecomastia by late puberty, and place the prevalence rate of carcinoma of the breast in this population at 9 in 1,000. They are careful to note that although this rate is above that for normal men and one-fifth the rate for women, the role of the extra X chromosome in this higher risk for carcinoma in KS is unknown.

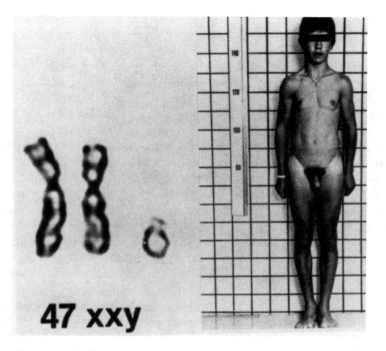

FIGURE 18.1. Patient with Klinefelter syndrome at age 13 years. (Courtesy K. Khoury; karyotype courtesy M. Rochon, Sherbrooke, Quebec, Canada.) From *Pediatric Neurology: Principles and Practice*, edited by K. F. Swaiman, 1989, St. Louis, MO: C. V. Mosby. Copyright 1989 by Mosby–Year Book, Inc. Reprinted by permission.

Severe gynecomastia is not improved with androgen therapy, and mastectomy is often recommended when there are significant physical or psychological concerns.

Neurological Development

Two hypotheses regarding neurological development have been put forth by Bender and Berch (1991) to explain the characteristics seen in sex chromosome disorders. One hypothesis is that the presence of a sex chromosome anomaly may alter normal patterns of brain growth, resulting in abnormal rates of brain tissue growth and maturation, which will then have an impact on functioning. This causal pattern, implicated in cases of extra X chromosomes, is that the extra chromosome interferes with left-hemisphere specialization for language, resulting in decreased language functioning. The second hypothesis involves the impact that hormones may have on brain growth and functioning. For example, the abnormal testosterone levels seen in individuals with KS may be related to their impairments in verbal ability. Bender and Berch were careful to point out, however, that neither hypothesis has been proven conclusively with physiological, empirical evidence. Some implications for differences in brain growth patterns have been made by studying dermal ridges. These may be used as indicators of prenatal growth because they become differentiated during midfetal development and remain constant from that point. Netley and Rovet (1982) found evidence for diminished dermal ridge counts in a group of KS children, indicating that their prenatal growth is slower.

Hemispheric specialization in individuals with KS has been studied by observing differences in their performance on verbal and nonverbal tasks. Netley and Rovet (1984) found that a group of boys with KS performed more poorly than controls on a number of tasks involving lateral presentation of material. For example, the KS boys did more poorly on dichotic stop consonants, although their performance was better than that of controls on dichotic melodies and half-field dots. The authors interpreted these findings to mean that boys with KS have difficulty in dealing efficiently with information normally preferentially processed by the left hemisphere, and that their right-hemispheric functions appear to play a larger role in both nonverbal and verbal processing. Overall, when compared to age-matched controls, children with KS were found to display diminished left-hemisphere specialization for language and enhanced right-hemisphere specialization for nonverbal processing (Netley, 1991). Their finding is supported by the fact that language deficits are also seen in females with XXX, particularly in expressive language and auditory processing (Walzer et al., 1986). A study examining dichotic listening performance found that for the KS group compared to a control group, left-hemispheric processing was impaired when they were presented with dichotic syllables (Theilgaard, 1984).

Still another hypothesis implicating hemispheric influences was advanced by Money (1993). After observing that the types of language difficulties often exhibited by these children involve some problem with temporal sequencing (e.g., narrative sequencing), he noted that these difficulties may be associated with anomalies found in the left hemisphere. Although Money's was not an empirical study, it does call into further question the role of the normal development of hemispheric specialization.

Cognitive Development

There are distinctions between the cognitive deficits seen in trisomies of the sex chromosomes and those associated with the autosomal trisomies. Individuals with sex chromosome trisomies may have normal or above-average intelligence, and if mental retardation is present, it is typically found to be in the mild range. Autosomal trisomies, on the other hand, usually result in profound mental retardation (Evans et al., 1996). Generally, research studies indicate that children with KS may display a wide range of intellectual ability, ranging from mild mental retardation to above-average intelligence. Bender and Berch (1991), commenting on the 23-year prospective Denver study done by Bender's group, note that the Full Scale IQs of individuals with KS are likely to be 10–15 points lower than those of controls, which would result in a slight increase in the possibility of a diagnosis of mental retardation. However, this finding using Full Scale IQs may mask discrepancies found between scores on Verbal and Performance scales. Another prospective study (Walzer et al., 1986) found that for a small group of boys with KS, their mean Full Scale IQ scores did not differ significantly from those of controls. However, they did exhibit significantly lower Verbal IQ scores.

One consistent finding among children with KS has been deficits in their verbal abilities. Verbal IQ scores on traditional measures (e.g., the Wechsler scales) are generally below average, while Performance IQ is normal (Ratcliffe et al., 1982a). On average, individuals with sex chromosome abnormalities have been described by some as mildly mentally retarded, but the average IQ for children with KS is estimated to be a standard score of 89 (Smith, 1981). Some have hypothesized that the presence of an extra X chromosome is what deflates the verbal skills, since females with an extra X chromosome also display impaired verbal ability (Netley & Rovet, 1982; Cohen & Durham, 1985). Others propose that the extra X chromosome represents a risk factor for a specific developmental reading disorder (Bender, Puck, Salbenblatt, & Robinson, 1986). In a small prospective study of the development of children with sex chromosome anomalies, Leonard and Sparrow (1986) found that boys with KS displayed variable intelligence. For example, one subject displayed average intelligence, while others fell in the below-average range. Netley (1987) sought to predict intellectual attainment in children with KS from the psychometric data of their siblings. He found that compared to their siblings, the boys with KS had lower intelligence, particularly in the verbal domain, although their IQ scores were highly correlated with those of their unaffected siblings. This would indicate that aptitude in young boys with KS could be predicted from that of their siblings.

In an exhaustive literature review on the cognitive profile of boys with KS, Rovet et al. (1996) concluded that a chronic cognitive deficit in verbal abilities and language processing was consistent across 27 independent research studies (see Table 18.1). A general pattern of underachievement in school and of risk for dyslexia was also evident in these children. Rovet et al. (1996) conducted their own longitudinal study of cognitive functioning in KS. They followed 36 boys and 33 sibling controls for 20 years. Their findings indicated that compared to controls, boys with KS demonstrated significantly depressed verbal ability contrasted with normal nonverbal ability. Walzer, Bashir, and Silbert (1990) found IQ to be 10–15 points lower than that of average peers in a group of 13 boys with KS. Of these, 11 had demonstrated problems in reading and spelling throughout their academic histories.

In cases of polysomies (e.g., XXXY, XXXXY), the level of intellectual impairment appears to increase with the number of additional X chromosomes. Mental retardation is frequent in those individuals who have four or more X chromosomes (Gardner & Sutherland, 1996). Behavioral difficulties also appear more frequently in this population. One case of a child with XXXXY was reported in which the child did not display severe mental retardation or abnormal social development (Sheridan & Radlinski, 1988). However, the authors noted that early intervention for learning and a supportive home environment may have contributed to this atypical presentation.

Language Development

Young boys with KS have also been noted to display delayed speech and language development. Specific deficits have been discovered in the areas of articulation, comprehension, verbal abstraction, sequencing, and expressing a story idea (Mandoki, Sumner, Hoffman, & Riconda, 1991). Language delays have been demonstrated up to 8 or 9 years of age, and some research indicates that it may continue through adulthood. In the longitudinal study mentioned above, Rovet et al. (1996) determined that males with KS had greater difficulty on tasks involving auditory memory, language comprehension, and language expression. This finding supports an earlier report by Leonard and Sparrow (1986), who found language delays in a small sample of males with KS. These subjects displayed delayed language development, limited vocabulary and syntax, difficulty with concepts, and lack of fluency. In the prospective study by Walzer et al. (1986), speech and language delays were evident by the third year of life. Specifically, parents reported problems with articulation, word finding, sentence formation, and expressive language. Assessment of these children indicated that although receptive language was age-appropriate, deficits existed in auditory memory and expressive language (e.g., syntax, dysnomia, and narrative production).

TABLE 18.1. Intelligence and Achievement Characteristics of Boys with Klinefelter Syndrome

Study	Country/city	n	Karyotype	Ascertainment	Age	Controls	Measures	Results	Conclusions
Nielsen et al. (1970)	Denmark/Aarhus	11	47,XXY 46,XY/47,XXY	CR	8.0–15.0	Yes	WISC WAIS School reports	Referred to psychiatric service due to problems at school, difficulty relating to other children. School problems in 82%.	Early diagnosis of SCA important so appropriate school placement, special teaching can be arranged.
Walzer & Gerald (1977)	USA/Boston, MA	13	47,XXY	NS	5.0–7.0	Yes	Bayley WPPSI	All XXY past Grade 1 given reading evaluations; 3 of 5 had moderate–severe reading, spelling, writing problems and LDs.	Developmental language deficits seen as expressive language problems (temporal sequencing, comprehension).
Funderburk & Ferjo (1978)	Sweden	11	47,XXY	CS	6.8–24.0	No	WISC WAIS	High frequency of speech and language problems, but normal intelligence. School underachievement in 9 (82%).	Appropriate educational intervention may diminish some long-term intellectual and psychiatric problems in some XXY males.
Leonard, Schowalter, Landy, Ruddle, & Lubs (1979)	USA/New Haven, CT	11	47,XXY 47,XYY 47,XXX 45,X	NS	8.0–9.5	Yes	School records	Grades repeated by 55% of SCA children, 0% of controls. Delayed language development, deficits in vocabulary, articulation.	Mild LDs and decreased achievement not attributed solely to SCA.

Study	Country	N	Karyotype		Age		Measures	Findings	Conclusions
Robinson, Lubs, & Bergsma (1979)	USA/Denver, CO	51	47,XXY 47,XYY 47,XXX	NS	5.0–11.0	Yes	School	School problems in 50% of XXY versus 32% of controls.	Possible increased risk for learning problems based on karyotype.
Stewart et al. (1979)	Canada/Toronto	47	47,XXY 47,XYY 47,XXX 47,XX male X/XX	NS	0.0–0.8	Yes	McCarthy WISC-R WRAT Rutter Parent Vineland	XXY deficits in reading and spelling, not arithmetic.	XXY similar to XXX, but less severe memory deficit in XXX.
Pennington, Bender, Puck, Salbenblatt, & Robinson (1982)	USA/Denver, CO	44	47,XXY 47,XXX 45,X Mosaics	NS	9.3–12.5	Yes	WPPSI PIAT School reports	School intervention in 69% of pure SCA children, 26% of controls. LDs in 60% of SCA subjects, 26% of mosaics and controls. Specific reading LDs in 27% of 47,XXY.	Depressed VIQ, reading and spelling delays in 47,XXY.
Ratcliffe, Bancroft, Axworthy, & McLaren (1982a)	UK/Edinburgh	12	47,XXY	NS	16.0–18.0	Yes	WISC-R WAIS BSRI HSPQ	No difference between XXY and controls until high school. Eight (67%) had learning, behavior problems, compared to 2 (17%) controls. Five (63%) did not pass school at ordinary grade; 6 (67%) controls passed at ordinary grade.	XXY boys at higher risk for problems with speech development, school performance, social adjustment.

(cont.)

415

TABLE 18.1. (cont.)

Study	Country/city	n	Karyotype	Ascertainment	Age	Controls	Measures	Results	Conclusions
Ratcliffe, Tierney, et al. (1982b)	UK/Edinburgh	67	47,XXY 47,XXX 47,XYY	NS	2.0–13.5	Yes	WISC-R Stanford–Binet Gesell Reynell	62% of XXY required remedial education versus 45% of XYY, 8.7% of male controls. Reading difficulty predominantly in XXY; lower VIQ than controls.	Higher incidence of language difficulties in all three SCA groups. XXX girls have greater cognitive deficits than XXY, XYY boys.
Nielsen, Sorensen, & Sorensen (1982)	Denmark/Aarhus	25	47,XYY 47,XXX 45,X	NS	7.0–11.9	Yes	WISC Bender Figure drawing Lateral dom. Rod and Frame GFW Aud. Dis.	40% of SCA group, 7% of controls had poor school achievement. None with poor math skills.	Extra-X or -Y children need special stimulation, support and teaching efforts in learning to read and write.
Evans, de von Flindt, Greenberg, Ramsay, & Hamerton (1982)	Canada/Winnipeg	12	47,XXY 47,XYY	NS	7.5–10.1	Yes	PIC Vineland WISC-R PPVT McCarthy WRAT	All XXYs one grade lower than expected for age, but no specific area of deficit.	XXY and XXX at greater risk than XYY for learning and school-related problems.

416

Study	Location	N	Karyotype		Age	Controls	Tests	Findings	Comments
Stewart et al. (1982); Stewart, Barley, Netley, Rovet, & Park (1986)	Canada/Toronto	51–53	47,XXY 47,XXX 47,XYY Mosaics 46,XX male	NS	9.0–12.0 12.5–16.5	Yes	WISC-R WRAT WJPB	XXY had significantly lower reading, spelling, arithmetic skills than controls; 59% of XXY, 16% of controls in special education.	Testosterone treatment did not produce any change in behavior or school performance in XXY. XXY subjects resemble other children with LDs. Extra-X children have limited short-term memory spans not accounted for by language impairment.
Walzer, Graham, Bashir, & Silbert (1982); Walzer et al. (1986)	USA/Boston, MA	13	47,XXY	NS	5.0–7.0	Yes	WRAT Bayley WPPSI WISC-R	89–92% required remedial help in reading, spelling. 77% of XXY, 11% of controls had early LDs and were in special ed. 88% of XXY with LDs had delays in speech and language development and significant VIQ–PIQ discrepancy.	Deficits in verbal ability associated with decreased achievement in reading and spelling tasks. Deficits in auditory memory and processing implicated in verbal and language impairments.

(cont.)

417

TABLE 18.1. (cont.)

Study	Country/city	n	Karyotype	Ascertainment	Age	Controls	Measures	Results	Conclusions
Leonard, Sparrow, & Schowalter (1982); Leonard & Sparrow (1986)	USA/New Haven, CT	11	47,XXY 47,XYY 47,XXX	NS	9.0–13.0 17.0–18.0	Yes	WISC-R VMI PPVT WRAT	All had some learning difficulties; 73% had repeated a grade, but 91% in regular classes. 64% had reading problems, 36% problems with math. Low-average, borderline intelligence levels.	Speech, language, and reading areas of most difficulty, but no mental retardation due to SCA alone.
Robinson et al. (1986)	USA/Denver, CO	48	46,XYY 47,XXX 45,X Mosaics	NS	9.0–19.0	Yes	VMI GFW Aud. Disc. Receptive Lang. Boston Naming	XXY lower reading and written language, WJ scores than controls; LDs requiring special education in 86% of XXY; 79% had a reading disability.	Slow cognitive processing, impaired language, verbal memory deficits in XXY. Deficits due to decreased processing speed, not lack of ability.
Ratcliffe, Jenkins, & Teague (1990); Ratcliffe, Butler, & Jones (1991)	UK/Edinburgh	67	47,XXY 47,XYY 47,XXX XX male	NS	8.0–15.0	Yes	WISC-R Burt Reading Bristol Soc. Adj. BSQ British Ability Scale	67% of XXY received special help, but had less severe cognitive deficits than XXX girls.	XXY increases risk of LDs.
Bender, Linden, & Robinson (1987)	USA/Denver, CO	46	47,XXY 47,XYY 47,XXX 45,X Mosaics	NS	10.5.15.5	Yes	Lang. Test Battery BOTMP Family dysfunction School reports	Language, school impairments more frequent in pure SCA karyotypes (21–66%) than controls (0–32%). More academic difficulties in pure SCA children from dysfunctional families.	Higher vulnerability to environmental stress in SCA children than controls.

Reference	Location	N	Karyotype		Age range		Measures	Findings	Comments
Graham, Bashir, Stark, Silber, & Walzer (1988)	USA/Boston, MA	14	47,XXY	NS	5.0–12.0	Yes	WISC-R Token Test TDA, ITPA Syntactic Comp. DLA, PPVT Boston Naming Repetition GFW Aud. Disc. Sentence Memory Gilmore GM (speed and accur.) Word Reading Schonell Spelling	Lower VIQ and decreased achievement in reading and spelling due to preexisting language disabilities. Problems in expressive language, auditory processing, and memory abilities correlated with reduced achievement.	Specific deficits in expressive language implicate left-hemisphere dysfunction.
Bender, Linden, & Robinson (1989)	USA/Denver, CO	32	47,XXY 47,XXX	NS	8.0–18.0	Yes	WISC-R Vocab. Thurstone WF PMA SR WJSR	47,XXY deficient in rapid retrieval of verbal information.	Additional time to learn or complete work required by 47,XXY.
Robinson, Bender, Linden, & Salbenblatt (1990)	USA/Denver, CO	46	47,XXY 47,XYY 47,XXX 45,X Mosaics	NS	12.5–20.0	Yes	WISC Language Test BOTMP School reports	LDs in 33 (87%) of nonmosaic SCA children. More LDs in males (90%) than females (75%), but LDs in nonmosaic females more global and severe. All three disorders (motor, language, learning) in 53% of SCAs, 0% of controls and mosaics.	SCAs affect development of CNS, as motor and cognitive abilities affected in nonmosaic SCA children.

(cont.)

TABLE 18.1. (cont.)

Study	Country/city	n	Karyotype	Ascertainment	Age	Controls	Measures	Results	Conclusions
Walzer, Bashir, & Silbert (1991)	USA/Boston, MA	24	47,XXY 47,XYY	NS	9.0–12.0	Yes	WISC-R Direct observation	Reading and spelling difficulties in 85% of 47,XXY; 36% with LDs in full-time special ed. Reading LDs in 11% of controls.	Severe reading and writing problems due to language deficits in both groups. XXY more impaired in expressive than receptive language.
Robinson, Bender, Linden, & Salbenblatt (1991)	USA/Denver, CO	41	47,XXY 47,XYY 47,XXX 45,X Mosaics	NS	14.0–24.0	Yes	BOTMP Self-esteem BDI BSRI PMA WF & SR WJSR PPVT WAIS-R	86% of XXY required help for learning difficulties, 79% for reading LDs. One XXY in university, 64% still in high school, one dropout.	Deficits based on karyotype and related types of LDs. 47,XXY had generally depressed language skills, 45X had deficits in spatial skills, and 47,XXX had globally reduced ability.
Leonard (1991)	USA/New Haven, CT	6	47,XXY 47,XXX 47,XYY	NS	20.0–21.0	No	Question-naires Interviews	All had some learning problems with speech and language delays; all required remediation, had to work hard to succeed. Four now employed in meaningful jobs and one in technical school.	After high school, subjects felt learning problems much less significant. More satisfactory development in children diagnosed prenatally rather than through screening.

Study	Country/City	N	Karyotype		Age		Measures	Findings	Implications
Stewart, Bailey, Netley, & Park (1991)	Canada/Toronto	38	47,XXY 47,XXX 46,XY/47,XXY 46,XX male	NS	18.0–21.0	Yes	WISC-R WAIS-R WRAT-R Educ. histories	XXY males below controls in reading, spelling, arithmetic. 61% of XXY, 17% of controls had special ed. in past 5 years. Of 3 mosaics, 1 mildly below average in intellectual ability and educational performance.	Ability to cope successfully in school has potential long-term implications for social adjustment in 47,XXY males.
Evans, de von Flindt, Greenberg, & Hamerton (1991)	Canada/Winnipeg	10	47,XXY 47,XYY 47,XXX Mosaics	NS	15.8–18.9	No	WISC-R WAIS-R WRAT	44% of SCA group had repeated a grade. Verbal deficits and VIQ–PIQ discrepancies frequently observed.	Best-functioning children from stable and supportive families.
Nielsen (1991); Nielsen & Wohlert (1991)	Denmark/Aarhus	25	47,XXY 47,XXX 47,XYY	NS	10.0–14.0 15.0–19.0	Yes	Parent interview School reports	All SCA children in normal school; no mental retardation; 63% below-average school performance. Remedial teaching in both math (42%) and reading (38%). Children average or above-average at school if good childhood conditions. Poor school performance behavior problems if poor childhood conditions.	Prevention of deviation from normal in school performance, behavior, and adjustment if appropriate social educational resources available and if parents willing to accept counseling and child's SCA.

(cont.)

TABLE 18.1. (cont.)

Study	Country/city	n	Karyotype	Ascertainment	Age	Controls	Measures	Results	Conclusions
Robinson, Bender, & Linden (1992)	USA/Denver, CO	29	47,XXY 47,XYY 47,XXX Mosaics	PS NS	7.0–14.0	Yes	Questionnaires School reports WISC-R Physician report	No language deficits or school problems in prenatal XXY boys. Learning problems in 11 (79%) of prenatally diagnosed XXYs. Fewer language, learning deficits in prenatal XXY boys, all postnatal in special education.	Confirms impressions that prenatally diagnosed SCA cohort may develop differently from postnatally screened children. Effect may be due to more supportive environment and higher SES in prenatal families.

Note. Abbreviations: *Ascertainment:* CR, case report; CS, clinic screening; NS, newborn screening; PS, prenatal screening. *Measures:* BDI, Beck Depression Inventory; BOTMR, Bruininks–Oseretsky Test of Motor Proficiency; BSQ, British Screening Questionnaire; BSRI, Bem Sex Role Inventory; DLA, Detroit Learning Attitudes; GFW Aud. Disc., Goldman–Fristoe–Woodcock Auditory Skills Test Battery; GM, Gates–McGinitie Speech and Accuracy subtests; HSPQ, High School Personality Questionnaire; ITPA, Illinois Test of Psycholinguistic Abilities; PIAT, Peabody Individual Achievement Test; PIC, Personality Inventory for Children; PMA SR, Primary Mental Abilities Spatial Relations Test; PMA WF, Primary Mental Abilities Word Fluency Test; PPVT, Peabody Picture Vocabulary Test; TDA, Templin–Dawley Articulation; Thurston WF, Thurstone Word Fluency; VMI, Developmental Test of Visual–Motor Integration; WAIS, Wechsler Adult Intelligence Scale; WISC, Wechsler Intelligence Scale for Children; WJPB, Woodcock–Johnson Psycho-Educational Battery; WJSR, Woodcock–Johnson Spatial Relations; WPPSI, Wechsler Preschool and Primary Scale of Intelligence; WRAT, Wide Range Achievement Test; YDE, Yale Developmental Exam. *Results* and *Conclusions:* CNS, central nervous system; LDs, learning disabilities; PIQ, Performance IQ; SCA, sex chromosome abnormality; SES, socioeconomic status; VIQ, Verbal IQ. Adapted from Rovet, Netley, Keenan, Bailey, and Stewart (1996). Copyright 1996 by PRO-ED. Adapted by permission.

BEHAVIORAL, ACADEMIC, AND EMOTIONAL PRESENTATION

Behavioral Presentation

Normally, behavioral development is felt to be the result of certain predispositions and environmental influences. With children who have genetic disorders, there are often physical consequences of their genetic abnormalities, which result in certain behaviors. However, as with all behaviors, the interaction between the children's characteristics and those of their environment must be considered in the etiology of their behavioral presentation (Hynd & Willis, 1988). Research studies conducted in the 1960s and even early 1970s with adult populations tended to find increased incidence of aggressiveness, alcohol and other substance abuse, arson, criminal behavior, depression, personality disorders, and schizophrenia (Schwartz & Root, 1991). However, as mentioned earlier in this chapter, these studies were methodologically flawed. Chiefly, they were limited to individuals who were already in psychiatric hospitals or penal institutions.

Interestingly, the behavioral characteristics associated with KS (e.g., low activity, high pliancy or manageability) have led some researchers to find that teachers may view these children as warm, likeable, anxious to please, and helpful. However, their tendency to withdraw in novel situations and to be less assertive may also tend to cause teachers to view these children as lazy, unmotivated, or unwilling to try (Walzer et al., 1986).

Academic Performance

Academic difficulties have been found in the areas of reading, spelling, and arithmetic; these are probably related to the specific language deficits in the area of auditory processing (Schwartz & Root, 1991). Mandoki et al. (1991) have also noted that poor school performance is typical in children with KS, particularly in reading and spelling. Difficulties with speech production, language processing, and sentence structuring are thought to interfere with both of these domains. Research on the development of reading and spelling in KS proposes that the course follows normal developmental patterns, but becomes arrested at some point (Seymour & Evans, 1988). Prospective and longitudinal research (Robinson et al. 1986; Walzer et al., 1986) indicates that children with KS are more likely to be referred for special education evaluations by their classroom teachers, and also more likely to be enrolled in a learning disability classroom. In the longitudinal study by Rovet et al. (1996), boys with KS were found to perform significantly worse on measures of word decoding, reading comprehension, spelling, written language skills, arithmetic and math problem solving, and the acquisition of conceptual knowledge in areas such as sciences and humanities. In addition, the boys with KS were found to perform lower on standardized achievement tests, and they tended to fall further behind grade and age level as they grew older. Interestingly, Rovet et al. (1996) noted that most of the boys with KS were equally impaired on measures of reading and arithmetic; however, they characterized the learning disability seen in KS as primarily language-based. The specific deficit demonstrated throughout all their findings appeared to reside in the area of auditory processing. This hypothesis is supported by earlier research demonstrating significant impairments in reading and auditory short-term memory in a group of boys with KS (Bender et al. 1986). Bender et al.'s sample was characterized by average intelligence, language dysfunction associated with slow processing and poor short-term memory, and a history of reading difficulty in school. In addition, impaired reading (i.e., low scores on the Passage Comprehension subtest of the Woodcock–Johnson Psycho-Educational Battery—Revised; Woodcock & Johnson, 1989) and poor short-term recall were noted.

Emotional Presentation

Data from the various prospective studies of this population characterize children with KS as less active, less assertive, and more susceptible to stress than controls (Bender & Berch, 1991). Temperamentally, these boys are also depicted as quieter and less sociable than controls. They have been described as pliant, withdrawn, and low in energy intensity (Netley, 1991). Specific temperamental characteristics were observed in a study of XXY males from birth to age 7 (Walzer et al., 1986). Interview and observational data were obtained on such variables as activity level, intensity of responding, pliancy, approach–withdrawal, adaptability, and capacity to relate. Compared to a control group, children with KS were consistently rated as lower in activity level, lower in intensity, more pliant, and more withdrawing in new situations.

On the Personality Inventory for Children (Lachar, 1982), boys with KS were found to differ significantly from controls on ratings of achievement, intelligence, and development, in addition to ratings of lower-than-average activity (Stewart, Bailey, Netley, Rovet, & Park, 1986) (see Table 18.2). Another study of the psychological nature of KS adults found them to be less teasing and sarcastic and more submissive than controls and a group of XYY men (Schiavi, Theilgaard, Owen, & White, 1984).

KEY ASSESSMENT ISSUES

Several issues are relevant to KS within the context of diagnosis and assessment. First, KS may be diagnosed at birth or shortly thereafter. If this is the case, early assessment of physiological development as well as learning problems can be made, and these can be monitored over the course of the child's schooling. However, a child may not be given a diagnosis at an early age, since many of the features most typical of KS (e.g., delayed puberty, diminished testes, diminished or absent secondary sex characteristics) do not appear until a child begins to enter adolescence. Therefore, parents, teachers, and other child care professionals should

TABLE 18.2. Scores on the Personality Inventory for Children of 47,XXY Boys versus Normal Males, Examined in a Test–Retest Reliability Study

	47,XXY ($n = 20$)		Comparison group ($n = 46$)			
	Mean	SD	Mean	SD	t	p
Achievement	58.60	10.72	50.6	9.7	2.86	<.01
Intellectual Screening	62.75	20.47	51.8	8.3	2.31	<.05
Development	56.80	9.28	49.9	10.9	2.63	<.02
Somatic Concern	58.30	16.91	52.8	11.1	1.33	NS
Depression	56.10	11.49	54.1	11.7	0.65	NS
Family Relations	54.10	10.73	50.3	10.7	1.32	NS
Delinquency	55.40	11.07	54.8	10.8	0.20	NS
Withdrawal	57.05	9.24	54.4	11.4	0.99	NS
Anxiety	54.00	10.05	55.9	13.1	0.64	NS
Psychosis	56.15	14.16	53.7	10.0	0.70	NS
Hyperactivity	43.40	8.41	52.1	12.9	3.25	<.01
Social Skills	53.60	10.50	53.5	10.9	0.04	NS

Note. NS, not significant. From Stewart, Bailey, Netley, Rovet, and Park (1986). Copyright 1986 by March of Dimes. Reprinted by permission.

be familiar with the characteristic learning, behavioral, and physical presentation of KS in order to refer these children for genetic evaluation. Finally, when an assessment is performed, it should include an evaluation of verbal abilities with an emphasis on expressive versus receptive language functioning, verbal memory, and auditory processing. Since these children are at special risk for reading and spelling disabilities, evaluators need to be aware of potentially important Verbal–Performance discrepancies and should be prepared to compare academic functioning with the most reliable estimate of cognitive function.

OPTIONS FOR TREATMENT OF PSYCHOSOCIAL, EDUCATIONAL, AND EMOTIONAL PROBLEMS

Psychosocial Problems

In a review of several studies regarding psychosocial adjustment in boys with KS (Robinson, Bender, Linden, & Salbenblatt, 1990), common personality descriptors included "shy," "immature," "restrained," "reserved," and "having poor peer relationships." The presence of a supportive and stable family environment was noted to have positive effects on psychosocial adjustment for these children. Other studies have described this population as cautious in new situations, low in motor activity, and possessing easy dispositions (Walzer et al., 1990). These authors commented that these characteristics predisposed children with KS to present as "low-key" children who were well liked by their teachers and who had few behavioral management problems. However, one problem with this study—a problem that plagues much research with the sex chromosome disorders—is that the study examined both XXY and XYY boys.

Bender, Linden, and Robinson (1991) described a high-risk profile for children with sex chromosome disorders, based on the results of a prospective study. The high-risk children tended to be those who had problems communicating with peers; academic problems marked by low achievement; few hobbies or little participation in extracurricular activities; behavioral immaturity; and social isolation. This profile was viewed as constituting a risk factor for increased problems with psychosocial functioning in youth, as well as adult psychopathology. The authors also recognized the importance of identifying environmental factors when predicting outcome.

Educational Problems

Given the difficulty of identifying infants with KS who may not display any abnormal features (e.g., congenital abnormalities), teachers may come across these children in the regular classroom. For example, Mandoki and Sumner (1991) described the case of a 14-year-old male who was diagnosed with KS only after suffering from years of academic failure, interpersonal problems, and emotional disturbance. Some physical features that may indicate KS include a small head circumference, greater-than-average height, small genitals, and disproportionately long legs (Mandoki et al., 1991). When these characteristics are coupled with learning difficulties specific to reading and spelling, a referral for diagnostic testing (i.e., by karyotype) may be in order. The most common presenting problems of boys with KS are school underachievement, poor peer relationships, impulsivity, aggressiveness, withdrawal, apathy, and immaturity. Some treatment with medication and hormones is available to address the abnormal sexual development and aggressive behaviors in these males (e.g., delayed pubertal development, reduced testicular size, female distribution of fat deposits). Although the learning disability will not be "cured" by this treatment, both medical and academic interventions are important for preventing these features from developing.

Some specific implications for interventions in the classroom have been offered by Rovet et al. (1996). Generally, they feel that intervention efforts should center on the language-based learning disability. Speech and language therapy is recommended, with a special emphasis on improving vocabulary, sentence understanding, comprehension skills, and word finding. Additional training to enhance memory functioning may be provided by presenting advance organizers for reading comprehension tasks, structuring lessons into smaller chunks to learn, and providing drilling on math facts.

Emotional Problems

The abnormal sexual characteristics as well as the academic difficulties of individuals with KS often result in low self-esteem and poor self-concept. A follow-up study indicated that adult males with KS are often lonely, immature, passive, and lacking in friends (Nielsen, Johnsen, & Sorensen, 1980). Testosterone treatment to enhance sexual development has also been found to improve problems stemming from low self-esteem (Schwartz & Root, 1991). Mazur and Clopper (1991) reviewed clinical cases they had seen with gynecomastia and determined that one of the greatest related concerns was the impact on psychosocial functioning. They reported that their patients had a history of being teased by peers regarding their breast development, which resulted in social isolation and withdrawal in approximately 70% of these children. Cases of anorexia nervosa have been described in conjunction with KS, with poor body image and problems with puberty implicated in the etiology (El-Badri & Lewis, 1991; Hindler & Norris, 1986). There are also accounts of schizophrenia in KS, with the hypothesis that the presence of an extra X chromosome and/or the abnormal hormonal levels during prenatal development are the cause of this association (Roy, 1981; Pomeroy, 1980). Other types of psychopathology, such as bipolar disorder, have been linked to KS, but there is less consensus regarding this relationship (Everman & Stoudemire, 1994). However, most accounts trace the etiology of the bipolar disorder to the presence of the extra X chromosome.

In an older study examining the sexual development of individuals with KS, these males were found to date and become sexually involved at a later age then their peers (Raboch, Mellan, & Starka, 1979). Considering the tendency toward withdrawal and negative peer interactions for this group, this relative delay is understandable. In a survey of men who were seen at an infertility clinic who were determined to have KS, they reported more problems with below-average school performance, little energy, poor relations with parents or siblings, and mental illness than a control group (Kessler & Moos, 1973). However, it should be noted that many of these individuals do marry and have successful relationships as adults.

ADOLESCENCE AND ADULTHOOD OUTCOMES

The onset of adolescence is typically not delayed in individuals with KS, but it is during this period that the major implications of this disorder become manifest. As discussed above, one of the chief signs is the smaller testes. An androgen deficiency may also be determined by testing blood levels, with typical treatments involving testosterone replacement. Although some authors recommend that this treatment begin at age 12 for all children with KS, this policy remains debated (Gardner & Sutherland, 1996). Beneficial results of this treatment include development of masculine sex characteristics, reduced breast size, improved self-esteem, and increased sexual interest (Pierce, 1990). A small study examining both physiological and psychological changes as a result of testosterone treatments found that the KS males not only began to develop a more masculine physique and secondary sex characteristics, but also had improved perceptions of body image, increased assertiveness and goal-directed behavior, and heightened sexual drive (Johnson, Myhre, Ruvalcaba, Thuline, & Kelley, 1970). Approximately 50% of adolescents with KS will display gynecomastia, which can be treated surgically.

Although infertility has been found to be the general rule among individuals with KS, some exceptions have been reported in the literature, as reviewed by Gardner and Sutherland (1996). They hypothesized that these reports were probably attributable to cases of mosaicism. A more important point made by these authors is that there is a lack of information regarding the risk of having children with sex chromosome anomalies for individuals with KS who may produce children. In other words, the probability of having children with KS is rare, and the risk of passing on the disorder is virtually unknown. Parents concerned that they may have another child with KS should be advised that there is a lack of evidence for any recurrence rate greater than normal risk estimates of having a child with a chromosomal disorder.

No current research supports the older contention that these individuals have higher rates of criminality or mental health problems. In a group of 24 adult males with KS, 4 had been imprisoned at some point, and 3 had been in a mental institution (Zuppinger et al., 1967). This supports other studies that found greater occurrences of KS in penal and psychiatric populations. For example, Murken (1973) concluded that due to a passive personality structure, low intelligence, and sexual difficulties, individuals with KS were unduly influenced by external forces and therefore were impelled to be social deviants. As noted throughout this chapter, however, these studies have methodological flaws (e.g., problems with sample size and selection bias) that more recent work has attempted to correct. As discussed above, there is a great variability in intelligence and also in adaptive skills, which can lead to a more positive picture than these earlier accounts suggested.

Genetic counseling for the family and the individual with KS can play an important role in education. The issue of sterility should be discussed with the parents and the male with KS. Robinson et al. (1986) found that parents of children with KS expressed worry about communicating information about the chromosomal abnormality and resulting infertility to their children. Furthermore, the parents felt a sense of loss and grief themselves regarding their children's probable infertility. An individual with KS should be educated early about the issue of sterility. In addition, alternatives such as adoption can be discussed as an option for raising children. Nielsen et al. (1980) found that within a group of individuals with KS, those who sought adoption or insemination by donor as alternatives were happier and had more stable marriages. Other interventions for infertility have begun to be explored. In a small study of non-mosaic Klinefelter adults, pregancy and birth were achieved using sperm retrieval through testicular fine needle aspiration and fertilized eggs via intracytoplasmic sperm injection (Reubinoff et al., 1998). The authors cautioned that prenatal diagnosis should be employed when these techniques are used, given the unknown risk of passing on KS to any offspring. In another small study (Staessen et al., 1996), pre-implantation diagnosis confirmed normal X and Y chromosome constitution in five embryos created from sperm recovered from three KS patients. Such procedures provide hope that medical advances will provide individuals with KS the chance to have children. Since it is not uncommon for individuals with KS to be discovered when infertility is the referral problem, marriage counseling may also be critical in these cases identified later.

ACKNOWLEDGMENT

The writing of this chapter was supported in part by a grant (No. R01-HD26890-03) to George Hynd from the National Institute of Child Health and Human Development.

REFERENCES

Abramsky, L., & Chapple, J. (1998). 47, XXY (Klinefelter syndrome) and 47,XYY: Estimated rates of and indication for postnatal diagnosis with implications for prenatal counseling. *Prenatal Diagnosis 18*, 303–304.

Bebb, G. G., Grannis, F. W., Jr., Paz, I. B., Slovak, M. L. & Chilote, R. (1998). Mediastinal germ cell tumor in a child with precocious puberty and Klinefelter syndrome. *Annals of Thoracic Surgery, 66*, 547–548.

Bender, B. G., & Berch, D. B. (1991). Overview: Psychological phenotypes and sex chromosome abnormalities. In D. B. Berch & B. G. Bender (Eds.), *Sex chromosome abnormalities and human behavior.* Boulder, CO: Westview Press.

Bender, B., Linden, M., & Robinson, A. (1987). Environment and developmental risk in children with sex chromosome abnormalities. *Journal of the American Academy of Child Psychiatry, 26*, 499–503.

Bender, B., Linden, M., & Robinson, A. (1989). Verbal and spatial processing efficiency in children with sex chromosome abnormalities. *Journal of the American Academy of Child and Adolescent Psychiatry, 25*, 577–579.

Bender, B. G., Linden, M., & Robinson, A. (1991). Sex chromosome abnormalities: In search of developmental patterns. In D. B. Berch & B. G. Bender (Eds.), *Sex chromosome abnormalities and human behavior.* Boulder, CO: Westview Press.

Bender, B. G., Puck, M. H., Salbenblatt, J. A., & Robinson, A. (1986). Dyslexia in 47,XXY boys identified at birth. *Behavior Genetics, 16*, 343–354.

Cohen, F. L., & Durham, J. D. (1985). Update your knowledge of Klinefelter syndrome. *Journal of Psychosocial Nursing and Mental Health Services, 23*, 19–25.

Drugan, A., Isada, N. B., Johnson, M. P., & Evans, M. I. (1996a). Genetics: An overview. In N. B. Isada, A. Drugan, M. P. Johnson, & M. I. Evans (Eds.), *Maternal genetic disease.* Stamford, CT: Appleton & Lange.

Drugan, A., Isada, N. B., Johnson, M. P., & Evans, M. I. (1996b). Parental chromosomal anomalies. In N. B. Isada, A. Drugan, M. P. Johnson, & M. I. Evans (Eds.), *Maternal genetic disease.* Stamford, CT: Appleton & Lange.

El-Badri, S. M., & Lewis, M. A. (1991). Anorexia nervosa associated with Klinefelter's syndrome. *Comprehensive Psychiatry, 32*(4), 317–319.

Elias, S., & Yanangi, R. M. (1981). Cardiovascular defects. In J. D. Schulman & J. L. Simpson (Eds.), *Genetic diseases in pregnancy: Maternal effects and fetal outcome.* New York: Academic Press.

Evans, J., de von Flindt, R., Greenberg, C., & Hammerton, J. (1991). Physical and psychological findings in adolescents with sex chromosome abnormalities ascertained in the Winnepeg cytogenetic study of newborns: 1970–1973. In J. Evans, J. Hamerton, & A. Robinson (Eds.), *Children and young adults with sex chromosome aneuploidy* (Vol. 26, pp. 189–200) New York: Alan R. Liss.

Evans, J., de von Flindt, R., Greenberg, C., Ramsay, S., & Hamerton, J. (1982). A cytogenetic survey of 14,069 newborn infants: IV. Further follow-up on the children with sex chromosome anomalies. In D. Stewart, J. Bailey, C. Netley, & E. Park (Eds.), *Children with sex chromosome aneuploidy: Follow-up studies* (Vol. 18, pp. 169–184). New York: Alan R. Liss.

Evans, M. I., Drugan, A., Pryde, P. G., & Johnson, M. P. (1996). Genetics and the obstetrician. In N. B. Isada, A. Drugan, M. P. Johnson, & M. I. Evans (Eds.), *Maternal genetic disease.* Stamford, CT: Appleton & Lange.

Everman, D. B., & Stoudemire, A. (1994). Bipolar disorder associated with Klinefelter's syndrome and other chromosomal abnormalities. *Psychosomatics, 35*, 35–40.

Forssman, H. (1970). The mental implications of sex chromosome aberrations. *British Journal of Psychiatry, 117*, 353–363.

Funderberk, S. J., & Ferjo, N. (1978). Clinical observations in Klinefelter (47,XXY) syndrome. *Journal of Mental Deficiency Research, 22*, 207–212.

Gardner, R. J. M., & Sutherland, G. R. (1996). *Chromosome abnormalities and genetic counseling* (2nd ed.). New York: Oxford University Press.

Gilbert, P. (1993). *The A–Z reference book of syndromes and inherited disorders.* London: Chapman & Hall.

Graham, J., Bashir, A., Stark, R., Silbert, A., & Walzer, S. (1988). Oral and written language abilities of XXY boys: Implications for anticipatory guidance. *Pediatrics, 81*, 795–806.

Hasle, H., Mellemgaard, A., Nielsen, J, & Hansen, J. (1995). Cancer incidence in men with Klinefelter syndrome. *British Journal of Cancer, 71*, 416–420.

Hindler, C. G., & Norris, D. L. (1986). A case of anorexia nervosa with Klinefelter's syndrome. *British Journal of Psychiatry, 149*, 659–660.

Hultborn, R., Hanson, C., Kopf, I., Verbiene, I., Warnhammar, E., & Weimarck, A. (1997). Prevalence of Klinefelter's syndrome in male breast cancer patients. *Anticancer Research, 17*, 4293–4297.

Humphreys, M., Lavery, P., Morris, C., & Nevin, N. (1997). Klinefelter syndrome and non-Hodgkin lymphoma. *Cancer Genetics and Cytogenetics, 97*, 111–113.

Hynd, G. W., & Willis, W. G. (1988). *Pediatric neuropsychology.* Needham Heights, MA: Allyn & Bacon.

Johnson, H. R., Myhre, S. A., Ruvalcaba, R. H. A., Thuline, H. C., & Kelley, V. C. (1970). Effects of testosterone on body image and behavior in Klinefelter's syndrome: A pilot study. *Developmental Medicine and Child Neurology, 12*, 454–460.

Kessler, S., & Moos, R. (1973). Behavioral aspects of chromosomal disorders. *Annual Review of Medicine, 24*, 89–102.

Klinefelter, H. F., Reifenstein, E. C., & Albright, F. (1942). Syndrome characterized by gynecomastia, aspermatogenesis without A-Leydigism, and increased excretion of follicle-stimulating hormone. *Journal of Clinical Endocrinology, 2*, 615–627.

Lachar, D. (1982). *The Personality Inventory for Youth—Revised.* Los Angeles: Western Psychological Services.

Leonard, M. (1991). A prospective study of development of children with sex chromosome anomalies: New Haven study V. Young adulthood. In J. Evans, J. Hamerton, & A. Robinson (Eds.), *Children and young adults with sex chromosome aneuploidy* (pp. 117–130). New York: Alan R. Liss.

Leonard, M., Schowalter, J. E., Landy, G., Ruddle, F., & Lubs, H. (1979). Chromosomal abnormalities in the New Haven newborn study: A prospective study of development of children with sex chromosome anomalies. In A. Robinson, H. Lubs, & D. Bergsma (Eds.), *Sex chromosome aneuploidy: Prospective studies on children* (Vol. 15, pp. 115–160). New York: Alan R. Liss.

Leonard, M., & Sparrow, S. (1986). Prospective study of development of children with sex chromosome anomalies: New Haven Study IV. Adolescence. *Birth Defects: Original Article Series, 22*, 221–249.

Leonard, M., Sparrow, S., & Schowalter, J. (1982). A prospective study of development of cihldren with sex chromsome anomalies—New Haven study III. In D. Stewart, J. Bailey, C. Netley, & E. Park (Eds.), *Children with sex chromosome aneuploidy: Follow-up studies* (Vol. 18, pp. 193–218). New York: Alan R. Liss.

Mandoki, M. W., & Sumner, G. S. (1991). Klinefelter syndrome: The need for early identification and treatment. *Clinical Pediatrics, 30*, 161–164.

Mandoki, M. W., Sumner, G. S., Hoffman, R. P., & Riconda, D. L. (1991). A review of Klinefelter's syndrome in children and adolescents. *Journal of the American Academy of Child and Adolescent Psychiatry, 30*, 160–172.

Mazur, T., & Clopper, R. R. (1991). Pubertal disorders: Psychology and clinical management. *Endocrinology and Metabolism Clinics of North America*, 20(1), 211–230.

Money, J. (1993). Specific neurocognitional impairments associated with Turner (45,X) and Klinefelter (47,XXY) syndromes: A review. *Social Biology*, 40(1–2), 147–151.

Murken, J. D. (1973). The XYY syndrome and Klinefelter's syndrome. In P. E. Becker, W. Lenz, F. Vogel & G. G. Wendt (Eds.), *Topics in human genetics* (Vol. 2). Stuttgart, Germany: Grammlich.

Nielsen, J. (1991). Follow-up of 25 unselected children with sex chromosome abnormalities to age 12. In J. Evans, J. Hamerton, & A. Robinson (Eds.), *Children and young adults with sex chromosome aneuploidy* (Vol. 26, pp. 201–208). New York: Alan R. Liss.

Nielsen, J., Bjarnason, S., Friedrich, U., Froland, A., Hansen, V., & Sorenson, A. (1970). Klinefelter's syndrome in children. *Journal of Child Psychology and Psychiatry, 11*, 109–119.

Nielsen, J., Johnsen, S. G., & Sorensen, K. (1980). Follow-up 10 years later of 34 Klinefelter males with karyotype 47,XXY and 16 hypogonadal males with karyotype 46,XY. *Psychological Medicine, 10*, 345–352.

Nielsen, J., Sorensen, A., & Sorensen, K. (1982). Follow-up until age 7 to 11 of 25 unselected children with sex chromosome abnormalities. In D. Stewart, J. Bailey, C. Netley, & E. Park (Eds.), *Children with sex chromosome aneuploidy: Follow-up studies* (Vol. 18, pp. 61–98). New York: Alan R. Liss.

Nielsen, J., & Wohlert, M. (1991). Chromosome abnormalities found among 34,910 newborn children: Results from a 13-year incidence study in Aarhus, Denmark. *Human Genetics, 87*, 81–83.

Netley, C. (1987). Predicting intellectual functioning in 47,XXY boys from characteristics of siblings. *Clinical Genetics, 32*, 24–27.

Netley, C. (1991). Behavior and extra X aneuploid states. In D. B. Berch & B. G. Bender (Eds.), *Sex chromosome abnormalities and human behavior*. Boulder, CO: Westview Press.

Netley, C., & Rovet, J. (1982). Verbal deficits in children with 47,XXY and 47,XXX karyotypes: A descriptive and experimental study. *Brain and Language, 17*, 58–72.

Netley, C., & Rovet, J. (1984). Hemispheric lateralization in 47,XXY Klinefelter's syndrome boys. *Brain and Cognition, 3*, 10–18.

Pei, D., Sheu, W. H., Jeng, C. Y., Liao, W. K., & Fuh, M. M. (1998). Insulin resistance in patients with Klinefelter's syndrome and idiopathic gonadotropin deficiency. *Journal of the Formosan Medical Association, 97*, 534–540.

Pennington, B. F., Bender, B., Puck, M., Salbenblatt, J., & Robinson, A. (1982). Learning disabilities in children with sex chromosome anomalies. *Child Development, 53*, 1182–1192.

Pierce, B. A. (1990). *The family genetic sourcebook*. New York: Wiley.

Pomeroy, J. C. (1980). Klinefelter's syndrome and schizophrenia. *British Journal of Psychiatry, 136*, 597–599.

Raboch, J., Mellan, J., & Starka, L. (1979). Klinefelter's syndrome: Sexual development and activity. *Archives of Sexual Behavior*, 8(4), 333–339.

Ratcliffe, S. G., Bancroft, J., Axworthy, D., & McLaren, W. (1982a). Klinefelter's syndrome in adolescence. *Archives of Disease in Childhood, 57*, 6–12.

Ratcliffe, S. G., Butler, G. E., & Jones, M. (1991). Edinburgh study of growth and development of children with sex chromosome abnormalities. In J. Evans, J. Hamerton, & A. Robinson (Eds.), *Children and young adults with sex chromosome aneuploidy* (Vol. 26, pp. 1–44). New York: Alan R. Liss.

Ratcliffe, S. G., Jenkins, J., & Teague, P. (1990). Cognitive and behavioural development of the 47,XYY child. In D. B. Berch and B. G. Bender (Eds.), *Sex chromosome abnormalities and behavior: Psychological studies* (pp. 161–184). Boulder, CO: Westview Press.

Ratcliffe, S., Tierney, I., Nshaho, J., Smith, L., Springblatt, A., & Webber, M. (1982). The Edinburgh study of growth and development of children with sex chromosome abnormalities. In D. Stewart, J. Bailey, C. Netley, & E. Park (Eds.), *Children with sex chromosome aneuploidy: Follow-up studies* (Vol. 18, pp. 41–60). New York: Alan R. Liss.

Reubinoff, B. E., Abeliovich, D., Werner, M., Schenker, J. G., Safran, A., & Lewin, A. (1998). A birth in non-mosaic Klinefelter's syndrome after testicular fine needle aspiration, intracyto-plasmic sperm injection and preimplantation genetic diagnosis. *Human Reproduction, 13,* 1887–1892.

Robinson, A., Bender, B. G., Borelli, J. B., Puck, M. H., Salbenblatt, J. A., & Winter, J. S. D. (1986). Sex chromosomal aneuploidy: Prospective and longitudinal studies. In S. G. Ratcliffe & N. Paul (Eds.), *Prospective studies on children with sex chromosome aneuploidy.* New York: Alan R. Liss.

Robinson, A., Bender, B., Linden, M. (1992). Prognosis of prenatally diagnosed children with sex chromosome aneuploidy. *American Journal of Medical Genetics, 440,* 365–368.

Robinson, A., Bender, B., Linden, M., & Salbenblatt, J. (1990). Sex chromosome aneuploidy: The Denver prospective study. *Birth Defects: Original Article Series, 26*(4), 59–115.

Robinson, A., Bender, B., Linden, M., & Salbenblatt, J. (1991). Sex chromosome aneuploidy: The Denver prospective study. In J. Evans, J. Hamerton, & A. Robinson (Eds.), *Children and young adults with sex chromosome aneuploidy* (Vol. 26, pp. 59–116). New York: Alan R. Liss.

Robinson, A., Lubs, H. A., & Bergsma, D. (Eds.). (1979). *Sex chromosome aneuploidy: Prospective studies on children* (Vol. 15). New York: Alan R. Liss.

Rovet, J., Netley, C., Keenan, M., Bailey, J., & Stewart, D. (1996). The psychoeducational profile of boys with Klinefelter syndrome. *Journal of Learning Disabilities, 29,* 180–196.

Roy, A. (1981). Schizophrenia and Klinefelter syndrome. *Canadian Journal of Psychiatry, 26,* 262–264.

Schiavi, R. C., Theilgaard, A., Owen, D. R., & White, D. (1984). Sex chromosome anomalies, hormones, and aggressivity. *Archives of General Psychiatry, 41,* 93–99.

Schroder, J., Chapelle, A., Hakola, P., & Virkkunen, M. (1981). The frequency of XYY and XXY men among criminal offenders. *Acta Psychiatrica Scandinavica, 63,* 272–276.

Schwartz, I. D., & Root, A. W. (1991). The Klinefelter syndrome of testicular dysgenesis. *Endocrinology and Metabolism Clinics of North America, 20*(1), 153–163.

Seymour, P. H. K., & Evans, H. M. (1988). Developmental arrest at the logographic stage: Impaired literacy functions in Klinefelter's XXXY syndrome. *Journal of Research in Reading. 11*(2), 133–151.

Sheridan, M. K., & Radlinski, S. (1988). Brief report: A case study of an adolescent male with XXXXY Klinefelter's syndrome. *Journal of Autism and Developmental Disorders, 18*(3), 449–456.

Smith, G. F. (1981). Genetics of mental retardation. In K. I. Abroms & J. W. Bennett (Eds.), *Issues in genetics and exceptional children.* San Francisco: Jossey-Bass.

Staessen, C., Coonen, E., Van Assche, E., Tournaye, H., Joris, H., Devroey, P., Van Steirteghem, A. C., & Liebaers, I. (1996). Preimplantation diagnosis for X and Y normality in embryos from three Klinefelter patients. *Human Reproduction, 11*(8), 1650–1653.

Stewart, D., Bailey, J., Netley, C., & Park, E. (1991). Growth, development, and behavioral outcome from mid-adolescence to adulthood in subjects with chromosome aneuploidy: The Toronto study. In J. Evans, J. Hamerton, & A. Robinson (Eds.), *Children and young adults with sex chromosome aneuploidy* (Vol. 26, pp. 131–188). New York: Alan R. Liss.

Stewart, D., Bailey, J., Netley, C., Rovet, J., & Park, E. (1986). Growth and development from early to midadolescence of children with X and Y chromosome aneuploidy: The Toronto study. *Birth Defects: Original Article Series, 22*(3), 119–182.

Stewart, D., Bailey, J., Netley, C., Rovet, J., Park, M., Curtiss, J., & Cripps, M. (1982). Growth and development of children with X and Y chromosomal aneuploidy from infancy to puberty. In D. Stewart, J. Bailey, C. Netley, & E. Park (Eds.), *Children with sex chromosome aneuploidy: Follow-up studies* (Vol. 18, pp. 99–154). New York: Alan R. Liss.

Stewart, D., Netley, C., Bailey, J., Haka-Ikse, K., Platt, J., Holland, W., & Cripps, M. (1979). Growth and development of children with X and Y chromosome aneuploidy: A prospective study. In A. Robinson, H. Lubs, & D. Bergsma (Eds.), *Sex chromosome aneuploidy: Prospective studies on children* (Vol. 15, pp. 75–114). New York: Alan R. Liss.

Styne, D. M. (1991). Puberty and its disorders in boys. *Endocrinology and Metabolism Clinics of North America, 20*(1), 43–69.

Swaiman, K. F. (Ed.). (1989). *Pediatric neurology: Principles and practice.* ST. Lewis, MO: C. V. Mosby.

Theilgaard, A. (1984). A psychological study of the personalities of XYY and XXY men. *Acta Psychiatrica Scandinavica, 69*(Suppl. 315), 1–132.

Tyler, C. V., Jr., Kungl, P. A., & Green, L. A. (1998). Genetic diagnosis in adulthood: A case report. *Journal of Family Practice, 47,* 227–230.

Walzer, S., Bashir, A. S., Graham, J. M., Silbert, A. R., Lange, N. T., DeNapoli, M. F., & Richmond, J. B. (1986). Behavioral development of boys with X chromosome aneuploidy: Impact of reactive style on the educational intervention for learning deficits. In S. G. Ratcliffe & N. Paul (Eds.), *Prospective studies on children with sex chromosome aneuploidy.* New York: Alan R. Liss.

Walzer, S., Bashir, A. S., & Silbert, A. R. (1990). Cognitive and behavioral factors in the learning disabilities of 47,XXY and 47,XYY boys. *Birth Defects: Original Article Series, 26,* 45–58.

Walzer, S., Bashir, A. S., & Silbert, A. R. (1991). Cognitive and behavioral factors in learning disabilities of 47,XXY and 47,XYY boys. In J. Evans, J. Hamerton, & A. Robinson (Eds.), *Children and young adults with sex chromosome aneuploidy* (pp. 45–58). New York: Alan R. Liss.

Walzer, S., & Gerald, P. S. (1977). A chromosome survey of 13,751 male neonates. In E. Hook & I. H. Porter (Eds.), *Population cytogenetics* (pp. 45–61). New York: Academic Press.

Walzer, S., Graham, J. M., Bashir, A., & Silbert, A. R. (1982). Preliminary observations on language and learning in XXY boys. In D. Stewart, J. Bailey, C. Netley, & E. Park (Eds.), *Children with sex chromosome aneuploidy: Follow-up studies* (Vol. 18, pp. 185–192). New York: Alan R. Liss.

Weatherall, D. J. (1991). *The new genetics and clinical practice* (3rd ed.). New York: Oxford University Press.

Wheeler, M. D. (1991). Physical changes of puberty. *Endocrinology and Metabolism Clinics of North America, 20*(1), 1–14.

Wollenberg, A., Wolff, H., Jansen, T., Schmid, M. H., Rocken, M., & Plewig, G. (1997). Acne conglobata and Klinefelter's syndrome. *British Journal of Dermatology, 136,* 421–423.

Woodcock, R. W., & Johnson, M. B. (1989). *Woodcock–Johnson Psycho-Educational Battery—Revised.* Allen, TX: DLM Teaching Resources.

Zollner, T. M., Veraart, J. C., Wolter, M., Hesse, S., Villemur, B., Wenke, A., Werner, R. J., Boehncke, W. H., Jost, S. S., Scharrer, I., & Kaufman, R. (1997). Leg ulcers in Klinefelter's syndrome—further evidence for an involvement of plasminogen activator inhibitor-1. *British Journal of Dermatology, 136,* 341–344.

Zuppinger, K., Engel, E., Forbes, A. P., Mantooth, L., & Claffey, J. (1967). Klinefelter's syndrome: A clinical and cytogenetic study in twenty-four cases. *Acta Endocrinologica, 54*(Suppl. 113), 5–48.

19

PHENYLKETONURIA

SUSAN E. WAISBREN

HISTORICAL AND THEORETICAL BACKGROUND

Religion, politics, geography, and genetics all pertain to the study of phenylketonuria (PKU). An isolated community in San'a, the capital of Yemen more than 300 years ago, was probably home to the bearer of an unusual gene for PKU. The Jews of Yemen were forbidden to marry persons of other faiths, and others were punished by death if they converted to Judaism. Consequently, the gene spread only within this community, and it has been possible to trace all cases of PKU in Israelis of Yemenite Jewish origin to the one family in San'a (Wright, 1990). Different mutations for PKU have been traced to the Vikings and to gene bearers in Japan, Italy, Denmark, Scotland, Ireland, Kuwait, South America, and South Africa. Each of these mutations leads to an obstruction in the metabolism of phenylalanine, an essential amino acid abundant in protein. As an autosomal recessive disorder, PKU is inherited from each parent and affects males and females at an equal rate. The mutant gene produces a defect in the liver enzyme phenylalanine hydroxylase, resulting in a block in the conversion of phenylalanine to tyrosine. The only cure presently available for this disorder is liver transplantation (Vajro et al., 1993). Given the risks inherent in liver transplantation, this "cure" is generally not considered. Moreover, a treatment exists that prevents mental retardation, the most severe consequence of PKU.

In 1934, Asbjorn Følling, a Norwegian physician, discovered PKU. A mother with two retarded children came to see him after consulting many other doctors. She insisted that both her children had a similar degree of mental retardation and patterns of behavior; in addition, she pointed out that both excreted urine with a unique odor. Følling, who had also trained in chemistry, studied the children's urine using a wide variety of agents until he discovered that it contained a large amount of phenylpyruvic acid. He knew that phenylpyruvic acid was a metabolite of phenylalanine, and he suspected that the defect in this disorder involves phenylalanine metabolism (Følling, 1934). Others demonstrated that the disorder is inherited and that excess phenylalanine is present in blood.

It was not until 1954, however, that a treatment was discovered. Again a persistent mother, this time in England, provided the impetus for the discovery (see Koch, 1997). She brought to a physician named Horst Bickel her 17-month-old daughter, who had the typical features of PKU: mental retardation, eczema, awkward gait, spastic reflexes, and no language abilities. She took no interest in her surroundings, moaned incessantly, and banged her head. The young doctor reasoned that perhaps if the child's phenylalanine intake were limited, the buildup of the toxic amino acid could be prevented. Along with Louis Woolf, in London, he created an amino acid mixture containing all the necessary parts of protein except for phenylalanine (Bickel, Gerrard, & Hickmans, 1954). He advised the mother to feed her daughter the special formula and to avoid all other protein foods or drinks. Two weeks later, the mother returned, claiming a miracle. The little girl had learned to crawl and pull herself to a stand, and was bright and cheerful instead of dull and irritable. Bickel prescribed continuation of the treatment, but this time added phenylalanine to the formula. The mother returned 2 days later to report that her daughter had reverted to the previous state and that the formula no longer worked (Gerrard, 1994). Through this experiment, Bickel proved that phenylalanine caused the neurological problems and that dietary treatment was beneficial. He also realized that the sooner the special diet could be started, the greater the benefit.

The scene then shifted to the United States, where Robert Guthrie met Robert MacCready at a meeting of the National Association for Retarded Children. Each was a father of a child with mental retardation. MacCready was also the director of the Diagnostic Division of the Massachusetts Public Health Laboratories in Boston, and Guthrie was a physician and microbiologist from Buffalo, New York. Guthrie told MacCready about a test he had invented, the now famous Guthrie bacterial assay for the filter paper blood test (Guthrie & Susi, 1963). From a drop of blood obtained from the heel of a newborn infant, PKU could be identified within the first few days of life. Treatment started at this early age prevented mental retardation. MacCready was so impressed by this new technology that he spent a week in Buffalo learning the test. He brought it back to Boston, installed it in the Bacteriology Laboratory, and started the first newborn screening program for PKU (MacCready, 1963).

Despite the straightforward results, the simplicity of the method, and the clear rationale for newborn screening, its acceptance was far from easy. With a persistence equal to that of the mothers from Norway and England, Guthrie lobbied in Washington and traveled throughout the United States arguing for mandatory, government-supported newborn screening (Koch, 1997). By 1964 they had succeeded in Massachusetts, and 11 years later 43 states had enacted a newborn screening law (Paul, 1999). Today laws mandating newborn screening for PKU exist throughout North America and most of Europe.

The reasons why PKU causes neurological problems remain unknown. Based on pathology reports, neuroimaging, research into biochemical pathways, and studies using animal models, three main theories exist to explain the pathology in PKU:

1. *Phenylalanine toxicity.* Phenylalanine or its metabolites in large quantities may be toxic to the brain by inhibiting myelin development (Scriver, Kaufman, Eisensmith, & Woo, 1995). Magnetic resonance imaging (MRI) studies suggest that when phenylalanine levels are high, myelination in the brain is reduced. In untreated or poorly treated children with PKU, myelination is delayed; in adults who discontinue the diet, dysmyelination occurs. Since, however, the degree of myelin in the brain has not been associated with IQ or clinical symptoms in PKU, the precise mechanism of phenylalanine toxicity is still unknown (Jones et al., 1995).

2. *Competition for transport.* Phenylalanine competes with several other essential amino acids (large neutral amino acids, or LNAAs) for transport across the blood–brain

barrier. Since the transporter across the blood–brain barrier tends to have a higher affinity for phenylalanine than for the other LNAAs in the presence of a high level of blood phenylalanine, other amino acids, such as tyrosine, fail to reach the brain (Miller, Braun, Pardridge, & Oldendorf, 1985). In a sense, phenylalanine "floods the system." This prevents other important amino acids—such as tyrosine and tryptophan, which are precursors of dopamine and serotonin, respectively—from entering the brain in their usual proportions (Güttler & Lou, 1986; Krause et al., 1985).

3. *Dopamine reduction*. Since phenylalanine cannot be metabolized to tyrosine in PKU, tyrosine is reduced, and the metabolites of tyrosine are also reduced. One of these metabolites is the neurotransmitter dopamine, and, as expected, dopamine levels are reduced in the cerebrospinal fluid of people with PKU. Treatment with large doses of tyrosine, however, do not prevent the neurological effects of PKU. Years ago, a child was not treated with the phenylalanine-restricted diet, but instead was treated only with high doses of tyrosine. Unfortunately, the treatment was unsuccessful, and the child became severely mentally retarded (Batshaw, Valle, & Bessman, 1981). In a more recent study, phenylketonuric adults who had discontinued or relaxed treatment were administered high doses of tyrosine or a placebo in a double-blind crossover study. Despite increases in plasma tyrosine (and presumed increases in brain dopamine) during tyrosine supplementation, no beneficial effects on any measure were noted (Pietz, Landwehr, Schmidt, de Sonneville, & Trefz, 1995). Thus high phenylalanine levels are still considered the most likely pathological agent in PKU. However, recent studies indicate that certain parts of the brain, specifically the prefrontal cortex, are highly sensitive to even modest reductions in dopamine. If this is found to be true, then specific functions related to these brain areas should be selectively impaired in patients with PKU (Diamond, Ciaramitaro, Donner, Djali, & Robinson, 1994).

Questions about the specific brain effects in PKU led investigators to search for animal models, where brain chemistry could be studied directly. Until recently, no monkeys, mice, rabbits, or any other animals with PKU could be found. It was possible to raise the blood phenylalanine levels of normal animals by loading the diet with phenylalanine, often in conjunction with an inhibitor of the phenylalanine hydroxylase enzyme. However, the conversion of phenylalanine to tyrosine could not be blocked sufficiently to prevent some increase in the tyrosine level; hence these experimental animals were never very similar to humans with PKU, who had chronically low levels of tyrosine. Using classical mutagenesis and selective breeding, researchers began to "create" the PKU mouse. When a known mutagen was fed to hundreds of pregnant mice, and when a phenylalanine-loaded diet was then fed to the offspring, mice suspected of being carriers for the mutant phenylalanine hydroxylase gene could be identified. After cross-breeding carriers for three generations, the researchers eventually created a strain of mice with PKU. These mice, when fed a normal-protein diet, had elevated phenylalanine levels and appeared mentally retarded; that is, they could not swim, while their littermates without PKU did so easily. Moreover, these mice had lighter-colored coats and were smaller in size—features corresponding to the lighter hair and small stature of children with untreated PKU. When fed a phenylalanine-restricted but otherwise nutritionally balanced diet, the mice began to look more like their non-PKU siblings. Some probably even learned to swim (McDonald, Bode, Dove, & Shedlovsky, 1990; Shedlovsky, McDonald, Symula, & Dove, 1993). With these mice, researchers are now investigating the actual levels of neurotransmitters in different parts of the brain, the degree of transport of the various amino acids across the blood–brain barrier, and the difference between the blood phenylalanine and tyrosine levels in these mice and the usual levels of these amino acids in the brain. The biochemical effects in the brain of restricting phenylalanine in the diet and supplementing with tyrosine can now also be directly measured.

Although devastating effects usually occur when PKU is untreated, and close-to-normal development is attained when PKU is treated within the first weeks of life, there are exceptions. A few individuals with untreated PKU and high phenylalanine levels have normal intelligence, and some individuals with well-treated PKU suffer neurological effects and have lower IQs than their siblings. Two individuals in the same family occasionally have dramatically different outcomes. None of the theories regarding the pathology in PKU can yet explain these exceptional cases.

GENETICS

The small warning label on diet soda cans containing the artificial sweetener aspartame reads, "Phenylketonurics: Contains phenylalanine." This warning has greatly increased the public awareness of PKU. In reality, PKU is one of the most common genetic disorders known. In the United States, 1 out of 50 people are carriers. Results of newborn screening of over 5 million neonates from throughout the world indicate varying rates. PKU is almost unknown among individuals of African descent, but fairly common among those of European descent, with prevalence rates ranging from 1 in 5,400 in Ireland to 1 in 11,000 in the United States and 1 in 16,000 in Switzerland (Woo, Lidsky, Güttler, Chandra, & Robson, 1983). As an autosomal recessive disorder, PKU is inherited from both parents. When both the mother and father are carriers, the chance of each child's inheriting PKU is 1:4.

The pattern of inheritance is not entirely simple, however. Soon after PKU was discovered, physicians and parents noted that not all children with PKU were the same in their phenylalanine levels when off diet, or in their tolerance for phenylalanine before their blood levels rose. People in Italy, for example, appeared to have a milder form of PKU than people in Ireland: They could tolerate more protein, they had lower blood phenylalanine levels, and they seemed to be less affected by their PKU. In the 1980s, the answer to this puzzling picture appeared. Woo et al. (1983) cloned the gene for phenylalanine hydroxylase, the enzyme responsible for the conversion of phenylalanine to tyrosine. When this gene is defective, the enzyme does not function or does not function completely; as a consequence, a rise in phenylalanine occurs. The investigators eventually realized that many mutations exist in the phenylalanine hydroxylase gene. Mapped to chromosome 12, the phenylalanine hydroxylase gene is 90 kb in length (q22–q24.2; 13 exons). Most children inherit two different mutations, resulting in substantial genetic heterogeneity in those with PKU (Scriver et al., 1995). By 1996, there were over 250 known mutations linked to PKU, and more are sure to be discovered (Guldberg et al., 1996).

Does genotype make a difference? The answer is yes and no. Studies (Trefz et al., 1993) suggest that patients with classic PKU, who have blood phenylalanine levels greater than 20 mg/dl on a normal diet and no activity of the phenylalanine hydroxylase enzyme, have genotypes differing from those of patients with mild PKU (with blood phenylalanine levels of 10–20 mg/dl and 5–15% residual activity of the enzyme) and of patients with non-PKU hyperphenylalaninemia (with blood phenylalanine levels of 2–10 mg/dl and an estimated 25% residual activity of phenylalanine hydroxylase).

The phenotype, however, depends primarily on the particular combination of genes inherited from the mother and father. For example, a patient with the genotype R408W/

IVS-12 will have a more severe biochemical defect (and probably a lower IQ) than a patient with the genotype R408W/Y414C, even though the two patients share the R408W gene. The reason is that although the R4O8W mutation confers no phenylalanine hydroxylase enzyme activity, the Y414C allows for enough of the enzyme activity to produce mild PKU, while the IVS-12 mutation also confers no phenylalanine hydroxylase activity and thus results in severe PKU. In addition to the genetic factors related to the phenylalanine hydroxylase genotype, however, other physiological and genetic factors affect the final phenotypic outcome in PKU (Ozalp et al., 1994).

An intriguing question is that of the persistence of PKU in the population. Some people have argued that the disease should have "died out," since until very recently almost all individuals with PKU were severely mentally retarded, and few reproduced. One explanation is that new mutations occur frequently enough to replace mutations that have disappeared through lack of reproduction (Levy, 1989). Others believe that there must be a selective advantage to carrier status for PKU (Kidd, 1987), possibly including a lower spontaneous abortion rate (Woolf, 1976). Most likely, carrier status is sufficiently high to remain constant, despite the rates at which affected individuals reproduce (Kirkman, 1982). Prenatal diagnosis is available for PKU (Scriver et al., 1995), but it is not commonly requested.

Gene therapy for PKU may one day be a reality. To date, researchers have successfully introduced into the liver of a PKU mouse a recombinant adenoviral vector containing a normal gene for phenylalanine hydroxylase. Within a week, the mouse was "cured" of PKU, but the effect did not persist. Moreover, mice once treated did not respond to repeated injections of the adenovirus vector (Fang et al., 1994; Eisensmith & Woo, 1994).

DEVELOPMENTAL COURSE

Untreated and Late-Treated PKU

Children with classic PKU, if untreated, develop mental retardation, eczema, seizures, ataxia, motor deficits, and behavioral problems. Childhood autism is often prominent. Although they appear normal until about age 6 months, infants with PKU gradually exhibit developmental problems. PKU produces a relentlessly progressive form of brain damage, probably beginning just after birth. Individuals with untreated PKU are some of the most difficult to manage in institutions for the mentally retarded, displaying self-mutilation, aggression, impulsivity, and psychosis (Penrose, 1972).

Parents and caretakers today now introduce the special phenylalanine-restricted diet to adults with untreated PKU when medications and behavioral programs fail to control psychotic symptoms, aggression, or self-abuse. Follow-up studies document little or no improvement in cognitive performance. However, case reports suggest moderate and sometimes even dramatic improvement in behavior if metabolic control is achieved and maintained on a long-term basis (Harper & Reid, 1987; Yannicelli & Ryan 1995; Baumeister & Baumeister, 1998).

Even today, an infant with PKU is occasionally missed in newborn screening because of laboratory or hospital errors. Not receiving the benefit of early dietary therapy, the child soon exhibits early signs of developmental delay. Most of these "missed" children are eventually diagnosed in early childhood. Treatment at this stage often results in improvement, with some children who neither walked nor talked at age 3 or 4 years gaining these developmental milestones shortly after restriction of their phenylalanine intake. Eventual developmental outcome in these children is variable, with a few attaining an IQ within the average range, but most others performing within the range of mild to moderate mental retardation. Late treatment such as this, however, is almost always associated with significant learning disabilities, even when IQ is within the average range.

Treated PKU

Treatment for PKU consists of a phenylalanine-restricted diet, including a special formula and foods low in phenylalanine. The formula contains all the necessary nutrients (amino acids) in protein, apart from phenylalanine. Unfortunately, amino acids in this form have a distinctive and strong taste and odor. Almost all infants accept the formula without difficulties; however, some children find it distasteful as they grow older, and many adults returning to the diet deem it unpalatable. The diet permits sugars, fats, measured amounts of fruits and vegetables, and special low-protein pastas, grains, and breads. Meats, fish, eggs, dairy products, nuts, soy products, regular grains, and corn are not allowed. When children or adults "cheat" or consume more than the allocated amount of protein, they do not immediately feel ill, although a few individuals report feeling tired or distracted. Most experience no side effects. It is only the cumulative effect of increased phenylalanine intake that is noticeable. Dietary control is monitored through frequent sampling of blood phenylalanine levels.

Until the 1980s, most clinics in North America and Europe recommended diet discontinuation during middle childhood (Schuett & Brown, 1984). At about age 5 or 6 years, most children with PKU were suddenly allowed to eat as much protein (phenylalanine) as they desired. Although it was known that their blood phenylalanine levels would rise, it was thought that their cognitive abilities would be unaffected. The fact that high phenylalanine levels are known to affect myelin in the brain, and that myelination is essentially complete after infancy, provided the rationale for this approach to treatment for PKU. Moreover, children who did not adhere to the diet despite medical recommendations did not become mentally retarded. Thus the policy of diet discontinuation was adopted.

Despite the early enthusiasm for considering PKU a disease of early childhood, evidence gradually mounted demonstrating that diet discontinuation resulted in diminished IQ in a sizable proportion of these children (Waisbren Schnell, & Levy, 1980). A North American PKU Collaborative Study was established to determine the effects of diet discontinuation in early-treated children with PKU (Koch, Azen, Friedman, & Williamson, 1982). The initial random assignment to diet continuation or discontinuation was abandoned, since some clinics came to consider it unethical to discontinue the diet for any child. At the same time, some children assigned to the diet continuation group failed to maintain metabolic control. The final sample included almost equal numbers of children considered on and off diet. The results of the follow-up study indicated that the age at which blood phenylalanine levels consistently exceeded 15 mg/dl was the best predictor of IQ and school achievement at ages 8 and 10 years (Holtzman, Kronmal, van Doorninck, Azen, & Koch, 1986). A retrospective study of 46 patients in Pennsylvania followed beyond age 12 years reported similar results (Legido et al., 1993). On the other hand, a policy of diet discontinuation at age 10 years was instituted in Scotland, and no declines in cognitive and motor functioning were noted after diet discontinuation in adolescents and young adults at a median age of 20 years. However, the individuals with PKU performed less well on all tests than age-matched subjects without PKU (Griffiths, Paterson, & Harvie, 1995).

Neuropsychological Effects despite Treatment

Early diagnosis and treatment for PKU unquestionably prevent mental retardation. Diet continuation, however, does not prevent all adverse effects from PKU. Despite the prevention of the severe neurological complications from PKU, more subtle psychological consequences have been exposed.

Visual–motor deficits are prevalent (Koff, Boyle, & Pueschel, 1977). Even early-treated children tend to have awkward pencil grips and poor handwriting. Fine motor speed is diminished, copying letters or figures is a laborious process, and work takes longer to complete. When asked to copy geometric designs, many children with PKU have notable difficulties, particularly when they are required to integrate figures. Visual demonstrations, diagrams, and models are less effective than verbal explanations. The children have difficulties remembering the location of objects in space. The "number line" may be incomprehensible for years after it has been taught in arithmetic class.

Also consistently noted in individuals with treated PKU have been problems in mental processing (Waisbren, Brown, de Sonneville, & Levy, 1994). This finding has led to increasing interest in the executive functioning of children with early-treated PKU (Pennington, van Doorninck, McCabe, & McCabe, 1985). "Executive functioning" is the ability to retain information and use it for problem solving. Planning, integrative processing skills (reasoning, comprehension, concept formation), and sustained attention depend on executive functioning. When information is presented slowly and simply, children with PKU learn and retain it as well as peers do. However, when the cognitive "load" is increased or a faster processing speed (reaction time) is required, the children often become confused and overwhelmed. Children without difficulties in executive functioning are able to increase their focus and adjust to the greater processing demands. When impaired in executive functioning, individuals often react more slowly and make more errors on tests related to mental processing (de Sonneville & Njiokiktjien, 1988). Results of neuropsychological testing in early-treated children with PKU demonstrate clear deficits in executive functioning and in reaction time (Brunner, Jordan, & Berry, 1983; Seashore, Friedman, Novelly, & Bapat, 1985; Welsh, Pennington, Ozonoff, Rouse, & McCabe, 1990; Krause et al., 1985; de Sonneville, Schmidt, Michel, & Batzler, 1990; Schmidt, Rupp, Burgard, & Pietz, 1992; Schmidt et al., 1994).

Factors Related to Neuropsychological Performance in Treated PKU

Many studies have focused on the blood phenylalanine level in treated PKU. Factors such as timing of treatment initiation, lifetime level of metabolic control, and current dietary status all have an impact. In most studies, if treatment is initially delayed past the first 3 months of life, a child performs less well than siblings with PKU who are treated earlier. If metabolic control is variable throughout childhood, the individual tends to have poorer mental processing skills, slower reaction time, diminished achievement, and a lower IQ. One study has documented IQ loss in early-treated adolescents with elevated phenylalanine levels (Beasley Costello, & Smith, 1994). By 18 years of age, 27% have an IQ less than 70. IQ is significantly related to the average phenylalanine control between birth and 14 years of age. The current blood phenylalanine level in an individual with PKU is also correlated with reaction time (Clarke, Gates, Hogan, Barrett, & McDonald, 1987; Schmidt et al, 1994) and is thought to reflect the level of brain phenylalanine (Jordan, Brunner,

Hunt, & Berry, 1985). If the child is currently off diet or in poor metabolic control, he or she demonstrates compromised neuropsychological functioning. For children and adults of normal intellectual abilities, resumption of diet and maintenance of good metabolic control result in improved reaction time and concentration. Although IQ remains essentially unchanged, functioning improves when blood phenylalanine levels are reduced.

Recommendations from the various PKU clinics vary with regard to what constitutes metabolic control in children over 6 years of age. The target for most clinics is now 2–6 mg/dl. However, due to the restrictiveness of the diet, fewer than half of teenagers are able to maintain levels within this range. In a follow-up study of children in the United Kingdom, only 12% of the children were following a strict diet by age 14 years, and only 4% were following a strict diet by age 18 years (Beasley et al, 1994). One research group suggests that levels as high as 15 mg/dl may be benign in teenagers and young adults (Griffiths et al., 1995). Other investigators contend that any elevation above 6 mg/dl may have adverse effects (Diamond, 1994).

The possibility exists that neuropsychological performance in treated PKU is related to the extent of the enzyme block. Individuals with natural blood phenylalanine levels in the range of non-PKU mild hyperphenylalaninemia perform at a higher level than early-treated individuals with mild PKU (also called "atypical PKU"), who in turn attain higher scores than those with classic PKU. In other words, the greater the activity of the phenylalanine hydroxylase enzyme, the better a person's functioning is.

Performances on neuropsychological tests suggest that there may be localization of brain effects in treated PKU, with a suspicion that the prefrontal cortex is involved (Welsh et al., 1990). If so, the possibility that dopamine has an important role in the cognitive limitations in PKU needs to be considered. Projections of dopaminergic neurons in the neocortex are found primarily in the frontal lobes (Porrino & Goldman-Rakic, 1982), and the prefrontal cortex has one of the highest levels of dopamine turnover in the brain (Diamond et al., 1994; Tam, Elsworth, Bradberry, & Roth, 1990). Investigations of individuals with PKU demonstrate that reductions in cerebrospinal fluid concentrations of dopamine and serotonin metabolites are associated with lower scores on reaction time tests (Lykkelund et al., 1988). With this information in mind, Diamond et al. (1994) and Diamond, Prevor, Callender, & Druin (1997) hypothesize that the prefrontal lobe is the most affected brain region in PKU, because it is most sensitive to mild reductions in dopamine.

Neuropsychological tests thought to be particularly sensitive to prefrontal cortical functioning—such as tests of motor planning, visual search, and verbal fluency; the Tower of Hanoi; the Stroop Color Word Test; and the Wisconsin Card Sorting Test—have been used to test this hypothesis. Diamond et al. (1997) reported that early and continuously treated children (with blood phenylalanine levels between 6 and 10 mg/dl) showed impaired performance on six tests that require working memory and inhibitory abilities dependent on the dorsolateral prefrontal cortex. Other investigations have supported these findings (Welsh et al., 1990; Weglage, Pietsch, Fünders, Koch, & Ullrich, 1996). Stemerdink (1996) found that in 36 older patients (aged 8 to 19 years) treated early and continuously, neuropsychological performance on three out of four prefrontal tasks was impaired. The same pattern has been found in adults with early-treated PKU (Ris, Williams, Hunt, Berry, & Leslie, 1994). Moreover, individuals with PKU attain lower standard scores on these tests than on control tests of parietal and temporal cortex functions.

Researchers have also found evidence for impairments in visual contrast sensitivity when blood phenylalanine levels are elevated. This is relevant, since it is hypothesized that the retina is also highly sensitive to moderate reductions in brain dopamine (Stemerdink, 1996; Diamond, 1994).

Not all studies, however, support the dopamine–prefrontal dysfunction hypothesis. Mazzocco et al. (1994), using the Tower of Hanoi and visual search tests, found that children aged 6 to 13 years who were treated early and continuously showed no deficits on the neuropsychological tests, despite a range of blood phenylalanine levels.

Variations on the dopamine hypothesis have also been proposed. Krause et al. (1985) have reported a correlation between increased reaction time and decreased urinary dopamine in patients with PKU. Since brain dopamine is concentrated in the corpus striatum, and since the choice reaction time test requires a motor response as well as integration of stimuli, they speculate that the nigrostriatal and corticostriatal pathways are affected. Faust, Libon, and Pueschel (1986–1987) obtained similar results; they suspect that the deficits are associated with complex areas of the brain, such as the anterior frontal regions, and in motor areas that represent less advanced functions.

Some studies have used MRI to investigate the relevance of myelin abnormalities in PKU. Reports conclude that the severity of the MRI changes is significantly and independently associated with the phenylalanine concentrations at the time of the investigation and the timing of diet discontinuation. When metabolic control improves, the MRI picture also improves. The area of the brain in which white matter abnormalities are most commonly noted is the parieto-occipital region. Despite the provocative nature of these results, MRI findings have not been found to correlate with IQ, neuropsychological functioning, or neurological symptoms (Thompson et al., 1993; Jones et al., 1995). One study suggests, however, that abnormal myelination neonatally disrupts the development of inter-hemispheric connections in early-treated PKU. Gourovitch, Craft, Dowton, Ambrose, and Sparta (1994) reported that children with early-treated PKU demonstrated slowed interhemispheric transfer from the left to the right hemisphere, compared to normal controls and to children with attention-deficit/hyperactivity disorder (ADHD). Age of treatment initiation and phenylalanine level at birth (but not concurrent blood phenylalanine levels) were correlated with reaction time on tests of interhemispheric transfer in this study.

Developmental Domains Usually Unaffected in PKU

Infants with early-treated PKU generally attain developmental milestones at the appropriate ages. Most sit up at about 6 months of age, walk at a year, and begin talking at 18 to 24 months. Although some do not want to give up the bottle, most graduate to a cup and demonstrate appropriate table manners. They learn to tie their shoes in kindergarten, ride a two-wheeler, count by twos, and recite the alphabet at the same time as most of their peers. Most do not have difficulties learning to read. They interact well with peers, try to please their teachers, and talk on the phone for hours as teenagers. And many children treated early and continuously show no impairments on a wide variety of tests of information processing (Stemerdink et al., 1995). Thus, in many respects, children with PKU are indistinguishable from other children their age.

BEHAVIORAL, ACADEMIC, AND EMOTIONAL PRESENTATION

Attention-Deficit/Hyperactivity Disorder

Often linked to the underlying neuropsychological deficits in PKU is ADHD. Researchers and clinicians have alluded to an increased prevalence of attentional problems in PKU (Lou,

1994; Burgard, Rey, Rupp, Avadie, & Rey, 1997). In one continuing study of 40 children, 25% of the boys, but none of the girls, with PKU have been diagnosed with ADHD (Waisbren, Varvogli, Warner-Rogers, & Levy, 1999). Results on parental checklists further indicate that 20–33% of the boys, but fewer than 15% of the girls, are rated as hyperactive or impulsive. The boys have a lower mean IQ (100) than the girls (113), and lower scores on the Freedom from Distractibility Scale of the Wechsler Intelligence Scale for Children—Revised (95 for the boys and 110 for the girls). If ADHD is truly associated with PKU, this disorder should be equally prevalent among girls and boys. However, the boys in this study have higher blood phenylalanine levels and are less likely to be rated by the nutritionist as being in good metabolic control. Elevated blood phenylalanine levels probably contribute to the incidence of ADHD, although gender stereotypes may help explain the greater frequency of ADHD among boys.

Methylphenidate (Ritalin) and other medications do not appear to result in significant improvements in attention and school achievement, although some parents report that their children exhibit greater self-control when on medication. However, careful studies of the effects of medications for ADHD in children with PKU need to be conducted.

School Achievement

Difficulties in arithmetic typify the learning profile among young children with PKU (Weglage, Fünders, Wilken, Schubert, & Ullrich, 1993). Achievement spans the full range, with some children placed in special programs, others struggling in regular classes, still others proceeding at the same rate as peers, and a few gaining honors in law school. Nonetheless, when children with PKU confront problems in school, they invariably falter in math class. The North American PKU Collaborative Study documents a steady decline in arithmetic scores in both diet-continued and diet-discontinued children from ages 6 to 10 years (Fishler, Azen, Henderson, Friedman, & Koch, 1987). By age 12 years, achievement scores in arithmetic fall again in 90% of children, regardless of dietary control (Azen et al., 1991).

With arithmetic, the underlying cause for difficulties seems to be twofold. First is the issue of spatial perception. Simply put, the children fail to perceive the number line in their "mind's eye." The concepts "more than" and "less than," equal distances between numbers, and fixed sequences are not secure ideas. One-to-one correspondence between numbers and objects comes slowly. Addition and subtraction can be drilled, but an intuitive sense of sums and differences may be forever lacking. Multiplication facts can be learned with considerable effort, but without frequent use, they are easily lost. Fractions present almost insurmountable obstacles, as do geometric shapes and formulas. A good sense of spatial arrangement is also needed to line up numbers for performing calculations with paper and pencil. Children with PKU commonly turn in disorganized papers, with wrong answers because numbers are lined up improperly. A second impediment to success in arithmetic is a weakness in executive functioning. Because of their difficulties maintaining information in memory, children with PKU struggle with calculations requiring more than one step. Word problems are especially challenging because they require a child to decide on the appropriate operation and to remember numbers for computing the answer.

As the children grow older, difficulties in reading comprehension become apparent. Decoding skills come readily to most children with PKU, and the first through third grades pass uneventfully. Fourth grade brings new demands for reading comprehension and application of rote skills. Suddenly many children with PKU fall behind their classmates and are referred for psychological evaluations. In actuality, the underlying weaknesses have always been there, but simple compensatory strategies have sufficed to keep the children at grade level. By fourth grade, too, problems in executive functioning and sustained attention interfere with the acquisition of new knowledge and the ability to master new skills. Science and social studies, as well as arithmetic and reading, become difficult subjects.

Spelling continues to be a strength for most of these children, although for some the sequencing issue hinders visualization of the correct order of letters. In fourth grade, homework increases, as does the amount of written work required. Again, the problems in visual–motor coordination that could once be overcome by hard work now overwhelm the children's coping mechanisms. Occupational therapy is sometimes recommended for children with poor visual–motor skills. If teachers do not recognize such a child's underlying learning difficulties, they may deem the child lazy, dull, inattentive, or obstinate. Even if teachers do suspect a learning disability, they may assume that the child has a typical form of dyslexia or ADHD. However, this may not be the case. Careful evaluation of the child is important to identify the specific pattern of deficits and the particular factors related to PKU that may have an impact on the child's behavior in the classroom. The child's level of PKU, treatment history, and current degree of metabolic control need to be considered, along with the psychosocial stresses the child may be experiencing.

Emotional Disturbances

The effects of PKU on personality and temperament were noted by early researchers (Fisch, Sines, & Chang, 1981). Measures of "persistence," "intensity," and "rhythmicity" were observed to be lower in children with PKU in one study (Schor, 1983). In another study, early-treated school children were rated as more clumsy, talkative, and hypersensitive than their peers (Siegel, Balow, Risch, & Anderson, 1968). On the other hand, patience, sociability, and obedience to the law were also attributed to the genetic defect. In untreated and late-treated PKU, bizarre behaviors were noted, including obsessive–compulsive rituals, self-abuse, and extreme tactile sensitivity. Although such attributions are rare today, they presaged interest in the effects of metabolic disequilibrium on personality and emotion. Today parents note that their children sometimes undergo personality changes when their phenylalanine levels rise (Schuett, 1997).

The long-term consequences of early-treated PKU are relatively unknown. Woolf (1979) speculated that if diet was discontinued in middle childhood an insidious process would begin, culminating in loss of IQ, antisocial behavior, and severe emotional disturbance (including frank psychosis). Although such consequences are rare, effects of a less serious nature are common. One study of young women with PKU revealed that they were less mature than their peers. They obtained a driver's license at a later age and tended to remain longer in their parents' homes (Waisbren, Hamilton, St. James, Shiloh, & Levy, 1995). Other studies of adolescents with PKU indicate that they are less independent, less achievement-oriented, lower in self-esteem, and more frustrated than peers (Weglage et al., 1992).

Agoraphobia has also been identified as a complication of elevated phenylalanine levels. Among five adults who experienced panic attacks and were unable to venture more than a short distance from their homes, the two who returned to the phenylalanine-restricted diet experienced dramatic improvement in symptoms (Waisbren & Levy, 1991).

In another study, adolescents and young women with PKU who either were late-treated (i.e., treatment was initiated after 90 days of age) or had terminated the diet for a period of at least 5 years were compared to women who were early-treated and had remained continuously on the diet. The women who had extended exposure to elevated phenylalanine levels evidenced significantly greater psychopathology as measured by the Minnesota Multiphasic Personality Inventory. The pattern of scores was remarkably consistent, with a tendency toward elevations on scales related to thought disorder and mood. Although they were not actively psychotic, the women who had experienced extended exposure to high blood phenylalanine levels were poor assessors of the emotions or expectations of others. They were also prone to feelings of alienation, depression, and social isolation, and had difficulties thinking and communicating (Waisbren & Zaff, 1994). For patients who remain on the diet, the future appears brighter, although few individuals maintain strict metabolic control as they grow older (Weglage et al., 1992).

Researchers from the German Collaborative Study (Pietz et al., 1997) report that the rate of psychiatric disorders in the adults with PKU is 35.7%, compared to 16.1% in controls. Patients with PKU show exclusively "internalizing" disturbances (especially depression and anxiety), whereas control subjects demonstrate both internalizing and externalizing (antisocial) symptoms. Females with PKU are more apt to experience depression than males. No correlation has been found between the severity or pattern of psychopathology and biochemical control. Moreover, no correlations between psychiatric symptoms and MRI abnormalities have been observed. However, a restrictive, controlling style of parenting is a risk factor for the development of psychiatric symptoms, prompting the authors to conclude that psychiatric disturbances in adults with PKU may be related to psychological factors rather than to biochemical or neurological sources.

MEDICAL COMORBIDITY

Case reports of a wide variety of syndromes associated with PKU have been reported. In the past, children with untreated PKU were often diagnosed with autism, and indeed presented with the hallmark features of this disorder (Koch, Acosta, Fishler, Schaeffler, & Wohlers, 1967). Even today, the few children in the United States missed by newborn screening and therefore not treated are often diagnosed as autistic, as well as developmentally delayed. Seizures, severe eczema, ataxia, and self-abusive behaviors are not infrequent in untreated PKU.

If "overtreated," with extreme limitation of protein intake resulting in phenylalanine depletion, a child with PKU can experience significant growth retardation, lethargy, and even death. Fortunately, the need to monitor metabolic status carefully to avoid overrestriction was recognized early in the history of treatment for PKU (Hanley, Linsao, Davidson, & Moes, 1970).

Some individuals who discontinue treatment experience dramatic consequences, including seizures, problems with balance, hallucinations, and paralysis of the legs. These reports, though quite alarming, do not represent the usual course of PKU in diet-discontinued individuals. Nonetheless, when they do occur, there is little doubt that phenylalanine toxicity is a contributing factor, since return to treatment alleviates (though it may not cure) the problems (Schuett, 1997).

Single-case reports of distinct medical conditions in association with PKU have also been published. These include anorexia nervosa (Clarke & Yapa, 1991), congenital hypothyroidism (Schmidt, Solberg, Diament, & Pimentel, 1981), diabetes (Webster & Wallace, 1995), Down syndrome (Fisch & Horrobin, 1968; Blehova, Pazoutova, & Subrt, 1970), Duchenne muscular dystrophy (Roth, Cohn, Berman, & Segal, 1976), Hartnup disease (Jonxis, 1957), hereditary fructose intolerance (Celiker, Dural, & Erdem, 1993), and histidinemia (Walker et al., 1981). Genetic linkages have been sought, but not found, between PKU and these disorders.

MATERNAL PKU

In a single generation, the benefits of newborn screening for PKU in terms of preventing mental retardation could be erased by the effects of maternal PKU (Kirkman, 1982). "Maternal PKU" refers to the risks to the fetus when the mother has PKU. The damage to the fetus occurs because of the intrauterine environment, since the fetus relies on the mother to metabolize phenylalanine. There are no particular risks inherent in paternal PKU, apart from the possibility of the child's having PKU if the mother is a carrier (Fisch, Matalon, Weisberg, & Michals, 1991). On the other hand, when the mother has classic PKU and does not receive treatment, her fetus is exposed to toxic levels of phenylalanine. Among the birth defects that result from phenylalanine exposure in untreated maternal PKU are mental retardation (95%), microcephaly (90%), and congenital heart disease (17%) (Lenke & Levy, 1980). The precise mechanism of fetal damage in maternal PKU is still unknown, although it is clear that the fetus is harmed by the abnormal intrauterine environment produced by the genetically abnormal mother (Ghavami & Levy, 1986; Levy & Ghavami, 1996).

The risks in maternal PKU are significantly reduced if the mother initiates strict dietary treatment prior to pregnancy and maintains metabolic control throughout pregnancy (Koch et al., 1990, 1994; Hanley, Clarke, & Schoonheyt, 1987; Lynch, Pitt, Maddison, Wraith, & Danks, 1988). Women with non-PKU mild hyperphenylalaninemia, whose natural blood phenylalanine levels are much less elevated than in women with PKU, incur little or no risk for adverse pregnancy outcomes (Levy & Waisbren 1983; Levy et al., 1994). This finding underscores the importance of metabolic control in maternal PKU.

Given the known benefits of dietary therapy, delivery of treatment for maternal PKU should be a straightforward process. However, this is not the case. Since the majority of young women with PKU terminated the diet during middle childhood, they must return to treatment. Many have difficulties resuming the highly restricted diet and tolerating the special formula. Many have not been followed by a metabolic clinic since childhood, and some may not even remember that they have PKU. Despite tracking and educational efforts, metabolic control is often not achieved adequately or in time to prevent damage to the fetus.

The International Collaborative Study of Maternal Phenylketonuria is a longitudinal, prospective study of the effects of dietary treatment during pregnancy in women with PKU in the United States, Canada, and Germany (Koch et al., 1993, 1994). The pregnant women receive ultrasound examinations, nutrition consultation, and metabolic monitoring as part of the study protocol. Offspring are developmentally evaluated in the neonatal period and at 12 and 24 months; thereafter, they are evaluated every 2 to 3 years through age 10 years. Although data analyses are incomplete, preliminary results strongly indicate that the number of gestational weeks until the mother reduces her blood phenylalanine level predicts the child's neonatal course, developmental quotient (DQ), and IQ. Birth head circumference is significantly related to maternal phenylalanine levels during weeks 8–12 of gestation (Rouse et al., 1997). Examiner ratings of infants on the Dubowitz Neurological Assessment of the Preterm and Full-Term Newborn Infant suggest that 29% evidence signs of abnormalities in muscle tone, head control, reflexes, and responsiveness. Those who attain abnormal ratings have poor responses on measures of axial tone: posterior head control, anterior head control, head lag, and ventral suspension. Scores on the Dubowitz Neurological Assessment are significantly influenced by the gestational age at which a mother with PKU attains metabolic control (Waisbren et al., 1998).

During infancy, the DQ of maternal PKU offspring whose mothers attain metabolic control by 20 weeks' gestation is within the average range, whereas the DQ of offspring whose mothers are not in metabolic control until after 20 weeks' gestation is in the borderline range (< 85). The mean IQ of these offspring follows a similar pattern: 93 for offspring whose mothers attain metabolic control by 10 weeks, 88 for those whose mothers attain metabolic control between 10 and 20 weeks, and 73 for those whose mothers are not in control until after 20 weeks (Hanley et al., 1996).

The neurodevelopmental picture of maternal PKU offspring is not yet complete. However, there are indications that it is similar to that found in fetal alcohol syndrome. Not only are there similarities in facial dysmorphology (Levy & Ghavami, 1996), but the neuropsychological profile may be similar, with increased rates of language deficits, hyperactivity, and deficient motor skills (Janzen, Nanson, & Block, 1995).

Thus, despite treatment, offspring from maternal PKU pregnancies often function developmentally and cognitively below normal levels (Koch et al., 1990). One reason for this is that more than 60% of women with PKU who become pregnant do so unintentionally and are not in metabolic control (Waisbren et al., 1995). Although this rate of unplanned pregnancies is similar to that in the general population in the United States (Harrison & Rosenfield, 1996), it has serious consequences for women with PKU (Koch et al., 1994; Hanley et al., 1987; Levy & Ghavami, 1996).

The factors found to be most highly correlated with adherence to medical recommendations in maternal PKU are social support and positive attitudes about the efficacy and acceptability of the treatment. Programs to enhance social support and positive attitudes are now being instituted, with promising results (Waisbren, Shiloh, St. James, & Levy, 1991; Waisbren et al., 1995, 1997; Levy & Waisbren, 1994). In addition, compliance can sometimes be improved through changes in the type of formula being used or the use of gelatin capsules containing the formula (Kecskemethy, Lobbregt, & Levy, 1993).

The deficits in offspring from treated maternal PKU pregnancies may also be caused in part by suboptimal home environments. Of concern are the limited intellectual abilities, reduced social resources, and emotional difficulties of women with PKU. In a study of adolescents and young adult women with PKU, the mean IQ was 85, and a substantial proportion of the women were of low socioeconomic status (Waisbren et al., 1995).

ASSESSMENT

Children with PKU require careful monitoring, especially during infancy and school years. As described earlier, even those children who maintain excellent metabolic control are at risk for learning disabilities. Annual testing in the preschool years should be followed with biennial testing during elementary school, preferably by a psychologist familiar with metabolic disorders. Thereafter, testing is recommended when a child experiences difficulties or when metabolic control changes. The frequency with which problems in executive functioning and attention occur suggests that neuropsychological testing should also be performed.

It is critical for the psychologist to communicate with the parents and schools about the specific learning profiles of students with PKU. Their difficulties in arithmetic may not be the same as the deficits noted in children without PKU. A recurring theme in the treatment of PKU is the importance of metabolic control. In almost all situations, the interpretation of test results must be done in association with the current blood phenylalanine level and the degree of metabolic control in previous years. Early history must also be taken into account.

Table 19.1 presents instruments that can be used to identify deficits common in PKU. In addition to neuropsychological testing, assessment techniques aimed at uncovering

TABLE 19.1. Instruments for Assessment of Various Domains Affected by PKU

Domain	Age group	Instrument
Infant development	6 months to 36 months	Bayley Scales of Infant Development, 2nd edition; Receptive–Expressive Emergent Language
Preschool cognitive development	2 years, 4 months to 8 years, 7 months	McCarthy Scales of Children's Abilities; Wechsler Preschool and Primary Scale of Intelligence—Revised
Achievement	5 years to 18 years, 11 months	Peabody Individual Achievement Test—Revised
Language development	4 years to 8 years, 11 months (Primary); 8 years, 6 months to 12 years, 11 months (Intermediate)	Test of Language Development, 2nd edition (Primary and Intermediate versions)
Behavior	2 years to 3 years (infant version); 4 years to 18 years (school-age version)	Achenbach Child Behavior Checklist; Conners Parent Rating Scale
Intelligence	6 years to 16 years, 11 months	Wechsler Intelligence Scale for Children, 3rd edition
Visual–motor skills	4 years to 17 years, 11 months	Developmental Test of Visual–Motor Integration
Self-esteem	8 years to 18 years	Piers–Harris Children's Self-Concept Scale
Adult intelligence	16 years to adults	Wechsler Adult Intelligence Scale, 3rd edition
Attentional skills, executive functioning	3 years to adults	Amsterdam Neuropsychological Tasks (de Sonneville, 1995)
Agoraphobia	Adults	Mobility Inventory for Agoraphobia (Chambless et al., 1987)
Personality	Adults	Minnesota Multiphasic Personality Inventory—2
Depression	Adults	Beck Depression Inventory

physiological correlates of functioning have been employed. Electroencephalographic examinations traditionally identified slow-wave abnormalities, but only in children who were late-treated or off diet. Evoked potentials appeared promising in the 1980s (Pueschel, Fogelson-Doyle, Kammerer, & Matsumiya, 1983), but more recent studies reveal no correlations between current clinical, biochemical, and neurophysiological parameters (Leuzzi, Cardona, Antonozzi, & Loizzo, 1994). Localized brain proton magnetic resonance spectroscopy (Johannik et al., 1994), and MRI of the brain (Jones et al., 1995; Cleary et al., 1994), have been used primarily for research purposes. The MRI examinations indicate that myelin reduction in PKU results from a reversible condition of reduced myelin synthesis rather than from excessive myelin loss. The term "dysmyelination" is more appropriate than "demyelination" for describing what occurs in PKU (Pearsen, Gean-Martin, Levy, & Davis, 1990). Moreover, the degree of myelin abnormalities appears to be irrelevant to level of functioning, with some of the children with the highest IQ scores having the most abnormal MRI findings.

TREATMENT

Treatment Adherence: Emotional and Developmental Issues

The biggest challenge in PKU is adherence to treatment. No matter how sophisticated the methods for monitoring development or biochemical status become, the outcome in PKU will unquestionably be determined by the affected individual's ability to restrict phenylalanine intake and consume an adequate amount of the formula. Maintaining metabolic control necessitates massive adjustments in daily life once a child is beyond infancy. Every social gathering, school lunch period, travel plan, summer activity, and nightly meal must be planned. Adolescents with PKU describe their social lives and emotional development as much more restricted than those of their peers (Weglage et al., 1992). Despite the best efforts of parents, most children and adolescents reject the formula or deviate from the diet at some periods. At different ages, the emotional issues vary, but the result is similar: a rise in blood phenylalanine levels and an increase in the risk for attentional, cognitive, and emotional problems.

The impact of PKU on neuropsychological functioning may lead to behaviors or personality styles in children that, in turn, elicit certain types of responses from parents or teachers. These responses may exacerbate the problem. For example, the hyperactive or impulsive behavior common in children with PKU may lead to poor self-control with the diet. This produces an anxious or overly controlling response from the parents, which may lead to an increase in poor dietary compliance and oppositional behavior in the children (Hendrikx, van der Schot, Slijper, Huisman, & Kalverboer, 1994).

When resistance to the diet occurs, various strategies may be employed. Usually parents can help their children regain equanimity, but sometimes psychological counseling is needed. The rebellious children who refuse formula, cheat on the diet, fuss, complain, and generally make their families miserable are well known to every clinic. These children frighten their parents and siblings by their nonchalant attitude about the consequences of elevated phenylalanine levels. Parents try rewards, punishments, and pleas. They ask doctors, nutritionists, and other professionals to talk to their children. They may drink the formula themselves to show that it is not distasteful. They may involve the children's friends to encourage dietary compliance. Nothing seems to alter the situation.

One interpretation of the time of rebellion is that it represents a struggle for identity, a sense of oneself apart from one's parents. This struggle can occur at many different ages. Some 2-year-olds go through this stage. Sometimes 10-year-olds or teenagers suddenly appear incorrigible with regard to the diet. The best strategy at this time is to validate the struggle for independence. The topic should be discussed in age-appropriate terms, and the need for greater autonomy should be acknowledged. Greater independence should then be granted in areas that are unrelated to food. For young children, this may mean later bedtimes or more choices about activities, friends, or clothing. In older children, encouragement to attend camp or to pursue a new hobby or skill may satisfy the need for independence without placing the children at risk. In every case, when the struggle for independence is at its height, there is a need to engage the child. This can be in the form of more special time with parents and extra support from professionals. A direct focus on the diet will be of little benefit, since the underlying issue is elsewhere.

For children who have generally been reasonable about the treatment but suddenly reject the diet, a cognitive approach may be best. A trip to the laboratory to see how blood specimens are analyzed, participation in PKU conferences, exposure to articles in newsletters or scientific journals, or discussions about the genetics and consequences of PKU may be helpful. Some children benefit from writing school reports on their disorder or from learning to cook low-protein foods, prepare the recipes, and maintain food records. A change in formula, a trial of using capsules, or a new schedule for drinking the formula can renew the commitment to the diet.

Suggestions for Developing Treatment Plans

An achievement protocol for knowledge and skills that each child needs in order to manage treatment better at a particular age can serve as a guide for parents and professionals. Below is an outline of one such protocol. This protocol can be referred to whenever a child or adolescent attends a clinic, in order to assess the level of knowledge and self-management that the young person has achieved.

Infants and toddlers (2–3 years)
1. Eats with the rest of the family at dinner
2. Names foods (in general)
3. Asks before eating uncertain foods
4. Shows awareness of difference in diet from family and friends
5. Has knowledge of "yes" and "no" foods
6. Has knowledge of procedural methods for blood sampling
7. Drinks formula out of a cup
8. Helps prepare formula—child can pour and stir/shake/blend
9. Begins to count food items
10. Reports foods consumed that day
11. Has basic knowledge of reasons for PKU diet

Preschool (4–6 years)
12. Handles social situations concerning food
13. Prepares formula (with assistance)
14. Can explain PKU and PKU diet in simple terms
15. Is knowledgeable about the daily schedule for formula intake
16. Takes blood sample with help
17. Has knowledge of basic reasons for his or her clinic visits
18. Understands basic number concepts necessary for measuring foods
19. Is knowledgeable about the daily phenylalanine allowance
20. Identifies and serves proper portions of allowed food

School age (7–10 years)
21. Prepares formula (with parents' supervision)
22. Is beginning to list foods on food record
23. Understands untreated versus poorly treated versus treated PKU
24. Acknowledges having PKU to peers
25. Has knowledge of PKU and PKU diet
26. Follows a low-phenylalanine recipe
27. Performs blood sampling with parental support
28. Monitors own blood levels and understands recommended range
29. Understands basic genetics of PKU
30. Can determine phenylalanine content of foods from manual or label

Adolescence (11+ years)

31. Prepares formula independently
32. Prepares a low-protein recipe
33. Performs blood sampling independently
34. Explains the genetics of PKU
35. Explains the rationale of dietary therapy
36. Understands whom to consult about PKU or the PKU diet
37. Demonstrates ability to cope with social pressures
38. Maintains diet record independently
39. (For a girl) Demonstrates knowledge of maternal PKU

Some clinics now offer a "PKU school," in which several children of similar age attend a clinic together and participate in a group learning activity, such as preparing a low-protein recipe or taking a finger stick blood specimen (Heffernan & Trahms, 1981). This provides social support as well as practical experience with some aspects of self-monitoring.

Recently, many young adults (both males and females) who discontinued treatment during middle childhood are returning to the diet. Many do so because of problems in concentration, emotional stability, or behavior. Others do so because of concerns for the future, although they have no obvious symptoms today. They, like younger children with PKU, achieve metabolic control more easily when social support programs are in place.

Camps and family retreat weekends are being offered in some parts of the United States and Europe to provide a more intensive social support experience (Waisbren et al., 1997). Activities include workshops, lectures, and group discussions, as well as recreational and social support programs. A manual on how to develop a maternal PKU camp has been developed that provides information on planning, fund raising, registering, and programming (Skitnevsky, Brown, & Waisbren, 1997).

In New England, the PKU Community Outreach Resource Programs (PKU CORPS) has provided social support activities for individuals with PKU and their families for several years. The PKU CORPS is composed of programs whose goals are to provide support, information, and practical assistance to help individuals and their families meet the challenges of treatment for PKU. This is accomplished through the joint involvement of peer support counselors, trained home visitors, other parents, and professional health care providers (Levy & Waisbren, 1994).

The first program of the PKU CORPS is called the PHE Buddy Program, through which peer counselors (mentors) are trained to work closely with younger children with PKU. These mentors, who are adolescents and young adults with PKU, encourage younger children to take more responsibility for their PKU. They advise them about ways to cope and provide them with support for maintaining metabolic control. Through the PHE Buddy Program, families are also linked together at weekend retreats and community outings. In this way, all individuals with PKU can have the opportunity for peer support even if they live in remote areas, far from the trained mentors.

The second program, the Resource Mothers Program, trains mothers of children with PKU to provide home visitation services to young women with PKU who are pregnant or planning a pregnancy. A pilot study of the Resource Mothers Program suggests that it is a promising approach to the problem of poor adherence to medical recommendations in women with PKU. Nineteen pregnancies in women who received the services of a resource mother were compared to 64 pregnancies in phenylketonuric women without resource mothers. Metabolic control was found to be achieved at a mean of 8 weeks after treatment began for participants in the Resource Mothers Program and at 16 weeks for women without resource mothers. Infants of participants had larger head circumferences at birth, and at 1 year of age they had a mean DQ of 108, compared to a mean DQ of 95 in the comparison group (St. James, Shapiro, & Waisbren, in press).

SUMMARY AND CONCLUSIONS

Despite the great amount of information learned in the past few decades, PKU exemplifies the challenges inherent in the study of neurodevelopment in genetic disorders. In one of nature's best-designed experiments (Roth, 1986), a defect in a single gene leads to disruptions in brain development that affect behavior, cognition, personality, social relationships, and even the health of the next generation. PKU is a disorder that has bred controversy since its discovery. Følling (1934), the doctor who first discovered the disorder, worked hard to convince colleagues that the musty smell noted in the urine of some mentally retarded children represented a metabolic disorder. Bickel et al. (1954), who discovered a treatment for PKU, fought skeptics who discounted their contention that high phenylalanine levels were harmful and that a low-phenylalanine diet could prevent brain damage in children with PKU. Guthrie, who discovered the simple bacterial assay to measure phenylalanine in filter paper blood specimens (Guthrie & Susi, 1963), and MacCready (1963), who worked for the Massachusetts Public Health Laboratories, at first faced ridicule for insisting on mandatory newborn screening. Later arguments arose over the safety of diet discontinuation, the value of dietary therapy for untreated adults with mental retardation, and the benefits of a return to diet for apparently well-functioning adults on a regular diet. Much still needs to be discussed about the theory that attributes deficits in frontal lobe functioning to moderate reductions of brain dopamine in children with PKU who are treated early and continuously. And, finally, debates continue about the meaning of abnormal MRI findings, the relevance of over 250 genotypes, and the feasibility of gene therapy.

A number of facts are indisputable:

1. PKU is an inherited disorder of phenylalanine metabolism, which inhibits the conversion of phenylalanine to tyrosine. In PKU, the gene controlling phenylalanine hydroxylase (the enzyme responsible for this conversion) is defective.

2. Treatment with a diet low in phenylalanine (and a synthetic protein supplement) prevents the most severe consequences of PKU if started within the first few weeks of life. Newborn screening provides the best means for identifying babies with PKU, so that the diet can be initiated before significant brain damage occurs.

3. Despite treatment, learning disabilities and deficits in neuropsychological functioning are common in children with PKU.

4. Some adolescents and young adults with PKU experience agoraphobia, depression, social withdrawal, and other emotional disturbances as a consequence of diet discontinuation.

5. Treatment for PKU must not be too strict or too lax. Since different individuals appear to have different tolerances for phenylalanine and varying responses to elevated levels, predictions about future complications are impossible. Some individuals experience dramatic consequences after diet discontinuation, while others appear to be unaffected. Occasionally other disorders have coexisted with PKU, but no genetic linkages have been discovered.

6. Damage to the fetus from untreated maternal PKU is caused by the intrauterine environment and results in microcephaly, congenital heart disease, low birth weight, and

mental retardation in the offspring. Treatment largely prevents these adverse outcomes. However, the majority of maternal PKU pregnancies continue to be inadequately treated because of psychosocial factors.

7. Assessment of children with PKU permits the early identification of learning difficulties and indicates directions for alternative teaching strategies. Particular attention needs to be given to visual–motor skills, information processing, arithmetic, and reading comprehension. The degree of metabolic control is usually correlated with neuropsychological outcome.

8. Neuropsychological testing, along with neuroimaging, can provide information about the brain effects associated with PKU. Neuropsychological testing suggests specific deficits in the prefrontal cortex, an area of the brain selectively sensitive to diminished levels of brain dopamine. MRI studies suggest myelin abnormalities that do not appear to be related to IQ or level of functioning.

9. Dietary compliance remains the critical factor in PKU treatment. Different strategies for maintaining metabolic control need to be employed, depending on the age and psychological issues of the child.

10. Treatment plans for PKU must address biochemical, nutritional, and psychosocial issues. Social support and positive attitudes toward treatment appear to be the most important factors associated with adherence to medical recommendations in PKU and maternal PKU.

The field remains open for more research to confront the controversies. With technological advances in genotyping, biochemical analysis, neuroimaging, and neuropsychological testing, answers should be forthcoming to some of the basic questions regarding the underlying pathology in PKU and the nature of optimal therapies for this disorder.

REFERENCES

Azen, C. G., Koch, R., Friedman, E. G., Berlow, S., Caldwell, J., Krause, W., Matalon, R., McCabe, E., O'Flynn, M., Petersen, R., Rouse, B., Scott, C. R., Sigman, B., Valle, D., & Warner, R. (1991). Intellectual development in 12-year-old children treated for phenylketonuria. *Amercan Journal of Diseases of Children, 145*, 35–39.

Batshaw, M. L., Valle, D., & Bessman, S. P. (1981). Unsuccessful treatment of phenylketonuria with tyrosine. *Journal of Pediatrics, 99*, 159–162.

Baumeister, A. A., & Baumeister, A. A., (1998). Dietary treatment of destructive behavior associated with hyperphenylalanineuria. *Clinical Neuropharmacology, 21*, 18–27.

Beasley, M. G., Costello, P. M., & Smith, I. (1994). Outcome of treatment in young adults with phenylketonuria detected by routine neonatal screening between 1964 and 1971. *Quarterly Journal of Medicine, 87*, 155–160.

Bickel, H., Gerrard, J., & Hickmans, E. M. (1954). The influence of phenylalanine intake on the chemistry and behavior of a phenylketonuric child. *Acta Paediatrica, 43*, 64–73.

Blehova, B., Pazoutova, N., & Subrt, I. (1970). Phenylketonuria associated with Down's syndrome. *Journal of Mental Deficiency Research, 14*, 274–275.

Brunner, R. L., Jordan, M. K., & Berry, H. K. (1983). Early-treated phenylketonuria: Neuropsychologic consequences. *Journal of Pediatrics, 102*, 831–835.

Burgard, P., Rey, F., Rupp, A., Avadie, V., & Rey, J. (1997). Neuropsychologic functions of early treated patients with phenylketonuria, on and off diet: Results of a cross-national and cross-sectional study. *Pediatric Research, 41*, 368–374.

Celiker, V., Dural, O., & Erdem, K. (1993). Anesthetic management of a patient with hereditary fructose intolerance and phenylketonuria. *Turkish Journal of Pediatrics, 35*, 127–130.

Chambless, D. L., Caputo, G. C., Jasin, S. E., Gracely, E. J., & Williams, C. (1987). The Mobility

Inventory for Agoraphobia. In K. Corcoran & J. Fischer (Eds.), *Measures for clinical practice.* (pp. 233–236). New York: Free Press.

Clarke, D. J., & Yapa, P. (1991). Phenylketonuria and anorexia nervosa. *Journal of Mental Deficiency Research, 35,* 165–170.

Clarke, J. T. R., Gates, R. D., Hogan, S. E., Barrett, M., & MacDonald, G. W. (1987). Neuropsychological studies on adolescents with PKU returned to phenylalanine-restricted diets. *American Journal of Mental Retardation, 92,* 255–262.

Cleary, M. A., Walter, J. H., Wraith, J. E., Jenkins, J. P. R., Alani, S. M., & Whittle, T. K. (1994). Magnetic resonance imaging of the brain in phenylketonuria. *Lancet, 344,* 87–90.

de Sonneville, L. M. J. (1995). *Amsterdam Neuropsychological Tasks (ANT).* (Available from SONAR [Sonneville Advice and Research], Amsterdanseweg 483, 1181 BR Amstelveen, The Netherlands)

de Sonneville, L. M. J., & Njiokiktjien, C. H. (1988). Aspects of information processing: A computer-based approach to development and disorders. *Pediatric Behavioural Neurology, 2,* Amsterdam Suyi Publ.

de Sonneville, L. M. J., Schmidt, E., Michel, U., & Batzler, U. (1990). Preliminary neuropsychological test results of the German Phenylketonuria Collaborative Study. *European Journal of Pediatrics, 149*(Suppl 1), S39–S44.

Diamond, A. (1994). Phenylalanine levels of 6–10 mg/dl may not be as benign as once thought. *Acta Paediatrica, 83*(Suppl. 407), 89–91.

Diamond, A., Ciaramitaro, V., Donner, E., Djali, S., & Robinson, R. M. (1994). An animal model of early-treated PKU. *Journal of Neuroscience, 14,* 3072–3082.

Diamond, A., Prevor, M. B., Callender, G., & Druin, D. P. (1997). Prefontal cortex cognitive deficits in children treated early and continuously for PKU. *Monographs of the Society for Research in Child Development, 62,* 1–208.

Eisensmith, R. C., & Woo, S. L. C. (1994). Gene therapy for phenylketonuria. *Acta Paediatrica, 83*(Suppl. 407), 124–129.

Fang, B., Eisensmith, R. C., Li, X. H. C., Shedlovsky, A., Dove, W., & Woo, S. L. C. (1994). Gene therapy for phenylketonuria: Phenotypic correction in a genetically deficient mouse model by adenovirus-mediated hepatic gene transfer. *Gene Therapy, 1,* 247–254.

Faust, D., Libon, D., & Pueschel, S. (1986–1987). Neuropsychological functioning in teated phenylketonuria. *International Journal of Psychiatry in Medicine, 16,* 169–177.

Fisch, R. O., & Horrobin, J. M. (1968). Down's syndrome with phenylketonuria. *Clinical Pediatrics, 7,* 226–227.

Fisch, R. O., Matalon, R., Weisberg, S., & Michals, K. (1991). Children of fathers with Phenylketonuria: An international survey. *Journal of Pediatrics, 118,* 739–741.

Fisch, R. O., Sines, L. K., & Chang, P. (1981). Personality characteristics of nonretarded phenylketonurics and their family members. *Journal of Clinical Psychiatry, 42,* 106–113.

Fishler, K., Azen, C. G., Henderson, R., Friedman, E., & Koch, R. (1987). Psychoeducational findings among children treated for phenylketonuria. *American Journal of Mental Retardation, 92,* 65–73.

Følling, A. (1934). Utskillelse av fenylpyrodruesyre i urinen som stoffskifteanomali i forbindelse med imbecillitet. *Nordisk Median Tikskiift, 8,* 1054–1059.

Gerrard, J. W. (1994). Phenylketonuria revisted. *Clinical and Investigative Medicine, 17,* 510–513.

Ghavami, M., & Levy, H. L. (1986). Prevention of fetal damage through dietary control of maternal hyperphenylalaninemia. *Clinical Obstetrics and Gynecology, 29,* 580–585.

Gourovitch, M. L., Craft, S., Dowton, S. B., Ambrose, P., & Sparta, S. (1994). Interhemispheric transfer in children with early-treated phenylketonuria. *Journal of Clinical and Experimental Neuropsychology, 16,* 393–404.

Griffiths, P., Paterson, L., & Harvie, A. (1995). Neuropsychological effects of subsequent exposure to phenylalanine in adolescents and young adults with early-treated phenylketonuria. *Journal of Intellectual Disability Research, 39,* 365–372.

Guldberg, P., Levy, H. L., Hanley, W. B., Koch, R., Matalon, R., Rouse, B. M., Trefz, F., de la Cruz, F., Friis, H. K., & Güttler, F. (1996). Phenylalanine hydroxylase gene mutations in the United States: Report from the Maternal PKU Collaborative Study. *American Journal of Human Genetics, 59,* 84–94.

Guthrie, R., & Susi, A. (1963). A simple phenylalanine method for detecting phenylketonuria in large populations of newborn infants. *Pediatrics, 32,* 338–343.

Güttler, F., & Lou, H. (1986). Dietary problems of phenylketonuria: Effect on CNS transmitters and their possible role in behaviour and neuropsychological function. *Journal of Inherited Metabolic Disease, 9*(Suppl. 2), 169–177.

Hanley, W. B., Clarke, J. T. R., & Schoonheyt, W. E. (1987). Maternal phenylketonuria (PKU): A review. *Clinical Biochemistry, 20,* 149–156.

Hanley, W. B., Koch, R., Levy, H. L., Matalon, R., Rouse, B., Azen, C. G., & de la Cruz, F. (1996). The North American Maternal Phenylketonuria Collaborative Study, developmental assessment of the offspring: Preliminary report. *European Journal of Pediatrics, 155*(Suppl. l), S169–S172.

Hanley, W. B., Linsao, L., Davidson, W., & Moes, C. A. (1970). Malnutrition with early treatment of phenylketonuria. *Pediatric Research, 4,* 318–327.

Harrison, P. F., & Rosenfield, A. (Eds.). (1996). *Contraceptive research and development: Looking to the future.* Washington, DC: National Academy Press.

Harper, M., & Reid, A. H. (1987). Use of a restricted protein diet in the treatment of behaviour disorder in a severely mentally retarded adult female phenylketonuric patient. *Journal of Mental Deficiency Research, 31,* 209–212.

Heffernan, J. F., & Trahms, C. M. (1981). A model preschool for patients with phenylketonuria. *Journal of the American Dietetic Association, 79,* 306–308.

Hendrikx, M. M., van der Schot, L. W., Slijper, F. M., Huisman, J., & Kalverboer, A. F. (1994). Phenylketonuria and some aspects of emotional development. *European Journal of Pediatrics, 153,* 832–835.

Holtzman, N. A., Kronmal, R. A., van Doorninck, W., Azen, C. G., & Koch, R. (1986). Effect of age at loss of dietary control on intellectual performance and behavior of children with phenylketonuria. *New England Journal of Medicine, 314,* 593–598.

Janzen, L. A., Nanson, J. L,. & Block, G. W. (1995). Neuropsychological evaluation of preschoolers with fetal alcohol syndrome. *Neurotoxicology and Teratology, 17,* 273–279.

Johannik, K., Van Hecke, P., Francois, B., Marchal, G., Smet, M. H., Jaeken, J., Breysem, L., Wilms, G., & Baert, A. L. (1994). Localized brain proton NRM spectorscopy in young adult phenylketonuria patients. *Magnetic Resonance in Medicine, 31,* 53–57.

Jones, S. J., Turano, G., Kriss, A., Shawkat, F., Kendall, B., & Thompson, A. J. (1995). Visual evoked potentials in phenylketonuria: Association with brain MRI, dietary state, and IQ. *Journal of Neurology, Neurosurgery and Psychiatry, 59,* 260–265.

Jonxis, J. H. P. (1957). Oligophrenia phenylpyruvica en de hartnupziekte. *Nederlands Tijdschrift voor Geneeskunde, 101,* 569–574.

Jordan, M. K., Brunner, R. L., Hunt, M. M., & Berry, H. K. (1985). Preliminary support for the oral administration of valine, isoleucine and leucine for phenylketonuria. *Developmental Medicine and Child Neurology, 27,* 33–39.

Kecskemethy, H. H., Lobbregt, D., & Levy, H. L. (1993). The use of gelatin capsules for ingestion of formula in dietary treatment of maternal phenylketonuria. *Journal of Inherited Metabolic Disease, 16,* 111–118.

Kidd, K. K. (1987). Population genetics of a disease. *Nature, 327,* 282–283.

Kirkman, H. N. (1982). Projections of a rebound in frequency of mental retardation from phenylketonuria. *Applied Research in Mental Retardation, 3,* 319–328.

Koch, J. H. (1997). *Robert Guthrie: The PKU story, a crusade against mental retardation.* Pasadena, CA: Hope.

Koch, R., Acosta, P., Fishler, K., Schaeffler, G., & Wohlers, A. (1967). Clinical observations on phenylketonuria. *American Journal of Diseases of Children, 113,* 6–15.

Koch, R., Azen, C. G., Friedman, E. G., & Williamson, M. L. (1982). Preliminary report on the effects of diet discontinuation in PKU. *Journal of Pediatrics, 100,* 870–875.

Koch, R., Hanley, W., Levy, W., Matalon, R., Rouse, B., de la Cruz, F., & Azen, C. G. (1990). A preliminary report of the Collaborative Study of Maternal Phenylketonuria in the United States and Canada. *Journal of Inherited Metabolic Disease, 13,* 641–650.

Koch, R., Levy, H., Matalon, R., Rouse, B., Hanley, W., & Azen, C. G. (1993). The North American Collaborative Study of Maternal Phenylketonuria: Status report, 1993. *American Journal of Diseases of Children, 147,* 1224–1230.

Koch, R., Levy, H. L., Matalon, R., Rouse, B., Hanley, W., Trefz, F., Azen, C. G., Friedman E. G., de la Cruz, F., Guttler, F., & Acosta, P. B. (1994). The International Collaborative Study of Maternal Phenylketonuria: Status report, 1994. *Acta Pediatrica, 83*(Suppl. 402), 111–119.

Koff, E., Boyle, P., & Pueschel, S. (1977). Perceptual–motor functioning in children with phenylketonuria. *American Journal of Diseases of Children, 131,* 1084–1087.

Krause, W., Halminski, M., McDonald, L., Dembure, P., Salvo, R., Freides, D., & Elsas, L. (1985). Biochemical and neuropsychological effects of elevated plasma phenylalanine in patients with treated phenylketonuria: A model for the study of phenylalanine and brain function in man. *Journal of Clinical Investigation, 75,* 40–48.

Legido, A., Tonyes, L., Carter, D., Schoemaker, A., Di George, A., & Grover, W. D. (1993). Treatment variables and intellectual outcome in children with classic phenylketonuria. *Clinical Pediatrics, 32,* 417–425.

Lenke, R. R., & Levy, H. L. (1980). Maternal phenylketonuria and hyperphenylalaninemia: An international survey of the outcome of untreated and treated pregnancies. *New England Journal of Medicine, 303,* 1202–1208.

Leuzzi, V., Cardona, F., Antonozzi, I., & Loizzo, A. (1994). Visual, auditory and somatosensorial evoked potentials in early and late treated adolescents with phenylketonuria. *Journal of Clinical Neurophysiology, 11,* 602–606.

Levy, H. L. (1989). Molecular genetics of phenylketonuria and its implications. *American Journal of Human Genetics, 45,* 667–670.

Levy, H. L., & Ghavami, M. (1996). Maternal phenylketonuria: A metabolic teratogen. *Teratology, 53,* 176–184.

Levy, H. L., Goss, B. S., Sullivan, D. K., Michals-Matalon, K., Dobbs, J. M., Guldberg, P., & Guttler, F. (1994). Maternal mild hyperphenylalaninemia: Results of treated and untreated pregnancies in two sisters. *Journal of Pediatrics, 125,* 467–469.

Levy, H. L., & Waisbren, S. E. (1983). Effects of untreated maternal phenylketonuria and hyperphenylalaninemia in the fetus. *New England Journal of Medicine, 309,* 1269–1274.

Levy, H. L., & Waisbren, S. E. (1994). PKU in adolescents: Rationale and psychosocial factors in diet continuation. *Acta Paediatrica, 83*(Suppl. 407), 92–97.

Lou, H. C. (1994). Dopamine precursors and brain function in phenylalanine hydroxylase deficiency. *Acta Paediatrica, 83*(Suppl. 407), 86–88.

Lykkelund, C., Nielsen, J. B., Lou, H. C., Rasmussen, V., Gerdes, A. M., Christensen, E., & Guttler, F. (1988). Increased neurotransmitter biosynthesis in phenylketonuria induced by phenylalanine restriction or by supplementation of unrestricted diet with large amounts of tyrosine. *European Journal of Pediatrics, 148,* 238–245.

Lynch, B. C., Pitt, D. B., Maddison, T. G., Wraith, J. E., & Danks, D. M. (1988). Maternal phenylketonuria: Successful outcome in four pregnancies treated prior to conception. *European Journal of Pediatrics, 148,* 72–75.

MacCready, R. A. (1963). Phenylketonuria screening programs. *New England Journal of Medicine, 269,* 52.

Mazzocco, M. M., Nord, A. M., Van Doorninck, W., Greene, C. L., Kovar, C. G., & Pennington, B. F. (1994). Cognitive development among children with early-treated phenylketonuria. *Developmental Neuropsychology, 10,* 133–151.

McDonald, J. D., Bode, V. C., Dove, W. F., & Shedlovsky, A. (1990). Pah[hph-5]: A mouse mutant deficient in phenylalanine hydroxylase. *Proceedings of the National Academy of Sciences USA, 87,* 1965–1967.

Miller, L., Braun, L. D., Pardridge, W. M., & Oldendorf, W. H. (1985). Kinetic constants for blood–brain barrier amino acid transport in conscious rats. *Journal of Neurochemistry, 45,* 1427–1432.

Ozalp, I., Coskum, T., Ozguc, M., Tokath, A., Yalaz, K., Vanh, L., Yilmaz, E., & Erbay, A. (1994). The PAH gene: Genetic and neurological evaluation of untreated and late-treated patients with phenylketonuria. *Journal of Inherited Metabolic Disease, 17,* 371.

Paul, D. B. (1999). PKU screening: Competing agendas, converging stories. In M. Fortun & E. Mendelsohn (Eds.), *The practices of human genetics* (pp. 185–195). Dordvecht, The Netherlands: Kluwer Academic Publishers.

Pearsen, K. D., Gean-Marton, A. D., Levy, H. L., & Davis, K. R. (1990). Phenylketonuria: MR imaging of the brain with clinical correlation. *Radiology, 177,* 437–440.

Pennington, B. F., van Doorninck, J. W., McCabe, L. L., & McCabe, E. R. B. (1985). Neuropsychological deficits in early treated phenylketonuric children. *American Journal of Mental Deficiency, 89,* 467–474.

Penrose, L. S. (1972). *The biology of mental defect* (4th ed.). London: Sidgwick & Jackson.

Pietz, J., Fatkenheuer, B., Burgard, P., Armbruster, M., Esser, G., & Schmidt, H. (1997). Psychiatric disorders in adult patients with early-treated phenylketonuria. *Pediatrics, 99,* 345–350.

Pietz, J., Landwehr, A., Schmidt, H., de Sonneville, L., & Trefz, F. K. (1995). Effect of high-dose supplementation on brain function in adults with phenylketonuria. *Journal of Pediatrics, 127,* 936–943.

Porrino, L. J., & Goldman-Rakic, P. S. (1982). Brain stem innervation of prefrontal and anterior cingulate cortex in the rhesus monkey revealed by retrograde transport of HRP. *Journal of Comparative Neurology, 205,* 63–76.

Pueschel, S. M., Fogelson-Doyle, L., Kammerer, B., & Matsumiya, Y. (1983). Neurophysiological, psychological and nutritional investigations during discontinuation of the phenylalanine-restricted diet in children with classic phenylketonuria. *Journal of Mental Deficiency Research, 27,* 61–67.

Ris, M. D., Williams, S. E., Hunt, M. M., Berry, H. K., & Leslie, N. (1994). Early-treated phenylketonuria: Adult neuropsychologic outcome. *Journal of Pediatrics, 124,* 388–392.

Roth, K. S. (1986). Newborn metabolic screening: A search for "nature's experiments." *Southern Medical Journal, 79,* 47–54.

Roth, K. S., Cohn, R. M., Berman, P., & Segal, S. (1976). Phenylketonuria and Duchenne muscular dystrophy: A case report. *Journal of Pediatrics, 88,* 689–705.

Rouse, B., Azen, C., Koch, R., Matalon, R., Hanley, W., de la Cruz, F., Trefz, F., Friedman, E., & Shifrin, H. (1997). Maternal Phenylketonuria Collaborative Study (MPKUCS) offspring: Facial anomalies, malformations, and early neurological sequelae. *American Journal of Medical Genetics, 69,* 89–95.

St. James, P. S., Shapiro, E., & Waisbren, S. E. (in press). The Resource Mothers Program for Maternal PKU: Program evaluation and implications. *American Journal of Public Health.*

Schmidt, B. J., Solberg, A. J., Diament, A. J. & Pimentel, H. (1981). Phenylketonuria in patients with congenital hypothyroidism. *Pediatric Research, 15,* 176.

Schmidt, E., Rupp, A., Burgard, P., & Pietz, J. (1992). Information processing in early treated phenylketonuria. *Journal of Clinical and Experimental Neuropsychology, 14,* 388.

Schmidt, E., Rupp, A., Burgard, P., Pietz, J., Weglage, J., & de Sonneville, L. M. J. (1994). Sustained attention in adult phenylketonuria: The influence of the concurrent phenylalanine-blood-level. *Journal of Clinical and Experimental Neuropsychology, 16,* 681–688.

Schor, D. P. (1983). PKU and temperament: Rating children three through seven years old in PKU families. *Clinical Pediatrics, 22,* 807–811.

Schuett ,V. E. (1997). Off-diet young adults with PKU: Lives in danger. *National PKU News, 8,* 1–5.

Schuett, V. E., & Brown, E. S. (1984). Diet policies of PKU clinics in the United States. *American Journal of Public Health, 74,* 501–503.

Scriver, C. R., Kaufman, S., Eisensmith, R. C., & Woo, S. L. C. (1995). The hyperphenylalaninemias. In C. R. Scriver, A. L. Beaudet, W. S. Sly, & E. Valle (Eds.), *The metabolic and molecular bases of inherited disease* (pp. 1025–1075). New York: McGraw-Hill.

Seashore, M. R., Friedman, E., Novelly, R. A., & Bapat, V. (1985). Loss of intellectual function in children with phenylketonuria after relaxation of dietary phenylalanine restriction. *Pediatrics, 75,* 226–232.

Shedlovsky, A., McDonald, J. D., Symula, D., & Dove, W. F. (1993). Mouse models of human phenylketonuria. *Genetics, 134,* 1205–1210.

Siegel, F., Balow, B., Risch, R. O., & Anderson, V. E. (1968). School behavior profile ratings of phenylketonuric children. *American Journal of Mental Deficiency, 72,* 937–943.

Skitnevsky, S. F., Brown, M., & Waisbren, S. E. (1997). *Make a world of difference: A manual for organizaing a maternal PKU camp.* (Available from S. E. Waisbren, IC Smith Bldg., Children's Hospital, 300 Longwood Avenue, Boston, MA 02115).

Stemerdink, B. A., van der Meere, J. J., van der Molen, M. W., Kalverboer, A. F., Hendrikx, M. M. T., Huisman, J., van der Schot, L. W. A., Slijper, F. M. E., van Spronsen, F. J., & Verkerk, P. H. (1995). Information processing in patients with early and continuously-treated phenylke-tonuria. *European Journal of Pediatrics, 154,* 739–746.

Stemerdink, N. (1996). *Early and continuously treated phenylketonuria: An experimental neuro-psychological approach.* Amsterdam: Academisch Proefschrift.

Tam, S. Y., Elsworth, J. D., Bradberry, C. W., & Roth, R. H. (1990). Mesocortical dopamine neu-rons: High basal firing frequency predicts tyrosine dependence of dopamine synthesis. *Journal of Neural Transmission, 81,* 97–110.

Thompson, A. J., Tillotson, S., Smith, I., Kendall, B., Moore, S. G., & Brenton, D. P. (1993). Brain MRI changes in phenylketonuria: Associations with dietary status. *Brain, 116,* 811–821.

Trefz, F., Burgard, P., Konig. T., Goebel-Schreiner, B., Lichter-Konecki, U., Konecki, D., Schmidt, E., Schmidt, H., & Bickel, H. (1993). Genotype–phenotype correlations in phenylketonuria. *Clinica Chimica Acta, 217,* 15–21.

Vajro, P., Strisciuglio, P., Houssin, D., Huault, G., Laurent, J., Alvarez, F., & Bernard, O. (1993). Correction of phenylketonuria after liver transplantation in a child with cirrhosis. *New En-gland Journal of Medicine, 329,* 363–366.

Waisbren, S. E., Brown, M. J., de Sonneville, L. M. J., & Levy, H. L. (1994). Review of neuropsy-chological functioning in treated phenylketonuria: An information processing approach. *Acta Paediatrica, 84*(Suppl. 408), 98–103.

Waisbren, S. E., Chang, P. N., Levy, H. L., Shifrin, H., Allred, E., Azen, C., de la Cruz, F., Hanley, W., Koch, R., Matalon, R., & Rouse, R. (1998). Neonatal neurological assessment of offspring in maternal PKU. *Journal of Inherited Metabolic Disease, 21,* 39–48.

Waisbren, S. E., Hamilton, B. D., St. James, P. J., Shiloh, S., & Levy, H. L. (1995). Psychosocial factors in maternal phenylketonuria: Women's adherence to medical recommendations. *Ameri-can Journal of Public Health, 85,* 1636–1641.

Waisbren, S. E., & Levy, H. L. (1991). Agoraphobia in phenylketonuria. *Journal of Inherited Metabolic Disease, 14,* 755–764.

Waisbren, S. E., Rokni, H., Bailey, I., Rohr, F., Brown, T., & Warner-Rogers, J. (1997). Social factors and the meaning of food in adherence to medical diets: Results of a maternal phenylke-tonuria summer camp. *Journal of Inherited Metabolic Disease, 20,* 21–27.

Waisbren, S. E., Schnell, R. R., & Levy, H. L. (1980). Diet termination in children with phenylke-tonuria: A review of psychological assessments used to determine outcome. *Journal of Inher-ited Metabolic Disease, 3,* 149–153.

Waisbren, S. E., Shiloh, S., St. James, P. J. ,& Levy, H. L. (1991). Psychosocial factors in maternal phenylketonuria: Prevention of unplanned pregnancies. *American Journal of Public Health, 81,* 299–304.

Waisbren, S. E., Varvogli, L., Warner-Rogers, J., & Levy, H. L. (1999). *Attention deficits and hy-peractivity in early treated phenylketonuria.* Manuscript in preparation.

Waisbren, S. E., & Zaff, J. (1994). Personality disorder in young women with treated phenylketo-nuria. *Journal of Inherited Metabolic Disease, 17,* 584–592.

Walker, V., Clayton, B. E., Ersser, R. S., Francis, D. E. M., Lilly, P., Seakins, J. W. T., Smith, I., & Whiteman, P. D. (1981). Hyperphenylalaninaemia of various types among three-quarters of a million neonates tested in a screening program. *Archives of Disease in Childhood, 56,* 759–764.

Webster, D. R., & Wallace, J. (1995). PKU and diabetes: Help requested. *Journal of Inherited Metabolic Disease, 18,* 649.

Weglage, J., Fünders, B., Wilken, B., Schubert, D., Schmidt, E., Burgard, P., & Ullrich, K. (1992). Psychological and social findings in adolescents with phenylketonuria. *European Journal of Pediatrics*, *151*, 522–525.

Weglage, J., Fünders, B., Wilken, B., Schubert, D., & Ullrich, K. (1993). School performance and intellectual outcome in adolescents with phenylketonuria. *Acta Paediatrica*, *81*, 582–586.

Weglage, J., Pietsch, M., Fünders, B., Koch, H. G., & Ullrich, K. (1996). Deficits in selective and sustained attention processes in early treated children with phenylketonuria: Result of impaired frontal lobe functions? *European Journal of Pediatrics*, *155*, 200–204.

Welsh, M. C., Pennington, B. F., Ozonoff, S., Rouse, B., & McCabe, E. R. B. (1990). Neuropsychology of early-treated phenylketonuria: Specific executive function deficits. *Child Development*, *61*, 1697–1713.

Woo, S. L. C., Lidsky, A. S., Güttler, F., Chandra, T., & Robson, K. J. H. (1983). Cloned human phenylalanine hydroxylase gene allows prenatal diagnosis and carrier detection of classical phenylketonuria. *Nature*, *306*, 151–155.

Woolf, L. I. (1976). A study of the cause of the high incidence of phenylketonuria in Ireland and west Scotland. *Irish Medical Journal*, *69*, 398–401.

Woolf, L. I. (1979). Late onset phenylalanine intoxication. *Journal of Inherited Metabolic Disease*, *2*, 19–20.

Wright, K. (1990, September). *Cradle of mutation*. Discover, pp. 22–23.

Yannicelli, S., & Ryan, A. (1995). Improvements in behaviour and physical manifestations in previously untreated adults with phenylketonuria using a phenylalanine-restricted diet: A national survey. *Journal of Inherited Metabolic Disease*, *18*, 131–134.

20

RETT SYNDROME

ROBERT T. BROWN
SARAH L. HOADLEY

Rett syndrome (RS) is a disorder that initially appears as a deterioration from apparently normal development in infancy or early childhood. It involves a slowdown in normal development; deceleration of head growth; lack of interest in the environment; deterioration of motor functioning, and loss of hand use and subsequently of locomotion; hand stereotypies (typically hand wringing or clapping); loss of expressive language; autistic and self-abusive behavior; and eventual severe to profound mental retardation. Prevalence estimates vary. Hagberg (1995b) has revised the estimate of prevalence of classic RS from 1 in 10,000 females to closer to 1 in 15,000. Cases have been reported in all parts of the world and in all ethnic groups (e.g., Moser & Naidu, 1991; Naidu, 1997).

Unique to RS is apparently normal initial development followed by rapid mental and physical deterioration, and then by stabilization or even reduction in some symptoms (e.g., Budden, 1997; Hagberg, 1995b). RS is unusual in several additional ways: (1) It apparently affects only women, whereas most gender-specific disorders affect only men; (2) it is manifested in part through loss of acquired function, but is apparently neurodevelopmental and not neurodegenerative (e.g., Glaze, 1995); (3) it is reflected in a fairly striking set of behavioral symptoms that have consistent developmental trends, but it was not initially described until 1966 and not brought to wide attention until 1983; (4) it is almost undoubtedly genetically based, but to date no marker for it has been identified; (5) although the subject of hundreds of articles, it is still relatively unknown in comparison to many other developmental disorders of comparable prevalence; and (6) it occurs in both classic and variant forms. Details on these and other features may be found in Hagberg, Anvret, and Wahlström (1993).

HISTORY AND BACKGROUND

Apparently owing to the structure of health services in Austria, Andreas Rett, a pediatrician at the University of Vienna, saw many Austrians who had severe or profound mental retardation in the early 1960s. One day in his clinic, he observed two thin girls sitting next to each other with their mothers; the girls were rocking back and forth in a virtually identical autistic-like fashion, and wringing their hands in a manner uncommon in those with severe mental retardation. In 1966, Rett published his observations on a number of patients, all girls, who had similar symptoms and developmental histories: After apparently normal development up to 6–18 months, the girls showed general deceleration of psychomotor development, cognitive and linguistic regression, and development of repetitive and stereotypic hand wringing or washing (see Hagberg, 1995b, for a summary of Rett's work). As it turned out incorrectly, Rett tied these symptoms to hyperammonema.

Although Rett's 1966 paper was followed by several other publications in German and at least one in an obscure source in English, his initial findings were largely overlooked until Hagberg, Aicardi, Dias, and Ramos (1983) published a major report on 35 cases in a journal in English. With the publication of Hagberg et al.'s 1983 article, RS became known throughout the world. Hagberg's seminal and continued work on the syndrome has led at least some authors (Gillberg, Ehlers, & Wahlström, 1990) to refer to it as Rett–Hagberg syndrome. RS is now studied in centers in many countries. Generally accepted criteria for diagnosis of the main disorder (classic RS), as well as several variants, have been developed. The criteria for classic RS are strict so as to maintain as homogeneous a group of diagnosed individuals as possible, in order to facilitate determination of the disorder's genetic basis.

DIAGNOSTIC CRITERIA: THE CLASSIC DISORDER AND VARIANTS

The diagnostic criteria for classic RS, established by the Rett Syndrome Criteria Work Group (1988), fall into three categories: necessary criteria, supportive criteria, and exclusionary criteria. The criteria have been modified by some authors (e.g., Glaze & Schultz, 1997; Hagberg, 1995b). Hagberg has also provided criteria for RS variants (e.g., Hagberg, 1995a, 1995b; Hagberg & Skjeldal, 1994). The criteria for classic RS and RS variants are listed in Tables 20.1 and 20.2, respectively.

As Table 20.1 indicates, necessary for diagnosis is apparently normal prenatal, perinatal, and early postnatal development, followed by sudden deceleration of head growth and loss of acquired skills (including hand use) and communication (including language), beginning in infancy or early childhood. Also required are evidence of mental retardation and the appearance of intense and persistent hand stereotypies. Girls who have developed walking must show gait abnormalities; some never develop walking. Electroencephalographic (EEG) abnormalities, seizure disorder, spasticity, marked scoliosis, and overall growth retardation are also typical.

In diagnosis, "a battery of clustered remarkable RS behavioral and other clinical oddities can be of considerable help" (Hagberg, 1996, p. 144). As described by Hagberg (1995b), this battery consists of the following:

1. *Stereotypic hand movements.* "The almost continuous repetitive wringing, twisting or clapping hand automatisms during wakefulness constitute the hallmark of the condition" (Hagberg, 1995b, p. 973). Adult females with mental retardation who show RS-type hand stereotypies should be considered potential cases and referred for diagnosis.

2. *Episodic hyperventilation and breath holding.* Characteristic are irregular episodes of hyperventilation, interrupted by breath holding for 30–40 seconds.

3. *Bloating.* Moderate air swallowing leading to some abdominal bloating is common, and severe bloating occurs in a small percentage of cases.

TABLE 20.1. RS: Necessary, Supportive, and Exclusionary Criteria

Necessary criteria

Apparently normal pre- and perinatal development
Apparently normal development until at least 5–6 months of age
Normal head circumference at birth
Deceleration of head growth, beginning from 3 months to 3 years of age
Loss of acquired skills, beginning from 3 months to 3 years of age
    Learned voluntary hand skills
    Verbal and nonverbal communication skills
Appearance of obvious mental retardation
Appearance of intense and persistent hand stereotypies
    Hand wringing/squeezing
    Hand washing/patting/rubbing
    Hand mouthing/tongue pulling
Gait abnormalities among ambulatory cases
    Gait apraxia/dyspraxia
    Jerky truncal ataxia/body dyspraxia
Diagnosis tentative until 2–5 years of age

Supportive criteria

Breathing dysfunction
    Periodic apnea during wakefulness
    Intermittent hyperventilation
    Breath-holding spells
    Forced expulsion of air or saliva
Bloating/marked air swallowing
EEG abnormalities
    Slow waking background and intermittent rhythmical slowing (3–5 Hz)
    Epileptiform discharges with or without clinical seizures
Epilepsy—various seizure forms
Spastic signs; later muscle wasting and/or dystonic traits
Peripheral vasomotor disturbances
Scoliosis of neurogenic type
Hypotrophic, small, cold feet
Growth retardation

Exclusionary criteria

Organomegaly or other signs of storage disease
Retinopathy or optic atrophy
Microcephaly at birth
Existence of metabolic or other hereditary degenerative disorder
Acquired neurological disorder resulting from severe infections or head trauma
Evidence of intrauterine growth retardation
Evidence of perinatally acquired brain damage

Note. Adapted from Hagberg, Goutieres, Hanefeld, Rett, and Wilson (1985) and Rett Syndrome Diagnostic Criteria Work Group (1988). Copyright 1985 by Elsevier Science, and 1988 by Lippincott Williams & Wilkins. Adapted by permission.

    4. *Bruxism.* A creaking sound made with the teeth, "similar to that when slowly uncorking a bottle" (Hagberg, 1995b, p. 973), is characteristic although not specifically diagnostic.

    5. *Night laughing.* Among the more common sleep disturbances, shown in 80–90% of preschool RS girls, are bouts of sometimes long and disturbing night laughing. These tend to become episodic over age, but may persist into adulthood.

6. *Hypoplastic, cold, red–blue feet.* Small, cold, red–blue feet are commonly, but not always, seen in RS.

7. *Scoliosis.* Neurogenic scoliosis is characteristic. Its degree is variable, but tends to progress relatively rapidly.

8. *Changed sensitivity to pain.* Pain perception is never absent, but it may be delayed or reduced.

9. *Intensive eye communication.* Eye communication, including eye pointing, appears in most RS girls after the regression stage described below.

The RS variant model in Table 20.2 was developed once it was realized that females with RS are much more heterogeneous than originally thought (Hagberg, 1995a, 1995b). Diagnosis of an RS variant should be made only in girls aged 10 years or older when at least three necessary and at least five supportive criteria are present. These behaviors may appear throughout childhood. Typically, girls who meet the criteria for an RS variant show less severe symptoms than those associated with classic RS. Both gross and fine motor control may be spared to a greater extent, and mental retardation is less severe. Girls with an RS variant may retain some language, although it tends to be abnormal and telegraphic. Those with language tend to have had a later and milder regression period.

Of importance, particularly for parents and therapists, is as accurate a diagnosis as early as possible. Some physicians may be reluctant to diagnose RS early, owing to the eventual severity of the disorder; however, as shown in our case descriptions below, many parents are frustrated by the lack of a diagnosis that fits their children's behaviors or has implications for treatment and care. For this reason, the term "potential RS" (Hagberg, 1995b) has been suggested for use with young cases.

DEVELOPMENTAL TREND

Classic RS develops through a fairly reliable four-stage sequence of behavioral and physical changes, first described by Hagberg and Witt-Engerström (1986) and since elaborated by many others. The age of onset and duration of the stages are highly variable, however, as is the duration of transition from one to another. Moreover, not all RS children show all the features of each stage. Major characteristics of early development and of each stage are described in this section, along with disorders from which RS needs to be differentiated at each stage. Except as specifically referenced, the information in this section comes from Budden (1997), Hagberg (1995b), Hagberg and Witt-Engerström (1986), and Naidu (1997).

Pre-Stage 1: Early Development

Much pre-Stage 1 development appears normal, and the necessary criteria for diagnosis include apparently normal development until at least 5–6 months of age. However, this normality may indeed be apparent and not actual, with subtle signs of RS appearing much earlier (see Kerr, 1995, for a review). Early motor skills appear, including reaching for objects. Self-feeding commonly develops, with infants being weaned onto solid foods. Many children will develop walking, but often with an unusual gait. However, appearance of many infant developmental milestones is delayed or absent. Medical records, parent interviews, and analyses of home videotapes suggest that feeding difficulties, floppiness, jerkiness, and delays in motor development may appear in early infancy. Infants have poor

TABLE 20.2. RS: The Variant Delineation Model

Necessary criteria

Female, at least 10 years of age, with mental retardation of unexplained origin and at least three of six primary criteria
  Loss of (partial or subtotal) acquired fine finger skill in late infancy/early childhood
  Loss of acquired single words/phrases/nuanced babble
  RS hand stereotypies, hands together or apart
  Early deviant communicative skills
  Deceleration in head growth of two standard deviations (even when still within normal limits)
  RS developmental profile: a regression period (Stage 2) followed by a period of limited recovery of contact and communication (Stage 3) rather than continued neuromotor regression to adolescence

Supportive criteria

In addition, at least 5 of 11 RS supportive criteria
  Breathing irregularities (hyperventilation and/or breath holding)
  Bloating/marked air swallowing
  Characteristic RS teeth grinding
  Gait abnormalities
  Neurogenic scoliosis or high kyphosis (ambulant girls)
  Development of abnormal lower limb neurology
  Small, blue/cold, impaired feet; autonomic/trophic dysfunction
  RS EEG abnormalities
  Unprompted sudden laughing/screaming spells
  Impaired/delayed nociception
  Intensive eye communication—"eye pointing"

Exclusionary criteria as presented in Table 20.1

Note. Adapted from Hagberg and Skjeldal (1994). Copyright 1994 by Elsevier Science. Adapted by permission.

mobility and may show high levels of repetitive limb movement (possible precursors of later motor coordination problems) and limited play. Kerr (1995) particularly notes repeated opening and closing of a hand with which the infant is attempting to grasp an object. Some slowing of brain growth may be seen in unusually low occipitofrontal circumference as early as 2 months of age. Repeated facial and mouth twitching in some infants at 2 or 3 months of age suggests the possibility of cortical abnormality (Kerr, 1995). Kerr (1995) points out that many of the infant skills survive intact into adulthood, suggesting that their neural substrate may be different from the ones affected by the disorder.

Many girls are reported to develop single-word communication, and a few use short phrases; however, according to Tams-Little and Holdgrafer (1996), most parents reported that their RS daughters had only developed an indiscriminate use of "mama" and "dada." Of interest from a potential early diagnostic standpoint, Tams-Little and Holdgrafer (1996) also found that the parents of only 1 of their 17 RS girls reported use of three gestures (giving, pointing, and showing) that normally appear at about 9–10 months of age and reflect a major developmental shift to intentional nonverbal communication.

Stage 1: Early-Onset Stagnation

The first stage begins from 6 to 18 months of age and has a duration of weeks or months. Although some advances may occur, particularly in gross motor control, in many ways an infant appears to hit a developmental wall. Many aspects of cognitive development cease. A deceleration of head growth leads to head circumference generally below average by the end of the second year of life (Kerr, 1995). Hypotonia, lack of interest in play and the environment, and loss of acquired hand functions and random hand movements are typical. No obvious pattern of abnormalities is apparent, however. Differential diagnoses include benign congenital hypotonia, cerebral palsy, Prader–Willi syndrome, and metabolic disorders.

Stage 2: Rapid Developmental Regression

Between 1 and 3 or 4 years of age, functioning begins to deteriorate so generally and rapidly that the onset may be taken for a toxic or encephalitic state (Hagberg & Witt-Engerström, 1986). Furthermore, Budden (1997, p. 2) reports that the onset "may be so acute that parents can sometimes give a specific date after which their child was no longer 'normal.'" General cognitive functioning, purposeful hand use, and expressive language deteriorate. The classic hand stereotypies, including hand wringing, washing, and mouthing, typically appear and may be continuous during waking hours. Walking may deteriorate or not develop. Gait abnormalities, particularly a spread-legged stance, are generally evident in girls who can walk. Hyperventilation and breath holding are common, as are behaviors characteristic of autism. Seizures and vacant spells resembling seizures may occur, and virtually all RS girls have abnormal EEGs. Differential diagnoses include autism, encephalitis, metabolic disorders (including inborn errors of metabolism), and neurodegenerative disorders.

Stage 3: Pseudostationary

Stage 3 has a highly variable age of onset, occurring at the end of the rapid deterioration, and lasts several years (generally until about 10 years of age). Hand stereotypies continue, and mobility may further deteriorate. Mental retardation in the severe to profound range is characteristic. On the other hand, autistic symptoms may diminish, and social interactions, hand use, communication, alertness, and self-initiated behavior may increase. Tremulousness, ataxia, teeth grinding (bruxism), hyperventilation or breath holding, and seizures may all occur. Overall rigidity is likely to increase and scoliosis to appear. Nonverbal communication through eye pointing may improve. Differential diagnoses include cerebral palsy and other motor disorders, Angelman and Lennox–Gastaut syndromes, and spinocerebellar degeneration.

Stage 4: Late Motor Deterioration

The final stage generally begins after age 10 years. Motor function decreases further, with increased rigidity, scoliosis, and muscle wasting. Mobility continues to decrease; many girls will be wheelchair-bound. Hands may be held in the mouth for long periods. Expressive language, if previously present, generally disappears, and receptive language decreases, although eye pointing as communication may continue. Chewing and swallowing may be lost, necessitating artificial feeding. Differential diagnosis is for unknown neurodegenerative disease. However, the final phenotypic characteristics of classic RS cases vary widely:

> With increasing age and advanced state of the disease, the final differences in severity of motor disability, pattern of neurology and degree of impairment are striking. Thus, in adulthood, there are ambulant RS females, certainly dyspraxic, but nonetheless not dissimilar to other

uncomplicated severely retarded patients. Other RS females have never learned to walk, some being completely helpless, with severe extrapyramidal syndromes, combined with neurogenic atrophies and secondary grotesque body deformities. (Hagberg, 1995b, p. 972)

Lifespan varies, but a number of deaths occur during sleep for unknown reasons before age 20 years. Overall survival is 70% at 35 years of age, considerably lower than the 98% of the female population at large, but higher than the 27% for the profoundly retarded overall (Naidu, 1997).

OVERALL INTELLECTUAL CHARACTERISTICS

Formal assessments indicate that RS girls function at a severe or profound level of mental retardation, but their actual cognitive functioning may be difficult to assess because of their motor and language impairments. Perry, Sarlo-McGarvey, and Haddad (1991) obtained Vineland Adaptive Behavior Scale data from interviews with parents of 28 RS girls, and administered the Cattell Infant Intelligence Scale to 15 of the girls when they averaged 9.4 years of age (range 2.9–19.5). Mean mental age on the Cattell was 3.0 months (range 0.4–7.8). Most of the subjects attended to visual and auditory stimuli, were interested in toys, and anticipated being fed. Only one appeared to have object permanence, however, and none succeeded on items requiring language or fine motor skills. Age equivalents on the Vineland were higher: Communication, mean 17.4 months (range 5–28); Daily Living Skills, mean 16.9 months (range 4–34); and Socialization, mean 25.9 months (range 14–36). The girls attended when spoken to and showed some understanding, but most did not speak or have any other communication system. Most could feed themselves, some with their fingers, and some could use a cup. Most were in diapers and did not perform other self-care tasks. They showed some interest in other people and could discriminate among them, but showed virtually no play behaviors. Cattell scores did not correlate with Vineland scores. Only Vineland Daily Living Skills correlated with age of onset and age at assessment. Cattell scores did not correlate with age at onset but showed a negative correlation with age at testing, indicating lower functioning in the older girls. As Perry et al. (1991) suggest, the higher scores on the Vineland may reflect a number of factors, including parental bias and the nature of scoring of the test, rather than actual higher functioning.

OVERALL EMOTIONAL CHARACTERISTICS

Many of the emotional characteristics of girls with RS have been described in the developmental section above, so this section summarizes those that occur commonly across a wide age range. Much of this information is taken from a mail survey of parents by Sansom, Krishnan, Corbett, and Kerr (1993), in response to requests by parents for clinical advice about their RS daughters' emotional and behavioral problems. At the time of the survey, the girls' mean age was 10.6 years (range 2.2–28.0). Although Sansom et al. (1993) reported the occurrence rates for various behaviors at four different age ranges, from below 5 to 16 years or older, the percentages of girls showing the behaviors differed little enough with age that overall figures can be given. Over 75% of the children showed anxiety, particularly in response to external situations. Most of the episodes were brief and consisted of screaming, hyperventilation, self-injury, frightened expressions, and general distress. Precipitating events included novel situations and people, sudden noises, some music, change

of routine, and high activity by others close to a child. Low mood, reflected partly in crying, occurred in 70% of the girls, but for extended periods in only a few. Almost 50%
showed self-injurious behaviors. Most were relatively mild, such as biting fingers or hands,
but more serious chewing of fingers, head banging, and hair pulling also occurred. Epilepsy was reported in 63%. Although over 75% of the children were reported to sleep well,
almost as many were reported to waken early, and nighttime laughing, crying, and screaming
were also commonly reported.

DIFFERENTIATION BETWEEN RS AND AUTISM

Many girls are initially diagnosed with autism who are later seen to have RS. RS and autism
do share certain characteristics, particularly at younger ages, but careful comparisons between groups of autistic and RS children suggest some differential diagnostic behaviors. A
review of differences between RS and other disorders is provided by Van Acker (1991),
who points out that the rarity of autism in females should alone lead to a consideration of
RS in young females showing autistic characteristics. This section mainly summarizes the
differential behaviors described by Olsson and Rett (1985). (For a fuller discussion of autism,
see Klin & Volkmar, Chapter 10, this volume.)

Olsson and Rett (1985) observed some behaviors only in RS children, some only in
autistic children, some always in RS children, and some always in autistic children. For
example, only RS children showed stereotyped hand movements with a broad-based stance,
stereotyped washing movements of hands and wetting of hands with saliva, problems in
chewing, and (at age 6 and older) slow movements and hypoactivity. All RS children in
addition showed few negative reactions to being touched or looked at, ataxia, greater time
looking at objects and people than handling objects, and no language development beyond
two-word phrases. Only autistic children showed a variety of swiftly alternating stereotyped movements that started and stopped rapidly; greater time handling objects than looking at objects and people; appropriate chewing, gripping, and gait; and no ataxia. Five
behaviors characteristic of autism were not observed in their RS children from ages
22 months to 20 years: "Predominate rejection of caressing and tenderness, Conspicuous
physical activity in terms of grabbing and concomitant locomobility, Excessive attachment
to certain objects, Rotation of small objects, [and] Stereotypic playing habits" (Olsson &
Rett, 1985, p. 287). Of potential interest, Smith, Klevstrand, and Lovaas (1995) closely
monitored three RS girls who participated in their treatment program for autistic children
(see section on treatment below). All three showed wide fluctuations in attention. Periods,
sometimes several days long, during which they were virtually unresponsiveness to social
and sensory stimuli alternated with periods during which they were much more responsive. Medical evaluations suggested that the periods of inattention could not be attributed
to seizures or other organic conditions. Smith et al. (1995) suggest that such swings in
attention are unusual in developmental disabilities (where general attention deficits are
common), and that they may be useful diagnostically.

GENETIC ASPECTS

In addition to the appearance of RS only in girls, other evidence indicates that it is a genetic disorder. Almost all monozygotic (MZ) twin pairs are concordant for the disorder

(in 9 of 10 pairs of MZ twins studied to date, where one twin has RS, the other does also), whereas almost all dizygotic (DZ) twin pairs are disconcordant (in 13 of 15 pairs of DZ twins studied thus far, where one twin has RS, the other does not). RS is familial in only about 1% of cases, so incidence among related individuals is rare; nevertheless, several cases have been reported, including seven sisters, two half-sisters, one aunt–niece pair, and one mother–daughter pair. Rett-like symptoms have been reported in a few males, but no cases of classic RS. (All of the genetic data just cited are from Percy, 1996.) However, in some pairs of concordant MZ twins, RS is more severe in one twin than in the other, suggesting that factors other than genetic ones may be involved. The disconcordance in one MZ pair adds to the genetic puzzle. Of interest, one family has been reported (Gillberg et al., 1990) in which three female maternal second cousins with the same great-grandparents all showed severe developmental disorders with infant onset. No one else in the three generations has any similar disorder. One of the three girls has autism with severe mental retardation, one has autism with mild retardation, and one has RS; this would suggest some genetic relationship between the disorders.

No clear genetic marker has been found to date, although, as would be expected, research has concentrated on the X chromosomes. An unusually high consanguinity rate has been found among the ancestors of a number of Swedish RS girls in both maternal and paternal lines. The ancestry of several could be traced to a small number of rural communities (Akesson, Hagberg, Wahlström, & Witt-Engerström, 1992). A more recent study extends the earlier findings and suggests that RS may involve both X chromosomes and an autosomal pair in which an ancestral premutation over generations results in a full mutation (Akesson, 1997). Some evidence suggests an X-linked dominant disorder, caused in all but the few familial cases by a spontaneous mutation in the RS gene in formation of the egg or sperm. Mutations occur more frequently in sperm than in eggs, and since women get one X chromosome from their fathers, more affected females than males would be expected (Thomas, 1996). If most cases of RS result from spontaneous mutation in formation of egg or sperm, then familial cases would be expected to be rare, as indeed they are. However, Akesson, Hagberg, and Wahlström (1997) have reported significantly fewer male siblings among RS girls than would be expected, which suggests that the gene causing RS is lethal to males prenatally. Since a male's X chromosome is received from his mother, maternal transmission is indicated in these cases. Various other genetic explanations, each with some supporting data, have been offered. Some suggest that the X chromosomes may not be primarily involved (Hagberg, 1995b; Naidu, 1997).

NEUROLOGICAL AND BIOCHEMICAL SEQUELAE

RS is associated with dramatic neurological, neurochemical, and neurophysiological effects. As these effects have been described in literally hundreds of reports, this section relies largely on recent reviews in an attempt to focus on some of the main and consistent findings. Not all findings are consistent. For example, the small neuronal size and increasing cell-packing density reported in many areas of RS girls' brains by Bauman, Kemper, and Arin (1995) were not found by Belichenko, Hagberg, and Dahlstrom (1997). As would be expected from the decreased head size in infancy, brain weight and size in RS girls are reduced by some 12–34% from those of age-matched controls. Recently, Subramaniam, Naidu, and Reiss (1997) compared the magnetic resonance imaging (MRI) findings of RS girls and age-matched normal girls. Size of the following brain areas was reduced between

20% and 30% in the RS girls: total cerebrum, total gray matter (and gray matter in cortex, caudate, putamen, and thalamus), total white matter, midbrain, and cerebellum. The pons did not differ in size, and cerebrospinal fluid volume was slightly increased in the RS girls. Interestingly, Subramaniam et al. (1997) also compared the MRIs of the pair of MZ twins discordant for RS. Generally, the brain of the RS twin was reduced compared to that of the unaffected twin (similar to the differences between the group data for RS and normal girls), although some differences were apparent. The thalamus of the RS twin was most reduced, whereas the white matter and cerebellar differences were smaller.

An absence of progressive neurological decreases with age (e.g., Subramaniam et al., 1997), and an absence of gliosis in brains of RS girls (e.g., Belichenko et al., 1997), support the concept of RS as neurodevelopmental rather than neurodegenerative (e.g., Glaze, 1995; Naidu, 1997; Percy, 1995, 1996). The frontal cortex, caudate, parts of the cerebellum, and midbrain show relatively greater reduction in size than occurs in the brain in general; the substantia nigra is hypopigmented, owing to reduction of melanin; and cell number in the nucleus basalis of Meynert is reduced (e.g., Belichenko et al., 1997; Naidu, 1997; Percy, 1995, 1996). Dendrites of pyramidal neurons are also disturbed, showing simplified dendrites and reduced arborizations, which again appear not to be progressive. Reductions are relatively greater in the frontal, motor, and inferior temporal cortices, but the arbors are preserved in the occipital cortex (Percy, 1996). Percy (1996) suggests that the latter finding could be related to the intense gaze that RS girls and women show. Simplified convolutions in the inferior olivary nucleus in the absence of any retrograde cell loss suggest that some abnormal development occurs before birth, since those convolutions develop between 28 and 32 weeks of gestation (Naidu, 1997). Other evidence summarized by Naidu (1997, p. 5) suggests "a disturbance in the early stages of neocortical maturation in RS." Gliosis and neural changes in the spinal cord may be involved in the scoliosis and lower-extremity dysfunction shown in RS (Budden, 1997; Naidu, 1997). Belichenko et al. (1997) have suggested that RS may be a postnatal synaptogenic developmental disorder.

Numerous neurochemical abnormalities have also been reported. "The clinical manifestations of abnormal movements, rigidity, and mental retardation have led to the consideration that altered neurotransmitters must play a role in RS secondary to disruption of dopaminergic striatonigral, mesocortical, and mesolimbic pathways from midbrain, and cholinergic basal forebrain projections to neocortex and hippocampus" (Naidu, 1997, p. 6). Neurotransmitter deficiencies include dopamine throughout the neocortex and basal ganglia, and acetylcholine in the neocortex, hippocampus, putamen, and thalamus. Experimental rodent models may help to clarify the underlying neurobiology of RS (e.g., Johnston, Hohmann, & Blue, 1995).

TREATMENT AND MANAGEMENT

No completely effective treatment regimen is available for RS, and the symptoms appear to follow an inexorable course. However, active intervention may delay the appearance of some symptoms and alleviate others: "A vigorous approach to caring for RS girls is advocated" (Glaze, 1995, p. 79). RS girls typically have very long latencies to respond to directions—an important consideration in all aspects of therapy. The delay in responding may be as long as a minute. Accurate diagnosis is important, both to ensure appropriate treatment and to avoid ineffective treatment. For example, three RS girls who had initially been diagnosed with autism have inadvertently been participants in Lovaas's intensive behavior modification program (Smith et al., 1995), which has been demonstrably effective with autistic children (e.g., Lovaas, 1987). The girls were 31 to 37 months old at the outset of treatment, which lasted from 8 months to 2 years. Their intellectual performance declined during treatment to such an extent that although each had been initially tested on the Bayley Scales of Infant Development, none could be tested at the end of treatment. Furthermore, except for a reduction in tantrums, gains tended to be offset by losses. One subject did proceed from echolalia to meaningful use of one word, but by the end of treatment, increasing articulation problems made her difficult to understand. Overall, the girls showed few if any changes that might not have occurred without treatment. However, the observations of their alternating periods of attention and nonresponsiveness may have important implications for therapy.

Individual differences in the degree of various impairments, and in responsiveness to, (as well as tolerance of) various interventions, necessitate individualized treatment programs (e.g., Van Acker, 1991). Owing to the multiplicity and diversity of problems associated with RS, a team approach is indicated.

Specialized behavior modification programs have successfully increased or decreased various behaviors in RS girls of different ages in several institutional settings. Age has not always been relevant to success. Using a variety of verbal and physical prompts and reinforcement (verbal praise), Piazza, Anderson, and Fisher (1993) attempted to teach five RS girls who initially had very limited self-feeding skills to scoop food onto a spoon, bring the spoon to their mouths, and put the spoon in their mouths. The girls showed improvement to varying degrees in self-feeding behaviors not only during the 8-week program, but in later follow-up. One girl was almost completely self-feeding 18 months after the end of the program. Through use of shaping, graduated guidance, and hand regulation, Bat-Haee (1994) increased self-feeding, ambulation, and use of an adaptive switch in a 24-year-old RS woman who at the outset of the program had been completely dependent on staff members.

Mechanical and computer-based devices have also been used to modify RS girls' behavior. A computer fitted with a touch-sensitive screen and voice synthesizer was used by Van Acker and Grant (1995) to present combined visual–auditory representations of favored foods, and (in a subsequent phase) new favored foods not initially presented and nonfavored foods, to three RS girls. In training, a picture of a favored food item appeared on the computer screen as the voice synthesizer asked, "Would you like some _____?" To varying extents, the girls learned, with some initial guidance, to touch the screen to receive a small amount of one or more of the pictured foods. Initial acquisition took some weeks at two sessions a day. In the later phase, two of the girls clearly discriminated between the new favored and nonfavored foods, learning relatively quickly to respond at a high rate for the favored foods, while maintaining a low rate of response to the nonpreferred foods. In subsequent generalization testing, the same two girls responded appropriately in lunchroom and home settings. Working with a nonambulatory, nonverbal, and very inactive 3-year-old RS girl, Sullivan, Laverick, and Lewis (1995) tried to increase contingent responding for music and musical toys. They fitted the girl's orthopedic chair with two pad switches, one behind her head and one between her hands. Pressing on either pad led to presentation of a toy for as long as the switch was depressed. The child rapidly acquired the head-pressing response, keeping the switch closed for minutes at a time. Hand responses also occurred, but at a lower frequency. Subsequent introduction of novel toys resulted in an increase in responding. After 6 months of training, the girl began to show positive anticipatory emotions at the outset of sessions and smiling, laughter, and vocalizations during sessions; after 9 months, she began to show positive emotions in anticipation of a session as her chair was being presented. One caution must be expressed, however, about the routine implementation of some of these programs, particularly by parents: Much effort, persistence, and tolerance for frustration are required, for the changes reported in some of these studies have been slow and even difficult to see. Indeed, Piazza et al. (1993) suggest that parents should be warned about the effort involved and the need to keep careful response records in order to see progress.

As apraxia is one of the main effects of RS, physical therapy is critical (e.g., Hanks, 1990). It helps RS girls to maintain or reacquire ambulation—"one of the critical skills to develop and maintain in persons with Rett syndrome" (Van Acker, 1991, p. 395)—and to develop or maintain the transitional behaviors needed to stand up from sitting or lying positions. Such therapy may involve use of a therapy ball and activities to stimulate balance, weight shifting and bearing, and gait. Gait is further impaired by rigidity in the heels of the feet, leading to toe walking. Ankle–foot orthoses and physical therapy help to maintain more normal walking (Budden, 1997). The stereotypic hand movements are involuntary, so behavior modification techniques designed to reduce them not only are likely to be ineffective, but may actually increase the movements by increasing anxiety. Several techniques, including restraints that prevent hand-to-mouth movements or simply holding a girl's hand, may be effective. Generally, whirlpool baths may be helpful. Some of the stereotyped hand clasping and other movements may be reduced by allowing a girl with RS to hold a favored toy. In one case, hand wringing was reduced by giving the girl a set of baby keys, which she would manipulate for long periods of time (Hanks, 1990).

Most RS girls begin to develop scoliosis before age 8, and many also show kyphosis (hunchback) (Huang, Lubicky, & Hammerberg, 1994). The disorders are basically neurogenic, but may be exacerbated by other factors such as loss of transitional motor skills and spatial perceptual orientation, postural misalignment, and rigidity (Budden, 1997). Physical therapy and careful positioning in seated positions may help slow the development of scoliosis, but corrective surgery is often required.

Although showing strong appetites, most RS girls show serious growth retardation, to the point of meeting criteria for moderate to severe malnutrition. Chewing and swallowing problems, as well as gastroesophageal reflux and digestive problems, contribute to this retardation. Speech therapy may be helpful not so much for retaining language as for facilitating chewing and swallowing. Supplementary tube feedings may be necessary to help increase growth (Glaze & Schultz, 1997). Further complicating feeding issues is the fact that constipation is common in RS. Although it is generally controllable through diet, laxatives or enemas may be necessary in some cases.

Seizures occur in most RS girls, and their control "is perhaps the most common problem facing the primary care provider or the treating neurologist" (Budden, 1997, p. 7). Seizures occur most commonly in Stage 3 (Glaze & Schultz, 1997). One commonly reported difficulty (e.g., Budden, 1997, Glaze & Schultz, 1997) is that parents overestimate seizure activity, some of which may be behaviorally based. On the other hand, parents may miss actual seizures, many of which occur during sleep. Most seizures can be controlled with antiseizure medication, most frequently carbamazepine and/or valproic acid. Occasionally, a ketogenic diet may be used in otherwise intractable cases (Budden, 1997), although it presents its own management problems.

Agitation, screaming, and tantrums are frequently reported. In fact, tantrums were among the first behaviors that caused alarm in one of the mothers in our case studies (see below). The rapid neurological and physical changes associated with the onset of the dis-

ease may understandably provoke emotional outbursts. RS girls frequently respond negatively to stimulus or routine change, so transitions from one setting or pattern to another
should be gradual and accompanied by a parent if possible. Agitation or screaming may
also reflect pain or irritation from a physical condition; in the absence of language or gestures, RS individuals may have no other way to signal such discomfort. Since the girls go
through puberty, caretakers need to be sensitive to their menstrual cycles. Some agitation
in older individuals may reflect premenstrual discomfort or some other gynecological disorder, which may be easily treatable (Budden, 1997). Again, various treatment approaches
have been used. Behavior modification may be helpful. As indicated above, tantrums were
the only behavior consistently affected by intensive intervention (Smith et al., 1995), being
eliminated in two and reduced in the third RS girl, and one of our parents also reported
that her use of behavior modification effectively reduced her daughter's tantrums. Since
the tantrums tend to decrease with age without intervention, however, one cannot be con-
fident that the observed changes actually resulted from the treatment, as Smith et al. (1995)
note. Other suggested treatments include medication (particularly at night), music, quiet
settings, massage, and Kellogg's (1903) favorite—hydrotherapy, particularly warm baths
(see e.g., Van Acker, 1991).

Owing to the lifelong impact of the disorder on parents and other family members,
ranging from home care issues to decisions about educational and other placement, counseling for them will be particularly important (Lieb-Lundell, 1988). Training the parents in behavior modification may help them in managing some aspects of their RS
daughter's behavior, including tantrums. Of importance, given the degree of care that
RS adults may require and their relative longevity, parents will eventually need to face
the issue of lifelong care and make financial arrangements for care of their daughter after
their deaths.

LIFE WITH AN RS CHILD: TWO CASE HISTORIES

The clinical description of RS does not capture the agonizing situation with which parents
and families of RS individuals are confronted. That they see their initially apparently normal daughter or sister stop developing and then show severe deterioration into a state of
multiple handicaps is obvious. But some of the problems as well as the other characteristics of individual RS children may best be seen in descriptions of individual cases. Here
described are two cases, involving children born 18 years apart.

Mary: From Infancy to Childhood

Mary was born in April 1992. Her early development appeared normal, such that at age
16 months she could point to body parts. When Mary was about two, the parents became
concerned because she was not developing language normally, was having sleeping problems, was drooling and chewing her tongue, was showing strange eye blinking, and was
screaming a lot. About 6 months later, Mary began to regress; she was no longer able to
point to body parts or stay on a swing. Her father commented, "She's plateaued."

Mary's mother consulted a psychologist, who, after viewing home videotapes, confirmed that Mary was not developing normally and recommended consultation with a
neurologist. When Mary was about 3, the neurologist diagnosed autism. The mother, who
worked for an autism center, questioned this diagnosis because she had never seen an au-

tistic child behave like Mary, who was now breathing heavily and easily excitable. A battery of tests, including MRI, EEG, and chromosomal analysis, revealed no abnormality. Mary continued to deteriorate, having what the mother described as "fading spells." She fell off things, lost the ability to climb stairs, began to crawl, and could sit only with assistance. A second EEG showed abnormalities but no seizures. The neurologist maintained the diagnosis of autism. On the recommendation of a pediatrician, the mother put Mary on the anticonvulsant carbamazepine (Tegretol). Within a week, Mary's behavior improved, her sleep problems decreased, and her balance returned. But lose of hand control continued, and Mary began making fists.

When Mary was almost 4, the director of the autism center where the mother worked told her that she and others at the center had been doing some reading and thought that the daughter might have RS. After the mother read one of the books, the proverbial "light bulb went off in my head," as she noted later. The Kennedy Krieger Institute at Johns Hopkins Medical Institutes confirmed RS; however, Dr. SakkuBai Naidu, a leading RS authority, indicated that it was probably not classic RS and that the family should continue therapy. The parents were relieved finally to have a diagnosis that both captured the child's behaviors and suggested some treatment. At about this time Mary suddenly started repetitive hand wringing, which the parents now could understand.

The mother told the original neurologist about the RS diagnosis, and he said that he avoided diagnosing RS before a child is 6 years old, since the disorder is so devastating and the diagnosis could be wrong. The mother told him that he should have given the diagnosis as early as possible, so that the parents would know what to expect. Mary spent 2 years at a United Cerebral Palsy center and is now at another special school. She not only has limited communication, can walk, can feed herself with her fingers, and can use a spoon with assistance, but has shown some recovery. She no longer drools and can stay seated in school. The mother credits physical therapy for these gains, and concentrates on helping Mary retain her current motor skills.

The parents have been affected in many ways. Because most people are unfamiliar with RS, they have difficulty accepting the extent of Mary's limitations, given her normal appearance. They occasionally think that behaviors such as throwing objects are purposeful. The parents are not as social as they were previously, since they must attend to Mary's needs. Until age 5, Mary would sleep by herself for an hour, which gave the parents some time for each other or for household chores. Now one of them sleeps with Mary every night, since she may waken 15 to 20 times, but goes back to sleep if a parent is with her. As the mother says, they "are not the same couple."

Jane: From Infancy to Adulthood

Jane was born in 1975, years before RS came to the attention of the English-speaking professional community. She was the firstborn child of a couple in which the father was in the military and frequently stationed outside the United States. Her mother kept a detailed journal of her development from birth, from which much of this information comes. Her early development appeared to be somewhat ahead of norms, as she sat at 4 months and could wind up toys by 7 months. She said her first proto-word at about 1 year, had a vocabulary of about 16 words at 16 months, and showed great interest in books. At about 12 months, however, she started having spontaneous tantrums. By 16 months, she started losing instead of gaining words, throwing toys or using them as weapons rather than playing with them, and putting everything she picked up (including dirt) into her mouth. Common words like "bye-bye" disappeared from her vocabulary. At 20 months of age, a younger sister was born; the pediatrician told the mother not to worry about Jane, since she was showing "normal regression." But although seeming to retain some comprehension, she was saying only "mama" and "papa."

Jane appeared to be extremely jealous of her sister, and pushed, hit, and scratched her severely enough to scar her face. She not only lost the ability to wind up toys, but by 24 months could not even pick one up. Growth retardation became prominent and continued. She entered an apparently autistic phase and began smearing feces on herself and her surroundings. At 28 months, she began to defecate in her hands and throw the feces at her mother. If the mother left her bed at night, she would scream and vomit. One of her grandmothers, insensitive to the possibility that she had a serious problem, urged Jane's mother simply to spank her more. But whenever the mother did spank her, Jane laughed, suggesting an insensitivity to pain. Some of Jane's behaviors were bizarre: She liked to chew ice, and several times she bit glasses and chewed the glass as though it were ice. Once she found a dead animal in the yard and started to eat it. When Jane was about 36 months old, she was hospitalized for assessment, which resulted in a diagnosis of either mental retardation or autism.

After moving to another base to be with her husband, the mother became so frantic that she was afraid she would become abusive. On the recommendation of a military base physician, the mother took an extensive course in behavior modification. Application of behavioral principles led to a cessation of vomiting and a reduction in many of Jane's other attention-getting behaviors. The mother credits the program with giving her a handle on Jane's behavior for the first time since infancy.

Physicians proposed various diagnoses, including schizophrenia, autism, mental retardation, childhood aphasia, and hyperactivity. Because the child was so small and did not gain weight, malnutrition was suggested, even though Jane ate a lot. At age 7, Jane was placed in a class for autistic children. A year later, she began to have what appeared to be generalized tonic–clonic seizures, which were not controlled by medication. At one point, even while on medication, she was having some 20 seizures daily. Tests indicated allergies to 43 substances, including lactose. Given interest at the time in the Feingold diet and other diets for such disorders as hyperactivity, one should not be surprised at the hypothesis that Jane's problems were caused by allergies, but dietary manipulation had few effects. At about age 9, she again began showing aggression toward herself and others. Once she slapped her own face so hard that she deformed her jaw and began to cry hysterically. When the mother tried to soothe her, Jane bit her and would not let go until the mother virtually pried her off. The parents considered residential treatment at this time because of the seizures and aggressive behavior. But Jane was admitted to a hospital for observation after having a severe seizure and falling down a flight of stairs. Her neurologist had just attended a conference on RS and finally diagnosed Jane appropriately. The mother, unsatisfied with the diagnoses suggested, had been doing a lot of reading on developmental disorders and had suspected RS for some time. After Jane was put on divalproex (Depakote), which had been found to be effective with RS girls, both the seizures and the aggressive behavior dissipated; she became again a "happy-go-lucky child," in her mother's words. The parents dropped plans for residential treatment, although she still showed severe mood swings. Speech therapy and physical therapy were provided. The speech therapy was ineffective, but the mother attributes Jane's continued walking to the efficacy of the physical therapy.

Jane showed virtually all of the current necessary and supportive criteria for RS, and apparently went through the four stages described earlier. Her cognitive development became largely arrested. She also developed the classic RS hand stereotypies—in her case, mainly hand mouthing, to such an extent that she developed infections on her hands. Although she maintained walking, her body movements became jerky, and she showed gait apraxia. She had surgery for scoliosis at age 15 years. Bruxism was common, as was air swallowing and breath holding. Growth retardation continued.

When Jane reached 19 years of age, the parents began to worry about her long-term future in light of their own ages. Jane now lives in a residential facility, which the parents describe to her as a college, but she goes home every weekend. She has a mental age of about 12 months and is still on seizure medication. The autistic behaviors have disappeared, and the mother describes her as loving and appreciative. However, she still occasionally lashes out, apparently to communicate pain caused by gastric distress. She communicates intensively with eye gaze, but has a long latency of response. She is still ambulatory, but her hands are now clasped at her mouth, which makes walking difficult owing to balance problems. She drools, which leaves her hands wet, interfering with treatment of a fungus. Jane apparently can still chew food but not swallow it, and is rapidly losing so much weight that she may have to be tube-fed.

Large parts of the lives of Jane's parents (particularly her mother) and siblings have been centered around dealing with and caring for Jane. The years of frustration before diagnosis are obvious, as are their remarkable tolerance and acceptance of her emotional outbursts and overall deterioration. So are the love and affection that they still have for her.

Comments on the Cases

RS has obviously become more widely known and researched between the births of Jane and Mary. As Jane's parents have said, they went from having a daughter for 10 years with a severe but undiagnosed condition, to having one of the first 250 or so diagnosed RS daughters worldwide, to the current situation where RS public service announcements appear on TV. But the two cases also show some striking similarities. Parents are frequently portrayed as "shopping" for a relatively favorable diagnosis. But Jane and Mary's parents were trying to determine for years what was wrong with their daughters; they knew that the initial diagnoses did not fit their daughters' characteristics. They were not looking for a favorable diagnosis, but an accurate one. Initially, Jane's mother had little success in convincing physicians that anything serious was wrong, and she was instrumental in the final diagnosis of RS. Both sets of parents have ended up describing RS to physicians. The evidence that parents seek the "best" diagnosis for their child, at least in the case of serious disorders, has never been strong and clearly does not apply to these cases. Although treatment of RS is relatively ineffective, knowledge of their children's condition was critical for both sets of parents in understanding what was happening to their daughters, in arranging care, and in knowing what to expect.

SUMMARY

RS is a severe, low-incidence neurodevelopmental disorder affecting only girls. Diagnositc criteria exist for both classic and variant forms of RS. It typically develops in a four-stage progression beginning in late infancy, although earlier signs may exist. RS is almost undoubtedly genetic, but its basis is unknown, although (as would be expected) research is focusing on an X chromosome abnormality. RS is associated with numerous neuroanatomical and neurochemical disturbances.

No effective treatment is available, but intense physical and speech therapy may delay or even reverse some of the deterioration in motor functioning. Bracing or surgery may be necessary to help to correct scoliosis, and medication generally controls seizures. Behavior modification may reduce tantrums and increase competence in specific areas. RS adults will need intensive caretaking throughout life, and residential placement for adults is common. Owing to the differential interventions used for RS and for autism, early diagnosis is important.

ACKNOWLEDGMENT

We express deep appreciation to the parents of our two RS cases for being so generous with their time and for sharing their experiences with their daughters with us.

REFERENCES

Akesson, H. O. (1997). Rett syndrome: The Swedish genealogic research project. New data and present position. *European Child and Adolescent Psychiatry*, 6(Suppl. 1), 96–98. (MEDLINE Abstract No. PMID 9452929)

Akesson, H. O., Hagberg, B., & Wahlström, J. (1997). Rett syndrome: Presumptive carriers of the gene effect. Sex ratio among their siblings. *European Child and Adolescent Psychiatry*, 6(Suppl. 1), 101–102. (MEDLINE Abstract No. PMID 9452931)

Akesson, H. O., Hagberg, B., Wahlström, J., & Witt-Engerström, I. (1992). Rett syndrome: A search for gene sources. *American Journal of Medical Genetics*, 42, 104–110.

Bat-Haee, M. A. (1994). Behavioral training of a young woman with Rett syndrome. *Perceptual and Motor Skills*, 78, 314.

Bauman, M. L., Kemper, T. L., & Arin, D. M. (1995). Microscopic observations of the brain in Rett syndrome. *Neuropediatrics*, 26, 105–108.

Belichenko, P. V., Hagberg, B., & Dahlstrom, A. (1997). Morphological study of neocortical areas in Rett syndrome. *Acta Neuropathologica*, 93, 50–61.

Budden, S. S. (1997). Understanding, recognizing, and treating Rett syndrome. *Medscape Women's Health*, 2(3), 1–11, on-line journal. http://www.medscape.com/Medscape/WomensHealth/journal/1997/v02.n03/w3185.budden.w3185.budden.html

Gillberg, C., Ehlers, S., & Wahlström, J. (1990). The syndromes described by Kanner and Rett–Hagberg: Overlap in an extended family. *Developmental Medicine and Child Neurology*, 32, 258–266.

Glaze, D. G. (1995). Commentary: The challenge of Rett syndrome. *Neuropediatrics*, 26, 78–80.

Glaze, D. G., & Schultz, R. J. (1997). Rett syndrome: Meeting the challenge of this gender-specific neurodevelopmental disorder. *Medscape Women's Health*, 2(1), 1–9, on-line journal. http://www.medscape.com/Medscape/WomensHealth/journal/1997/v02.n01/w223.glaze/w223.glaze.html

Hagberg, B. (1995a). Clinical delineation of Rett syndrome variants. *Neuropediatrics*, 26, 62.

Hagberg, B. (1995b). Rett syndrome: Clinical peculiarities and biological mysteries. *Acta Paediatrica*, 84, 971–976.

Hagberg, B. (1996). Rett syndrome: Recent clinical and biological aspects. In A. Arzimanoglou & F. Goutières (Eds.), *Trends in child neurology* (pp. 143–146). Paris: John Libbey Eurotext.

Hagberg, B., Aicardi, J., Dias, K., & Ramos, O. (1983). A progressive syndrome of autism, dementia, ataxia, and loss of purposeful hand use in girls: Rett's syndrome. Report of 35 cases. *Annals of Neurology, 14,* 471–479.

Hagberg, B., Anvret, M., & Wahlström, J. (Eds.). (1993). *Rett syndrome: Clinical and biological aspects* (Clinics in Developmental Medicine No. 127). London: MacKeith.

Hagberg, B., Goutieres, F., Hanefeld, F., Rett, A., & Wilson, J. (1985). Rett syndrome: Criteria for inclusion and exclusion. *Brain and Development, 7,* 272–273.

Hagberg, B., & Skjeldal, O. H. (1994). Rett variants: A suggested model for inclusion criterion. *Pediatric Neurology, 11,* 5–11.

Hagberg, B., & Witt-Engerström, I. (1986). Rett syndrome: A suggested staging system for describing impairment profile with increasing age toward adolescence. *American Journal of Medical Genetics, 24*(Suppl. 1), 47–59.

Hanks, S. (1990). Motor disabilities in the Rett syndrome and physical therapy strategies. *Brain and Development, 12,* 157–161.

Huang, T.-J., Lubicky, J. P., & Hammerberg, K. W. (1994). Scoliosis in Rett syndrome. *Orthopaedic Review, 23,* 931–937.

Johnston, M. V., Hohmann, C., & Blue, M. E. (1995). Neurobiology of Rett syndrome. *Neuropediatrics, 26,* 119–122.

Kellogg, J. H. (1903). *Rational hydrotherapy* (2nd ed.). Philadelphia: Davis.

Kerr, A. M. (1995). Early clinical signs in the Rett syndrome. *Neuropediatrics, 26,* 67–71.

Lieb-Lundell, C. (1988). The therapist's role in the management of girls with Rett syndrome. *Journal of Child Neurology, 3*(Suppl.), S31–S34.

Lovaas, O. I. (1987). Behavioral treatment and normal educational and intellectual functioning in young autistic children. *Journal of Consulting and Clinical Psychology, 55,* 3–9.

Moser, H. W., & Naidu, S. (1991). The discovery and study of Rett syndrome. In A. J. Capute & P. J. Accardo (Eds.), *Developmental disabilities in infancy and childhood* (pp. 325–333). Baltimore: Paul H. Brookes.

Naidu, S. (1997). Rett syndrome: A disorder affecting early brain growth. *Annals of Neurology, 42,* 3–10.

Olsson, B., & Rett, A. (1985). Behavioral observations concerning differential diagnosis between the Rett syndrome and autism. *Brain and Development, 7,* 281–289.

Percy, A. K. (1995). Rett syndrome. *Current Opinion in Neurology, 8,* 156–160.

Percy, A. K. (1996). Rett syndrome: The evolving picture of a disorder of brain development. *Developmental Brain Research, 9,* 180–196.

Perry, A., Sarlo-McGarvey, N., & Haddad, C. (1991). Brief reports: Cognitive and adaptive functioning in 28 girls with Rett syndrome. *Journal of Autism and Developmental Disorders, 21,* 551–556.

Piazza, C. C., Anderson, C., & Fisher, W. (1993). Teaching self-feeding skills to patients with Rett syndrome. *Developmental Medicine and Child Neurology, 35,* 991–996.

Rett, A. (1966). Uber ein eigenartiges Hirnatrophisches Syndrom bei Hyperammonamie im Kindes alter. [On an unusual brain atropic syndrome with hyperammonemia in childhood]. *Wiener Medizinische Wochenschrift, 116,* 425–428.

Rett Syndrome Diagnostic Criteria Work Group. (1988). Diagnostic criteria for Rett syndrome. *Annals of Neurology, 23,* 425–428.

Sansom, D., Krishnan, V. H. R., Corbett, J., & Kerr, A. (1993). Emotional and behavioural aspects of Rett syndrome. *Developmental Medicine and Child Neurology, 35,* 340–345.

Smith, T., Klevstrand, M., & Lovaas, O. I. (1995). Behavioral treatment of Rett's disorder: Ineffectiveness in three cases. *American Journal of Mental Retardation, 100,* 317–322.

Subramaniam, B., Naidu, S., & Reiss, A. L. (1997). Neuroanatomy in Rett syndrome: Cerebral cortex and posterior fossa. *Neurology, 48,* 399–407.

Sullivan, M. W., Laverick, D. H., & Lewis, M. (1995). Brief report: Fostering environmental control in a young child with Rett syndrome. A case study. *Journal of Autism and Developmental Disorders, 25,* 215–221.

Tams-Little, S., & Holdgrafer, G. (1996). Early communication development in children with Rett syndrome. *Brain and Development, 18,* 376–378.

Thomas, G. H. (1996). High male:female ratio of germline mutations: An alternative explanation for postulated gestational lethality in males in X-linked dominant disorders. *American Journal of Human Genetics, 58,* 647–653.

Van Acker, R. (1991). Rett syndrome: A review of current knowledge. *Journal of Autism and Developmental Disorders, 21,* 381–406.

Van Acker, R., & Grant, S. H. (1995). An effective-computer-based requesting system for persons with Rett syndrome. *Journal of Childhood Communication Disorders, 16,* 31–38.

21

LESCH–NYHAN SYNDROME

PAMILLA C. MORALES

Lesch–Nyhan syndrome is a rare genetic disorder characterized by severe dystonia, spasticity, speech impairment, gout, renal disease, varying degrees of cognitive deficit, and compulsive self-injury (Nyhan & Wong, 1996). Lesch–Nyhan syndrome is an X-linked recessive disorder of the enzyme hypoxanthine–guanine phosphoribosyltransferase (HPRT). The syndrome was first reported by Michael Lesch and William L. Nyhan in 1964, when they described two affected brothers (Lesch & Nyhan, 1964). The defective gene is recessive and carried on the X chromosome, creating a syndrome that typically affects only males. Although there have been two documented cases of females with Lesch–Nyhan syndrome, these are extremely rare; females almost never exhibit the various characteristics of the syndrome, but may be carriers (Yamada, Goto, Yukawa, Akazawa, & Ogasawara, 1994; Yukawa et al., 1992).

There are 17 identified independent enzyme mutations resulting in HPRT deficiency; however, only one is identified as Lesch–Nyhan syndrome, making a definitive early diagnosis difficult (Davidson et al., 1991; Tarle et al., 1991). Recent research in this area has found that a possible mechanism underlying this dysfunction is deficient dopaminergic neurons and impaired differentiation of HPRT (Zheng & Howard, 1998). Lesch–Nyhan syndrome appears to be distributed evenly among races and geographic locales, and occurs in approximately 1 of every 380,000 births (Nyhan & Wong, 1996). Because of its rarity, there are only several hundred individuals with Lesch–Nyhan syndrome currently living in the United States. Congenital errors of metabolism are extremely rare; however, Lesch–Nyhan syndrome is actually one of the more common congenital errors of metabolism, second only to phenylketonuria (Nyhan & Wong, 1996).

PHYSIOPATHOLOGY

Lesch–Nyhan syndrome is a congenital disorder of uric acid metabolism associated with a nearly complete absence of the enzyme HPRT. Enzymes are complex proteins that are capable of inducing chemical changes in other substances without being changed themselves. They can also increase the rate at which specific chemical reactions take place.

478

Enzymes are very specific in their action and will only act upon a certain substance or a group of closely related chemical substances. The structure and functioning of each enzyme are determined by a specific gene. When an individual inherits a defective enzyme gene, as is the case with Lesch–Nyhan syndrome, the result is a partially or completely absent or nonfunctioning enzyme. The molecule normally converted by that particular enzyme builds up, while the molecule normally produced by that enzyme becomes scarce. The outcome is either an accumulation of a toxic substrate or a deficiency in the product, either of which is detrimental to survival and/or functioning of the individual (Mateos-Anton & Garcia-Puig, 1994).

In Lesch–Nyhan syndrome the enzyme HPRT, which normally metabolizes hypoxanthine and guanine into uric acid, is deficient. This deficiency causes an almost complete absence of HPRT activity in the cells of affected patients, and thus creates a vacuum in the metabolic pathway. HPRT and its availability to the metabolic pathway are essential for the maintenance, metabolic function, and integrity of cells. HPRT normally catalyzes the conversion of hypoxanthine and guanine into their respective nucleotides in DNA and RNA, inosinic acid and guanylic acid, and then into uric acid. Uric acid is a waste product within a class of chemical compounds known as "purines." Purines are the parent compounds of purine bases (e.g., adenine, guanine, xanthine, caffeine, and uric acid). Many different metabolic pathways exist for making purines, converting purine compounds, reusing purines consumed in the diet, and disposing of excess purines.

Purines have four basic functions that are vital to the life process: (1) They convert the energy produced by the oxidation of food molecules into a structure that cells can utilize; (2) they serve as nerve conductors and muscle contractors, and thus act as messengers; (3) they rid cells of excess nitrogen; and (4) they act as antioxidants, protecting cells from cancer-causing agents (Tu, 1994). Purines share a basic nine-member ring structure and are synthesized from small molecules such as the amine nitrogen of glutamine, glycine, and bicarbonate in an elaborate 11-step process (Fuscoe & Nelson, 1994; Nyhan & Wong, 1996).

The synthesizing process requires a considerable amount of energy. Each process must contain the intermediates ribose and phosphate along with two molecules of adenosine triphosphate for each molecule of necleotide synthesized (Fuscoe & Nelson, 1994). Employing a salvage pathway, HPRT and adenine phosphoribosyltransferase reuse preformed bases that result from cell turnover and metabolism. In Lesch–Nyhan syndrome, because there is little or no HPRT activity, the salvage pathway is not utilized; this results in excessive synthesis of purine nucleotides, which then causes enormous overproduction of uric acid in the body. The positive symptoms for Lesch–Nyhan syndrome are the results of this extreme overproduction; they include the manifestations of gout, renal dysfunction, hyperuricemia, uricosuria, tophaceous gouty arthritis, urinary tract calculi, and urate nephropathy (Fuscoe & Nelson, 1994; Jenkins, Hallett, & Hull, 1994; Rosenfeld, Preston, & Salvaggi-Fadden, 1994).

NEUROLOGICAL COMPROMISE

The neurological presentations of Lesch–Nyhan syndrome are unaccompanied by anatomical abnormalities in the brain, such as lesions and/or tumors; this suggests that the pathogenesis must be neurochemical in nature (Buitelaar, 1993). Some of the other clinical features of Lesch–Nyhan syndrome are also present in gout and are the direct consequences of hyperuricemia and metabolic abnormality, but the pathogenesis of the central nervous system abnormalities remains unclear (Buitelaar, 1993). It is hypothesized that the disruption of the salvage pathway and the accumulation of phosphoribosylpyrophosphate cause cells in the brain to be unable to synthesize required nucleotides (Tohyama, Nanba, & Ohno, 1994; Zoref, Bromberg, Brosh, Sidi, & Sperling, 1993). A conservative interpretation would associate the corticospinal dysfunction seen in this syndrome with the following structures: The spasticity would be linked to the basal ganglia, and the ataxia and dyskinesia with the cerebellum. Lesch–Nyhan syndrome is clearly a disorder of the extrapyramidal system.

The extrapyramidal system reaches segmental levels of distribution with neuronal chains synaptically grounded in the basal ganglia, subcortical ganglia, and reticular areas. This system consists of three layers of integration: cortical, striatal, and tegmental. The principal functions of this system are movement, postural adjustments, and autonomic integration. Because of the athetosis, chorea, and spasticity seen in Lesch–Nyhan syndrome, it is believed that the foci of damage are the caudate nucleus, putamen of the striate bodies, basal ganglia, and midbrain nuclei.

In addition to the characteristics just mentioned (ataxia, dyskinesia, spasticity, etc.), the neurological features of Lesch–Nyhan syndrome include mental retardation, delayed motor development, and opisthotonos (Ernst et al., 1996; Hunter et al., 1996; Wong et al., 1996; Sivam, 1996). Perhaps the strangest and most disturbing feature of all is the characteristic behavior of patients with the syndrome, which is described as aggressive, compulsive, and self-injurious (Buitelaar, 1993; Christie et al., 1982). However, the term "aggressive" should be used with caution, as many believe that it is not an accurate description of individuals with Lesch–Nyhan syndrome (Matthews, Solan, & Barabas, 1995). One of the bizarre characteristics of the neurobehavioral manifestations is that patients are unable to control their behavior. It is not unusual for individuals with Lesch–Nyhan syndrome to act aggressively toward care providers, spitting, cursing, hitting, and biting them, while simultaneously apologizing for their behavior (Matthews et al., 1995).

Among the most salient features of self-injurious behavior for individuals with Lesch–Nyhan syndrome is self-biting, which has been reported in the majority of these patients (Anderson & Ernst, 1994). The biting and other forms of self-mutilation may be so severe that they result in serious lacerations, loss of tissue, and amputation of the fingertips (Eguchi, Tokioka, Motoyoshi, & Wakamura, 1994; Nyhan & Wong, 1996; Wurtele, King, & Drabman, 1984). Individuals with Lesch–Nyhan syndrome are not insensitive to pain, and many individuals possess the intellectual capacity to understand their actions. However, they continue to act compulsively in their self-injurious behavior, often asking for physical restraint as the only means of intervention, as they appear unable to restrain themselves (Anderson & Ernst, 1994).

There are no clear indications that the disordered purine metabolism is responsible for these self-injurious manifestations (or, if so, how), but there is substantial evidence of abnormalities in neurotransmitters—specifically, irregularity in dopaminergic function in the basal ganglia (Ernst et al., 1996; Hunter et al., 1996; Wong et al., 1996; Sivam, 1996). Lloyd, Hornykiewicz, and Davidson (1981) autopsied three Lesch–Nyhan patients and revealed that levels of dopamine, homovanillic acid, and dopa decarboxylase in the basal ganglia were 10% of normal levels. Silverstein, Johnston, Hutchinson, and Edwards (1985) found dopaminergic aberrations that were consistent over a broad age range for patients with Lesch–Nyhan syndrome; these researchers suggested that the alteration in dopamine metabolism is not solely responsible for the self-injury and other neurological manifestations, but reflects an impact of the inborn error of metabolism on a sensitive target population of neurons. However, it is not known how the Lesch–Nyhan mutation reduces dopamine levels, or what specific chemicals and/or structures are involved in the characteristic behaviors of compulsive self-injury.

Dopamine is a neurotransmitter synthesized by the adrenal gland and is the immediate precursor in the synthesis of norepinephrine. Neurotransmitters are chemical messenger substances that activate the brain and are produced by nerve cells. These substances stimulate the sending of microelectric signals/information from neuron to neuron, which in turn allows the nervous system to function as a unit. Dopamine is crucial, as it helps activate epinephrine and norepinephrine, is a regulator of mood, and controls motor movement and coordination. The mesotelencephalic dopamine system consists of the ascending projections of dopamine-releasing neurons from the mesencephalon into various regions of the telencephalon, and continues through the lateral hypothalamus as part of the medial forebrain bundle. The neurons that compose the mesotelencephalic dopamine system have their cell bodies in two different midbrain nuclei, the substantia nigra and the ventral tegmental area. Their axons project to a variety of telencephalic sites, including specific regions of prefrontal neocortex and limbic cortex, the olfactory tubercle, the nucleus accumbens, the amygdala, the septum, and the striatum. It is this system that appears to be functioning at a reduced rate in individuals with Lesch–Nyhan syndrome.

The possible role of the dopamine system in Lesch–Nyhan syndrome suggests the need for intensive examination of this disorder with the many new imaging techniques available. Positron emission tomography and single-photon emission computed tomography have been successfully employed to study neuronal loss in Parkinson disease in nonhuman primates (Wong et al., 1996). Functional magnetic resonance imaging has been used to image blood flow and blood volume, but it may also be able to provide indirect measurements of biochemical abnormalities. High-temporal-resolution techniques may be of future use in the understanding of metabolic disorders such as Lesch–Nyhan syndrome (Wong et al., 1996). Cocaine analogues, which bind tightly to the presynaptic dopamine transporter, have increasingly been used to measure neuronal integrity—not only in Lesch–Nyhan syndrome, but also in Parkinson disease (Wong et al., 1996). These various techniques may lead to better methods of identifying and monitoring therapies for both diseases.

Ernst et al. (1996) conducted research on the dopaminergic system of Lesch–Nyhan syndrome patients, using positron emission tomography to measure presynaptic accumulation of fluorodopa F 18 tracer in the dopaminergic regions of the brain. This procedure measures dopa decarboxylase activity and provides an indicator of neuronal dopamine activity. The results of their research indicated that the fluorodopa F 18 ratio was significantly lower in the patients with Lesch–Nyhan syndrome than in the normal subjects, indicating decreases in dopamine activity of 31–57% in the putamen, caudate nucleus, frontal cortex, substantia nigra, and ventral tegmentum. The authors concluded that patients with Lesch–Nyhan syndrome have abnormally few dopaminergic nerve terminals and cell bodies, and that the abnormality involves all dopaminergic pathways and is not restricted to the basal ganglia.

The findings of Ernst et al. (1996) are consistent with those of Wong et al. (1996), who used *in vivo* imaging to study dopaminergic function in Lesch–Nyhan syndrome. These researchers used the ligand WIN-35,428, which binds to dopamine transporters, to estimate the density of dopamine-containing neurons in the caudate and putamen of 6 patients with Lesch–Nyhan syndrome, 10 control subjects, and 3 patients with Rett syndrome. Results indicated that in the Lesch–Nyhan syndrome patients there was a 50–63% reduction of the binding to dopamine transporters in the caudate, and a 64–75% reduction in the putamen, compared to the control group. These findings indicate that there is a major reduction in the intensity of dopamine-containing neurons or terminals in Lesch–Nyhan syndrome patients. It has been hypothesized that this dopamine reduction in Lesch–Nyhan patients changes the growth of nerve cell branches in the developing brain, creating neurological impairment in the growing child.

Although the specific neurobiological basis of self-injurious behavior in Lesch–Nyhan syndrome remains unclear, researchers have begun exploring the dopaminergic system as an explanation for the compulsive self-mutilating acts that characterize the disorder. Sivam (1996) reviewed the data on self-injurious behavior in Lesch–Nyhan syndrome induced by the dopamine uptake inhibitor GBR-12909, and compared these data to the neurochemical data on self-injurious behavior in neonatal 6-hydroxydopamine lesioned rats. The animal data indicated that a substantial reduction of dopamine accompanied by an increase in serotonin turnover may be highly conducive to the occurrence of self-injurious behavior. In addition, this phase is either superimposed upon or followed by a D1 and/or D2 dopamine-receptor-linked activation of striatonigral tachykinin neurons, resulting in enhanced tachykinin biosynthesis and release, which may sustain the self-injurious behavior. Thus a dynamic interplay among dopamine, serotonin, and tachykinin neuronal systems in the basal ganglia appears to influence the genesis and/or expression of self-injurious behavior. New advances in animal models have begun to link dopamine and serotonin systems to self-injurious behavior. Jinnah et al. (1999) have found that age and strain has a negative influence on striatal dopamine loss in rat models. Stodgell, Loupe, Schroeder, and Tessel (1998) discovered that neonatal 6-OHDA-induced neostriatal catecholamine depletion could be antagonized in rat models by experiential change causing higher incidence rates of self-injurious behavior. Risperidone has also been found to consistantly antagonize self-mutilation in rat models indicating that serotonergic systems may be useful in the treatment of Lesch–Nyhan syndrome (Allen, Freeman, & Davis, 1998). These new lines of research suggest that drugs may be useful in altering the dopamine and/or serotonergic systems in early life, which may eventually lead to easing or preventing the symptoms of Lesch–Nyhan syndrome. Drugs that affect the development of the dopamine system in early life may one day be used to ease or prevent the symptoms of Lesch–Nyhan syndrome.

CARRIER AND PRENATAL DIAGNOSIS

Because individuals with Lesch–Nyhan syndrome experience neurological complications and renal failure, few such individuals survive into their second decade. Genetic testing has great value in being able to predetermine genetic risk for possible carriers before pregnancy, and also to aid in the prenatal diagnosis of Lesch–Nyhan syndrome, so that early intervention can help lessen the effects of renal decline and malfunction (Mateos-Anton & Garcia-Puig, 1992; Mateos-Anton et al., 1991; Zheng & Howard, 1998). Unfortunately, no current treatment is capable of affecting the central nervous system presentations of Lesch–Nyhan syndrome— the self-injurious behavior, ataxia, spastic cerebral palsy, and choreoathetosis (Nyhan, 1996).

Genetic testing is the analysis of human DNA, RNA, chromosomes, proteins, or other gene products to detect disease-related genotypes, mutations, phenotypes, or karyotypes. Its purposes include predicting disease risks, identifying carriers, monitoring, establishing a diagnosis or prognosis, and establishing genetic identity. Recombinant DNA techniques were discovered in the 1970s, and their applications to mapping and sequencing the entire genome have greatly accelerated the discovery of genes that, when altered by germline or somatic mutations, result in disease or in increased risk of disease. The analyses can be performed on DNA from any nucleated somatic cell in the body from the earliest stages of the embryo onward. Other new techniques facilitate examining gene products, such as messenger RNA or proteins, in a wide range of cell types (Hunter et al., 1996). These new techniques have allowed researchers to screen carriers and confirm prenatal diagnosis in Lesch–Nyhan syndrome.

Alford, Redman, O'Brien, and Caskey (1995) demonstrated 100% sensitivity for the detection of mutations in the HPRT gene of affected males, and highly efficient carrier testing of at-risk females. The identification of the mutation in the index case of each family permits precise carrier diagnosis, using polymerase chain reaction (PCR) amplification of HPRT gene sequences and automated DNA sequencing. This research illustrates the utility and precision of molecular methodologies for carrier and prenatal diagnosis of Lesch–Nyhan syndrome, and also illustrates that molecular diagnostic studies of affected males and carrier testing prior to pregnancy can clarify genetic risk predictions and eliminate unnecessary prenatal procedures.

Mansfield et al. (1993) used complementary fluorescence-based PCR assays to analyze disease-causing mutations and found that two polymorphic small tandem repeats (STRs)—HPRTB [AGAT]n, mapping within intron 3 of the HPRT gene, and the CA-repeat at DXS294—can be used to establish linkage to Lesch–Nyhan syndrome. In addition, they utilized a cycle-sequencing strategy employing dye-labeled dideoxy terminators and a laser-activated, fluorescence emission DNA sequence in order to define carrier status in 10 family members at risk for Lesch–Nyhan syndrome, due to a splice donor mutation in intron 7. They were able to corroborate STR inheritance patterns in the family, which could possibly be used to facilitate rapid diagnosis of the various Lesch–Nyhan disease-causing mutations.

Many medical problems that were mysterious only a few years ago, including various errors of body chemistry, can now be treated or prevented both postnatally and prenatally through the use of gene therapy. The identification of genes is the first step toward developing specific treatment in which a healthy gene is used to replace one that is missing or malfunctioning. For instance, research has tentatively identified genes in some families linked to depression, alcoholism, and schizophrenia (Hornykiewicz, 1993). Understanding and knowing the locations and functions of genes will provide information about how they become flawed, and perhaps about how to treat or replace them before they cause damage. Because Lesch–Nyhan syndrome is the first disorder specifically linked to a gene defect that causes a specific behavior (i.e., compulsive self-injury; Ernst et al., 1996; Nyhan, 1996), Jinnah and Friedmann (1995) have suggested the use of gene therapy as a potentially effective treatment strategy for Lesch–Nyhan syndrome. In theory, the gene treatment would replace the defective gene with a functioning gene that would then encode the purine salvage enzyme HPRT. To date, research in gene therapy with animal models and *in vitro* systems has been positive. In a recent study, Lapchak, Araujo, Hilt, Sheng, and Jiao (1997) found that virally delivered GDNF promotes the recovery of nigral dopaminergic tone and improves behavioral performance in rodents with extensive nigrostriatal dopaminergic denervation. This area of research may eventually have applications in the area of neurodegenerative diseases and defective gene replacement.

DEVELOPMENTAL CONSIDERATIONS

Pregnancies that have resulted in individuals with Lesch–Nyhan syndrome are generally reported as normal, and the neonatal period is often described as unremarkable (Alford et al., 1995). The earliest presentations of Lesch–Nyhan syndrome begin to occur between 10 and 30 days of age, with orange crystals appearing in the diapers indicating renal insufficiency, and in some cases tophi in the hands and feet (Alford et al., 1995; Lesch & Nyhan, 1964). "Tophi" are deposits of sodium biurate in tissues near a joint, in the ear, or in bone, and are not as prevalent as the other signs of renal dysfunction. Crystalluria, hematuria, or renal tract stone disease may develop during the first 3 months of life; however, these also vary and are not specific presentations in all patients. Within the first 3 months of development, the neurological examination is negative in most children, and very few demonstrate cerebral presentations (Nyhan, 1976; Lesch & Nyhan, 1964).

Neurological symptoms begin to appear in infants after 3 months of age (Crawhall, Henderson, & Kelley, 1972). Prior to this, children with Lesch–Nyhan syndrome are reported to develop normally, beginning to smile at 4 weeks and being able to roll from a prone to a supine position at 3 months. At approximately 3–6 months of age, severe developmental delays begin to be present, with poor motor development or episodes of motor movement indicating possible neuromotor dysfunction (Crawhall et al., 1972; Nyhan, 1976; Lesch & Nyhan, 1964). Abnormal muscle tone or spasticity generally begins between the ages of 3 and 5 months; so does athetosis, which is described as a slow, irregular, twisting movement seen in the upper extremities (especially in the hands and fingers) and performed involuntarily (Crawhall et al., 1972; Nyhan, 1976; Lesch & Nyhan, 1964). Infants who had previously been sitting and holding their heads up will begin to lose these abilities. Many children are not yet specifically diagnosed with Lesch–Nyhan syndrome, however, with the most common diagnosis at this time being cerebral palsy.

Early neurological findings are alterations in muscle tone, which is generally recorded as hypotonic (i.e., the normal muscle tone is decreased; Crawhall et al., 1972; Nyhan, 1976; Lesch & Nyhan, 1964). Hypotonic muscles feel soft and flabby and offer less than normal resistance to passive movement. A change occurs between 6 and 12 months of age: Lesch–Nyhan syndrome patients become markedly hypertonic (i.e., normal muscle tone is increased), with spasticity, rigidity, and flexor spasms. In spasticity, there is increased resistance to sudden passive movements, and after the initial resistance there may be muscle relaxation (often referred to as the "clasp-knife phenomenon"). Flexor spasms are involuntary contraction of large groups of muscles, such as the arm, leg, or neck muscles. In rigidity, there is increased resistance on passive motion in any direction, usually unrelated to speed or direction of movement, due to steady contraction of flexors and extensors. Most Lesch–Nyhan syndrome patients are spastic, with choreoathetoid cerebral palsy being the most consistent feature. The characteristic movements of Lesch–Nyhan syndrome patients are opisthotonic spasms—episodic arching of the back, with the head bending back on the neck, the heels bending back on the legs, and the arms and hands flexing rigidly at the joints (Christie et al., 1982; Crawhall et al., 1972; Nyhan, 1976; Lesch & Nyhan, 1964). In some patients there is torticollis, which is an abnormal condition in which the head is inclined to one side as a result of the contraction of the muscles on that side of the neck.

Often the motor defects eventually become so severe that individuals with Lesch–Nyhan syndrome are unable to sit or stand without support and are only able to sit in a wheelchair if they are appropriately restrained and securely fastened around the chest. The most severe alterations in muscle tone occur between 8 and 11 years of age (Crawhall et al., 1972; Nyhan, 1976; Lesch & Nyhan, 1964). The severity for some individuals progresses to contractures and to dislocation of the hips and scissoring in the lower extremities. As patients get older, these spasms begin to appear to be at least semivoluntary. Caution must be exercised with these patients if they are placed on a hard surface, as they can lacerate or otherwise injure their heads (Crawhall et al., 1972; Nyhan, 1976; Lesch & Nyhan, 1964)

Speech in Lesch–Nyhan syndrome individuals is characterized by athetoid dysarthria, with the development of communication being hampered by poor articulation as a result of pseudobulbar palsy and obstructed air flow (Nyhan, 1976; Lesch & Nyhan, 1964). As the patients get older, these problems in communication become particularly frustrating, and their frustration increases the dysarthria still further (Christie et al., 1982; Nyhan, 1976; Lesch & Nyhan, 1964). Athetoid dysphagia is another problem in Lesch–Nyhan syndrome and can sometimes be life-threatening, as often individuals have great difficulty swallowing and can be very difficult to feed (Nyhan, 1976; Lesch & Nyhan, 1964). They are also reported to vomit and aspirate frequently, to have difficulty with pneumonia, and to be underweight. As a result of the many difficulties with digestion and the eating process, many patients have delayed skeletal maturation, and anemia is observed with some frequency (Christie et al., 1982; Nyhan, 1976; Lesch & Nyhan, 1964).

Cognitive impairment is present in many individuals, but to varying degrees. The testing of patients with Lesch–Nyhan syndrome is often very difficult as a result of their severe physical disabilities, combined with the self-abusive tendencies and the need for constant restraint (Anderson, Ernst, & Davis, 1992; Matthews et al., 1995; see below for further discussion). It has been reported that because of the difficulty of testing Lesch–Nyhan syndrome patients, they may be more intelligent than test scores indicate (Matthews et al., 1995).

A unique aspect of Lesch–Nyhan syndrome, as noted earlier, is the self-mutilating behavior that is reported in almost all patients; in many cases, this is what distinguishes the syndrome from other neurological disorders. The average age at which self-mutilating behavior begins in most patients is approximately 26 months. The mutilation begins with the lips, fingers, and hands, with the biting breaking the skin and causing lacerations. The self-mutilating behaviors escalate in violence and harm as a child grows older and becomes not only more physically capable of inflicting self-injury, but more cognitively capable of conceiving new methods of self-injury (Ball, Datta, Rios, & Constantine, 1985; Bull & LaVecchio, 1978; Gilbert, Spellacy, & Watts, 1979). Permanent loss of tissue is a regular consequence of biting with many Lesch–Nyhan syndrome patients; the self-amputation of fingers or tongue, and extensive loss of lip tissue, often occur. Many types of behavioral techniques have been tried with Lesch–Nyhan patients, but none have been successful in eradicating the self-mutilating behavior.

To date, the only methods that have been successful in controlling the self-mutilating behavior have been extensive restraints (see below). Many individuals with Lesch–Nyhan syndrome have had their teeth extracted to prevent mutilation of the lips and tongue. Although self-mutilation is not uncommon in populations of retarded children (often demonstrated as picking, beating, biting, or hitting at some part or parts of their bodies), the resulting damage is usually a lesion of hypertrophy, callus, or swelling, rather than loss of tissue. Rarely do these forms cause the severe damage that is seen in Lesch–Nyhan syndrome (Nyhan, 1976). As described above, it has been hypothesized that the self-mutilation in Lesch–Nyhan syndrome patients is related to neurotransmitter abnormalities, in particular derangements in dopamine or serotonin metabolism (Ernst et al., 1996; Hunter et al., 1996; Wong et al., 1996). Pain perception in Lesch–Nyhan syndrome patients appears normal, and sensations appear to be intact (Nyhan, 1976). They will scream in pain while they bite themselves, and only feel safe and happy when they are securely protected from themselves by physical restraint (Nyhan, 1976).

PSYCHOSOCIAL COMPROMISE

The psychosocial issues for Lesch–Nyhan syndrome individuals are complex because of the various neurological manifestations, which leave patients unable to care for themselves or perform even the simplest of self-care tasks. Because individuals with Lesch–Nyhan syndrome display spastic cerebral palsy in varying degrees, many are unable to stand or sit unassisted, and are able to sit in wheelchairs only if they are securely restrained. The cognitive compromise that is often present further impedes their interactions with their environments; however, there is a wide variation in presentation, ranging from normal intelligence levels to severe mental retardation (Anderson et al., 1992; Christie et al., 1982; Matthews et al., 1995). As noted above, there can also be abnormalities in breathing, sucking, and swallowing, causing difficulties in eating.

The renal system manifestations of Lesch–Nyhan syndrome are similar in all patients and include hyperuricemia, gout, uric acid stones, and urate nephropathy. Although these types of symptoms can be controlled, they require systematic medical management. Lesch–Nyhan syndrome patients are treated with allopurinol, which inhibits xanthine oxidase activity; this decreases the levels of uric acid in the patients' bodies, prevents renal and musculoskeletal manifestations, and generally prolongs life. Another aspect of daily maintenance is diet, which must be monitored and kept purine-free as a result of the enzyme deficiency and the inability to process many types of foods.

The often extreme neurological compromise in Lesch–Nyhan syndrome individuals generally requires that these patients be fed. This presents still another difficulty in daily management, because they are very difficult to feed as a result of athetoid dysphagia. Vomiting is a persistent problem, and many individuals have difficulty chewing and swallowing. The lack of adequate nutrition combined with the enzyme deficiency often creates developmental issues, with most patients having shortness of stature and delayed bone age or skeletal maturation (Nyhan, 1976). Their weight also tends to be disproportionately lower than their height in relation to standards for the patients' age (Nyhan, 1976).

The most difficult psychosocial component of Lesch–Nyhan syndrome is the extreme self-mutilating behavior. In addition to the severe self-biting described earlier, they often engage in head banging, arm and leg banging, rubbing various body parts until raw, nose gouging, and eye gouging (Anderson & Ernst, 1994; Anderson, Dancis, & Alpert, 1979; Ashkenazi, Shahar, Brand, Bartov, & Blumenthal, 1992; Christie et al., 1982; Eguchi et al., 1994; Evans, Sirikumara, & Gregory, 1993; Letts & Hobson, 1975; Nyhan, 1976). As noted above, the self-injurious behavior escalates in violence as they grow older and are able to create new ways to injure themselves (Anderson & Ernst, 1994; Ashkenazi et al., 1992; Christie et al., 1982; Nyhan, 1976). The physical presentation of these individuals can be distressing as a result of the missing tissue. It is not uncommon for these patients to have missing fingers or lips, and often their teeth are removed to prevent further tissue damage and loss. Again, these patients are able to feel pain and often scream in pain and distress when they inflict self-injurious behavior; once they are physically restrained and the self-injurious behavior contained, they become calm and at ease. It is reported that many of these children will scream all night until their parents or guardians are taught how to restrain them securely in bed, because of their fears of self-injurious behavior and inability to control themselves (Anderson & Ernst, 1994; Christie et al., 1982; Eguchi et al., 1994; Evans et al., 1993; Nyhan, 1976). Nyhan (1976) has found that the severity of self-injury does not change over the years and that the age of onset is a predictor of outcome (the earlier the age of onset, the worse the self-injury eventually becomes).

Research with Lesch–Nyhan syndrome patients has found that behavioral modification and pharmacological treatment has provided mixed results in controlling the self-mutilating behavior. Kirkpatrick-Sanchez, Williams, Gualtieri, and Raichman (1998) found that dose dependent reductions in self-injurious behavior occurred with paroxetine and sertraline combined with behavioral treatment and physical restraints in one 6-year-old subject. Allen and Rice (1996) found a reduction in self-mutilation in one subject after the application of risperidone. Roach, Delgado, Anderson, and Iannaccone (1996) found in their study of four patients that carbamazepine reduced self-mutilation and the need for constant restraint in three out of the four patients. This research was unable to confirm sensory neuropathy, and the researchers concluded that any effect of carbamazepine was likely to occur in the CNS. What continues to be the most effective treatment in the majority of patients in terms of controlling self-mutilating behavior have been mechanical restraints, including gloves, masks, and helmets (Anderson & Ernst, 1994; Christie et al., 1982; Eguchi et al., 1994; Evans et al., 1993; Nyhan, 1976; Obi, 1997). The focus in mechanical restraints has been on designing comfortable and functional constraints that do not become further instruments for self-injury (Anderson & Ernst, 1994; Christie et al., 1982; Eguchi et al., 1994; Evans et al., 1993; Nyhan, 1976). Lesch–Nyhan syndrome individuals are often so determined in their self-mutilating behavior that extreme forms of restraint management are necessary in order to protect them from self-harm (Nyhan, 1996). The use of protective devices in Lesch–Nyhan syndrome differs from that in other types of self-injurious behavior, as Lesch–Nyhan patients do not fight the restraints; instead, they desire and request their application because of their inability to restrain themselves (Anderson & Ernst, 1994; Anderson et al., 1979; Ashkenazi et al. 1992; Christie et al., 1982; Eguchi et al., 1994; Evans et al., 1993; Letts & Hobson, 1975; Nyhan, 1976). Physical restraints have often been viewed as restrictive; however, in the case of Lesch–Nyhan syndrome they reduce the stress and fear of self-injury, and allow the individuals to concentrate on constructive activity (Nyhan, 1996; Christie et al., 1982). Nyhan (1976) found that if individuals with Lesch–Nyhan syndrome lose trust in their care providers' ability to keep them safe, the increased stress will result in a higher frequency and intensity of self-injury. Although no cure and no medical management of the self-abusive behavior are possible, it appears that a multidisciplinary approach in supportive treatment has been effective (Anderson et al., 1992; Christie et al., 1982; Matthews et al., 1995).

Families who attempt to take care of children with this syndrome require a great deal of support and assistance. The many difficult conditions that accompany Lesch–Nyhan syndrome (chronic illness, mental compromise, spastic cerebral palsy, compulsive self-injury, difficulty with nutrition, etc.) can result in stressful conditions for an individual's family. These can include extreme financial burdens, along with the emotional and physical toll taken by the huge amount of care and constant supervision that the patient requires. Families will often place these children in long-term medical facilities or other institutions because of the degree of management they require. In many cases these individuals cannot be left alone for any significant amount of time, and require physical restraint even while asleep. Individuals with Lesch–Nyhan syndrome not only are unable to take care of themselves or live independently, but require assistance with even the smallest of self-care tasks, such as bathing and toileting.

Another very difficult aspect of providing care to individuals with Lesch–Nyhan syndrome is that their destructive behavior is not limited to themselves, but is often projected upon caregivers. Many of these patients frequently attempt to hit other people. Other types of aggressive actions include spitting at others and vomiting on them. They are only limited in their aggression against others by their motor defects, and they will bite others if given the opportunity, with the majority of injuries occurring while they are being bathed or being moved from physical restraints. It appears that these individuals do not want to injure or otherwise abuse others, but are unable to control these behaviors any more than they can control the self-injurious behaviors. Unfortunately, this means that they strike out at those people they care for the most, such as parents, teachers, and aides (Nyhan &

Wong, 1996; Nyhan, 1976). As they get older and learn speech, they become verbally aggressive as well. Other examples of abusive behavior demonstrated by pinching and grabbing at caregivers' genitals and related areas, individuals with Lesch–Nyhan syndrome include kicking and head butting while being dressed or bathed, cursing without provocation, and spilling drinks (Nyhan, 1976). After performing such behaviors, an individual will characteristically apologize profusely, only to repeat the behaviors shortly thereafter (Nyhan, 1976). These aggressive behaviors often cause caregivers to become angry or frustrated, which can result in patients' being punished or emotionally mistreated.

Research has found that although behavioral techniques have proved ineffective in preventing self-injurious behaviors, these techniques have been found to reduce the aggressive and abusive behaviors toward others (Nyhan & Wong, 1996). Many hospital reports that they employ a behavioral technique they term "selective ignoring." The goal of this technique is to act as if the aggressive behavior is not happening, with no physical or verbal recognition of it, and to continue with whatever was happening prior to the aggressive behavior.

Effective methods of modifying aggressive behaviors toward others have been those that take into account a subject's level of cognitive ability and self-awareness (Anderson et al., 1992). Some parents have been able to disrupt the behaviors by holding, talking to, and playing with younger children, along with providing toys and television (Anderson et al., 1992). Older boys want to be included in conversation and decision making; for example, they like to choose a television channel or learn the scores of a ball game (Anderson et al., 1992). The most commonly used method for managing problem behavior is the adjustment of restraints, with most individuals becoming content when they are well restrained (Anderson et al., 1992).

Stress elicits self-injury and generalized agitation in Lesch–Nyhan syndrome patients. The highest rates of self-injury are associated with the removal of restraints during bathing. Self-injurious behavior tends to increase with illness, new people, or new situations (Anderson et al., 1992; Christie et al., 1982). Anderson et al. (1992) asked parents and caregivers open-ended questions about situations that decreased self-injury. The parents and caregivers listed interesting activities and social interactions that kept the patients occupied and concentrating on a task; behavioral techniques that the respondents did not find useful included ignoring, time out, or taking away a beloved object, which often only increased the self-destructive behavior (Anderson et al., 1992).

In spite of their many difficulties, Lesch–Nyhan syndrome individuals are described as engaging persons when they are restrained, with a good sense of humor and the ability to laugh easily. They are often described as being favorites in hospitals or institutions where they are receiving care (Nyhan, 1976).

SPECIFIC NEUROPSYCHOLOGICAL IMPAIRMENTS

Cognitive Deficits

One of the cardinal features of Lesch–Nyhan syndrome has been mental retardation (Nyhan, 1976). Because of the extreme neurological compromise, standardized testing of individuals with Lesch–Nyhan syndrome has been difficult, and the assessment of cognitive abilities has relied on general estimations and inference (Anderson et al., 1992). Research in this area has shown that the cognitive status of these individuals may not be as severely compromised as was once believed; instead, there appears to be a great deal of individual variation (Anderson et al., 1992; Christie et al., 1982; Matthews et al., 1995). The largest study of cognitive abilities to date involve 42 individuals with Lesch–Nyhan syndrome, and a nonstandardized instrument that relied on parent self-report was used to collect data (Anderson et al., 1992). This study indicated wide variation in cognitive compromise, and it provided information on cognitive skills rather than standardized estimates of intelligence. The next largest study involved nine subjects and utilized the Peabody Picture Vocabulary Test as a standardized instrument of cognitive ability, which indicated a mean IQ of 58 (Christie et al., 1982). One study had a sample size of one and did not report using any type of test instrument, but indicated a standardized IQ of 70–74 (Wood, Fox, Vincent, Rye, & O'Sullivan, 1972). The remaining studies each had one subject and utilized either the Peabody, the Wechsler Intelligence Scale for Children, Revised, or the Stanford–Binet Intelligence Scale; collectively, they indicated a standardized IQ of between 54 and 91 (Ball et al., 1985; Bull & LaVecchio, 1978; Gilbert et al., 1979; Scherzer & Illson, 1969; Wurtele et al., 1984).

Attention and Concentration

Matthew et al. (1995) found that individuals with Lesch–Nyhan syndrome had difficulty with multistep reasoning and were unable to comprehend complex patterns with multiple features or to consider two strands of thought simultaneously. It appears that the mental flexibility, sequential skills, and environmental monitoring required for attention and concentration may be somewhat impaired; however, it is unclear whether this is a function of the syndrome itself or a psychosocial effect, resulting from the patients' limited exposure to varied stimuli and physical restraint. However, Anderson et al. (1992) found in their study that individuals with Lesch–Nyhan syndrome had a high level of concentration, a strong sense of observation, and a good attention span. All individuals in this study were fully oriented to time, place, and person; were able to recognize and name the persons who took care of them; and were able to tell the day of the week and the time of day.

Academic Achievement

Like standardized estimates of cognitive ability, standardized estimates of academic achievement have been difficult to obtain in Lesch–Nyhan syndrome patients as a result of the severe muscular involvement that leaves them incapable of coordinated movement and intelligible speech (Blakely & Poling, 1986; Buzas, Ayllon, & Collins, 1981; Carter, 1975; Nyhan, 1976). Anderson et al. (1992) found that 58% of subjects older than 4 years of age could read a little, but that only 13% were reading at their appropriate grade level.

The self-injurious behavior displayed by Lesch–Nyhan syndrome patients makes the educational process a challenge, because often their restraints cannot be removed, and they require a great deal of individualized attention and supervision. Teachers must become creative in the educational planning for these patients. In order to control their self-injurious behaviors, individuals with Lesch–Nyhan syndrome often have their hands wrapped, which restricts hand and finger movements and consequently the ability to play with peers and to complete schoolwork. Another feature to be considered is that stress and anxiety can either create or exacerbate the self-injurious behavior, which then must be controlled with the application of physical restraints and/or with the termination or modification of the activity. Speech is usually dysarthric and difficult to understand, but, depending on their cognitive abilities, Lesch–Nyhan syndrome patients may be able to attend schools for the physically and mentally handicapped (Anderson et al., 1992).

Christie et al. (1982) have stated that educational management of Lesch–Nyhan syndrome patients must be considered on an individual basis, and that performance should be assessed via oral examinations because of the patients' inability to control motor movement and their self-injurious behavior, which both result in their being unable to write. For most individuals with Lesch–Nyhan syndrome, school experience is possible, and operant conditioning can be successfully employed to modify many socially objectionable behaviors (e.g., spitting, aggressive actions, and vomiting; Nyhan, 1976). However, it is important to remember that the self-injurious behavior will continue unless an individual is physically restrained, and that neither behavioral management, operant conditioning, nor pharmacological intervention has been successful at eliminating or decreasing this behavior.

Sensory, Motor, Visual–Spatial, and Perceptual Skills

Sensory, visual–spatial, and perceptual skills provide individuals with awareness of sensations such as sights, sounds, and touches, and with the ability to recognize these stimuli and to interpret their meaning in our environment. Lesch–Nyhan syndrome patients appear to have few impairments in their abilities to attend to, and understand relationships among, visual and auditory stimuli (Anderson et al., 1992). However, it is difficult to discern whether these and other skills in this area are compromised, and what types of sensations and perceptions patients are able to interpret, because of the variation in cognitive compromise. In addition, the need for physical restraints certainly limits the patients' ability to experience tactile sensation, and often specific areas have been damaged, such as the hands, tongue, and lips.

Christie et al. (1982) found that individuals with Lesch–Nyhan syndome do appear to have subtle deficits in visual–motor integration. Matthews et al. (1995) found that Lesch–Nyhan syndrome patients seem to have intact visual percepts for spatial orientation and visual detail, with one exception: They seem to have difficulty with complex features, such as the combination of size, shape, and shading. Their performance on visual tasks also appears to be compromised when a task requires simultaneous consideration of visual information and memory and the integration of both. However, they are able to complete one- and two-feature items, which suggests that they are quick processors of visual information (Matthews et al., 1995).

Motor skills, by contrast, are profoundly impaired in these individuals (Nyhan & Wong, 1996). For most Lesch–Nyhan syndrome patients, their severe cerebral palsy has a major impact on both gross and subtle motor skill. The impairments consist of spasticity; involuntary contraction of large groups of muscles, such as the arm, leg, or neck muscles; and choreiform movements, which are extremely variable, purposeless, coarse, quick, and jerky. These movements begin suddenly and show no rhythmicity, with the involved muscles becoming atonic until the next one begins.

Language Skills

The development of communication in Lesch–Nyhan syndrome is hampered by poor articulation due to pseudobulbar palsy and obstructed air flow. It appears that in most individuals with Lesch–Nyhan syndrome, language impairments are the results of motor difficulties rather than of specific hemisphere compromise. In other individuals, cognitive compromise is the major factor in the problems with language and language skills (Matthews et al., 1995). Once again, because of the diffuseness of the syndrome, it is difficult to assess the specific focus of the language impairment. However, it appears that even the most affected children appear to comprehend language well. Anderson et al. (1992) found that of the 42 individuals with Lesch–Nyhan syndrome they studied, 93% were able to communicate through talking and gesturing, and 53% had the ability to communicate their needs very well.

Another factor often adding to language impairment is the self-injurious behavior. In many cases individuals have bitten off their lips, and tips of the tongue, which have resulted in the removal of their teeth to protect the remaining tissue. Many must wear mouthpieces or mouthguards to restrict the uncontrollable biting. These factors often restrict language and hamper communication. Sugahara, Mishima, and Mori (1994) found that when soft acrylic mouthguards were constructed on the impressions of patients' teeth, these were very effective in the facilitation of communication skills and language development, as they allowed unencumbered conversation and effectively controlled the self-injurious behavior.

Organization, Sequencing, Learning, and Memory

Christie et al. (1982) found that many of their subjects with Lesch–Nyhan syndrome appeared to have grasped the concepts of addition, subtraction, and multiplication and were able to recall arithmetical facts with variable success, but were unable to respond to questions concerning fractions or division. Errors on items of addition, subtraction, and multiplication typically stemmed from problems with keeping track of the information or with inflexibility of thought. The overall pattern of response across subjects of varying abilities and ages suggested a limited capacity for mental manipulation and abstract thought. Christie et al.'s (1982) subjects also appeared to have a response pattern suggesting deficits in short-term verbal recall and difficulty in processing complex grammar. These skills appeared to be influenced by age and the extent of distractibility.

Matthews et al. (1995) found that subjects were able to process three to five units on the Memory for Digits Test (corresponding to mental ages of 3 to 7 years), but were unable to perform more complex tasks of memory. They appeared unable to hold verbally presented stimuli and then to repeat or transform the information as required for the Digits Backward subtest. However, Anderson et al. (1992) reported that their subjects were able to remember team records and batting averages, were able to recall names and facts concerning a large number of friends and acquaintances, remembered where to find misplaced objects, and were able to give directions while riding in the car. Anderson et al. (1992) suggested that individuals with Lesch–Nyhan syndrome may have greater memory capacity when contextual cues are available or when the subject matter has some personal relevance to the subjects.

Executive Functions

"Executive functions" are those operations that direct and control thought and behavior. These functions appear to be severely impaired for Lesch–Nyhan individuals. It appears that for these individuals, perception of visual and auditory stimuli is intact; however, attention, concentration, and higher intellectual functions are impaired. Matthews et al.

(1995) found that their subjects were limited in the amount of information that they could attend to and organize or integrate, and that they had difficulty sustaining memory traces for the purpose of mental manipulation. There were also conceptual limitations evident in the subjects' failure to grasp the concepts of division and fractions and in their pattern of impairment in short-term memory functions. Matthews et al. (1995) also found a pattern of cognitive development in which younger subjects consistently attained higher intellectual functioning scores, whereas the older subjects had lower and more uniform scores.

Anderson et al. (1992) found that their subjects could plan for and anticipate their own actions, and that many could tell when they were going to participate in self-injurious behavior. They were often able to anticipate others' feelings and reactions; they were also conscious of their syndrome and were able to express a desire to be normal. Furthermore, these individuals were able to understand higher-level concepts such as illness and death, and could respond appropriately in most social interactions. Finally, Anderson et al. (1992) stated that four of the children had taught themselves the rules of their favorite sport, were curious about people and events, and were eager to be included in social events.

ASSESSMENT

Should Standardized Testing Be Employed?

Opinions about the standardized testing of individuals with Lesch–Nyhan syndrome have varied widely. Some authors argue that it is inappropriate (Anderson et al., 1992); others contend that it is essential (Scherzer & Ilson, 1969). The extreme motor compromise of individuals with Lesch–Nyhan syndrome creates difficulties with standardized testing, and such testing is generally not an effective way of helping to determine individual educational plans, career and occupational possibilities, or grade levels for these individuals (Matthews et al., 1995). However, standardized testing may provide limited information about an individual's full functional capacity and future performance, in addition to data on specific skill areas (Matthews et al., 1995). Another way of using standardized testing of individuals with Lesch–Nyhan syndrome may be the establishment and monitoring of baselines in order to assess the effects (if any) of medical treatment programs on intellectual, behavioral, and functional status, as well as to assess change in the individuals' profiles over time (Matthews et al., 1995).

Other Key Issues in Assessment

The neuropsychological assessment of children with Lesch–Nyhan syndrome is a unique challenge for the examiner, as a result of the complexity of the behavioral manifestations, possible mental retardation, and other neurological issues. The examiner must possess not only a clear understanding of the normal developmental emergence of intellect, memory, language, and motor functioning, but a thorough understanding of the deviations from patterns of normal development seen in Lesch–Nyhan syndrome. Cognitive compromise for children with this syndrome fluctuates from individual to individual, as does other symptomatology. As a result of the individuality of the syndrome, the assessment should be flexible.

Neuropsychological assessments conducted on individuals with Lesch–Nyhan syndrome must be modified as a result of the neurological impairments. The evaluation should focus on verbal skills and other skills that do not require physical manipulation of objects indeed, any assessment instruments that require controlled hand movements will be unusable for most of these individuals. Because stress often increases self-injurious behavior, the examiner must be prepared either to discontinue the testing (at least for the time being) or to move on to items that are less strenuous if there is an increase in aggressive or self-injurious behavior. Matthews et al. (1995) found that self-abusive behavior often emerged as items became more difficult or the individuals became anxious or stressed, with subjects poking at their eyes, writhing, cursing, spitting, or flailing their arms. However, these behaviors were often reduced or eliminated by structuring the test setting, providing simple reassurances, or introducing easier items (Matthews et al., 1995). Testing sessions should also be kept brief, as these individuals are easily fatigued; it is recommended that sessions be limited to 20 minutes once or twice a week until the testing is completed.

An assessment for a child with Lesch–Nyhan syndrome should cover three specific domains: (1) the biological domain, (2) the social–interpersonal domain, and (3) the educational domain. Within the biological domain, the examiner is seeking knowledge about the current progression of the disease, the degree of motor impairment, the child's response to medical treatment, physical restraints currently utilized, and current self-injurious behavior. Important assessment instruments for general development that may be utilized include the Childhood Development Inventory (Ireton & Glascoe, 1995) and the Vineland Adaptive Behavior Scales (Sparrow, Balla, & Cicchetti, 1984). The social–interpersonal domain involves exploration of behavior problems manifested by the child. An instrument that may be utilized to assess this is the Child Behavior Checklist (Achenbach, 1991a, 1991b). Within the educational domain it will be important to measure intellectual functioning, utilizing such instruments as the Stanford–Binet (Thorndike, Hagen, & Sattler, 1986) or the Wechsler Intelligence Scale for Children (Wechsler, 1991), with appropriate modifications. As a result of their many difficulties, children with Lesch–Nyhan syndrome may not have been placed in traditional educational settings; therefore, an individualized achievement test such as the Woodcock–Johnson Psycho-Educational Battery—Revised (Woodcock & Johnson, 1989) may be needed to assess specific competencies or to determine grade placement.

Essential Elements of a Neuropsychological Examination

An essential element of a neuropsychological assessment is a thorough clinical interview conducted with the child's primary caregiver. Prior to this interview, the neuropsychologist should review all of the patient's medical records and prior medical treatments. The clinical interview should develop a history of the child and family from the following perspectives: medical/neurological, psychological/emotional, and developmental/educational. The use of Anderson et al.'s (1992) questionnaire is very helpful for patients with Lesch–Nyhan syndrome, as it was developed specifically for such patients and systematizes caregivers' observations of the subjects' behavior during a wide variety of daily events. This instrument also assesses nine different aspects of cognitive skills, which may be helpful in addition to the more structured instruments.

Neuropsychological testing should cover all aspects of intelligence/cognitive functioning, with both verbal and nonverbal memory and learning. The assessment of language will be a vital component of testing, but it will be very difficult because of the extreme motor involvement of most patients and the inability to control fine motor movement, combined with self-inflicted injuries to the tongue and lips in many cases. Another problem is that many individuals are difficult to understand because of their inability to control the muscles responsible for vocal production. It is suggested that comprehensive speech and language assessment be referred to a speech pathologist, as often the types of presentations seen in Lesch–Nyhan syndrome individuals require specific training to evaluate.

The evaluation of motor movements, both fine and gross, may not be as important in the neurological assessment of patients with Lesch–Nyhan syndrome as it is for other individuals, because of the obvious evidence of severe motor impairment. It will also be difficult to test visual–motor skills as a result of the restraints that are necessary to prevent the individual from participating in self-injurious behavior. Visual–spatial functions should be assessed within the areas of analysis, synthesis, and construction. Frontal executive functions should be assessed for the following; attention, speed of responding, response inhibition, tracking, and abstraction. The assessment of educational achievement and social and emotional functioning should be comprehensive, covering both past and present. The nature of the various problem areas (e.g., motor functioning, cognitive ability, and language) should be described in detail, and then this information should be related to achievement and social–emotional functioning. This will provide guidance for educational planning and for the development of caregiver strategies to enhance a child's ability to interact with the environment.

The testing and assessment of Lesch–Nyhan syndrome patients require a great deal of adaptability, as noted above; therefore, a flexible battery approach should be utilized, which incorporates a core battery of tests with additional tests to address the developmental and intervention needs of these individuals. The examiner also needs to be familiar with the specific primary, secondary, and tertiary effects of this syndrome, and to be able to make needed adjustments in the clinical assessment along with modifications in testing procedures. There will be no normative data available, as Lesch–Nyhan syndrome is so rare and its symptoms vary from individual to individual. This type of approach will allow the examiner to follow both a nomothetic approach and an idiographic approach to addressing the child's needs.

CURRENT TREATMENT AND FUTURE DIRECTIONS IN TREATMENT AND PREVENTION

There is currently no treatment for the motor impairment of Lesch–Nyhan syndrome, or for the self-injurious behavior other than physical restraint. Allopurinol is used to treat the symptoms of gout, renal dysfunction, hyperuricemia, uricosuria, tophaceous gouty arthritis, urinary tract calculi, and urate nephropathy; as noted earlier, this is able to prolong life, allowing individuals to live into their second decade.

Despite all that has been learned about Lesch–Nyhan syndrome, effective treatment has been elusive. Although allopurinol is effective in reducing the renal system manifestations, it has absolutely no effect on the neurobehavioral or other neurological manifestations of the disease. At the present time, the only method for prevention for Lesch–Nyhan syndrome appears to be the early identification of carriers and genetic counseling. In the future, gene therapy may be utilized; perhaps a functioning gene could be introduced into Lesch–Nyhan syndrome patients' cells, resulting in stable expression of HPRT and normal cell functioning. This therapy, though promising, remains in the realm of theory, as animal models have not yet been successful.

In addition, the emerging research into abnormalities in dopaminergic function in Lesch–Nyhan syndrome may lead to new pharmacological approaches that can interrupt the abnormal cycles and provide treatment for the self-injurious patterns of behavior and neurological impairments. Functional imaging of the central nervous system abnormalities also appears to be a promising approach and could possibly aid in the development of interventions to treat and prevent the metabolic injuries in the brains of patients with Lesch–Nyhan syndrome.

SUMMARY

Lesch–Nyhan syndrome is an X-linked recessive disorder of purine metabolism caused by the absence or near-absence of the enzyme HPRT. It is characterized by cognitive compromise in most individuals; severe dystonia, spasticity, and other neuromuscular difficulties; speech impairment; renal disease; and compulsive self-injury (most often in the form of mutilation of fingers, lips, and tongue by biting). Hyperuricemia and the effects of serum uric acid can be managed to a degree with allopurinol, but most individuals die of urate nephropathy in their teens. Allopurinol has no effect on the neurological complications of the syndrome, but it inhibits xanthine oxidase activity, thus decreasing uric acid levels and preventing the renal and musculoskeletal manifestations.

Many experimental therapies have been tried to combat the compulsive self-injury, but currently there is no effective treatment for this syndrome. Aggressive behavior toward others has been decreased by behavioral techniques. Pharmacological attempts at eliminating self-mutilation have been unsuccessful. In addition, traditional medication has not significantly reduced crying, screaming, or spasticity. Neuropsychological assessment is helpful in maintaining a baseline and in developing educational plans.

REFERENCES

Achenbach, T. M. (1991a). Manual for the Child Behavior Checklist/2–3. Burlington, VT: University of Vermont, Department of Psychiatry.

Achenbach, T. M. (1991b). Manual for the Child Behavior Checklist/4–18. Burlington, VT: University of Vermont, Department of Psychiatry.

Alford, R. L., Redman, J. B., O'Brien, W. E., & Caskey, C. T. (1995). Lesch–Nyhan syndrome: Carrier and prenatal diagnosis. *Prenatal Diagnosis, 15*(4), 329–338.

Allen, S. M., Freeman, J. N., & Davis, W. M. (1998). Evaluation of risperidone in the neonatal 6-hydroxydopamine model of Lesch–Nyhan syndrome. *Pharmacology, Biochemistry and Behavior, 59*(2), 327–330.

Allen, S. M., & Rice, S. N. (1996). Risperidone antagonism of self-mutilation in a Lesch–Nyhan patient. *Progress in Neuro-Psychopharmacology and Biological Psychiatry, 20*(5), 793–800.

Anderson, L., Dancis, J., & Alpert, M. (1979). Behavioral contingencies and self-mutilation in Lesch–Nyhan disease. *Journal of Consulting and Clinical Psychology, 46*, 529–536.

Anderson, L. T., & Ernst, M. (1994). Self-injury in Lesch–Nyhan disease. *Journal of Autism and Developmental Disorders, 24*(1), 67–81.

Anderson, L. T., Ernst, M., & Davis, S. V. (1992). Cognitive abilities of patients with Lesch–Nyhan disease. *Journal of Autism and Developmental Disorders, 22*(2), 189–203.

Ashkenazi, I., Shahar, E., Brand, N., Bartov, E., & Blumenthal, M. (1992). Self-inflicted ocular mutilation in the pediatric age group. *Acta Paediatrica, 81*(8), 649–651.

Ball, T. S., Datta, P. C., Rios, M., & Constantine, C. (1985). Flexible arm splints in the control of a Lesch–Nyhan victim's finger biting and a profoundly retarded client's finger sucking. *Journal of Autism and Developmental Disorders, 15*, 177–184.

Blakely, E., & Poling, A. (1986). Lesch–Nyhan syndrome and its treatment. *Mental Retardation and Learning Disability Bulletin, 14*(1), 20–34.

Breese, G. R., Criswell, H. E., & Mueller, R. A. (1990). Evidence that lack of brain dopamine during development can increase the susceptibility for aggression and self-injurious behavior by influencing D1-dopamine receptor function. *Progress in Neuro-Psychopharmacology and Biological Psychiatry, 13,* 65–80.

Buitelaar, J. K. (1993). Self-injurious behaviour in retarded children: Clinical phenomena and biological mechanisms. *Acta Paedopsychiatrica, 56*(2), 105–111.

Bull, M., & La Vecchio, F. (1978). Behavior therapy for a child with Lesch–Nyhan syndrome. *Developmental Medicine and Child Neurology, 20,* 368–375.

Buzas, H. O., Ayllon, T., & Collins, R. (1981). A behavioral approach to eliminate self-mutilative behavior in a Lesch–Nyhan patient. *Journal of Mind and Behavior, 2,* 47–56.

Carter, J. L. (1975). Auditory discrimination and training effects for educable retarded children. *Education and Training of the Mentally Retarded, 10*(2), 94–95.

Christie, R., Bay, C., Kaufman, I. A., Bakay, B., Border, M., & Nyhan, W. L. (1982). Lesch–Nyhan disease: Clinical experience with nineteen patients. *Developmental Medicine and Child Neurology, 24,* 293–306.

Crawhall, J. C., Henderson, J. F., & Kelley, W. N. (1972). Diagnosis and treatment of the Lesch–Nyhan syndrome. *Pediatric Research, 6,* 504–513.

Davidson, B. L., Tarle, S. A., Van-Antwerp, M., Gibbs, D. A., Watts, R. W., Kelly, W. N., & Palella, T. D. (1991). Identification of 17 independent mutations responsible for human hypoxanthine-guanine phosphoribosyltransferase (HPRT) deficiency. *American Journal of Human Genetics, 48*(5), 951–958.

Eguchi, S., Tokioka, T., Motoyoshi, A., & Wakamura, S. (1994). A self-controllable mask with helmet to prevent self finger-mutilation in the Lesch–Nyhan syndrome. *Archives of Physical Medicine and Rehabilitation 75*(6), 709–710.

Ernst, M., Zametkin, A. J., Matochik, J. A., Pascualvaca, D., Jons, P. H., Hardy, K., Hankerson, J. G., Doudet, D. J., & Cohen, R. M. (1996). Presynaptic dopaminergic deficits in Lesch–Nyhan disease. *New England Journal of Medicine, 334*(24), 1568–1572.

Evans, J., Sirikumara, M., & Gregory, M. (1993). Lesch–Nyhan syndrome and the lower lip guard. *Oral Surgery, Oral Medicine, Oral Pathology, 76*(4), 437–440.

Fuscoe, J. C., & Nelson, A. J. (1994). Molecular description of a hypoxanthine phosphoribosyltrasferase gene deletion in Lesch–Nyhan syndrome. *Human Molecular Genetics, 3*(1), 199–200.

Gilbert, S., Spellacy, F., & Watts, R. W. E. (1979). Problems in the behavioral treatment of self-injury in the Lesch–Nyhan syndrome. *Developmental Medicine and Child Neurology, 21,* 795–800.

Hornykiewicz, O. (1993). Parkinson's disease and the adaptive capacity of the nigrostriatal dopamine system: Possible neurochemical mechanisms. *Advances in Neurology, 60,* 140–147.

Hunter, T. C., Melancon, S. B., Dallaire, L., Taft, S., Skopek, T. R., Albertini, R. J., & O'Neill, J. P. (1996). Germinal HPRT splice donor site mutation results in multiple RNA splicing products in T-lymphocyte cultures. *Somatic Cell and Molecular Genetics, 22*(2), 145–150.

Ireton, H., & Glascoe, F. P. (1995). Assessing children's development using parents' reports: The Child Development Inventory. *Clinical Pediatrics, 34*(5), 248–255.

Jenkins, E. A., Hallett, R. J., & Hull, R. G. (1994). Lesch–Nyhan syndrome presenting with renal insufficiency in infancy and transient neonatal hypothyroidism. *British Journal of Rheumatology, 33*(4), 392–396.

Jinnah, H. A., & Friedmann, T. (1995). Gene therapy and the brain. *British Medical Bulletin, 51*(1), 138–148.

Jinnah, H. A., Jones, M. D., Wojcik, B. E., Rothstein, J. D., Hess, E. J., Friedmann, T., & Breese, G. R. (1999). Influence of age and strain on striatal dopamine loss in a genetic mouse model of Lesch–Nyhan disease. *Journal of Neurochemistry, 72*(1), 225–229.

Kirkpatrick-Sanchez, S., Williams, D. E., Gualtieri, C. T., & Raichman, J. A. (1998). Case report: The effects of serotonergic reuptake inhibitors combined with behaviorl treatment on self-injury associated with Lesch–Nyhan syndrome. *Journal of Developmental and Physical Disabilities, 10*(3), 283–290.

Lapchak, P. A., Araujo, D. M., Hilt, D. C., Sheng, J., & Jiao, S. (1997). Adenoviral vector-mediated GDNF gene therapy in a rodent lesion model of late stage Parkinson's disease. *Brain Research, 777*(1–2), 153–160.

Lesch, M., & Nyhan, W. L. (1964). A familial disorder of uric acid metabolism and central nervous system function. *American Journal of Medicine, 36,* 561–570.

Letts, R. M., & Hobson, D. A. (1975). Special devices as aides in the management of child self-mutilation in the Lesch–Nyhan syndrome. *Pediatrics, 55,* 852–855.

Lloyd, K. G., Hornykiewicz, O., & Davidson, L. (1981). Biochemical evidence of dysfunction of brain neurotransmitters in the Lesch–Nyhan syndrome. *New England Journal of Medicine, 350,* 1106–1111.

Mansfield, E. S., Blasband, A., Kronick, M. N., Wrabetz, L., Kaplan, P., Rappaport, E., Sartore, M., Parrella, T., Surrey, S., & Fortina, P. (1993). Fluorescent approaches to diagnosis of Lesch–Nyhan syndrome and quantitative analysis of carrier status. *Molecular and Cellular Probes, 7*(4), 311–324.

Mateos-Anton, F., & Garcia-Puig, J. (1992). Diagnostico prenatal del sindrome de Lesch–Nyhan [Prenatal diagnosis of Lesch–Nyhan syndrome]. *Neurologia, 7*(4), 63–69.

Mateos-Anton, F., & Garcia-Puig, J. (1994). Purine metabolism in Lesch–Nyhan syndrome versus Kelly–Seegmiller syndrome. *Journal of Inherited Metabolic Disease, 17*(1), 138–142.

Mateos-Anton, F., Garcia-Puig, J., Ramos, T. H., Jimenez, J. L., Romera, N. M., & Gonzalez, A. G. (1991). Prenatal diagnosis of Lesch–Nyhan syndrome by purine analysis of amniotic fluid and cordocentesis. *Advances in Experimental Medicine and Biology, 309,* 47–50.

Matthews, W. S., Solan, A., & Barabas, G. (1995). Cognitive functioning in Lesch–Nyhan syndrome. *Developmental Medicine and Child Neurology, 37*(8), 715–722.

Nyhan, W. L. (1976). Behavior in the Lesch–Nyhan syndrome. *Journal of Autism and Childhood Schizophrenia, 6,* 235–252.

Nyhan, W. L., & Wong, D. F. (1996). New approaches to understanding Lesch–Nyhan disease. *New England Journal of Medicine, 334*(24), 1602–1604.

Obi, C. (1997). Restraint fading and alternative management strategies to treat a man with Lesch–Nyhan syndrome over a 2 year period. *Behavioral Interventions, 12*(4), 195–202.

Roach, E. S., Delgado, M., Anderson, L., & Iannaccone, S. T. (1996). Carbamazepine trial for Lesch–Nyhan self-mutilation. *Journal of Child Neurology, 11*(6), 476–478.

Rosenfield, D. L., Preston, M. P., & Salvaggi-Fadden, K. (1994). Serial renal sonographic evaluation of patients with Lesch–Nyhan syndrome. *Pediatric Radiology, 24*(7), 509–512.

Scherzer, J. E., & Ilson, J. B. (1969). Normal intelligence in the Lesch–Nyhan syndrome. *Pediatrics, 41,* 71–90.

Silverstein, F. S., Johnston, M. V., Hutchinson, R. J., & Edwards, N. L. (1985). Lesch–Nyhan syndrome: CSF neurotransmitter abnormalities. *Neurology, 36,* 907–911.

Sivam, S. P. (1996). Dopamine, serotonin and tachykinin in self-injurious behavior. *Life Sciences, 58*(26), 2367–2375.

Sparrow, S. S., Balla, D. A., & Cicchetti, D. V. (1984). *Vineland Adaptive Behavior Scales, Interview Edition: Survey form manual.* Circle Pines, MN: American Guidance Services.

Stodgell, C. J., Loupe, P. S., Schroeder, S. R., & Tessel, R. E. (1998). Cross-sensitization between footshock stress and apomorphine on self-injurious behavior and neostriatal catecholamines in a rat model of Lesch–Nyhan syndrome. *Brain Research, 783*(1), 10–18.

Sugahara, T., Mishima, K., & Mori, Y. (1994). Lesch–Nyhan syndrome: Successful prevention of lower lip ulceration caused by self-mutilation by use of mouth guard. *International Journal of Oral–Maxillofacial Surgery, 23*(1), 37–38.

Tarle, S. A., Davidson, B. L., Wu, V. C., Zidar, F. J., Seegmiller, J. E., Kelly, W. N., & Palella, T. D. (1991). Determination of the mutations responsible for the Lesch–Nyhan syndrome in 17 subjects. *Genomics, 10*(2), 499–501.

Thorndike, R. L., Hagen, E. P., & Sattler, J. M. (1986). *The Stanford–Binet Intelligence Scale* (4th ed.). Chicago: Riverside.

Tohyama, J., Nanba, E., & Ohno, K. (1994). Hypoxanthine guanine phosphoribosyltransferase

(HPRT) deficiency: Identification of point mutations in Japanese patients with Lesch–Nyhan syndrome and hereditary gout and their permanent expression in an HPRT deficient mouse cell line. *Human Genetics, 93*(2), 175–181.

Tu, J. B. (1994). Theory and practice of psychopharmacogenetics. *American Journal of Medical Genetics, 54*(4), 391–397.

Wechsler, D. (1991). *Wechsler Intelligence Scale for Children* (3rd ed.). New York: Psychological Corporation.

Wong, D. F., Harris, J. C., Naidu, S., Yokoi, F., Marcenco, S., Dannals, R. F., Ravert, H. T., Yaster, M., Evans, A., Rousset, O., Bryan, R. N., Gjedde, A., Kuhar, M. J., & Breese, G. R. (1996). Dopamine transporters are markedly reduced in Lesch–Nyhan disease *in vivo. Proceedings of the National Academy of Sciences USA, 93*(11), 5539–5543.

Wood, M. H., Fox, R. M., Vincent, L., Rye, C., & O'Sullivan, W. J. (1972). The Lesch–Nyhan syndrome: Report of three cases. *Australian and New Zealand Journal of Medicine, 2*, 57–64.

Woodcock, R. W., & Johnson, M. B. (1990). *Woodcock–Johnson Psycho-Educational Battery— Revised.* Allen, TX: DLM Teaching Resources.

Wurtele, S. K., King, A. C., & Drabman, R.S. (1984). Treatment package to reduce SIB in a Lesch–Nyhan patient. *Journal of Mental Deficiency Research, 28*, 227–234.

Yamada, Y., Goto, H., Yukawa, T., Akazawa, H., & Ogasawara, N. (1994). Molecular mechanisms of the second female Lesch–Nyhan patient. *Advances in Experimental Medicine and Biology, 370*, 337–340.

Yukawa, T., Akazawa, H., Miyake, Y., Takahashi, Y., Nagao, H., & Takeda, E. (1992). A female patient with Lesch–Nyhan syndrome. *Developmental Medicine and Child Neurology, 34*(6), 543–536.

Zheng, Y. J., & Howard, S. (1998). Impaired differentiation of HPRT-deficient dopaminergic neurons: A possible mechanism underlying neuronal dysfunction in Lesch–Nyhan. *Journal of Neuroscience Research, 53*(1), 78–85.

Zoref, S. E., Bromberg, Y., Brosh, S., Sidi, Y., & Sperling, O. (1993). Characterizations of the alterations in purine nucleotide metabolism in hypoxanthine–guanine phosphoribosyltransferase-deficient rat neuroma cell line. *Journal of Neurochemistry, 61*(2), 457–463.

22

SEIZURE DISORDERS

MAILE HO-TURNER
THOMAS L. BENNETT

Seizures are relatively common in infants, children, and adolescents. Hauser (1994) estimated that 30,000 newly diagnosed cases of juvenile epilepsy occurred in the United States in 1990 alone. Lechtenberg (1984) estimated the occurrence of at least one seizure in 8 of every 1,000 children. Cowan, Bodensteiner, Leviton, and Doherty (1989) conducted a retrospective epidemiological study that estimated prevalence rates of epileptic disorders (more than one seizure episode) at between 4% and 8%. Recurrent seizure disorders sometimes dissipate as children mature, but in over 80% of adults with epilepsy, their syndrome began in childhood. Childhood epilepsy syndromes have long been clinically observed to have some genetic or hereditary component. It has not been until recently that solid pathological and neurodevelopmental data supporting these observations have been linked to clinical observations (e.g., see Schwartzkroin, MoshÄ, Noebels, & Swann, 1995).

Furthermore, a child's immature brain is not simply a miniature of an adult brain; it is both anatomically and physiologically different. Thus, one needs to look to, and specifically study, the immature brain in order to understand childhood epilepsy disorders. The appearance of epilepsy through different stages of cortical development in the fetus and through early childhood years has differential implications and manifestations, as well as outcome prognoses and treatment implications.

What we do know about childhood epilepsy is that many factors appear to contribute to seizure thresholds. Seizure thresholds have a major impact on the child's propensity to develop a recurrent seizure disorder (epilepsy), which will in turn have resulting cognitive deficits associated with the epileptic syndrome. Three major factors affecting the occurrence of seizures are (1) genetic predisposition/familial history, (2) age at onset, and (3) environmental stressors. The effect of these factors is cumulative. That is, a child of a particular age who has a familial history of epilepsy and who is exposed to environmental stressors (e.g., fever) has a greater chance of developing a seizure disorder than a child of the same age without the familial history and/or the environmental stressors.

MAJOR PRECIPITATING FACTORS

Genetics

As early as 1960, Lennox and Lennox noted a strong concordance rate for childhood absence epilepsy in identical twins and the higher incidence rates of electroencephalographic (EEG) spike and wave patterns in families with a family history of epilepsy. Since then, both partial and generalized seizure types have been linked to genetic causes. Animal studies in which genetic mutations result in familial strain occurrences of epilepsy have also contributed to the increased awareness of the contribution of genetics to epilepsy syndromes. However, the exact effects of these mutations and inheritances on the neuroanatomical development and physiology of the brain and seizure thresholds are still unclear.

The occurrence and development of some forms of epilepsy have been definitively linked to genetic inheritance, while others have a weaker connection. Febrile seizures, childhood absence epilepsy, juvenile myoclonic epilepsy, Rasmussen syndrome, generalized tonic–clonic epilepsy, and complex partial seizures, among others, have all been shown to have definite genetic contributions in their development. That is, a familial history increases the occurrence of these seizure types, although it is not the sole determinant of its manifestation.

Age at Onset

Newborns have a very high cortical threshold, and elicitation of a seizure response is very difficult. However, as children progress into infancy and toddlerhood (up to about age 2), they have a much higher susceptibility to febrile and other seizures; in other words, their seizure threshold has lowered. This is the time period when most childhood epilepsy syndromes begin, although each epilepsy syndrome has its own peak incidence age ranges. Through childhood and adolescence (age 2 years and beyond), the seizure threshold increases proportionally until it reaches adult levels.

Environmental Stressors

Environmental stressors include fever spiking, fatigue, excitement, ionic concentrations/metabolism, and other factors. Fevers as a precipitating agent to seizures are especially notable in febrile seizures, as their name implies. The rate of rise and amplitude of the fever are directly related to the seizure onset and intensity.

This chapter continues with a brief description of the stages of neurodevelopment and associated neuropathologies that have been recently linked together to provide a better understanding of childhood epilepsy. We then describe the various classification schemes of childhood seizures and epilepsy syndromes. Finally, the manifestation of childhood seizure syndromes and their behavioral, cognitive, and neuropsychological issues are considered.

NEURODEVELOPMENTAL AND NEUROPATHOLOGICAL ASPECTS

There are four relatively distinct stages of neural development, which can each serve as a point of disruption and which have specific implications for the appearance of seizure disorders. The first three stages of neural development (regional determination and segmentation, cytogenesis, and cell migration) are completed by the end of the second trimester of pregnancy. The last stage of development (growth and differentiation) begins late in the second trimester and continues through the early years of postnatal development, when many epilepsy syndromes manifest themselves. Generally, the earlier the pathology occurs, the graver the outcome.

Deviance in the earliest stages of neural development is so grave, in fact, that the fertilized egg may not even be implanted in the uteral lining for development, or miscarriage may occur. Fetuses that do survive the first stage of regional determination and segmentation with deviant neural development often do not survive to term. If such a fetus does survive to term, the infant usually has severe malformations of the cerebrum. Any further neural development is also deviant and probably will produce seizure disorders. Deviance in the cytogenic and migratory stages of development is more survivable than earlier deviance, but it produces neuroanatomical anomalies that are grossly and microscopically apparent. Displaced neural tissue (heterotopia) defects such as agyria and microgyria occur in these stages. Also possible with deviant development in these stages, but not grossly visible, is the clustering of neurons in the wrong areas of the brain (microdysgenesis).

Generally, these heterotopic and microdysgenetic disorders are due to defects in the development of the neuronal guidance tracts (also known as [a.k.a.] radial glides) or the migrating neurons themselves. Microdysgenetic patterns have been histologically linked to childhood epileptic disorders and to various cognitive problems in childhood (e.g., dyslexia, mental retardation, etc.). Cell transformations and interactions to produce a mature brain are the major activities in the last stage (growth and differentiation) of development. Again, this stage begins only after the first three stages of development are complete and continues through infancy until about age 2. This is the "fine-tuning" stage. Of notable interest here is that many childhood epilepsy syndromes appear in infancy and up to age 2, although recent research indicates that this stage of cortical development may be largely complete by the first year of life.

Dudek, Wuarin, Tasker, Kim, and Peacock (1995) have recently provided evidence of cortical maturity levels by age 1 that are capable of supporting the mechanisms of synaptic transmission, and therefore epileptogenesis. Moreover, tissue from children with the most catastrophic epilepsies still had normal synaptic transmission capabilities within their resected or "diseased" tissue.

A long series of studies of neuropathologies associated with childhood epilepsy syndromes was conducted by Meencke in the 1980s and his findings appear strikingly parallel to the findings regarding the developmental stages of the fetal brain (Meencke, 1985, 1989). Meencke studied the brains of infants and children with a variety of childhood epilepsies, including infantile spasms (a.k.a. West syndrome), Lennox–Gastaut syndrome, and primary generalized seizure disorders (including childhood and juvenile myoclonic epilepsies). From the observed patterns of pathologies he observed, Meencke drew the following inferences: (1) Pathoanatomical abnormality of the brain is reflective of an increased likelihood of epilepsy, and vice versa; (2) the younger the child is at the age of onset, the greater the gravity of the pathoanatomical disruption; and (3) the younger the child is at the age of onset, the more aggressive the syndrome is, and the greater the gravity of the seizure disorder and behavioral disability.

The conclusion that is beginning to emerge is that epileptic syndromes are largely genetically based, and that their etiologies and pathologies may eventually be explained in terms of inherited or acquired neurodevelopmental anomalies. These genetically acquired, anomalous developmental sequences of the brain may have long-term repercussions in the form of (frequently) lifelong epileptic syndromes.

CLASSIFICATION SCHEMES

In general, a "seizure" may be conceptualized as a sudden discharge of electrical activity in the brain that results in alterations of sensation, behavior, or consciousness. "Epilepsy" is a condition of recurrent seizures. An "epileptic syndrome" is characterized by a recurrence of consistent symptoms and behavioral manifestations.

There are three major ways in which childhood seizures and epilepsy can be studied and classified. In this section we discuss seizure classification by (1) the cause of the seizure, (2) the seizure syndrome presentation, and (3) the epilepsy syndrome (this type of classification is generally more age- and behavior-based). These methods of classifying seizures are not mutually exclusive, and terms from more than one scheme are frequently used concurrently to discuss a single epileptic syndrome.

Classification by Cause of Seizure

Symptomatic Seizures

Symptomatic seizures and epileptic syndromes have a known cause, such as trauma, metabolic imbalance, developmental abnormality, or fever. Symptomatic seizures are also called "reactive" or "provoked" seizures when they occur in response to some irritation (e.g., fever or trauma) to the brain. The cause of a symptomatic seizure, therefore, can be either developmental in nature or acquired.

Cryptogenic Seizures

Cryptogenic seizures have a cause that is undetermined but that appears to be related in occurrence to some other neurological or cognitive condition. The seizures are presumed to be symptomatic, but their exact cause is as yet hidden.

Idiopathic Seizures

Idiopathic seizures are those for which the cause is completely unknown and there is no evidence of an underlying abnormality. The child with epilepsy is essentially normal except for the occurrence of the seizures. Idiopathic seizures are presumed to be inherited and are defined by age-related onsets.

Classification by Seizure Syndrome Presentation

Prenatal Seizures

Prenatal seizures are extremely rare. The only prenatal seizures that are readily recognizable (by the mother) are those induced by pyridoxine dependence, which results in a generalized tonic–clonic seizure of the fetus. Even massive cortical damage to the fetal brain will rarely produce recognizable seizures in the fetus. However, the fact that seizure manifestations in a newborn (discussed next) are so different from adult seizures leads to speculation that seizures in the fetus may occur more frequently than suspected, but that they are undiscernible to the mother or otherwise mistaken for normal fetal movement unless they are generalized tonic–clonic seizures.

Neonatal Seizures

A neonatal seizure can occur from birth up to about 1 month of age. The occurrence of neonatal seizures is higher in newborns with a familial history of epilepsy (Quattlebaum, 1979; Ryan, Wiznitzer, & Hollman, 1991), and benign neonatal seizures are associated with familial autosomal dominant inheritance. Approximately 14% of infants with benign neonatal seizures that are inherited will develop some other childhood epilepsy syndrome. The vast majority, however, experience a spontaneous resolution within the first few months of life. Benign familial neonatal seizures usually begin 2 or 3 days after birth and spontaneously resolve by 6 months of age. No intellectual or cognitive sequelae are known to result. Nonfamilial neonatal seizures are extremely rare after 2 months of age, and the neonatal seizure is always symptomatic of some central nervous system (CNS) disturbance (e.g., neurodevelopmental anomalies, withdrawal from maternal drug addiction, pyridoxine dependence, etc.). Diagnosis of neonatal seizures is difficult, because it is very dependent on astute and careful behavioral observation.

Based on his observations and clinical studies, Volpe (1987, 1989) proposed a separate neonate seizure classification based on the newborn's limited behavioral repertoire and resulting seizure manifestation. The neonate not only has a more limited behavioral repertoire than the older child, but also has a vastly different level of cortical maturity. This neuronal immaturity has implications for the newborn brain's ability to propagate, spread, and inhibit abnormal firing that could result in a seizure. Neurodevelopmental aspects of seizures in the neonate are also evidenced by the differential manifestation of seizures in full-term versus premature infants. In general, the younger the neonate is (neurodevelopmentally speaking) the more primitive is the seizure manifestation.

There are four major classes of neonatal seizures (subtle, tonic, clonic, and myoclonic). Subtle seizures appear to be the most commonly observed type of neonatal seizures. Subtle seizures can be subclassified, according to their manifestations, into those with motor, oral–buccal, eye, or apneic involvement. Subtle motor seizures manifest themselves as repetitive swimming, rowing, and pedaling behaviors of the upper or lower extremities. Subtle oral–buccal seizures are manifested as lip-smacking, chewing, and sucking behaviors. Subtle eye seizures manifest themselves as deviant horizontal eye movements and sustained blinking or opening of eyes. Subtle seizures that are manifested as apnea are very rare but may accompany other oral seizures (Murphy & Dehkharghani, 1994). Schulte (1966) postulated the cause of such primitive behaviors to be a disinhibition of subcortically controlled, primitive reflexes. Tonic, clonic, and myoclonic neonate seizures may be subclassified into focal and generalized seizures, and myoclonic seizures may also be multifocal. There is some limited evidence of lesional relationships to seizure manifestation. Focal clonic seizures in the neonate may occur with local cortical lesions (Levy, Abroms, Marshall, & Rosquete, 1985). Widespread cortical lesions may result in generalized tonic or multifocal clonic seizures. Myoclonic seizures are also observed in the neonate, and generalized tonic–clonic seizures are very rarely observed. The classification of neonatal seizures proposed by Volpe (1989) and diagnostic notes are presented in Table 22.1.

International Classification of Seizures

The international classification scheme is the most widely accepted and utilized format for clinical classification of epileptic seizure disorders. Its rough division of seizure types was first conceived by Gowers in 1885 (see the reprinted original—Gowers, 1885/1964), but was further developed and refined by the International League Against Epilepsy's Com-

TABLE 22.1. Neonatal Seizure Classification

Seizure type	Behavioral manifestation and general diagnostic notes
Subtle	Stereotyped and involuntary movements; normal EEG
Motor	Swimming, rowing, pedaling in upper or lower extremities
Oral	Lip smacking, chewing, sucking
Eyes	Horizontal deviation, blinking, sustained open eyes
Apneic	Rare on their own but may occur with subtle oral seizures
Clonic	Abnormal EEG associated with underlying pathology
Focal	Rhythmic unilateral involvement of the limbs, face, or trunk
Generalized	Bilateral or shifting involvement
Tonic	More common in premature infants; normal EEG
Focal	Sustained posturing of one limb
Generalized	Sustained posturing of all limbs
Myoclonic	
Focal	Sudden flexion or extension of large muscle groups; normal EEG
Multifocal	More than one muscle group involved; normal EEG
Generalized	All muscle groups; may be accompanied by abnormal EEG

Note. Adapted from Volpe (1989). Copyright 1989 by *Pediatrics*. Modified by permission of *Pediatrics*.

mission on Classification and Terminology in 1989. In this conceptualization, seizures are broadly classified as being either partial or generalized, and then further subclassified according to their behavioral manifestations. Although many variations of this classification system exist, one such variation is presented here as Table 22.2.

Partial seizures (previously referred to as "focal" or "local" seizures) are initially limited to one hemisphere. The onset of the seizure and most of its initial manifestation are limited. Partial seizures can be further subclassified into simple and complex partial seizures, depending on whether consciousness is altered. When consciousness remains intact, the seizure is termed a "simple partial seizure." The manifestations of these types of seizures can then be further subclassified into those affecting motor skills or those involving sensory symptoms. Complex partial seizures affect consciousness.

Seizures whose onset involves both hemispheres are termed "primary generalized seizures." These seizures can be convulsive or nonconvulsive and can also be subclassified into absence (petit mal or staring spells), myoclonic, and tonic–clonic (grand mal) seizures. Partial seizures of any type may become generalized seizures and are thus termed "secondarily generalized seizures" or "secondary generalizations."

Classification by Specific Childhood Epilepsy Syndromes

The third method of classification is probably the most useful when one is considering childhood epilepsy, because virtually all of these syndromes are age-related. Table 22.3 provides a quick reference of childhood epilepsy syndromes, along with the peak onset ages and hallmark features of each syndrome.

Infantile Spasms/West Syndrome

Infantile spasms usually appear between the ages of 4 and 7 months. They rarely occur before 2 months of age or after 1 year. Etiology may be genetic (e.g., an inherited condi-

TABLE 22.2. International Classification of Seizures

I. Partial/focal epilepsies
  A. Symptomatic (Note that as imaging technology improves, more and more epilepsies are being reclassified as being symptomatic)
    1. Rasmussen syndrome
    2. Syndromes characterized by seizures with specific modes of precipitation
    3. Partial epilepsies with a lobe of origin (e.g., temporal lobe epilepsy)
  B. Idiopathic (including, but not limited to the following)
    1. Benign childhood epilepsy with centrotemporal spike
    2. Childhood epilepsy with occipital paroxysms
    3. Primary reading epilepsy
  C. Cryptogenic

II. Generalized epilepsies
  A. Symptomatic (Note that as imaging technology improves, more and more epilepsies are being reclassified as being symptomatic)
    1. Nonspecific etiologies
    2. Specific etiologies
  B. Idiopathic
    1. Benign neonatal convulsions (familial and nonfamilial)
    2. Benign myoclonic epilepsy in infancy
    3. Childhood absence epilepsy
    4. Juvenile absence epilepsy
    5. Juvenile myoclonic epilepsy
  C. Cryptogenic
    1. Infantile spasms (West syndrome)
    2. Lennox–Gastaut syndrome
    3. Epilepsy with myoclonic–astatic seizures
    4. Epilepsy with myoclonic absences

III. Epileptic syndromes with undetermined focal or generalized seizures
  A. Neonatal seizures (see Table 22.1)
  B. Severe myoclonic epilepsy in infancy

IV. Special syndromes
  A. Febrile seizures
  B. Status epilepticus
  C. Seizures in reaction to specific environmental stressors

Note. Adapted from Commission on Classification and Terminology (1989). Not all syndromes addressed by the Commission are included here.

tion called tuberous sclerosis), or it may be attributable to a host of other etiologies, including metabolic imbalances or aminoacidurias. Although two-thirds of infantile spasms are generally considered to be symptomatic of brain lesions and the remaining cases are considered idiopathic, new imaging techniques are quickly reclassifying the vast majority as symptomatic in etiology.

Infantile spasms are characterized by a very specific seizure manifestation. The infant experiences a sudden flexion of the entire body, with knees flexed, arms extended, and head tucked. This position is held for a couple of seconds and is repeated every few seconds. The spasms occur in definite sets of 5, 10, or 15. That is, the alternations between flexion and relaxation (separated by a few seconds) occur in sets of 5, 10, or 15. They most often occur in the transitional period between sleep and wakefulness. These seizures are most often treated with antiepileptic drugs (AEDs), and if uncontrolled, the child's

TABLE 22.3. Childhood Epilepsy Syndromes, Their Peak Onset Range, and Hallmark Features

Epilepsy syndrome	Peak age at onset	Hallmark features
Infantile spasms	4 to 7 months	Definite sets (5, 10, or 15) of flexion–extension
Infantile myoclonic epilepsy	1 to 2 years	Flexion–extension in single or cluster events, not sets
Febrile seizures	6 to 24 months	Precipitated by a high fever with a fast rise
Myoclonic–astatic epilepsy	2 to 3 years	Manifestation is complex and can include all seizure types
Lennox–Gastaut syndrome	3 to 4 years	Specific triad: tonic–clonic seizures, abnormal EEG, mental retardation
Rasmussen syndrome	3 to 10 years	Focal seizures that move to produce a series of distinct focal seizures; moderate intellectual decline
Benign rolandic epilepsy	4 to 10 years	Seizure occurrence during sleep or onset; remits in adolescence
Epilepsy with myoclonic absences	6 to 7 years	Absence seizures with bilateral clonic jerks
Childhood absence epilepsy	7 years	Frequent staring spells daily
Juvenile absence epilepsy	12 to 13 years	Less frequent staring spells, fewer than one per day
Juvenile myoclonic epilepsy	14 to 15 years	Bilateral, irregular jerking on awakening from sleep; frequently elicited by sleep deprivation and fatigue

epilepsy will evolve into the Lennox–Gastaut syndrome (at about age 3 or 4). The uncontrolled infantile spasm progressing into Lennox–Gastaut syndrome can result in severe mental retardation and a regression in developmental milestones.

Infantile Myoclonic Epilepsy

Infantile myoclonic epilepsy occurs in children during their first or second year of life who are otherwise normal in development but who have a familial history of epilepsy. Its etiology is usually symptomatic of some CNS abnormality but may remain cryptogenic for some time.

The seizure manifestation, as its name suggests, involves brief episodes of muscular contractions that can occur as one brief episode or in clusters. The classic form of it consists of a sudden flexion or extension of the trunk and/or limbs. It is differentiated from infantile spasms by the lack of dependable serial clustering in contractions. The EEG is often normal unless prolonged recordings are conducted that demonstrate hypsarrhythmia. Intellectual development may be mildly delayed, and some minor personality change may occur (Commission on Classification and Terminology 1989), but the general outlook is good.

Febrile Seizures

Up to 4% of all children will experience at least one febrile seizure, and Hauser (1994) reported 100,000 occurrences of febrile seizures in the United States in 1990. The onset of febrile seizures most commonly occurs between the ages of 6 months and 2 years. They are uncommon before 6 months of age, and after the age of 2, the occurrence rate drops steadily. Febrile seizures are rare after 5 years of age. They are reliably elicited by a rapidly evolving and very high fever, but their occurrence is also dependent on age and cortical maturity, as well as familial history/genetic predisposition (Degan, Degan, & Hans, 1991). Thus febrile seizures are often considered the paradigm for age-dependent epilepsies because of their consistent and direct interdependence on three factors: age, genetics, and environmental factors.

Febrile seizures can be subclassified into simple and complex categories, although the use of the terms "simple" and "complex" can be misleading. A simple febrile seizure is a purely reactive, single, uncomplicated febrile seizure episode. Complex febrile seizures start with a focal seizure, and the seizure episode lasts longer than 15 minutes and occurs repeatedly within a 24-hour period.

Febrile seizures are not associated with an increased risk of mental retardation or other long-lasting, detrimental effects. Therefore, treatment of febrile seizures with AEDs is often discouraged unless a second episode occurs. This is based on the observations that there are no increased risk factors for developmental stunting from such a seizure itself. However, the AEDs used to control seizures may have adverse effects on behavior, cognitive processes, and intellectual development, as well as other health factors (e.g., liver damage).

Up to 30% of all children who experience a febrile seizure will experience a second febrile seizure (depending on their predisposing factors). Between 2% and 10% of children who experience febrile seizures will develop a nonfebrile seizure disorder (epilepsy).

Myoclonic–Astatic Epilepsy

Myoclonic–astatic epilepsy has a complex seizure manifestation, which can include myoclonic, astatic, myoclonic–astatic, tonic absence, clonic absence, and tonic–clonic seizures. It occurs in children between the ages of 7 months and 6 years, but incidence rates peak in children between the ages of 2 and 5 years. Myoclonic–astatic epilepsy occurs in genetically predisposed children who have developed normally up to that point. The progression of the syndrome is variable, but status frequently occurs, and the progression into a tonic epilepsy syndrome is not associated with a favorable prognosis.

Lennox-Gastaut Syndrome

The Lennox–Gastaut syndrome usually appears in children at about age 3 or 4 (but spans the ages from 1 to 8) who have previously experienced uncontrolled infantile spasms. However, the syndrome can also appear in otherwise healthy children and adolescents without any apparent precursor. The onset of the syndrome may be accompanied by a cessation of intellectual development. Development after onset for some children may be severely arrested; for other affected children, it may be less severely affected. The syndrome is accompanied by a very abnormal and easily recognizable EEG of spike and wave discharge superimposed on abnormal background activity. Thus it is characterized by a specific triad: seizures, abnormal EEG, and mental retardation.

The seizure manifestation is similar to infantile spasms (sudden flexion of the body), but does not appear in definitive series. The child, who is now walking, experiences the sudden body flexion (a.k.a. myoclonic, atonic, or akinetic seizures) and often falls to the ground. The syndrome is severe and appears to be a combination of seizure types, including focal and/or multifocal generalized tonic, tonic–clonic, myoclonic, atonic, and absence seizures. These seizures are unpredictable, are difficult to control, and occur with increased frequency as the syndrome progresses. Thus many children with this syndrome are very sheltered and wear protective headgear.

It is notable, however, that although most of the literature supports this severe sequence of events associated with Lennox–Gastaut syndrome, there have been reports of less severe developmental sequelae. Recent longitudinal following of children with this syndrome indicates that they may be capable of attaining a low average intellect, although they do have multiple attention and learning difficulties. Nonetheless, these children can fare reasonably well with a combination of educational, psychosocial, and pharmaceutical intervention (S. Goldstein, personal communication, September 22, 1997).

Progressive Unilateral Encephalopathy/Rasmussen Syndrome

Rasmussen syndrome is a devastating syndrome that appears in healthy and normally developed children between the ages of 3 and 10. It strikes without warning, and the initial episode is usually a severe generalized seizure that has no precipitating incident. A child then experiences focal seizures that increase in frequency. These focal seizures will gradually become more intense (but will not become multifocal), until more than half of these children experience a continuous focal seizure (epilepsy partialis continua).

The syndrome then progresses to surrounding areas of the initial foci and will spread in concentric circles until the entire hemisphere is involved. Note, however, that the seizure does not generalize. Rather, the focal seizure will move from the initial loci to a conjoining area, and the function associated with that cortical area will become the manifestation of the seizure. The manifestation will eventually change again to whatever behavior or function is associated with the area adjoining the second foci.

The progressive intellectual deterioration occurring with Rasmussen syndrome usually results in moderate mental retardation. Its progression appears unstoppable, but some children have responded well to radical hemispherectomy. Such children often experience some improvement in intellectual functioning. Recent research has pointed to the cause of Rasmussen encephalopathy as being an autoimmune disorder in which antibodies bind to and overstimulate glutamate receptors in the brain. Promising research has indicated that effective treatment may be found in techniques such as plasma exchange, in which the antibodies are filtered from the blood ("Antibodies Linked to Rare Epilepsy," 1995). Thus far, however, this treatment has had limited success, and patients have relapsed after a few months. In the meanwhile, radical hemispherectomy continues as the best viable option; children respond better when the surgery is performed at younger ages (Freeman & Vining, 1991).

Benign Rolandic Epilepsy

The onset of benign rolandic epilepsy typically occurs between the ages of 4 and 10. It is thought to be an autosomal dominant inherited disorder. Seizures most frequently occur at night, during sleep or sleep onset, and can be partial or generalized seizures that are accompanied by centrotemporal spikes in the EEG. The seizure disorder usually remits on its own in adolescence.

Epilepsy with Myoclonic Absences

The combination of absence seizures interspersed with bilateral clonic jerks defines epilepsy with myoclonic absences. Seizures occur frequently throughout a typical day, but are usually not accompanied by other seizures. AED therapy is difficult, and cognitive impairment and progression to other forms of epilepsy (such as Lennox–Gastaut syndrome) may occur. The EEG is strikingly characteristic in that the abnormal activity, similar to that of childhood absence epilepsy, is characterized by reliably occurring bilateral synchronous spike and wave discharges.

Childhood Absence Epilepsy

Childhood absence epilepsy (a.k.a. pyknoepilepsy, petit mal epilepsy) typically occurs in children between the ages of 4 and 8, with peak manifestation between the ages of 6 and 7. Its etiology significantly notable for genetic factors, and prevalence rates for childhood absence epilepsy are much higher in children with a familial history of epilepsy. Concordance studies in monozygotic twins have been reported at 65–75% for seizures, and up to 84% for spike and wave patterns of discharge (Berkovic, 1993). The prevalence is also higher in females than in males. Several absences (staring spells) a day are experienced, and EEG study may reveal spike and wave activity superimposed on a normal background. Generalized tonic–clonic seizures may surface during adolescence in approximately 40% of children with absence seizures.

Juvenile Absence Epilepsy

The seizure manifestation of juvenile absence epilepsy looks very much like that of childhood absence epilepsy, but the frequency of seizure occurrence is much lower. Seizures typically are fewer than one per day. Onset occurs between the ages of 10 and 17, with a peak onset at about age 12. Seizures may be accompanied by generalized tonic–clonic seizures or absence seizures. Generalized tonic–clonic seizures also frequently precede the onset of a juvenile absence epilepsy syndrome. EEG study may reveal spike and wave discharges that are greater than 3 Hz in frequency.

Juvenile Myoclonic Epilepsy

Juvenile myoclonic epilepsy is characterized by bilateral, irregular jerking in the upper extremities upon awakening that appears at about puberty in normal adolescents and frequently becomes a lifelong disorder. It typically manifests itself between the ages of 12 and 18, with a peak onset between the ages of 14 and 15. Juvenile myoclonic epilepsy is frequently accompanied by generalized tonic–clonic seizures (75–90%; Wolf, 1985; Serratosa & Delgado-Escueta, 1993) and much less frequently by absence seizures (about 30%). It has a fairly strong familial occurrence rate, with autosomal recessive inheritance suspected. Twenty-five percent of adolescents who develop juvenile myoclonic epilepsy have a relative with some form of epilepsy (Panayiotopoulos & Obeid, 1989; Delgado-Escueta et al., 1990). Sleep deprivation is an overwhelmingly significant precipitating factor. Panayiotopoulos, Obeid, and Tahan (1994) found that 90% of JME seizures were attributable to sleep deprivation and 74% to fatigue. The prognosis for intellectual development is good. The presence of intellectual or neurological decline should lead one to suspect progressive myoclonic epilepsy rather than juvenile myoclonic epilepsy.

NEUROPSYCHOLOGICAL SEQUELAE ASSOCIATED WITH EPILEPSY

Intellectual and cognitive impairments in people with epilepsy, especially memory deficits, were observed and noted in the literature over 100 years ago. Unfortunately, there is increasing evidence that cognitive deficits result not only from seizures themselves, but from the use of many, if not most, AEDs. Therefore, AEDs may thereby compound the cognitive difficulties and behavioral problems seen in persons with epilepsy (Bellur & Hermann, 1984; Blumer & Benson, 1982; Committee on Drugs, American Academy of Pediatrics, 1985; Corbett, Trimble, & Nichol, 1985; Himmelhock, 1984; Reynolds & Trimble, 1985; Walker & Blumer, 1984; Wilson, Petty, Perry, & Rose, 1983). The following discussion has been adapted in large part from Bennett (1992) and Bennett and Ho (1997). The specific cognitive effects of AEDs are not addressed here, and the interested reader is referred to Bennett and Ho (1997) for specific information.

The apparent association between cognitive impairment and epilepsy has been observed for several centuries. Dewhurst (1980) uncovered a reference in Thomas Willis's 17th-century lectures at Oxford University to the losses in memory, intellect, and reality that persons experience during and after seizures. Physicians continued to note the frequent concomitant occurrence of cognitive impairment with epilepsy throughout the 19th century and into the middle of the 20th century. As research continued on the relationship of epilepsy and cognitive impairment, it became apparent that intellectual decline was not as pervasive as was formerly believed. Various sampling errors and design methodology oversights (e.g., studying institutionalized patients, lack of control for medication types and levels, lack of control for type of seizures studied) were proffered as explanations. Another major issue was the rather primitive means of assessing cognitive functioning available in that era. Early studies largely depended on IQ testing as their major objective measure. Although IQ testing can provide a relatively sound measure of a person's biological level of adaptive functioning, it is highly dependent on achievement. In addition, IQ testing is not sensitive to the cognitive effects of brain injury, and the relationship of recurrent seizure disorders to brain injury is obvious.

Neuropsychological Assessment in Childhood Epilepsy

Rather than using IQ as a measure of cognitive functions, recent research has used a cognitive process approach in evaluating cognitive abilities in epileptic populations. The cognitive processes investigated have included sensory functions, attention and sustained concentration, learning and memory, language skills, perceptual abilities, conceptualization and reasoning, and motor abilities. The majority of studies have not investigated all of these processes, and within a given process such as attention, one is struck by the fact that few investigators use the same task. Second, a test may not evaluate what it purports to evaluate; thus, a "test of memory" may require high levels of attention for success. Poor performance may also be a consequence of impaired language or conceptualization processes.

This last difficulty can potentially be circumvented by utilizing a comprehensive battery approach in assessment, such as the Halstead–Reitan Neuropsychological Test Battery (Reitan & Wolfson, 1985). Reitan (1974) believed that this approach would be sensitive to the aggregate of cognitive impairments that might characterize a particular type of epilepsy under investigation. Carl Dodrill has further refined the battery approach in the assessment of individuals with epilepsy (see, e.g., Dodrill, 1978, 1981) by expanding the Halstead–Reitan Battery to optimally assess cognitive deficits associated with epilepsy. His Neuropsychological Battery for Epilepsy uses 16 measures of performance (as well as other psychosocial and empirically pertinent measures, such as familial history of seizure disorders), and he has established norms that reliably distinguish the performance of patients with epilepsy from that of closely matched control subjects. Dodrill's battery, and the general application of neuropsychological test battery approaches to evaluate the cognitive effects associated with epilepsy, represent advances. Unfortunately, the most common approach still remains narrow, and the majority of inquiries on this topic have continued to focus on a single type, or only a few types, of cognitive ability.

When competently provided, the neuropsychological assessment can be a valuable aid in establishing the severity of cognitive impairments and monitoring the effects of treatments for the seizure disorder. Although the vast majority of epileptic children retain normal levels of intellectual functioning, they are disproportionately skewed toward the lower end of normal IQ levels. This is presumably due to the underlying pathophysiology of the epileptic syndrome.

The importance of understanding a child's intellectual capabilities is key to being able to decipher underlying causes of poor academic performance. Material beyond a child's difficulty level, or boredom with material beneath his or her level, can each lead to poor academic performance. Frustration with these academic difficulties and with misplaced parental and teacher expectations can lead the child to behave in improper manners during school and thus to be classified as a behaviorally problematic child. Pressures to perform at unrealistic levels by parents and teachers may be alleviated early in the child's academic career by recognizing the contributions and appropriateness of intelligence testing to academic placement and performance. Learning problems due to interrupted auditory or visual information processing secondary to the seizure activity are common. Lack of concentration and distractibility are also more common to children with epilepsy than children without such conditions. Particular care must be taken to evaluate the possible influences of AEDs on learning and attentional deficiencies, as they all can cause problems (Freeman, Vining, & Pillas, 1990). Such sequelae are common causes of academic difficulties in children with epilepsy, and careful evaluation of the causes of academic problems must be made.

A Neuropsychological Model of Brain Functioning

To appreciate fully the effects of epilepsy on cognitive processes, it is helpful to consider these processes within a theoretical or conceptual model of the behavioral correlates of brain functioning. In our own conceptualizations, we have found it helpful to expand on and modify the model presented by Reitan and Wolfson (1985), which denotes six categories of brain–behavior relationships. Bennett (1988) has expanded the number of categories to seven, in order to separate attention from memory and to emphasize the dependence of memory on attention and concentration. He has also expanded on their level of logical analysis and renamed it "executive functions." Note that this is a process model, not an anatomical model. With the exceptions of (1) language skills and (2) visual–spatial skills, visual construction, and manipulospatial (i.e., perceptual–motor) skills—which are primarily represented in the left and right hemispheres, respectively—these processes are bilaterally represented. This model is diagrammed in Figure 22.1.

According to this model, the first level of neuropsychological processing is input to the brain via one of the sensory systems. It should be remembered that input can also arise endogenously from within the brain. The input must be attended to or concentrated on for information processing to occur and for the significance of the input to be ascertained (second level). Determining the significance of the stimulus or remembering it for later reference requires involvement of the memory system (third level).

The interdependence of attention and memory illustrates the fact that this neural system is dynamic, with activity flowing in both directions. In general, if information is to be

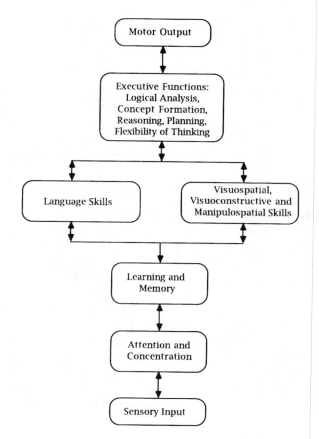

FIGURE 22.1. Conceptual model of the behavioral correlates of brain functioning (after Reitan & Wolfson, 1985). From Bennett (1988). Copyright 1988 by *Journal of Cognitive Rehabilitation*. Reprinted by permission.

remembered, it must be attended to (although, on the other hand, attention is no guarantee for memory). Similarly, attention is dependent on memory in terms of attentional processes' being involved in such activities as habituation and filtering of gated-out, nonrelevant information.

Input material that is verbal in nature requires the processing activities of a fourth neuropsychological category, language skills. Nonverbal material similarly requires processing mechanisms of a fifth category—visual–spatial skills, visual construction, and manipulospatial (perceptual–motor) skills.

Executive functions represent the highest level of information processing. These activities are involved in logical analysis, conceptualization, planning, self-monitoring, and flexibility of thinking. Poor performance on tests of executive functions can result from a primary deficit to those functions themselves, or it can result from a primary deficit to one of the lower levels of processing on which executive functions depend. Executive functions quickly become quite impaired in the person who is distractible, forgetful, and/or language-impaired, or who cannot perform higher-level perceptual processes.

Motor functions are the basis for responding and represent the final common path of the neuropsychological processes. They reflect the output capabilities of the system. This is the rationale for placing motor output at the top of the diagram. With this neuropsychological model as a backdrop, the effects of epilepsy on specific cognitive processes can be discussed.

Effects of Epilepsy on Specific Cognitive Processes

Sensory Input

Both impairment and exaggeration of sensory input can be said to result from seizures. Absence or petit mal attacks are generalized nonconvulsive seizures that occur particularly in children. They are characterized by brief episodes of loss of consciousness lasting approximately 5 to 15 seconds. During these episodes, the child seems to be unaware of his or her surroundings, and stares with a vacant expression. Sensory input occurring during these periods is neither attended to nor registered.

Complex partial seizures, on the other hand, may be manifested as sensory misperceptions and/or hallucinations. Misperceptions are often visual and complex. They typically involve distortions in depth perception or size. Size misperceptions can result in objects' being perceived as much smaller (micropsia) or larger (macropsia) than they are. Visual misperceptions reflect a posterior temporal lobe seizure focus. For example, they were observed to occur in a patient of ours prior to discovery of a right temporal lobe astrocytoma, and they diminished following its removal.

Misperception of voices results from a focal discharge of the anterior temporal lobe neocortex, especially from the left hemisphere. Voices may be perceived as too high or too low in pitch, or as being too loud or too soft. The patient may complain that the voices around him or her sound as if they are "coming out of a tunnel."

Hallucinations or auras that are experienced by patients with complex partial seizures are typically simple. In general, olfactory–gustatory sensations, which are often quite displeasing, result from a focal discharge in the uncus of the hippocampus. Our patients who experience these auras most typically report salty or bitter taste sensations, and/or olfactory sensations best described as "burning flesh" or "putrid." One patient—whose seizures were particularly refractory to AED therapy, and who experienced secondary generalized seizures that correlated with menstruation—was anosmic except when she experienced olfactory auras just prior to and during menstruation each month.

Abdominal and epigastric sensations typically arise from an amygdala focus. Simple auditory phenomena, such as buzzing, ringing, and hissing sounds, are produced by focal activity on the surface of the temporal lobe, especially the primary auditory reception area. Complex visual hallucinations, although uncommon, arise from the temporal–parietal–occipital junction (Rodin, 1984).

Cephalgic auras reflect discharge originating in the central regions of the temporal lobes. They consist of severe, sharp, stabbing knife-like head pains that are often associated with the head's feeling too big, too small, or off the body. Cephalgic auras will occasionally be misdiagnosed as migraine headaches and subsequently incorrectly medicated.

An important feature of auras is that they are passive experiences. The patient feels like an observer of these ictal (seizure-related) events, dissociated from the actual experience. This is different from the experience of a schizophrenic, who firmly believes that his or her hallucinations are "real" experiences. The ictal events are unrelated to the environment, except for rare seizures triggered by specific stimuli (e.g., musicogenic seizures, sexual seizures). We once had a patient whose seizures were reliably triggered whenever he played the arcade game Foosball! More typically for the patient with complex partial seizures, the ictal events begin spontaneously with an arrest of all activity, and the aura and/or psychomotor responses follow. Finally, while attention is usually paid to the most salient attribute of the epileptic patient's aura, the dream-like quality of the epileptic aura will often encompass many experiences. For example, a patient of ours regularly experienced a series of events including epigastric sensations, time distortion, detachment from her surroundings, and olfactory sensations as components of her seizure episodes.

Attention and Concentration

Impairment of attention and concentration, in the absence of overt clinical seizures, has been documented by several writers. Teacher and caretaker ratings for children with epilepsy frequently note marked inattentiveness and the detrimental effects of epilepsy-associated inattention on academic success (Bennett-Levy & Stores, 1984; Wilson, Ivani-Chalain, Besag, & Bryant, 1993).

Williams et al. (1996) studied 84 children with epilepsy of varying etiologies and found that attention may be subtly affected. In addition, the children who were being treated with polydrug therapy exhibited more problems with both attention and memory than children who were treated with only one AED. Williams and Haut (1995) also found attentional difficulties in children with epilepsy relative to controls.

Specific attentional difficulties in epilepsy appear related to seizure type. Patients with generalized seizures are more impaired on measures of sustained attention than are patients with focal seizures. It has been argued that this occurs because generalized seizures are more likely than focal seizures to affect the central subcortical structures that are responsible for maintaining attention.

In contrast, it appears that patients with focal seizures are more impaired on selective attention than are patients with generalized seizures (Loiseau, Signoret, & Strube, 1984). Loiseau et al. demonstrated that individuals with focal seizures and generalized seizures performed significantly worse on tests of selective attention than nonepileptic individuals did. The worst performance was seen in the group with focal seizures. Stores (1984) explain this phenomenon by indicating that subcortical structures are important in determining what to pay attention to (selective attention). Focal seizures in the cortex thus produce inattentiveness by disrupting selective attention.

Learning and Memory

Deficits in epileptic children's ability to learn and remember material on a daily basis have been noted by teachers and parents for many years. Wilson et al. (1993) have used a children's version of the Rivermead Behavioural Memory Test to demonstrate everyday memory difficulties encountered by children with severe epilepsies. Not only do children with epilepsy have more overall memory difficulties than their normal peers, but they also exhibit more verbal memory difficulties than children with substance abuse problems or other psychiatric problems (Williams & Haut, 1995).

Evidence has accumulated associating memory deficits with temporal lobe epilepsy foci. In an early study that compared cognitive abilities in patients with generalized seizures to patients with focal complex partial seizures of temporal lobe origin, Quadfasel and Pruyser (1955) found that memory impairment was significant only in the focal group. This is probably related to the anatomical location of the hippocampus in the temporal lobe and its role in the consolidation of memories.

It is well established in both adults and children that focal seizures of left temporal lobe origin yield greater verbal than nonverbal deficits, and that the opposite pattern is obtained with right temporal lobe dysfunction (Cohen, 1992; Jambaque, Dellatolas, Dulac, Ponsot, & Signoret, 1993; Majdan, Sziklas, & Jones-Gotman, 1996; Masui et al., 1984; Mayeux, Brandt, Rosen, & Benson, 1980). Long-term memory appears to be more significantly affected than short-term memory. Delaney, Rosen, Mattson, and Novelly (1980) reported similar findings in patients with right versus left temporal lobe foci who were matched for age of onset, duration of epilepsy, and seizure frequency. This lateralizing effect on memory is also supported when concurrent EEG recordings are utilized (Kasteleijn-Nolst Trenite, Smit, Velis, Willemse, & van Emde Boas, 1990). Therefore, the pattern of memory deficits exhibited by the individual continues to be an aid in determining the laterality of a temporal lobe seizure focus.

A study of the differences in qualitative aspects of verbal memory between left and right temporal foci epileptic patients on the one hand, and patients with nonepileptic seizures on the other, was reported by Bortz, Prigatano, Blum, and Fisher (1995). Their results demonstrated significant qualitative (response bias) differences individuals with seizures of epileptic and nonepileptic origin on the California Verbal Learning Test. Their report, however, also indicates some trends in the data that may differentiate epileptic patients according to lateralization of seizure origin. Patients with left temporal lobe seizure foci exhibited more intrusion errors on the delayed- and free-recall tasks, as well as a bias toward false-positive recognition of nontarget words. Patients with right temporal lobe seizure foci did not demonstrate a response bias. This pattern of deficits is frequently seen in other populations that have primary difficulties in consolidating new materials, and it indicates a poverty in the initial learning of the verbal materials in patients with left temporal foci. This lack of learning and consolidation produces a resultant inability to recognize materials accurately. Patients with right temporal foci did not demonstrate the same bias in recognition responding, indicating that their verbal learning skills and resulting recognition were relatively intact.

Additional difficulty in detecting and addressing memory difficulties experienced by epileptic populations is evidenced by their lack of insight into their own memory difficulties. This "metamemory" deficit in association with temporal lobe seizure foci was noted by Prevey, Delaney, and Mattson (1988), who observed that persons with left temporal foci had poorer insight and self-monitoring skills with respect to verbal memory. Nonverbal metamemory difficulties were observed in higher frequency in persons with right temporal foci.

Taken together, these studies suggest a significant impairment of memory functions in patients with seizures of temporal lobe origin. A word of caution comes from the work of Mayeux et al. (1980), who have published findings indicating that dysnomia contributes greatly to the interictal memory impairment seen in patients with complex partial seizures. The vast research on memory processes alone illustrates the difficulties encountered in attempting to evaluate specific cognitive processes for patients with epilepsy.

Language Skills

Both experimental inquiry and clinical observation have long indicated that epilepsy may adversely affect language skills and reading skill acquisition. Williams et al. (1996) found that children with uncontrolled seizures (absence or complex partial) had more difficulty with complex verbal materials than children whose seizures were well controlled. An interesting case has recently been reported by Vargha-Khadem et al. (1997), in which an 8½-year-old child with uncontrolled seizures underwent radical hemispherectomy of the left hemisphere. Prior to his surgery, the child was mute and had the language comprehension skills of a 3- to 4-year-old. Not only did his seizures remit following the surgery, but he spontaneously regained language development a month after withdrawal of AEDs! These results prompt new questions regarding whether the mechanisms of seizure control (usually AEDs) actually have detrimental effects on language skills as severe as those of the epilepsy itself. Rapidly progressing research in the basic sciences and clinical sciences will undoubtedly continue to shed light on the specific mechanisms of cognitive impairment.

Regardless of the mechanisms by which language skills are affected, it is well established that specific language skills can also be affected. Dysarthria was noted in two-thirds of children with severe epilepsy studied by Harvey, Goodyer, and Brown (1988). As indicated earlier, Mayeux et al. (1980) demonstrated that dysnomia was prominent in their patients whose complex partial seizures had a left temporal lobe focus, as indexed by scores on the Boston Naming Test. They wrote that "the relative anomia demonstrated in temporal lobe epilepsy patients may have been interpreted by these patients and their relatives as poor memory" (p. 123). The authors further suggested that the verbosity and circumstantiality observed in some patients with complex partial seizures (e.g., Bennett, 1987) may be the expression of a compensatory mechanism for dysnomia.

Circumstantiality is seen in both the spoken and written communication of these patients. Their communications are often overinclusive and include excessive background detailing, precise times, clarifications, and other nonessentials (Bear, Freeman, & Greenberg, 1984); these can prevent conversations from reaching a normal end. This interpersonal communication style can lead to such patients' being shunned.

Hypergraphia (i.e., a tendency toward excessive and compulsive writing) is also often seen in patients with complex partial seizures; it was first well documented in these patients by Waxman and Geschwind (1980). It is often characterized by verbosity and circumstantiality, but it facilitated the writing of the complex partial seizure victim and legendary author Feodor Dostoievsky (Geschwind, 1984).

Perceptual–Motor Skills

There has not been a great deal of research investigating the effects of epilepsy on perceptual–motor skills, but the following has been reported. As noted earlier, Dodrill (1978, 1981) found that total time, memory, and localization scores from the Tactual Performance Test were sensitive measures of the effects of epilepsy on cognitive processes. The total time score is a measure of perceptual–motor (manipulospatial) ability. A deficit in spatial memory can be evaluated via the localization score if a significant discrepancy exists between the localization score and the memory score from this task.

Morgan and Groh (1980) reported greater impairment on the Frostig Test of Developmental Visual Perception in children with focal seizures than in those with generalized seizures. Poorer Bender–Gestalt performances in children with epilepsies have also been reliably reported.

Executive Functions

Because of their dependence on lower-level neuropsychological functions, executive functions of the brain involved in such processes as conceptualization, logical analysis, reasoning, planning, sequential thinking, flexibility of thinking, and self-monitoring are especially sensitive to dysfunction, including that associated with epilepsy. As indicated earlier in this chapter, executive functions will typically be impaired in the person who is distractible, has a poor memory, is language-impaired, and/or has difficulty with perceptual–motor skills. In a general sense, executive functions are the basis for a person's ability to meet the demands of his or her environment effectively. Although these impairments may be easily overlooked, they are commonly seen in individuals with epilepsy as indicated by performance on such tests as the Trail Making Tests, the Wisconsin Card Sorting Test (WCST), and the Category Test.

An interesting study by Hermann, Wyler, and Richey (1988) investigated WCST performance (a test of frontal lobe functions) in patients with complex partial seizures of temporal lobe origin. Performance was studied in individuals whose seizures arose from the dominant versus nondominant temporal lobe, as well as in an epilepsy control group composed mainly of patients with primarily generalized seizures. Thirty-seven percent of the dominant temporal lobe group and 79% of the nondominant temporal lobe group were impaired on this task, suggesting frontal lobe involvement. Only 17% of the epilepsy controls were impaired. It was suggested that these findings reflected dysfunction of the frontal lobes because of epileptic discharge ("neural noise") being propagated from a temporal lobe–hippocampal epileptic focus. Pathways that could transmit such temporal–frontal discharges are well known. After partial resection of the epileptogenic temporal lobe, WCST performance improved, presumably because of a significant diminuation of neural noise. A similar explanation was used to account for the finding by Novelly et al. (1984) that patients who underwent unilateral temporal lobectomy experienced a postoperative improvement in material-specific memory mediated by the hemisphere contralateral to the resection.

Corcoran and Upton (1993) conducted a follow-up study to that of Hermann et al. (1988), utilizing a modified WCST with patients who had hippocampal sclerosis associated with temporal lobe epilepsy. They postulated that working memory may play a significant role in WCST performance after the hippocampally sclerotic patients (particularly the right foci patients) performed more poorly than those with frontal lobe seizure foci (Upton & Corcoran, 1995). The debate surrounding the Hermann et al. (1988) study has continued, and there is wide variability in regard to the tasks utilized to reflect frontal or "executive" functions, as well as in the conceptualization of executive functions. In fact, the "central executive" functions conceptualized and referred to by many authors often overlap with working memory. Cowey and Green (1996) conducted a methodologically eloquent study of temporal lobe epileptics with left or right foci, epileptics with frontal lobe foci, and normal controls on tests of the "central executive" functions. In their study, patients with frontal dysfunction performed the most poorly on a dual-task paradigm (originated by Baddeley, Bressi, Della Sala, Logie, & Spinnler, 1991) that requires the individual to perform two tasks simultaneously, and thus can be conceptualized to require planning, judgment, and allocation skills.

Thus, amidst the ongoing debates concerning conceptualization and testing of executive functions, there still is no consensus regarding the effects of epilepsy on executive functions independent of other cognitive functions.

Motor Output

Decreased reaction time and psychomotor speed are common difficulties for individuals with epilepsy, especially when the epilepsy is associated with spike and wave activity that is more than 3 seconds in duration. McGuckin (1980) has proposed that lack of speed is one of four main barriers to competitive employment faced by adults with epilepsy, and this same lack of speed may also be conceptualized as a barrier to academic success in children and adolescents (Bennett-Levy & Stores, 1984).

ETIOLOGICAL FACTORS IN THE COGNITIVE DEFICITS ASSOCIATED WITH EPILEPSY

The same factors that influence the development of epilepsy (age, genetics, environmental stressors) are also related to the cognitive sequelae associated with epilepsy. In addition, the etiology and type of seizures associated with a child's epileptic syndrome have some differential effects on cognition. These differential cognitive sequelae are discussed here.

In general, more significant effects are thought to result if the seizure disorder starts at an early age, if a patient has poor seizure control, if the individual has had the disorder for a relatively long period of time, and if the person exhibits multiple seizure types. Complex partial seizures, particularly those of temporal lobe origin, are typically believed to produce more obvious cognitive and behavioral changes than most other seizure types.

Etiology of the Seizure Disorder

Of the intellectual correlates associated with epilepsy and the variables that alter them, the most predictable is that of seizure etiology and its relationship to IQ. IQ scores of individuals whose seizures are idiopathic have long been established to be significantly higher than scores attained by patients whose seizures have known etiologies; this is true of both institutionalized and noninstitutionalized children and adults.

Etiology can significantly confound attempts to study neuropsychological processes in persons with epilepsy. For example, Fowler, Richards, Berent, and Boll (1987) utilized a modified Halstead–Reitan Neuropsychological Test Battery to assess cognitive impairments in persons with epilepsy, and investigated the correlation between deficits on these tests and EEG indices of focus localization. They were able to demonstrate cognitive impairments on most of the measures employed and, where applicable, to correlate these findings with EEG localization. For example, persons scoring low on tests of verbal comprehension usually had a left temporal lobe focus. However, approximately half of the subjects in this study knew the origin of their seizure disorder. Etiologies included head injury, infectious disease (e.g., encephalitis), intracranial tumors, and cerebrovascular disease (e.g., stroke). Given that brain damage alone can severely impair cognitive functioning and that the Halstead–Reitan Neuropsychological Test Battery is highly sensitive to the effects of these conditions, it would seem impossible to sort out the cognitive impairments due to epilepsy from those due to the disorders underlying the epilepsy in this inquiry.

Research in our laboratory on the cognitive effects of epilepsy in adults with clear evidence of focal left versus right temporal lobe seizures, but without prior head injury or neurological disease, indicated that no lateralized deficits were observed (Haynes & Bennett, 1991). The only trend that appeared was that the subjects with epilepsy as a group exhibited generalized deficits in the areas of psychomotor speed, selective attention, and reasoning ability. This study emphasizes the importance of ruling out underlying cerebral pathology due to head injury or other neurological disease in studying cognitive processes in persons with epilepsy per se.

Seizure Type and Frequency

In addition to seizure etiology, the type and frequency of seizures constitute important variables influencing the nature and extent of intellectual and cognitive dysfunction. A number of studies have shown generalized tonic–clonic seizures to be associated with greater intellectual and cognitive impairment than other types of seizures. Studies over the years have also repeatedly demonstrated, in both children and adults, that frequent generalized seizures are associated with the highest levels of cognitive impairment (vs. less frequent seizures and other types of seizures). The detrimental effect of frequency of seizures on intellectual and cognitive functioning has been shown to be consistent across all seizure types.

Farwell, Dodrill, and Batzel (1985) evaluated a large group of children whose ages ranged from 6 to 15 years. Within each seizure type studied, lower seizure frequency was associated with higher scores on the Wechsler Intelligence Scale for Children—Revised (WISC-R). In addition, seizure type was found to be a discriminating factor when both IQ and neuropsychological functions were evaluated. The minor motor and atypical absence groups showed statistically significant lower IQ scores than all other groups. However, children with partial or generalized tonic–clonic seizures demonstrated WISC-R Full Scale IQ scores comparable to those observed in the control group. When considered together, children with epilepsy showed significantly greater neuropsychological impairment than controls, as measured by the age-appropriate Halstead–Reitan Battery. Overall, neuropsychological impairment was found to differentiate between seizure types with greater sensitivity than did WISC-R Full Scale IQ. Children with minor motor or atypical absence seizures demonstrated no detectable neuropsychological impairment, but when seizure types were mixed (classical absence plus generalized tonic–clonic), impairment was again evident.

Early studies also found seizure type to affect selected cognitive functions differentially. Regardless of seizure type, the performance of children with epilepsy was below that of the control group. Of greater interest, however, were the findings that children with left temporal lobe foci showed learning and memory deficits on measures that required delayed recall of verbal material, whereas children with right temporal lobe foci had greater difficulty with recall tasks involving visual–spatial abilities. Significant differences between performance on measures of recent memory were not evident between groups. Furthermore, children whose seizures were centrencephalic in nature performed at a significantly lower level on tasks of sustained attention than did the temporal lobe groups, but they did not demonstrate either short-term or long-term memory impairment.

Patterns of intellectual performance on the Wechsler Adult Intelligence Scale—Revised (WAIS-R) or WISC-R that varied with seizure type were observed by Giordani et al. (1985). Adults and children with partial seizures performed better on Digit Span, Digit Symbol (or Coding), Block Design, and Object Assembly than did patients with either generalized or partial secondarily generalized seizures, although significant differences between groups on Full Scale IQ scores were not present.

Studies by Delaney et al. (1980) and Loiseau et al. (1984) have not shown a clear relationship between frequency of seizures and greater intellectual impairment. O'Leary et al. (1983) found only one variable that showed a significant difference in performance between groups of children with differing seizure disorders: Children with partial seizures performed significantly better on the Tactual Performance Test (total time) than children with generalized seizures. The partial seizure group in this study, however, was composed of children with simple partial, complex partial, and partially secondarily generalized seizure types, and this wide variation of seizure types within one group may have accounted for the limited differences seen when groups were compared.

Because seizure classifications and their inclusion criteria have not been consistent, particularly in the earlier studies, and populations tested have not been uniform across investigations (institutionalized versus noninstitutionalized), direct comparisons between studies are not always possible. The study of seizure type and frequency and its effect on intellectual and cognitive functioning is further complicated by the severity of seizures and the levels of AEDs necessary to achieve adequate seizure control. It is also possible that in some cases, the association between observed cognitive deficits and frequency of seizures is due to the extent of cerebral damage that is responsible for both. When considered as a whole, however, current studies suggest that the extent of intellectual and cognitive dysfunction in epilepsy varies with the type of seizure and increases with greater seizure frequency.

Age at Onset and Duration of Disorder

The relationship between early onset of seizure disorder and poor prognosis for mental functioning has been noted for over a century, and current research continues to support this observation. Studies of intellectual and neuropsychological functions in children with epilepsy, regardless of seizure type, indicate that onset of seizures early in life and a consequently long duration of seizure disorder place children at higher risk for cognitive dysfunction.

O'Leary et al. (1983) studied the effects of early onset of epilepsy in children 9 to 15 years of age with partial versus generalized seizures. Results indicated that both groups of children with early seizure onset performed more poorly on measures of neuropsychological abilities than children whose seizures began at a later age. Dodrill (1993) also found the same detrimental relationship between age at onset and intellectual ability in an archival study of 510 files from his own clinic. These findings remain consistent with observations of the effect of seizure onset by Farwell et al. (1985), who studied a variety of seizure types, and Scarpa and Carassini (1982), who studied children with partial seizures.

Dodrill (1993) is careful to point out the need for careful consideration of other possible factors that contribute to the poorer intellectual outcome associated with early onset, such as the fact that a lower age at onset usually means a much higher number of total seizure occurrences. In fact, Dodrill (1986) has previously found evidence that the total number of tonic–clonic seizures a person experiences may be as important as, if not more important than, the age at onset.

SUMMARY

Childhood epilepsy syndromes are wide and varied. Their seizure and behavioral manifestations span the possibilities of syndromes classified by the International League Against Epilepsy (listed in Table 22.2). Moreover, childhood epilepsies have been shown to exist both neonatally and (on rare occasions) prenatally. Seizures at these age ranges have their own manifestation and classification. What we know to be common about most childhood epilepsy disorders is that their onset, whether a single seizure occurrence or a long-lasting epileptic disorder, usually has some genetic component (i.e., a close relative experienced some sort of seizure disorder). We know more about the genetic inheritance modes of some epileptic disorders than we do about others. We also know more about the cognitive and neuropsychological consequences of some syndromes than we do about others. However, it does appear that the age at which the disorder began, the duration of the disorder, and the frequency and duration of the seizures are all factors in a child's long-term outcome. As basic and applied scientists continue to collaborate and compare notes, we come closer to reaching answers about the neurodevelopmental and physiological underpinnings of epilepsy and their impact on cognitive development.

REFERENCES

Antibodies linked to rare epilepsy. (1995). *Science*, *268*, 362–363.

Baddeley, A. D., Bressi, S., Della Sala, S., Logie, R., & Spinnler, H. (1991). The decline of working memory in Alzheimer's disease. *Brain*, *114*, 2521–2542.

Bear, D. M., Freeman, R., & Greenberg, M. (1984). Behavioral alterations in patients with temporal lobe epilepsy. In D. Blumer (Ed.), *Psychiatric aspects of epilepsy* (pp. 197–227). Washington, DC: American Psychiatric Press.

Bellur, S., & Hermann, B. P. (1984). Emotional and cognitive effects of anticonvulsant medications. *International Journal of Clinical Neuropsychology*, *6*, 21–23.

Bennett, T. L. (1987). Neuropsychological aspects of complex partial seizures: Diagnostic and treatment issues. *International Journal of Clinical Neuropsychology*, *9*, 37–45.

Bennett, T. L. (1988). Use of the Halstead–Reitan Neuropsychological Test Battery in the assessment of head injury. *Journal of Cognitive Rehabilitation*, *3*, 18–24.

Bennett, T. L. (1992). Cognitive effects of epilepsy and anticonvulsant medications. In T. L. Bennett (Ed.), *The neuropsychology of epilepsy*. New York: Plenum Press.

Bennett, T. L., & Ho, M. R. (1997). The neuropsychology of pediatric epilepsy and antiepileptic drugs. In C. R. Reynolds & E. Fletcher-Janzen (Eds.), *Handbook of clinical child neuropsychology* (2nd ed., pp. 517–538). New York: Plenum Press.

Bennett-Levy, J., & Stores, G. (1984). The nature of cognitive dysfunction in school-children with epilepsy. *Acta Neurologica Scandinavica*, *69*(Suppl. 99), 79–82.

Berkovic, S. F. (1993). Childhood absence epilepsy and juvenile absence epilepsy. In E. Wyllie (Ed.). *The treatment of epilepsy: Principles and practice* (pp. 547–551). Philadelphia: Lea & Febinger.

Blumer, D., & Benson, D. F. (1982). Psychiatric manifestations of epilepsy. In D. F. Benson & D. Blumer (Eds.), *Psychiatric aspects of neurological disease* (Vol. 2, pp. 25–48). New York: Grune & Stratton.

Bortz, J. J., Prigatano, G. P., Blum, D., & Fisher, R. S. (1995). Differential response characteristics in nonepileptic and epileptic seizure patients on a test of verbal learning and memory. *Neurology*, *45*, 2029–2034.

Commission on Classification and Terminology, International League Against Epilepsy. (1989). Proposal for revised classification of epilepsies and epileptic syndromes. *Epilepsia*, *30*, 389–399.

Committee on Drugs, American Academy of Pediatrics. (1985). Behavioral and cognitive effects of anticonvulsant therapy. *Pediatrics*, *76*, 644–647.

Cohen, M. (1992). Auditory/verbal and visual/spatial memory in children with complex partial epilepsy of temporal lobe origin. *Brain and Cognition*, *20*, 315–326.

Corbett, J. A., Trimble, M. R., & Nichol, T. C. (1985). Behavioral and cognitive impairments in children with epilepsy: The long-term effects of anticonvulsant therapy. *Journal of the American Academy of Child Psychiatry*, *24*, 17–23.

Corcoran, R., & Upton, D. (1993). A role for the hippocampus in card sorting? *Cortex*, *29*, 293–304.

Cowan, L. D., Bodensteiner, J. B., Leviton, A., & Doherty, L. (1989). Prevalence of the epilepsies in children and adolescents. *Epilepsia*, *30*, 94–106.

Cowey, C. M., & Green, S. (1996). The hippocampus: A "working memory" structure? The effect of hippocampal sclerosis on working memory. *Memory*, *4*, 19–30.

Degan, R., Degan, H. E., & Hans, K. A. (1991). A contribution to the genetics of febrile seizures: Waking and sleeping EEG in siblings. *Epilepsia*, *32*, 515–522.

Delaney, R. C., Rosen, A. J., Mattson, R. H., & Novelly, R. A. (1980). Memory function in focal epilepsy: A comparison of non-surgical, unilateral temporal lobe, and frontal lobe samples. *Cortex*, *15*, 103–117.

Delgado-Escueta, A. V., Greenberg, D., Weissbecker, K., Liu, A., Treiman, L., Sparkes, R., Park, M. S., Barbetti, A., & Terasaki, P. I. (1990). Gene mapping in idiopathic generalized epilepsies: Juvenile myoclonic epilepsy, childhood absence epilepsy, epilepsy with grand-mal seizures, and early childhood myoclonic epilepsy. *Epilepsia*, *31*(Suppl. 3), S19–S29.

Dewhurst, K. (1980). *Thomas Willis' Oxford lectures*. Oxford: Sanford.

Dodrill, C. B. (1978). A neuropsychological battery for epilepsy. *Epilepsia, 19*, 611–623.

Dodrill, C. B. (1981). Neuropsychology of epilepsy. In S. B. Filskov & T. J. Boll (Eds.), *Handbook of clinical neuropsychology* (pp. 366–395). New York: Wiley.

Dodrill, C. B. (1986). Correlates of generalized tonic-clonic seizures with intellectual, neuropsychological, emotional, and social function in patients with epilepsy. *Epilepsia, 27*, 399–411.

Dodrill, C. B. (1993). Neuropsychology. In J. Laidlaw, A. Richens, & D. Chadwick (Eds.), *A textbook of epilepsy* (4th edition., pp. 459–473). New York: Churchill Livingstone.

Dudek, F. E., Wuarin, J. P., Tasker, J. G., Kim, Y. I., & Peacock, W. J. (1995). Neurophysiology of neocortical slices resected from children undergoing surgical treatment for epilepsy. *Journal of Neuroscience Methods, 59*, 49–58.

Farwell, J. R., Dodrill, C. B., & Batzel, L. W. (1985). Neuropsychological abilities in children with epilepsy. *Epilepsia, 26*, 395–400.

Fowler, P. C., Richards, H. C., Berent, S., & Boll, T. J. (1987). Epilepsy, neuropsychological deficits, and EEG lateralization. *Archives of Clinical Neuropsychology, 2*, 81–92.

Freeman, J. M., & Vining, E. P. G. (1991). Hemispherectomy: The ultimate focal resection. In H. Lüders (Ed.), *Epilepsy surgery* (pp. 111–118). New York: Raven Press.

Freeman, J. M., Vining, E. P. G. & Pillas, D. J. (1990). *Seizures and epilepsy in childhood: A guide for parents*. Baltimore: Johns Hopkins University Press.

Geschwind, N. (1984). Dostoievsky's epilepsy. In D. Blumer (Ed.), *Psychiatric aspects of epilepsy* (pp. 325–334). Washington, DC: American Psychiatric Press.

Giordani, B., Berent, S., Sackellares, J. C., Rourke, D., Seidenberg, M., O'Leary, D. S., Dreifuss, F. E., & Boll, T. J. (1985). Intelligence test performance of patients with partial and generalized seizures. *Epilepsia, 26*, 37–42.

Gowers, W. R. (1964). *Epilepsy and other chronic convulsive disorders* (American Academy of Neurology Reprint Series). New York: Dover. (Original work published 1885)

Harvey, I., Goodyer, I. M., & Brown, S. W. (1988). The value of a neuropsychiatric examination of children with complex severe epilepsy. *Child: Care, Health, and Development, 14*, 329–340.

Hauser, W. A. (1994). The prevalence and incidence of convulsive disorder in children. *Epilepsia, 35*(Suppl. 2), S1–S6.

Haynes, S., & Bennett, T. L. (1991). Cognitive impairment in adults with complex partial seizures. *International Journal of Clinical Neuropsychology, 12*, 74–81.

Hermann, B. P., Wyler, A. R., & Richey, E. T. (1988). Wisconsin Card Sorting Test performance in patients with complex partial seizures of temporal lobe origin. *Journal of Clinical and Experimental Neuropsychology, 10*, 467–476.

Himmelhock, J. M. (1984). Major mood disorders related to epileptic changes. In D. Blumer (Ed.), *Psychiatric aspects of epilepsy* (pp. 271–294). Washington, DC: American Psychiatric Press.

Jambaque, I., Dellatolas, G., Dulac, O., Ponsot, G., & Signoret, J. (1993). Verbal and visual memory impairment in children with epilepsy. *Neuropsychologia, 31*, 1321–1337.

Kasteleijn-Nolst Trenite, D. G. A., Smit, A. M., Velis, D. N., Willemse, J., & van Emde Boas, W. (1990). On-line detection of transient neuropsychological disturbances during EEG discharges in children with epilepsy. *Developmental Medicine and Child Neurology, 32*, 46–50.

Lechtenberg, R. (1984). *Epilepsy and the family*. Cambridge, MA: Harvard University Press.

Lennox, W. G., & Lennox, M. A. (1960). *Epilepsy and related disorders*. Boston: Little, Brown.

Levy, S. R., Abroms, I. F., Marshall, P. C., & Rosquete, E. E. (1985). Seizures and cerebral infarction in the full-term newborn. *Annals of Neurology, 17*, 366–390.

Loiseau, P., Signoret, J. L., & Strube, E. (1984). Attention problems in adult epileptic patients. *Acta Neurologica Scandinavica, 69*(Suppl. 99), 31–34.

Majdan, A., Sziklas, V., & Jones-Gotman, M. (1996). Performance of healthy subjects and patients with resection from the anterior temporal lobe on matched tests of verbal and visuoperceptual learning. *Journal of Clinical and Experimental Neuropsychology, 18*, 416–430.

Masui, K., Niwa, S., Anzai, N., Kameyama, T., Saitoh, O., & Rymar, K. (1984). Verbal memory disturbances in left temporal lobe epileptics. *Cortex, 20*, 361–368.

Mayeux, R., Brandt, J., Rosen, J., & Benson, F. (1980). Interictal and language impairment in temporal lobe epilepsy. *Neurology, 30*, 120–125.

McGuckin, H. M. (1980). Changing the world view of those with epilepsy. In R. Canger, F. Angeleri, & J. K. Perry (Eds.), *Advances in Epileptology: XIth Epilepsy International Symposium, 1980* (pp. 205–208). New York: Raven Press.

Meencke, H. J. (1985). Neuron density in the molecular layer of the frontal cortex in primary generalized epilepsy. *Epilepsia, 26,* 450–454.

Meencke, H. J. (1989). Pathology of childhood epilepsies. *Cleveland Clinic Journal of Medicine, 56*(Suppl. 1), S111–S120.

Morgan, A., & Groh, C. (1980). Changes in visual perception in children with epilepsy. In B. Kulig, H. Meinardi, & G. Stores (Eds.), *Epilepsy and behavior, 1979.* Lisse, The Netherlands: Swets & Zeitlinger.

Murphy, J. V., & Dehkharghani, F. (1994). Diagnosis of childhood seizure disorders. *Epilepsia, 35*(Suppl. 2), S6–S17.

Novelly, R. A., Augustine, E. A., Mattson, R. H., Glaser, G. H., Williamson, P. D., Spencer, D. D., & Spencer, S. S. (1984). Selective memory improvement and impairment in temporal lobectomy for epilepsy. *Annals of Neurology, 15,* 64–67.

O'Leary, D. S., Lovell, M. R., Sackellares, J. C., Berent, S., Giordani, B., Seidenberg, M., & Boll, T. J. (1983). Effects of age of onset of partial and generalized seizures on neuropsychological performance in children. *Journal of Nervous and Mental Disease, 171,* 624–629.

Panayiotopoulos, C. P., & Obeid, T. (1989). Juvenile myoclonic epilepsy: An autosomal recessive disease. *Annals of Neurology, 25,* 440–443.

Panayiotopoulos, C. P., Obeid, T., & Tahan, A. R. (1994). Juvenile myoclonic epilepsy: A 5-year prospective study. *Epilepsia, 35,* 285–296.

Prevey, M. L., Delaney, R. C., & Mattson, R. H. (1988). Metamemory in temporal lobe epilepsy: Self monitoring of memory functions. *Brain and Cognition, 7,* 298–311.

Quadfasel, A. F., & Pruyser, P. W. (1955). Cognitive deficits in patients with psychomotor epilepsy. *Epilepsia, 4,* 80–90.

Quattlebaum, T. G. (1979). Benign familial convulsions in the neonatal period and early infancy. *Journal of Pediatrics, 95,* 257–259.

Reitan, R. M. (1974). Psychological testing of epileptic patients. In O. Magnus & L. de Haas (Eds.), *Handbook of clinical neurology: Vol. 15. The epilepsies* (pp. 559–575). Amsterdam: Elsevier.

Reitan, R. M., & Wolfson, D. (1985). *The Halstead–Reitan Neuropsychological Test Battery: Theory and clinical interpretation* (2nd ed.). Tucson, AZ: Neuropsychology Press.

Reynolds, E. H., & Trimble, M. R. (1985). Adverse neuropsychiatric effects of anticonvulsant drugs. *Drugs, 29,* 570–581.

Rodin, E. (1984). Epileptic and pseudoepileptic seizures: Differential diagnostic considerations. In D. Blumer (Ed.), *Psychiatric aspects of epilepsy* (pp. 179–195). Washington, DC: American Psychiatric Press.

Ryan, S. G., Wiznitzer, M., & Hollman, C. (1991). Benign familial neonatal convulsions: Evidence for clinical and genetic heterogeneity. *Annals of Neurology, 29,* 469–473.

Scarpa, P., & Carassini, B. (1982). Partial epilepsy in childhood: Clinical and EEG study in 261 cases. *Epilepsia, 23,* 333–341.

Schulte, F. J. (1966). Neonatal convulsions and their relation to epilepsy in early childhood. *Developmental Medicine and Child Neurology, 8,* 381–392.

Schwartzkroin, P. A., MoshÄ, S. L., Noebels, J. L. & Swann, J. W. (1995). *Brain development and epilepsy.* New York: Oxford University Press.

Serratosa, J. M., & Delgado-Escueta, A. V. (1993). Juvenile myoclonic epilepsy. In E. Wyllie (Ed.). *The treatment of epilepsy: Principles and practice* (pp. 552–570). Philadelphia: Lea & Febinger.

Upton, D., & Corcoran, R. (1995). The role of the right temporal lobe in card sorting: A case study. *Cortex, 31,* 405–409.

Varga-Khadem, F., Carr, L. J., Isaacs, E., Brett, E., Adams, C., & Mishkin, M. (1997). Onset of speech after left hemispherectomy in a nine-year-old boy. *Brain, 120,* 159–182.

Volpe, J. J. (1987). *Neurology of the newborn* (2nd ed.). Philadelphia: W. B. Saunders.

Volpe, J. J. (1989). Neonatal seizures: Current concepts and revised classification. *Pediatrics, 84,* 422–428.

Walker, A. E., & Blumer, D. (1984). Behavioral effects of temporal lobectomy for temporal lobe epilepsy. In D. Blumer (Ed.), *Psychiatric aspects of epilepsy* (pp. 295–323). Washington, DC: American Psychiatric Press.

Waxman, S. A., & Geschwind, N. (1980). Hypergraphia in temporal lobe epilepsy. *Neurology, 30,* 314–317.

Williams, J., & Haut, J. S. (1995). Differential performances on the WRAML in children and adolescents diagnosed with epilepsy, head injury, and substance abuse. *Developmental Neuropsychology, 11,* 201–213.

Williams, J., Sharp, G., Lange, B., Bates, S., Griebel, M., Spence, G. T., & Thomas, P. (1996). The effects of seizure type, level of seizure control, and antiepileptic drugs on memory and attention skills in children with epilepsy. *Developmental Neuropsychology, 12,* 241–253.

Wilson, A., Petty, R., Perry, A., & Rose, R. C. (1983). Paroxysmal language disturbance in an epileptic treated with clobazam. *Neurology, 33,* 652–654.

Wilson, B. A., Ivani-Chalain, R., Besag, F. M. C., & Bryant, T. (1993). Adapting the Rivermead Behavioural Memory Test for use with children aged 5 to 10 years. *Journal of Clinical and Experimental Neuropsychology, 15,* 474–486.

Wolf, P. (1985). Juvenile myoclonic epilepsy. In J. Roger, C. Dravet, M. Bureau, F. E. Dreifuss, & P. Wolf (Eds.), *Epileptic syndromes in infancy, childhood and adolescence* (pp. 247–258). London: John Libbey.

23

PRADER–WILLI SYNDROME

ELISABETH M. DYKENS
SUZANNE B. CASSIDY

Prader–Willi syndrome is a complex, multisystem disorder whose intriguing genetic and behavioral features have attracted renewed interest from researchers and clinicians alike. The major manifestations of Prader–Willi syndrome include hypotonia; early failure to thrive, followed by later excessive appetite and obesity; hypogonadism; short stature; characteristic appearance; developmental disability; and significant behavioral dysfunction. Approximately 1 in 10,000 to 15,000 individuals is diagnosed with Prader–Willi syndrome (Burd, Vesely, Martsolf, & Kerbeshian, 1990), and it occurs in both sexes and all races.

Prader–Willi syndrome was first described in 1956 (Prader, Labhart, & Willi, 1956). Twenty-five years later, the syndrome captured the interest of human geneticists because it was the first syndrome that was found to be caused by a small missing piece of chromosomal material called a "microdeletion"; this discovery was made by researchers using the newly developed technique of high-resolution chromosome analysis (Ledbetter et al., 1981). Prader–Willi syndrome is now known to be one of the most common microdeletion syndromes, one of the most frequent disorders seen in genetics clinics, and the most common recognized genetic form of obesity.

Prader–Willi syndrome is also the first recognized human disorder in which it was appreciated that the relevant genes are expressed differently, depending upon whether they are inherited from the mother or the father (Nicholls, Knoll, Butler, Karam, & Lalande, 1989). This phenomenon of differential gene expression is known as "genomic imprinting." In addition, Prader–Willi syndrome is distinctive in being caused by several different genetic alterations of the relevant chromosomal region, which is the long arm of chromosome 15. Prader–Willi syndrome thus occupies an important place in the contemporary history of human genetic disorders.

Clinical diagnostic criteria for Prader–Willi syndrome have been developed (Holm et al., 1993), and accurate, specific genetic testing has recently become available (American Society of Human Genetics [ASHG] & American College of Medical Genetics [ACMG],

1996). However, the diagnosis is still delayed in many cases because of a failure to recognize the syndrome's characteristic physical and behavioral manifestations. In addition to a distinctive physical phenotype, Prader–Willi syndrome has a characteristic behavioral phenotype, which includes a blend of unusual cognitive findings, psychiatric vulnerabilities, and maladaptive behaviors (e.g., temper tantrums and argumentativeness). These features are as important to quality of life and morbidity as are some of the syndrome's medical problems, and they are often the focus of intervention and treatment (Cassidy, 1984; Holm et al., 1993; Dykens, Hodapp, Walsh, & Nash, 1992b; Dykens & Cassidy, 1995).

Since its identification over 40 years ago, then, Prader–Willi syndrome has emerged as a complicated disorder that highlights the need for a multidisciplinary approach to research and management. This chapter reviews many aspects of Prader–Willi syndrome, including its medical, genetic, cognitive, behavioral, developmental, and psychiatric features. As appropriate management often has a positive impact on the health and quality of life of people affected with Prader–Willi syndrome, the chapter also summarizes commonly used medical and behavioral interventions, especially those aimed at controlling the syndrome's characteristic obesity and behavioral/psychiatric dysfunction.

CLINICAL FINDINGS AND NATURAL HISTORY

Although many of the physical manifestations of Prader–Willi syndrome are related to functional hypothalamic deficiency, the disorder's clinical appearance in infancy differs considerably from that in childhood and adulthood.

Hypotonia

Hypotonia of prenatal onset is nearly uniformly present and is the likely cause of decreased fetal movement, frequent abnormal fetal position, and difficulty at the time of delivery, often necessitating cesarean section (Cassidy, 1984; Holm et al., 1993). The neonatal central hypotonia is almost invariably associated with poor suck, with consequent failure to thrive and the necessity for gavage or other special feeding techniques. Infantile lethargy, with decreased arousal and weak cry, are also prominent findings, often leading to the necessity to awaken the child to feed. Reflexes may be decreased or absent. Neuromuscular electrophysiological and biopsy studies are normal or nonspecific, and the hypotonia gradually improves. Delayed motor milestones are evident; the average age of sitting is 12 months and of walking is 24 months. Adults remain mildly hypotonic, with decreased muscle bulk and tone.

Hypogonadism

Hypogonadism is prenatal in onset (Lee, 1995), and is evident at birth as small genitalia. Males generally have undescended testes; a small, hypopigmented, and poorly rugated scrotum; and sometimes a small penis. In females, the labia minora and clitoris are small. These findings persist throughout life, though spontaneous descent of testes has been observed up to adolescence. There is also evidence of hypogonadism in abnormal pubertal development. Although pubic and axillary hair may develop early or normally, the remainder of pubertal development is delayed and usually incomplete. Adult males only occasionally have voice change, male body habitus, or substantial facial or body hair. In females, breast development generally begins at a normal age, but menstrual periods are either absent or infrequent (and, if occurring, they are late in onset). In both males and females, sexual activity is relatively rare, and infertility is the rule.

The hypogonadism is hypothalamic in origin, and both pituitary and gonadal hormones are generally deficient (Cassidy, 1984; Lee, 1995). Since the pituitary gland and gonads are normal but understimulated, treatment with pituitary or gonadal hormones can increase the development of secondary sex characteristics.

Obesity

Obesity is the major cause of morbidity and mortality in Prader–Willi syndrome, and longevity may be nearly normal if obesity is avoided (Greenswag, 1987; Cassidy, Devi, & Mukaida, 1994). Significant weight excess, if allowed to occur, follows the early period of failure to thrive; the onset of excessive eating, or hyperphagia, typically begins between 1 and 6 years of age. Food-seeking behaviors are common, including hoarding or foraging for food; eating unappealing substances such as garbage, pet food, and frozen food; and stealing food or money to buy food. Low muscle tone and a disinclination to exercise add to the effects of the drive to eat excessively. A high threshold for vomiting may complicate bingeing on spoiled food from the garbage or items such as boxes of sugar or frozen uncooked meat. Toxicity has occurred from ineffective ipecac used to induce vomiting.

As shown in Figure 23.1, the obesity in Prader–Willi syndrome is central in distribution, with relative sparing of the distal extremities; even individuals who are not overweight tend to deposit fat on the abdomen, buttocks, and thighs. Cardiopulmonary compromise results from excessive obesity, as can type II diabetes mellitus, hypertension, thrombophlebitis, and chronic leg edema. Sleep apnea occurs at increased frequency.

The hyperphagia in Prader–Willi syndrome is due to a hypothalamic abnormality resulting in lack of satiety (Zipf & Bernston, 1987; Holland et al., 1993). In addition, there is a decreased caloric requirement (Holm & Pipes, 1976), probably related to hypotonia and decreased activity.

Facial Features

Characteristic facial features are either present from birth or evolve over time (Aughton & Cassidy, 1990). As shown in Figure 23.2, facial features include narrow bifrontal diameter, almond-shaped palpebral fissures, narrow nasal bridge, and downturned mouth with a thin upper lip. Small, narrow hands with a straight ulnar border and sometimes tapering fingers are usually present by age 10, as are short, often broad feet, with an average adult female shoe size of 3 and male shoe size of 5 (Hudgins, McKillop, & Cassidy, 1991). African Americans with Prader–Willi syndrome are less likely to have small hands and feet, and they may also lack the typical facial phenotype (Cassidy, Geer, Holm, & Hudgins, 1996).

A characteristic body habitus, including sloping shoulders, heavy midsection, and genu valgus with straight lower leg borders, is usually present from toddlerhood (see Figure 23.1). Fairer coloring than other family members, manifested as lighter skin, hair, and eye color,

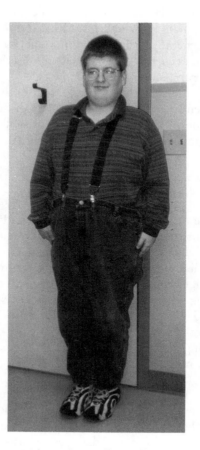

FIGURE 23.1. A 27-year-old man with Prader–Willi syndrome. Note the narrow bifrontal diameter and typical body habitus, with central obesity and small hands. Photograph used by permission of the patient and his family.

occurs in about a third of affected individuals (Butler, 1989). Strabismus is often present. Scoliosis, kyphosis, or both are common; the former can occur at any age, and the latter develops in early adulthood.

Short Stature

Birth weight and length are usually within normal limits, but the early period of failure to thrive may mean that both weight and length fall below the 3rd centile. Short stature, if not apparent in childhood, is almost always present by the second half of the second decade, associated with lack of a pubertal growth spurt. Average height is 155 cm for males and 148 cm for females. African Americans tend to be taller (Cassidy et al., 1996). Growth hormone deficiency has been demonstrated in most tested patients with Prader–Willi syndrome, and treatment with growth hormone increases height and lean body mass, often resulting in decreased body mass index (Lee, 1995; Angulo et al., 1996).

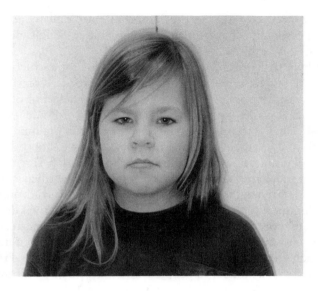

FIGURE 23.2. Face of a typical 10-year-old girl with Prader–Willi syndrome. Note the relatively narrow bifrontal diameter, almond-shaped eyes, and downturned corners of the mouth. Photograph used by permission of the patient's family.

Other Medical Issues

Numerous more minor physical findings characterize this condition, including thick, viscous saliva that may predispose to dental caries and contribute to articulation abnormalities; high pain threshold; skin picking; and high threshold for vomiting. Sleep disturbances, especially excessive daytime sleepiness and oxygen desaturation in rapid-eye-movement sleep, are common even in the absence of obesity (Hertz, Cataletto, Feinsilver, & Angulo, 1995). Osteoporosis is also frequent.

Despite the multisystem nature of Prader–Willi syndrome, people with this condition generally enjoy good health if morbid obesity is avoided. Indeed, parents often report that their child with Prader–Willi syndrome is healthier than the child's unaffected siblings.

ORIGIN AND GENETIC BASIS

Since the first description of Prader–Willi syndrome, it has been apparent that many of its features arise from insufficient function of the hypothalamus. Thus many of the functions of this part of the brain are disturbed in Prader–Willi syndrome, including control of homeostatic functions such as hunger, thirst, sleep–wake cycles, and temperature regulation. The hypothalamus also releases hormones that travel to the pituitary gland, controlling the release of other hormones such as growth hormone, the sex hormones (gonadotropins), and thyroid-stimulating hormones (which regulate basal metabolic rate). Studies of the destruction of the hypothalamus in animals, particularly cats, show that many of the functional abnormalities seen in Prader–Willi syndrome occur in these animals. Prader–Willi syndrome symptoms are seen as well in cases of previously normal persons with acquired damage to the hypothalamus due to an injury, stroke, or tumor. Even the personality characteristics seen in Prader–Willi syndrome, including the temper tantrums, may result.

Because the hypothalamus was a logical place to look for a structural defect in Prader–Willi syndrome, the few reported autopsy studies have focused on that part of the brain. Unfortunately, no visible gross or microscopic structural defect or other abnormality has been documented that could explain the clinical features of Prader–Willi syndrome. The hypothalamic deficiency is thus likely to be functional, with preliminary findings suggesting altered function of oxytocin-secreting neurons (putative satiety cells) in the hypothalamic paraventricular nucleus (Swaab, Purba, & Hofman, 1995).

Although the exact hypothalamic deficit has yet to be identified, considerable progress has been made in identifying the genetic basis of Prader–Willi syndrome. At the end of the 1970s, a new technique, high-resolution chromosome banding, was developed for analyzing chromosomes in more detail than was previously possible. This technique operates by capturing the chromosome in an earlier stage of the cell cycle, when it is more elongated, thus allowing much greater visibility of fine chromosome structure. Prior to this time, researchers had noted that a number of people with Prader–Willi syndrome had a rearrangement of the chromosomes that involved chromosome 15. Using the new technique of high-resolution chromosome analysis, Ledbetter et al. (1981) reported the presence of a small deletion within the long arm of chromosome 15—called del 15(q11–13) in standard chromosome nomenclature—in about half the people with Prader–Willi syndrome whom they studied. This deletion was found to represent a new change in the affected individual (*de novo* deletion), since neither parent was found to have it. Subsequently, many workers studied series of patients to further delineate the exact location and frequency of the deletion, which is now known to occur in approximately 70% of those with Prader–Willi syndrome (ASHG & ACMG, 1996; Butler, 1996). With a few exceptions, the remainder of patients with Prader–Willi syndrome have normal-appearing chromosomes under the microscope.

The development of molecular genetic technology in the late 1980s allowed determination of the basis for Prader–Willi syndrome in patients with normal chromosomes. First, molecular techniques allowed investigators to confirm the observation previously made under the microscope that the deletion, when it was found, occurred solely in the paternally inherited chromosome 15, even though the blood chromosomes of the father were normal (Butler, 1990; Nicholls et al., 1989). Second, as expected, it was determined that some people who did not have a deletion visible with chromosomal techniques did have a deletion with the more accurate molecular techniques (Delach et al., 1994). However, this was the case in only a small proportion of individuals without a visible deletion. More interestingly, a seminal study by Nicholls et al. (1989) found via molecular techniques that most of the remaining patients without a deletion had two maternally derived chromosome 15s and no paternally derived chromosome 15—a situation called "uniparental disomy" (UPD). Thus, instead of inheriting one paternal and one maternal chromosome 15 (which is the usual situation), people with Prader–Willi syndrome who do not have a deletion have the syndrome because they have received no paternal chromosome 15, but instead have two maternal chromosome 15s. The chromosomes themselves are normal in number and structure, but the inheritance pattern is wrong.

In effect, whether there is a paternal deletion or maternal UPD, Prader–Willi syndrome results from the lack of paternal contribution to the specific region of chromosome 15's long arm associated with this disorder. Sometimes a person with Prader–Willi syndrome due to maternal UPD has two copies of the same member of the maternal chromosome 15 pair (isodisomy), sometimes both members of the maternal chromosome 15 pair (hetero-disomy), and sometimes a complicated combination of the two. However, the composition of the maternal chromosomes really does not affect the end result, since all the chromosome 15s are normal.

The genetic findings in Prader–Willi syndrome can be explained by a phenomenon called "genomic imprinting." This is a process whereby genes or groups of neighboring genes are modified differently, and thereby expressed differently, depending upon the sex of the parent from whom they were inherited. The genes themselves are not altered, since imprinting is a reversible process. Rather, some genes are inactivated or switched off, so that they no longer produce RNA and then protein in the process of decoding that consti-tutes gene expression. Although imprinting has been recognized for several years in some genes of other animals and plants, Prader–Willi syndrome was the first human disorder in which it was recognized. Several other human conditions have subsequently been found to be related to imprinting. The maternally derived copies of chromosome 15 in the region critical for Prader–Willi syndrome are inactivated in the normal situation, and only the paternally derived region is expressed in cells. When the paternal copy of this region is missing—by deletion or by complete absence, as in maternal UPD—there is no active copy of the genetic information and an abnormality in development therefore results in Prader–Willi syndrome (Nicholls, 1993).

Thus, again, Prader–Willi syndrome is caused by the absence of the normally active paternally inherited genes at chromosome 15(q11–13). In about 70% of cases, it is due to a deletion; in most individuals the deletion is of the same size, with the same breakpoints on the chromosome. Most of the remaining patients have maternal UPD for chromosome 15 (Nicholls et al., 1989; Robinson et al., 1991; Mascari et al., 1992). Approximately 5% of patients with Prader–Willi syndrome have a translocation or other structural abnor-mality involving chromosome 15 that has caused either a deletion or maternal UPD for the critical region. UPD usually affects the whole chromosome 15, but it is only the small region of imprinted genes related to Prader–Willi syndrome where it matters which parent the chromosome comes from.

Approximately 1–5% of patients with Prader–Willi syndrome—including virtually all studied families in which there has been a recurrence of Prader–Willi syndrome—have neither deletion nor UPD, but rather have a very small deletion in the center controlling the imprinting process within 15q11–13 (Buiting et al., 1994; Saitoh et al., 1997). Methyl-ation is one mechanism by which genomic imprinting can occur, and methylation has been demonstrated for several genes identified within the Prader–Willi critical region. Interest-ingly, a clinically very different disorder, Angelman syndrome, is the result of an oppo-sitely imprinted gene in the same region of chromosome 15 (Williams et al., 1995). In contrast to Prader–Willi syndrome, people with Angelman syndrome typically have severe to profound mental retardation, limited expressive language, seizure disorder, an ataxic gait, and bouts of inappropriate laughter.

Several genes have been mapped within the Prader–Willi/Angelman region, and oth-ers that are not maternally inactivated have been mapped between the common deletion breakpoints. The first mapped gene, considered an important candidate gene, is small nuclear ribonucleoprotein N (*SNRPN*). This gene is expressed from the paternally inher-ited chromosome only (Ozcelik et al., 1992; Glenn et al., 1996), and is expressed abun-dantly in the brain. The other identified genes are currently of unknown function. The nonimprinted *P* gene, which also resides in this region, codes for tyrosinase-positive albi-nism, and its deletion probably causes the hypopigmentation seen in one-third of patients with Prader–Willi syndrome (Spritz et al., 1997).

Recently, some clinical differences have been reported between patients with Prader–Willi syndrome due to deletion versus UPD (Gillessen-Kaesbach et al., 1995; Mitchell et al., 1996; Cassidy et al., 1997). Perhaps the most clinically significant of these are that patients with UPD may lack the typical facial phenotype (Cassidy et al., 1997), and that they may have delayed diagnosis (Gunay-Aygun & Cassidy, 1997).

DIAGNOSIS, DIFFERENTIAL DIAGNOSIS, AND DIAGNOSTIC TESTING

Prior to the availability of complete sensitive and specific laboratory testing, diagnostic criteria for Prader–Willi syndrome were developed through a consensus process (Holm et al., 1993). These criteria, listed in Table 23.1, are still extremely valuable in suggesting the diagnosis and indicating the need for diagnostic testing. It should be emphasized that no one individual will have all the manifestations of the disorder, and that there is considerable variability in the severity of each of the findings.

The differential diagnosis for Prader–Willi syndrome in infancy includes many causes of neonatal hypotonia, particularly neuromuscular disorders. Later in childhood and adulthood, a number of conditions involving mental retardation with associated obesity may be included in the differential diagnosis, including Bardet–Biedl syndrome, Albright hereditary osteodystrophy, and Cohen syndrome (see Gunay-Aygun, Cassidy, & Nicholls, 1997, for a review). Mental retardation disorders in which obesity is an occasional finding, such as fragile X, Smith–Magenis, and Angelman syndromes, may also be confused with Prader–Willi syndrome. Acquired hypothalamic injury from accidents, tumors, or surgical complications can closely mimic Prader–Willi syndrome.

TABLE 23.1. Summary of the Clinical Diagnostic Criteria for Prader–Willi Syndrome

Major criteria (1 point each)	Minor criteria (½ point each)	Supportive criteria (no points)
Infantile central hypotonia	Decreased fetal movement and infantile lethargy	High pain threshold
Infantile feeding problems/failure to thrive	Typical behavior problems	Decreased vomiting
Rapid weight gain between 1 and 6 years	Sleep disturbance/sleep apnea	Temperature control problems
Characteristic facial features	Short stature for the family by age 15 years	Scoliosis and/or kyphosis
Hypogonadism: genital hypoplasia, pubertal deficiency	Hypopigmentation	Early adrenarche
Developmental delay/mental retardation	Small hands and feet for height, age	Osteoporosis
	Narrow hands with straight ulnar border	Unusual skill with jigsaw puzzles
	Esotropia, myopia	Normal neuromuscular studies
	Thick, viscous saliva	
	Speech articulation difficulties	
	Skin picking	

Note. The diagnosis should be strongly suspected in children under 3 years of age with 5 points, 3 from major criteria; or in those above 3 years with 8 points, 4 from major criteria. The original diagnostic criteria, developed before the availability of sensitive and specific genetic testing, included a major criteria of chromosome 15 deletion or other chromosome 15 anomaly. Items from Holm et al. (1993).

Two important organizations in genetic research, the ASHG and the ACMG, published a statement in 1996 regarding the status of genetic testing for Prader–Willi and Angelman syndromes. Currently, the most efficient molecular diagnostic test for Prader–Willi syndrome examines the parent-specific methylation pattern within the Prader–Willi/Angelman region, using Southern hybridization and methylation-sensitive probes (*SNRPN* and *PW71*) (ASHG & ACMG, 1996). If the methylation pattern is characteristic of maternal-only inheritance, Prader–Willi syndrome is confirmed; if not, Prader–Willi due to deletion, UPD, or an imprinting mutation is ruled out. Knowing whether the Prader–Willi syndrome is due to deletion, UPD, or an imprinting mutation is important for genetic counseling purposes, as well as for identifying those few cases with a translocation or inherited microdeletion. High-resolution cytogenetic analysis can often detect the 15q11–13 deletion; however, this technique has unacceptably high false-negative and false-positive rates, and it is no longer considered sufficient for diagnostic purposes. The definitive diagnostic test for the common size deletion causing Prader–Willi syndrome is fluorescent *in situ* hybridization (FISH), using probes within the Prader–Willi/Angelman critical region (*SNRPN* or *D15S11*). UPD can be detected with polymerase chain reaction, using informative microsatellite markers from the Prader–Willi/Angelman region by studying both parents and the child. Additional markers from other chromosomes can confirm correct paternity.

Prenatal detection of Prader–Willi syndrome is now possible. FISH is indicated when a cytogenetic 15q deletion is suspected after chorionic villus sampling (CVS) or amniocentesis. If trisomy 15 is detected on CVS and the fetus survives, parent-of-origin studies (methylation analysis or microsatellite marker) are indicated and validated (Christian et al., 1996; Kubota et al., 1996). FISH and parent-of-origin studies are also indicated if an inherited or *de novo* translocation involving chromosome 15 is detected prenatally. Parents should be studied in cases with an identified imprinting mutation, since a healthy parent can carry this abnormality and be at increased risk for recurrence (Saitoh et al., 1997). Prenatal detection is possible through identification of the mutation or maternal-only methylation pattern in a fetus (Kubota et al., 1996).

Prader–Willi syndrome due either to the large deletion in the absence of a structural chromosome abnormality or to UPD has not been reported to recur, though a theoretical recurrence risk of approximately 1% or less is appropriate for genetic counseling purposes. UPD is caused by nondisjunction, as evidenced by advanced maternal age in this group (Robinson et al., 1991; Mascari et al., 1992), and by documentation of cases of trisomy 15 on CVS and maternal UPD at birth. Since nondisjunction can recur, a recurrence risk of 1% is appropriate for genetic counseling. In families with an imprinting mutation, a recurrence risk of up to 50% pertains, as this probably involves a dominant mutation in the paternal grandmother's germ line.

In many ways, then, Prader–Willi syndrome is a model genetic disorder—the source of remarkable new genetic discoveries. Now cast as the most common recognized genetic form of obesity, Prader–Willi has also made genetic history by being the first recognized human disease associated with UPD, with genomic imprinting, and with a clinically distinct yet genetically related "sister" syndrome (Angelman syndrome). Furthermore, the search for specific genes in the Prader–Willi/Angelman critical region is now well underway.

In contrast to these genetic advances, we know much less about Prader–Willi's complex cognitive and behavioral phenotype. Findings to date, however, suggest that Prader–Willi syndrome is also a promising condition for studying behavioral phenotypes of mental retardation syndromes in general (Dykens, 1995). As described in the remainder of the chapter, many people with Prader–Willi syndrome show a blend of unusual cognitive styles, maladaptive behaviors, and psychiatric vulnerabilities that may prove unique, and that open up specific avenues of treatment and intervention.

COGNITIVE, ADAPTIVE, AND BEHAVIORAL PHENOTYPE

Cognitive and Adaptive Functioning

Cognitive and Adaptive Levels

The average IQ reported in most studies of people with Prader–Willi syndrome is about 70 (e.g., Dykens, Hodapp, Walsh, & Nash, 1992a). The mean IQ in Prader–Willi syndrome is thus high relative to those in other genetic disorders, including prevalent conditions such as fragile X syndrome (Dykens, Hodapp, & Leckman, 1994) or Down syndrome (Hodapp, 1996), and less prevalent disorders, such as 5p– syndrome (Dykens & Clarke, 1997) or Smith–Magenis syndrome (Dykens, Finucane, & Gayley, 1997).

Although on average people with Prader–Willi syndrome show mild levels of mental retardation, their IQ scores range from average to profoundly mentally retarded. Extrapolating IQ data from 575 subjects in 57 published studies, Curfs (1992) found that 34% showed mild mental retardation, 27% had moderate delays, and only 6% showed severe to profound levels of impairment. Approximately one-third of subjects were relatively high-functioning, or with IQs above 70; 27% showed borderline levels of intelligence (IQs of 70 to 84); and 5% showed average IQ scores.

Even high-functioning individuals, however, rarely perform adaptively at a level commensurate with their IQs. Adaptive functioning is typically viewed as the performance of behaviors required for personal or social sufficiency (Sparrow, Balla, & Cicchetti, 1984). Clinical observations in Prader–Willi syndrome often suggest impaired adaptive functioning, yet only one study has formally assessed adaptive behavior in this population. Dykens et al. (1992b) administered a standardized assessment instrument, the Vineland Adaptive Behavior Scales (Sparrow et al., 1984), to caregivers of 21 adolescents and young adults with Prader–Willi syndrome. These subjects showed adaptive behavior composite standard scores that ranged from 20 to 50, all in the moderate to severe range of delay. The mean Vineland composite standard score was 37, which fell more than two standard deviations (31 points) below subjects' mean IQ of 68. As discussed later, low adaptive performance is probably associated with interference from significant behavioral dysfunction and a persistent drive to eat.

Cognitive Level and Weight

Early work in Prader–Willi syndrome suggested a significant inverse correlation between IQ and weight (Crnic, Sulzbacher, Snow, & Holm, 1980), with lower IQ scores associated with increased weight. It was even suggested that prevention of obesity might also prevent mental retardation. Yet common lore in the Prader–Willi syndrome community actually suggests the opposite relation—that brighter individuals may be more clever or ingenious about obtaining food, and are thus at increased risk of obesity. Recent data do not support either hypothesis: Dykens et al. (1992a) found no significant relations between IQ and body mass index (a measure of obesity). Persons with relatively high versus low IQ scores thus seem similarly vulnerable to the syndrome's problems with obesity.

Cognitive Profiles

Early clinical observations suggested that many children with Prader–Willi syndrome showed significant relative strengths in reading and weaknesses in arithmetic (e.g., Holm, 1981; Sulzbacher, Crnic, & Snow, 1981). These informal observations led to the idea that cognition in Prader–Willi syndrome was best characterized by uneven academic performance, as found in youngsters with learning disabilities.

Achievement studies, however, do not provide overwhelming support for a specific learning disability profile in Prader–Willi syndrome. Administering the Kaufman Assessment Battery for Children (K-ABC; Kaufman & Kaufman, 1984) to 21 adolescents and adults with Prader–Willi syndrome, Dykens et al. (1992a) found a nonsignificant discrepancy in age-equivalent scores in arithmetic versus reading (7.68 years vs. 8.55 years, respectively). Furthermore, Taylor (1988) examined an unspecified number of individuals with Prader–Willi syndrome, and reported a mean standard achievement test score of 70 in math and 73 in reading. Such findings only hint at uneven academic performance. Clearly, more studies are needed on the extent to which individuals with Prader–Willi syndrome show discrepancies across areas of academic achievement, as well as between achievement and IQ.

Only a few studies have moved beyond academic achievement to identify other aspects of cognitive processing in people with Prader–Willi syndrome. Examining global cognitive patterns on Wechsler-based tests, Borghgraef, Fryns, and Van den Berghe (1990) reported "great differences" (p. 148) in Verbal versus Performance IQ scores in 8 of their 12 subjects with Prader–Willi syndrome. Three of these individuals showed at least a 15-point discrepancy in favor of the Verbal IQ. Significant Verbal versus Performance IQ differences were also found in a study of 26 children with Prader–Willi syndrome, aged 7 to 15 years; 10 subjects showed elevations in the Performance IQ, and 3 in the Verbal IQ (Curfs, Wiegers, Sommers, Borghgraef, & Fryns, 1991). Findings are thus inconsistent, with perhaps a slight favoring of the Performance IQ.

More detailed studies of specific cognitive processes shed some light on these inconsistent findings. Table 23.2 summarizes these studies. Taylor (1988) compared Wechsler subtests in an unspecified number of subjects with Prader–Willi syndrome to a sample of obese, mentally retarded individuals without Prader–Willi syndrome. The two groups showed comparable subtest scores, with just one exception: Relative to the obese controls, subjects with Prader–Willi syndrome showed significantly higher scores on Block Design, a task tapping visual–motor integration. Similarly, Curfs et al. (1991) found that one-half of their sample showed significant WISC-R subtest scatter, and that 9 of these 13 children had relative strengths in Block Design. These findings suggest strengths in some individuals in perceptual–spatial organization and visual–motor integration.

Consistent with these strengths, many people with Prader–Willi syndrome show an unusual facility with jigsaw puzzles. This skill is so striking that it is noted as a supportive finding in the consensus diagnostic criteria for Prader–Willi syndrome (Holm et al., 1993). Clinically, we observe as well that many adolescents and young adults have a strong propensity for "word search" puzzles, often carrying their word-finding books with them to school or work. We also found that subject performance on a visual memory task was correlated with parental reports of subject interest and facility with jigsaw and word search puzzles. Additional studies are needed that better relate facility with puzzles to cognitive profiles, and that determine exactly how widespread puzzle-solving skills are in the Prader–Willi population.

Visual processing strengths are also suggested by Gabel et al. (1986), who administered a battery of attentional, visual–spatial, and psychomotor tasks to 15 children with

TABLE 23.2. Summary of Cognitive and Adaptive Studies in People with Prader–Willi Syndrome

Study	Number and age of subjects	Key findings
Cognitive processing		
Curfs et al. (1991)	26 PWS, 7–15 years	WISC-R Performance IQ > Verbal IQ in 10 subjects. Verbal IQ > Performance IQ in 3 subjects. Block Design high in 9 subjects.
Dykens et al. (1992a)	21 PWS, 13–26 years 31 PWS, 5–30 years	K-ABC Simultaneous Processing > Sequential Processing. Strengths: Visual perceptual. Weaknesses: Visual–motor short-term memory. Stable IQ in childhood and adulthood.
Gabel et al. (1986)	15 PWS, *M* = 12 years 15 normal controls	Normals exceeded PWS on all measures. For PWS on Detroit Test of Learning Aptitude, visual recall of objects, letters > auditory recall of words.
Taylor (1988)	Unspecified PWS Obese, retarded controls	On WISC-R, PWS > controls on Block Design only.
Warren & Hunt (1981)	11 PWS, age unknown 12 nonspecific, matched on age and IQ	On pictorial memory tasks, PWS < nonspecific in visual short-term memory; PWS had no improvements in Performance with increasing age or IQ; PWS on par with nonspecific in long-term memory for well-known information.
Adaptive behavior		
Dykens et al. (1992b)	21 PWS, 13–26 years	On Vineland, strengths in Daily Living Skills (especially domestic skills), weaknesses in Socialization (especially coping skills); modest increases in adaptive skills with advancing age.

Note. PWS, Prader–Willi syndrome; WISC-R, Wechsler Intelligence Scale for Children—Revised; K-ABC, Kaufman Assessment Battery for Children.

Prader–Willi syndrome and 15 age- and sex-matched normal children. Not surprisingly, the Prader–Willi group scored consistently lower than the normal controls; however, they also showed discrepancies in scores on subtests of the Detroit Tests of Learning Aptitude (Baker & Leland, 1967). Specifically, the Prader–Willi subjects had relatively low scores on tasks assessing auditory attention and recall for words, and high scores on tasks measuring visual attention and recall for objects and letters. Gabel et al. (1986) conclude that youngsters with Prader–Willi syndrome may have strengths in visual processing relative to auditory processing.

Further work clarifies and expands certain aspects of the apparent strengths in visual processing. In the administration of the K-ABC to 21 subjects, Dykens et al. (1992a) found that Simultaneous Processing was better developed than Sequential Processing. High scores were noted in tasks assessing perceptual closure, long-term memory, spatial organization, attention to visual detail, and visual–motor integration. Among the Sequential Processing tasks, which rely on short-term memory, subjects showed particular difficulties with visual–motor and auditory–visual short-term memory. A profile is thus suggested for some individuals with Prader–Willi syndrome: relative strengths in perceptual organization, and difficulties in visual and other short-term memory tasks.

Indeed, visual processing strengths may not always be readily apparent, especially in short-term memory tasks. In a series of studies assessing pictorial short-term memory, Warren and Hunt (1981) compared 11 children with Prader–Willi syndrome to age- and

IQ-matched mentally retarded children with nonspecific etiologies. Relative to their mentally retarded counterparts, children with Prader–Willi syndrome showed more difficulties with immediate visual memory, no improvements in recall of stimuli with either increasing mental or chronological age, and a greater loss of information over time. In contrast to these short-term memory deficits, the Prader–Willi children performed on par with the nonspecific group in a long-term memory task assessing how quickly subjects recalled well-known information. Interestingly, parents often report that their offspring with Prader–Willi syndrome can recall well-known or more obscure facts with a remarkable level of detail (e.g., where people parked as they arrived for a family party years ago). As suggested by Warren and Hunt's (1981) findings, however, this type of recall is not likely to prove unique to Prader–Willi syndrome.

In summary, then, some people with Prader–Willi syndrome show relative strengths in spatial–perceptual organization and visual processing. Relative weaknesses may be apparent in short-term memory, including visual, motoric, and auditory short-term processing. Although findings suggest a distinctive cognitive profile, not all persons with Prader–Willi syndrome show this profile. Studies are needed that identify the range of cognitive profiles seen in Prader–Willi syndrome, including how variables such as age or IQ may relate to different cognitive patterns. Cognitive profiles identified to date in Prader–Willi syndrome may be shared among people with other genetic syndromes or with nonspecific etiologies. Additional comparative studies are thus necessary to settle the issue of whether Prader–Willi syndrome is associated with a unique profile of cognitive or academic strengths or weaknesses.

Adaptive Profiles

Deficits in specific domains of adaptive behavior are salient in the definition and diagnosis of mental retardation (see Hodapp & Dykens, 1994, for a review). Despite their nosological prominence, however, little is known about the adaptive strengths and weaknesses of people with specific syndromes, including those with Prader–Willi syndrome (Dykens, 1995). In one study of adolescents and adults with Prader–Willi syndrome, relative strengths were found on the Daily Living Skills domain of the Vineland Scales, especially in domestic skills such as cooking and cleaning (Dykens et al., 1992b). As noted in Table 23.2, these same subjects showed significant relative weaknesses in the socialization domain, notably in the coping skills subdomain.

Although distinctive, these profiles are not unique to Prader–Willi syndrome. Males with fragile X syndrome, for example, show relative strengths in Daily Living Skills on the Vineland (Dykens, Hodapp, & Leckman, 1994), and females with fragile X syndrome have relative weaknesses in Socialization (Freund, Reiss, & Abrams, 1993). However, the reasons for these similar profiles are likely to be different across syndromes. In individuals with Prader–Willi syndrome, strengths in cooking or cleaning seem consistent with interests in food, whereas these same skills in fragile X males may be related to the repetitive, rote nature of these daily living tasks (Dykens, Hodapp, & Leckman, 1994). The weaknesses in coping skills seen in Prader–Willi syndrome are likely to be associated with the impulsivity, temper tantrums, and compulsive tendencies that characterize this syndrome (Dykens & Cassidy, 1995). Among fragile X females, however, problems with Socialization are seen primarily in the interpersonal subdomain, and are probably related to that syndrome's proneness to shyness, gaze aversion, and social anxiety (Freund et al., 1993). Although Vineland profiles may thus be similar across these or other syndromes, the factors associated with these profiles are likely to be different.

Linguistic Profiles

Language development in children with Prader–Willi syndrome is typically delayed, though expressive vocabulary and language may eventually emerge as areas of strength for many youngsters with the syndrome. To date, only two studies have examined speech/language issues in people with Prader–Willi syndrome, and neither has found a distinctive linguistic profile. Branson (1981) found no common features in the language profiles of 21 children with Prader–Willi syndrome. Similarly, various linguistic profiles were observed in 18 children by Kleppe, Katayama, Shipley, and Foushee (1990). Differences were seen across subjects' severity of speech and language problems, and in the range of their intelligibility, fluency, and voice problems. Kleppe et al. (1990) did, however, find some common speech/language characteristics, primarily hypernasality, errors with certain speech sounds and complex syntax, and reduced vocabulary skills relative to age expectations. The speech and articulation difficulties are likely to be associated with hypotonia, and perhaps with thick, viscous saliva (Kleppe et al., 1990). Speech problems, primarily with articulation and intelligibility, were also noted by 33 out of 43 parents of children with Prader–Willi syndrome aged 4 to 19 years (Dykens & Kasari, 1997). In addition, individuals with Prader–Willi syndrome often talk too much and verbally perseverate on a narrow range of topics (Dykens, Leckman & Cassidy, 1996). It remains unknown, however, how perseveration relates to such linguistic features as pragmatics, discourse, and the social uses of language.

Cognitive and Adaptive Development

Data are limited on how cognition in people with Prader–Willi syndrome changes over the course of development. An early study of eight children with Prader–Willi syndrome reported that IQ declined in early childhood (Dunn, 1968). It was unclear, however, whether these declines were assessed by formal IQ tests or by a failure to achieve certain developmental milestones.

Using standardized IQ scores, Dykens et al. (1992a) conducted both cross-sectional and longitudinal analyses of IQ change in children and adults. IQ scores were cross-sectionally examined in 21 adolescents and adults, and longitudinal analyses included 31 subjects aged 5 to 30 years who had been given the same IQ test twice. IQ scores showed nonsignificant fluctuations in both cross-sectional and longitudinal analyses, with no evidence of IQ declines in childhood or early adulthood. Overall IQ scores thus appear relatively stable in school-age children with Prader–Willi syndrome, reflecting slow and steady gains in mental age that then stabilize in the adult years.

Regarding their levels of adaptive skills, adolescents and young adults with Prader–Willi syndrome seem to show steady gains in certain aspects of their adaptive behavior, primarily their daily living and socialization skills (Dykens et al., 1992b). Longitudinal studies are necessary to clarify these preliminary findings, as well as to identify how gains in adaptive skills relate to age, IQ, residential placement, and educational or vocational programming.

Findings to date thus point to a different course of cognitive and adaptive development in people with Prader–Willi syndrome, compared to people with some other genetic syndromes. Some children with Down syndrome, for example, show alternating periods of growth and stability in their cognitive, adaptive, and linguistic development (Dykens, Hodapp, & Evans, 1994; Hodapp & Zigler, 1990). Many males with fragile X syndrome show slow, steady gains in cognitive and adaptive functioning that seem to stabilize in late childhood or early adolescence, resulting in a plateau in mental age scores and decline in

IQ and adaptive behavior standard scores (Dykens, Hodapp, & Leckman, 1994). Different trajectories across Prader–Willi and other syndromes call into question the idea that people with mental retardation are uniform in their course of slowed development, regardless of their etiology (Silverstein, 1982).

In addition to comparative studies, longitudinal work is sorely needed that relates cognitive and adaptive development to the onset of hyperphagia in young children with Prader–Willi syndrome. No studies have yet been done that examine how the onset or severity of hyperphagia affects a young child's developing cognitive or behavioral schemas. Given the central role of hyperphagia in Prader–Willi syndrome, we suspect that this effect is far-reaching. It may be, for example, that the young child with Prader–Willi syndrome develops cognitive or behavioral schemas to accommodate to hyperphagia, such as more attention to some stimuli than to others, or tantrums or anxiety when food is denied. These strategies may then stay with the child over time; may spill over into areas unrelated to food; and ultimately contribute to the perseverative, compulsive-like behaviors, tantrums, and other problems that characterize Prader–Willi syndrome.

Maladaptive Behavior and Psychopathology

Range of Maladaptive Behavior

Most behavioral work in Prader–Willi syndrome focuses on maladaptive features and psychopathology. These problems are often severe, and they immediately capture our attention as both clinicians and researchers. Although the behavioral dysfunction is compelling, studies of it have been accomplished at the expense of research on the personality and psychosocial strengths of people with Prader–Willi syndrome. Although studies of strengths in people with Prader–Willi syndrome are now underway, at this time we know very little about how social competencies or personality strengths relate to behavioral dysfunction and psychopathology.

Anecdotally, young children with Prader–Willi syndrome are described as pleasant, friendly, social, and somewhat placid (Cassidy, 1984). These features do not necessarily disappear, but older children and adults are routinely described as showing a host of negative or maladaptive behaviors. Often these behaviors are more difficult to manage than food seeking, and they pose multiple challenges to families, teachers, and clinicians (Dykens & Hodapp, 1997).

Characteristic behavior problems are noted as minor criteria in the consensus diagnostic criteria for Prader–Willi syndrome (Holm et al., 1993), with often-noted problems including temper tantrums, stubbornness, oppositionality, rigidity, lying, and stealing. Many persons with Prader–Willi syndrome are also described as quite clever and manipulative, especially in regard to obtaining food.

The frequency and severity of maladaptive behaviors were recently examined in more detail in two different samples of subjects with Prader–Willi syndrome. We administered the Child Behavior Checklist (CBCL; Achenbach, 1991) to parents and caregivers of 91 subjects with Prader–Willi syndrome subjects were aged 4 to 47 years). Maladaptive behaviors that occurred in 50% or more of the sample are summarized in Table 23.3. Certain behaviors were seen in 75% to almost 100% of subjects, including skin picking, argumentativeness, stubbornness, obsessions, tantrums, underactivity, excessive sleep, compulsions, and anxiety.

We administered a different measure, the Reiss Screen for Maladaptive Behavior, to parents and caregivers of 61 adolescents and adults with Prader–Willi syndrome (subjects

TABLE 23.3. Frequently Occurring CBCL Behaviors in 91 Prader–Willi Subjects Aged 4–47 Years

Behavior	%	Behavior	%
Skin picking	97	Mood changes	76
Argues a lot	95	Excessive sleep	75
Stubborn	95	Steals (food)	72
Obsessions	94	Compulsions	71
Overeating	93	Worried, anxious	70
Tantrums	88	Talks too much	68
Underactive	87	Prefers being alone	67
Overtired	81	Can't concentrate	66
Clumsy	80	Gets teased a lot	65
Disobedient	78	Speech problems	65
Demands attention	78	Peers don't like	60
Lies (food-related)	78	Hoards	55
Overweight	77	Withdrawn	53
Impulsive	76	Unhappy, sad	51

were aged 13 to 49) years (Dykens & Cassidy, 1995). Certain behaviors were remarkably consistent across samples and measures, including temper tantrums (84%), overeating (81%), impulsivity (74%), and aggression (64%).

The majority of subjects in both samples had scores that reached clinically significant levels. Among the 91 children and adults, 82% had CBCL T-scores consistent with those of Achenbach's (1991) clinically referred sample. Among the 61 adolescents and adults, 85% had one or more clinically elevated subtest scores on the Reiss Screen, with most (72%) showing two or more clinical elevations (Dykens & Cassidy, 1995). Maladaptive behaviors thus often reach a point where further clinical evaluation and interventions are necessary (Dykens & Hodapp, 1997).

Specificity of Maladaptive Features

Although certain behaviors are both salient and clinically significant in Prader–Willi syndrome, studies have yet to compare these features to those of other persons with mental retardation. In particular, we do not know which maladaptive features are specific to Prader–Willi syndrome, which are shown by many persons with mental retardation, and which are shared by persons with only a few other etiologies of mental retardation.

At first glance, hyperphagia appears a unique aspect of Prader–Willi syndrome. Although some people with mental retardation show increased interests in food or propensities to being overweight (Prasher, 1995), these generally do not occur to the same degree as in Prader–Willi syndrome. Other behaviors, such as temper tantrums, argumentativeness, or stubbornness, are seen in many persons with mental retardation in general.

Although persons with Prader–Willi syndrome are not unique in all aspects of maladaptive behavior, certain behaviors may be more common in this population than in others with mental retardation. Dykens and Kasari (1997) compared 43 subjects with Prader–Willi syndrome aged 4 to 19 years to age- and sex-matched subjects with Down syndrome and nonspecific mental retardation. On the CBCL (Achenbach, 1991), subjects with Prader–Willi syndrome showed significantly higher levels of internalizing, externalizing, and overall problem behaviors. The Prader–Willi syndrome group was also more apt to overeat and be overweight; to be teased by peers, and to show skin picking, argumentativeness, verbal perseveration, obsessions, compulsions, fatigue, sleep problems, underactivity, and stealing at home (primarily food or money to buy food).

A discriminant-function analysis of these CBCL data suggested a relatively distinct Prader–Willi syndrome behavioral phenotype, with 91% of Prader–Willi syndrome cases correctly classified, and just 3 of the 86 comparison group subjects mistakenly assigned to the Prader–Willi syndrome group. As shown in Table 23.4, seven behaviors best discriminated the three groups, with the Prader–Willi group being singularly high in skin picking, fatigue, obsessions, and talking too much. Thus a blend of certain maladaptive behaviors appears quite distinctive to Prader–Willi syndrome, and may be highly predictive of this disorder. Overeating, food obsessions, and sleep disturbances are salient in Prader–Willi syndrome; yet other obsessions and repetitive, compulsion-like behaviors also seem to be central distinguishing features of this syndrome.

Correlates of Maladaptive Behavior

Most studies do not find significant gender differences in the maladaptive behavior of people with Prader–Willi syndrome. Three other variables, however, do relate to maladaptive behavior, sometimes in unexpected ways: IQ scores, weight, and family stress.

IQ Scores. A central issue is whether people with relatively high IQ scores are somehow protected from some of the syndrome's more troublesome maladaptive behaviors. A high IQ often emerges as a protective factor in children who are at risk for delay or adjustment problems, or who are experiencing psychosocial adversities (Garmezy, Masten, & Tellegen, 1984, although see also Luthar, 1991). We (Dykens & Cassidy, 1995) tested this possibility by comparing 43 subjects with relatively high IQs (mean IQ of 79) to 43 subjects with lower IQs (mean IQ of 59). No significant differences were found in either the type or severity of maladaptive behavior across groups.

These data, which are consistent with clinical observations of patients with Prader–Willi syndrome, have important implications for service delivery. In particular, state or other agencies that use low IQ scores (usually below 70) as a service eligibility requirement may exclude higher-functioning persons whose treatment needs are similar to those of lower-functioning persons. In Prader–Willi syndrome, then, IQ may be a less meaningful entry point into state or other systems of care than are the behavioral needs of the persons being served.

TABLE 23.4. Seven Behaviors That Discriminated Children with Prader–Willi Syndrome from Those with Down Syndrome and Nonspecific Mental Retardation with 91% Accuracy

Behavior	Prader–Willi syndrome	Down syndrome	Nonspecific mental retardation
Skin picking	High	Low	Low
Overtired	High	Low	Low
Obsessions	High	Low	Low
Impulsivity	High	Low	High
Speech problem	High	Low	Low/High[a]
Hyperactive	Low	Low	High

Note. Items from Dykens and Kasari (1997).

[a]Lower than subjects with Prader–Willi syndrome, higher than subjects with Down syndrome.

Weight. Unlike IQ, maladaptive behavior may be related to weight, but in a way that is opposite to general expectations. We (Dykens & Cassidy, 1995) found that thinner adults (i.e., those with lower body mass indices) had significantly higher maladaptive behavior scores than heavier persons (i.e., those with higher body mass indices), notably in internalizing symptoms. Specifically, thinner subjects showed more distressful affect and problems in thinking—confused and distorted thinking, anxiety, sadness, fearfulness, and crying. These findings need to be further explored, including how they relate to the stress of losing weight, as well as to changes in brain chemistry and physical activity level.

Family Stress. Finally, maladaptive behaviors are significantly related to heightened levels of familial stress (Dykens et al., 1996; Hodapp, Dykens, & Masino, 1997). Behavior problems in offspring with Prader–Willi syndrome (especially externalizing problems, such as tantrums and aggression) are the best predictors of familial stress, even as compared to such features as the offspring's age, sex, IQ level, or degree of obesity. Furthermore, stress in families with children with Prader–Willi syndrome is high relative to stress in families with offspring with other types of mental retardation (Hodapp et al., 1997). Although parents are often most concerned about their children's tantrums and compulsiveness, these problems probably interact with hyperphagia and the lifelong need for dietary management to create high levels of stress.

Development of Maladaptive Behavior

It is not yet clear how maladaptive features in persons with Prader–Willi syndrome shift and change over the course of development. The beginning of hyperphagia in early childhood is often associated with the onset or worsening of such behaviors as temper tantrums and aggression. These behaviors then seem fairly stable across the developmental years. We (Dykens & Cassidy, 1995) found similar rates of tantrums and other "externalizing" behaviors in young children (aged 4 to 7 years) and in older children (aged 8 to 12 years). Yet advancing age in these same children was correlated with heightened internal distress and features of depression, including withdrawal, isolation, negative self-image, and pessimism.

Some clinical reports note that behavioral problems increase in the adolescent and adult years, due to growing physical and psychosocial pressures (Greenswag, 1987; Whitman & Accardo, 1987). In contrast, others observe clinically that behavioral and emotional problems lessen with advancing age, and that older adults with Prader–Willi syndrome may be more amenable to intervention (Waters, 1990).

Yet changes in maladaptive behavior may not follow a simple linear function. Instead, these behaviors may wax and wane throughout adulthood (Dykens & Cassidy, 1995; Dykens et al., 1992b). Whereas some behaviors may increase with age, others may improve or remain fairly stable. Examining 21 adolescents and adults cross-sectionally with the CBCL, Dykens et al. (1992b) found that underactivity and fatigue increased with age, while certain "externalizing" difficulties (e.g., running away and destroying property) decreased from adolescence to adulthood. Still other behaviors seemed to be fairly stable, such as temper tantrums, stubbornness, skin picking, and hoarding (Dykens et al., 1992b).

The waxing and waning of behavior problems may sometimes be associated with specific psychosocial stressors. Many young adults, for example, experience increased behavioral difficulties when they leave home and move into a group home setting, or when they make the transition from one job to another. In other persons, however, psychosocial precipitants for behavioral shifts are not apparent.

Psychiatric Features

The vast majority of studies in "dual diagnosis," or co-occurring mental retardation and psychiatric illness, have used heterogeneous groups of subjects with mixed or unknown etiologies (Dykens, 1996). As a result, more is known about psychiatric illness in the general, heterogeneous population of people with mental retardation than in persons whose mental retardation has specific genetic etiologies.

Partly because of this mixed-group approach, little is yet known about the prevalence rates of psychiatric disorders in the population of persons with Prader–Willi syndrome. Although population-based prevalence studies have yet to be done, clinically we find that certain psychiatric disorders occur infrequently. For example, although many people with Prader–Willi syndrome steal food, and are impulsive and distractible, rates seem low for full-blown conduct disorder or attention-deficit/hyperactivity disorder. Tic disorders, dementia, and schizophrenia also appear relatively infrequently in this population. Recently, however, Clarke (1993) and Clarke, Webb, and Brachmann-Clarke (1995) reported on psychotic episodes in four young adults with Prader–Willi syndrome; all cases showed a paternal deletion of chromosome 15. These patients had a sudden onset of hallucinations and other psychotic symptoms, with no obvious precipitating events. All showed good outcome following milieu and pharmacological treatment. These cases suggest a need for large-scale studies that can identify whether Prader–Willi syndrome involves a particular vulnerability to schizophrenia-spectrum disorders, above and beyond the risk associated with mental retardation.

Furthermore, Prader–Willi syndrome does not appear to include a heightened risk of autism or pervasive developmental disorder not otherwise specified (PDD NOS), beyond the risk due to mental retardation. Of the handful of patients with Prader–Willi syndrome and co-occurring autism or PDD NOS that we have seen in the clinical setting, however, all had maternal UPD of chromosome 15. These clinical observations are consistent with those of Rogan et al. (1994), who suggest increased risks of autism or other, rare disorders in Prader–Willi syndrome cases involving maternal UPD of chromosome 15.

However, several other psychiatric disorders may occur with increased frequency in persons with Prader–Willi syndrome. These include affective disorders and obsessive-compulsive disorder (OCD). Depressive features such as sadness and low self-esteem, as well as anxiety, fears, and worries, have all been noted in several studies of maladaptive behavior in Prader–Willi syndrome (e.g., Dykens et al., 1992b; Dykens & Cassidy, 1995; Dykens & Kasari, 1997; Stein, Keating, Zar, & Hollander, 1994; Whitman & Accardo, 1987). Among 91 children and adults assessed with the CBCL, for example, we found that 76% showed mood lability; 70% were worried or anxious; and 51% showed sadness, depression, and withdrawal.

Yet no studies have examined samples with Prader–Willi syndrome using formal *Diagnostic and Statistical Manual of Mental Disorders*, fourth edition (DSM-IV; American Psychiatric Association [APA], 1994) or *International Classification of Diseases*, 10th revision (ICD-10) diagnostic criteria for depressive disorders, or for anxiety disorders other than OCD. It thus remains unknown to what extent the sadness or worry shown by some persons with Prader–Willi syndrome might lead to full-blown cases of these disorders. It is also unclear what factors might predispose some persons with the syndrome to be more or less susceptible to affective disorders.

Increased risks of OCD have been found in persons with Prader–Willi syndrome. Compulsive-like symptoms have long been hallmark features of Prader–Willi syndrome, primarily skin picking, food preoccupations, and repetitive food-seeking behaviors (e.g.,

Dykens et al., 1992b; Hellings & Warnock, 1994; Holm et al., 1993; Stein et al., 1994). Yet many persons show repetitive thoughts and compulsive behaviors not related to skin picking or food.

Recently, we (Dykens et al., 1996) identified a wide range of non-food-related obsessions and compulsions in 91 children and adults with Prader–Willi syndrome. As measured by the Yale–Brown Obsessive–Compulsive Scale (Goodman et al., 1989), prominent compulsions in this sample included hoarding items such as paper, pens, trash, and toiletries (58%); rewriting and redoing things (37%); and concerns with symmetry, exactness, ordering, and arranging (35–40%). Over half of the subjects (53%) also had to tell, ask, or say things, often perseverating on a narrow range of topics. Relatively fewer subjects had cleaning, contamination, or checking symptoms (15–24%). Thus, for instance, many subjects in this study often ordered and arranged toys or objects according to specific rules based on size, shape, or color, or simply until they were "just right." Others rewrote letters or words until they were just right, or could not tolerate slight imperfections in the environment.

Furthermore, as specified in the DSM-IV criteria for OCD (APA, 1994), a remarkably high proportion of subjects had moderate to severe levels of obsessive and compulsive symptomatology. Indeed, 64% showed at least a moderate level of symptom-related distress, and 80% had symptom-related adaptive impairment. Other ties between Prader–Willi syndrome and OCD were found by comparing 43 adults with Prader–Willi syndrome to age- and sex-matched nonretarded adults with OCD (Dykens et al., 1996). As shown in Table 23.5, the matched Prader–Willi and nonretarded OCD groups showed similar levels of symptom severity, similar numbers of compulsions, and more areas of symptom similarity than difference.

Increased risks of OCD are thus strongly indicated in persons with Prader–Willi syndrome; these individuals exhibit a wide range of severe symptoms, and are similar to nonretarded adults with OCD. In contrast, studies with heterogeneous groups of persons with mental retardation find that only 1–3% meet criteria for OCD (e.g., Meyers, 1987; Vitiello, Spreat, & Behar, 1989). It may be that one or more genes associated with this increased vulnerability to OCD will be found in the Prader–Willi critical region on chro-

TABLE 23.5. Comparison of Compulsions in 43 Adults with Prader–Willi Syndrome versus Age- and Gender-Matched Adults with OCD

	PWS		OCD		
Y-BOCS features	M	SD	M	SD	F
Number of compulsions	3.75	2.11	4.02	2.81	NS
Severity of compulsions	10.77	3.90	9.09	4.44	NS
Specific symptoms	%		%		χ^2
Cleaning	33%		37%		NS
Checking	16%		55%		21.16**
Repeating rituals	40%		54%		NS
Counting	19%		28%		NS
Ordering/arranging	29%		28%		NS
Hoarding	79%		7%		46.75**
Need to tell, ask	51%		23%		7.16*

Note. Y-BOCS, Yale–Brown Obsessive–Compulsive Scale; NS, nonsignificant. Items from Dykens, Leckman, and Cassidy (1996).

*$p < .01$; **$p < .001$.

mosome 15, or that the pathogenesis of Prader–Willi syndrome in some way predisposes individuals to obsessive and compulsive behaviors.

Further work needs to identify the extent to which Prader–Willi syndrome also involves heightened risks of affective, impulse control, or psychotic disorders, above and beyond the risks associated with mental retardation per se. It also remains unknown how any of these psychiatric features relate to molecular genetic status. Behavioral or cognitive differences have generally not been found between subjects with chromosome 15 paternal deletion versus maternal UPD (Cassidy et al., 1997). Although deletion cases may be more prone to repetitive skin picking and perhaps other compulsive symptoms (Cassidy, 1995), and maternal UPD cases may be more prone to autism or PDD symptoms (Rogan et al., 1994), more research is needed to clarify these preliminary observations.

INTERVENTIONS: MEDICAL AND BEHAVIORAL

Managing Prader–Willi syndrome's characteristic obesity and significant behavioral/psychiatric dysfunction constitutes a major treatment challenge, requiring cooperative input from geneticists, primary care physicians, endocrinologists, nutritionists, psychologists, psychiatrists, educators, families, group home staff members, and other care providers. It is often helpful for a health or mental health professional to follow an individual with Prader–Willi syndrome on a long-term basis, to help maintain continuity of care and to coordinate services. Table 23.6 summarizes many of the intervention recommendations discussed below. More detailed information on the management of Prader–Willi syndrome

TABLE 23.6. Salient Treatment Recommendations in Prader–Willi Syndrome

- Maintain well-balanced, reduced-calorie diet (1,000–1,200 kilocalories/day), assuring adequate calcium intake.
- Encourage regular, sustained exercise (30 minutes daily).
- Restrict access to food (e.g., locked cabinets, refrigerator).
- Provide close supervision, especially in the school cafeteria, at work, and in the community.
- Maintain external food supports even when people lose weight or have high IQs.
- Be aware of possible conflict between food restrictions and choice/personal rights.
- Assess feasibility of growth hormone treatment.
- Consider over-the-counter products to increase saliva production.
- Appreciate impact of tantrums and other maladaptive behaviors on family stress.
- Provide clear behavioral expectations and limits, beginning at an early age; apply consistent limits across home and school or work.
- Maintain consistency in daily routines.
- Assess for increased risks of OCD, impulse control problems, and depressive disorders.
- Determine whether compulsive tendencies lead to getting stuck, and provide extra support with transitions.
- Check for sadness even in persons with adequate weight control.
- Ensure appropriate special education, and be sure that IEPs address needs for speech and physical therapies, as well as needs for increased physical activity.
- Provide ample planning for school-to-work transition; consider need for food supports in transition plans; assess feasibility of dedicated group homes versus other living settings.

may be found in an edited volume written for care providers of all types, now in its second edition (Greenswag & Alexander, 1995).

Medical Management

Obesity

With good reason, weight and dietary management have long been targets of intervention in Prader–Willi syndrome. Experience in over 18 years of managing Prader–Willi syndrome in an interdisciplinary clinic has demonstrated that obesity prevention or weight reduction and maintenance can be achieved with the following:

- A well-balanced, low-calorie diet of about 1,000–1,200 kilocalories/day (assuring adequate calcium intake).
- Periodic weigh-ins (e.g., once a week).
- Regular exercise to increase muscle mass and thus efficiently burn calories (30 minutes per day is an appropriate goal).
- Environmental modification as needed, such as locking kitchen cabinets and the refrigerator.
- Close supervision to minimize access to food (e.g., supervision of spending money; supervision of meals in the school cafeteria, on the job, or in the community).

Although these techniques are considered state-of-the-art in treating hyperphagia in Prader–Willi syndrome, they are increasingly viewed by advocates in the developmental disability field as being too restrictive, and as limiting the personal rights and choices of adults with Prader–Willi syndrome (see Dykens, Goff, et al., 1997, for a discussion). Clinicians thus need to be aware of possible conflicts between some interventions (e.g., locking the refrigerator or limiting spending money) with their clients' right to food and to their paychecks. Furthermore, external food supports and interventions should be continued even when people lose weight or show needs for less supervision in the non-food-related parts of their lives.

To date, no medication has shown long-term effectiveness in controlling appetites in people with Prader–Willi syndrome, despite the widespread interest in such a medication in the Prader–Willi syndrome community. Therefore, behavioral approaches continue to be of considerable value in helping parents and other care providers set limits concerning food, and supporting them in the lifelong effort to prevent the health consequences of obesity (Dykens & Cassidy, 1995).

Other Medical Concerns

Management of other physical problems associated with Prader–Willi syndrome is largely problem-oriented. Although the use of growth hormone in Prader–Willi syndrome is still somewhat controversial, ongoing controlled studies suggest great benefit from growth hormone replacement therapy. Not only does such treatment result in increased height; perhaps more importantly, it causes an improvement in body composition and increased muscle mass, thus decreasing the body mass index (Angulo et al., 1996).

Sex hormone replacement therapy will increase the development of secondary sex characteristics and theoretically may improve osteoporosis, but testosterone treatment is sometimes associated with an increase in aggressive behavior. No controlled trials of treatment with sex hormones have yet been published.

Products to increase saliva production have proved of benefit in treating the dry mouth associated with Prader–Willi syndrome, and are also likely to improve dental hygiene and perhaps articulation as well. Speech therapy can be beneficial to people with Prader–Willi syndrome of all ages to address speech production abnormalities, and physical and occupational therapies have also proven helpful in treating hypotonia and poor coordination.

Educational, Behavioral, and Psychiatric Management

Educational and Vocational Management

Most children with Prader–Willi syndrome need special education services that address their unique cognitive and behavioral needs (Levine & Wharton, 1993). Although individualized education plans (IEPs) should be based on a careful assessment of each student's cognitive strengths and weaknesses, most IEPs include speech/language and physical therapies; supervision around food; and extra physical education classes or other ways of increasing physical activity during the school day (e.g., walking). Many students do well with "hands-on" lessons and techniques that capitalize on their visual–spatial strengths, and that minimize their weaknesses in auditory–verbal short-term memory and sequential processing.

Students with Prader–Willi syndrome are placed in both inclusive and specialized or segregated educational settings; often a combination of these settings works well. Parents of students with Prader–Willi syndrome tend to view their children's ideal educational placement as specialized rather than inclusive (Hodapp, Freeman, & Kasari, in press). Compared to parents of children with Down syndrome, parents of students with Prader–Willi syndrome request more specialized services (e.g., speech or physical therapies), even if this means leaving their local neighborhood school; they are also more concerned with the transition from school to work in the adolescent years (Hodapp et al., in press).

Adults with Prader–Willi syndrome need careful vocational planning. Successful job placements typically require job coaches and extra support to address food seeking and other behavioral difficulties. Many adults also do well in group homes, especially ones designed specifically for persons with Prader–Willi syndrome. Compared to family homes or less supervised community settings, group homes dedicated to adults with Prader–Willi syndrome appear to be the most effective in reducing and maintaining weight over time, as well as in managing behavioral difficulties (Cassidy et al., 1994; Greenswag, 1987).

Behavioral and Psychiatric Management

Clinicians need to be aware that even though food-related behavior is a significant issue in Prader–Willi syndrome, other maladaptive behaviors are likely to be the major reasons why many families seek professional help. We have noted earlier that even as compared to food issues, obesity, age, or IQ level, the best predictors of family stress are maladaptive behaviors such as temper tantrums, compulsion, and needs for sameness in routine (Dykens et al., 1996; Hodapp et al., 1997).

Improved behavior both at home and at school is often the result of strict reinforcement of behavioral limits, clear delineation of behavioral expectations, and establishment of regular routines. Establishing clear limits regarding food and behavior is especially important with the emergence of hyperphagia in the toddler or preschool years. Clinically, we find that setting behavioral limits at a young age paves the way for more successful responses to limit setting over the developmental and adolescent years.

But families often have difficulty adhering to and enforcing behavioral and food limits over the long term. Some families benefit from occasional or more sustained support from behavioral, family, and other therapists, as well as from the support of other families with a Prader–Willi syndrome member. Ongoing parent support groups are now offered through the state chapters of the Prader–Willi Syndrome Association and through the Prader–Willi Foundation; toll-free numbers for these organizations are (800) 926-4797 and (800) 253-7993, respectively. Support groups can also be accessed through state and national meetings, as well as the Internet. These formal and informal parent-to-parent support mechanisms are often of enormous help to families.

In addition to behavioral interventions and family support, many persons with Prader–Willi syndrome need extra help getting "unstuck" from their obsessions and compulsions. Indeed, tantrums and stubbornness in persons with Prader–Willi syndrome often seem related to their being "stuck" and unable to move from one activity or thought to the next. Consistent limit setting across home and school settings often helps reduce tantrums, as do predictable daily routines. Other tantrums may be circumvented by distraction and by giving individuals ample warning about transitions, including special auditory or visual transitional cues. If tantrums are inevitable, it is typically helpful for parents or teachers to avoid talking about the issue until well after the individual has settled down.

Although the prevalence of affective disorders remains unknown in the Prader–Willi syndrome population, depressive features need to be carefully assessed in clients with Prader–Willi syndrome. As they develop, children may be particularly vulnerable to increased negative self-evaluation, isolation, and withdrawal (Dykens & Cassidy, 1995); these features may reflect the child's growing awareness of his or her differences from peers. Depressive features and disorganized thinking may also be heightened among adolescents and adults who have achieved adequate weight control (Dykens & Cassidy, 1995). Many children and adults benefit from school, clinic, or recreational programs that target improved self-esteem, social skills, and peer relations (Dykens & Cassidy, 1995; Levine & Wharton, 1993).

In addition, pharmacology is often used to address depressive or obsessive–compulsive features, as well as severe aggression and temper tantrums. Several case studies report that selective serotonin reuptake inhibitors (SSRIs) have helped some individuals gain better control of tantrums and compulsive symptoms such as skin picking (Benjamin & Bout-Smith, 1993; Dech & Budow, 1991; Hellings & Warnock, 1994; Warnock & Kestenbaum, 1992). Although SSRIs are currently quite popular in the Prader–Willi syndrome community, controlled studies have yet to be published.

NEXT STEPS

Although Prader–Willi syndrome was identified just over 40 years ago, research on it is accumulating at a growing rate, particularly on the genetic aspects of this disorder. Work is now well underway that aims to identify specific genes in the Prader–Willi /Angelman critical region, as well as mechanisms associated with genomic imprinting. In comparison, research on Prader–Willi syndrome's behavioral phenotype lags behind. This gap is probably attributable to the predominant practice in behavioral studies of using heterogeneous groups of subjects with mental retardation (Dykens, 1995; Dykens, 1996; Hodapp &

Dykens, 1994). We thus know more about behavior and development in people with mental retardation in general than we do about people with distinctive etiologies such as Prader–Willi or other syndromes.

With its genetic and behavioral complexities, Prader–Willi syndrome is an ideal condition to pave the way for more syndrome-specific behavioral research. Although studies on maladaptive behavior and psychiatric problems are now emerging, research is also needed on the strengths and competencies of people with this disorder. Furthermore, approaches are needed that tie together genetics and behavior in Prader–Willi syndrome. Studies might, for example, systematically compare behavior, development, and hypothalamic function across persons with deletions as opposed to UPD. Finally, treatment outcome research is sorely needed, including studies of how early diagnosis and intervention affect subsequent health, mental health, and quality of life. Such research offers much promise for improving the long-term success of people with Prader–Willi syndrome and their families.

ACKNOWLEDGMENTS

We are grateful to the families of patients affected with Prader–Willi syndrome for their continuing support and participation in Prader–Willi Syndrome Clinics and clinical research. Particular appreciation goes to those who are willing to have photographs published. We are grateful as well to the many professionals who help run the Prader–Willi Syndrome Clinics at the University of Connecticut, the University of California at Los Angeles, and Case Western Reserve University. We also thank Robert M. Hodapp for his helpful comments on this chapter. This work was supported in part by Grant No. 03008 from the National Institute of Child Health and Human Development.

REFERENCES

Achenbach, T. M. (1991). *Manual for the Child Behavior Checklist/4–18 and 1991 Profile.* Burlington: University of Vermont, Department of Psychiatry.

American Psychiatric Association (APA). (1994). *Diagnostic and statistical manual of mental disorders* (4th ed.). Washington, DC: Author.

American Society of Human Genetics (ASHG) & American College of Medical Genetics (ACMG). (1996). Diagnostic testing for Prader–Willi and Angelman syndromes: Report of the ASHG/ACMG Test and Technology Transfer Committee. *American Journal of Human Genetics, 58,* 1085–1088.

Angulo, M., Castro-Magana, M., Mazur, B., Canas, J. A., Vitollo, P. M., & Sarrantonio, M. (1996). Growth hormone secretion and effects of growth hormone therapy on growth velocity and weight gain in children with Prader–Willi syndrome. *Journal of Pediatric Endocrinology and Metabolism, 9,* 393–400.

Aughton, D. A., & Cassidy, S. B. (1990). Physical features of Prader–Willi syndrome in neonates. *American Journal of Diseases of Children, 144,* 1251–1254.

Baker, H. J., & Leland, B. (1967). *Detroit Tests of Learning Aptitude.* Indianapolis, IN: Bobbs-Merrill.

Benjamin, E., & Buot-Smith, T. (1993). Naltrexone and fluoxetine in Prader–Willi syndrome. *Journal of the American Academy of Child and Adolescent Psychiatry, 32,* 870–873.

Borghgraef, M., Fryns, J. P., & Van den Berghe, V. D. (1990). Psychological profile and behavioral characteristics in 12 patients with Prader–Willi syndrome. *Genetic Counseling, 38,* 141–150.

Branson, C. (1981). Speech and language characteristics of children with Prader–Willi syndrome. In V. A. Holm, S. Sulzbacher, & P. Pipes (Eds.), *The Prader–Willi syndrome* (pp. 179–183). Baltimore: University Park Press.

Buiting, K., Saitoh, S., Gross, S., Dittrich, B., Schwartz, S., Nicholas, R. D., & Horsthemke, B. (1994). Inherited microdeletions in the Angelman and Prader–Willi syndromes define an imprinting centre on human chromosome 15. *Nature Genetics, 9,* 395–400.

Burd, L., Vesely, B., Martsolf, J., & Kerbeshian, J. (1990). Prevalence study of Prader–Willi syndrome in North Dakota. *American Journal of Medical Genetics, 37,* 97–99.

Butler, M. G. (1989). Hypopigmentation: A common feature of the Prader–Labhart–Willi syndrome. *American Journal of Human Genetics, 45,* 140–146.

Butler, M. G. (1990). Prader–Willi syndrome: Current understanding of cause and diagnosis. *American Journal of Medical Genetics, 35,* 319–332.

Butler, M. G. (1996). Molecular diagnosis of Prader–Willi syndrome: Comparison of cytogenetic and molecular genetic data including parent of origin dependent methylation DNA patterns. *American Journal of Medical Genetics, 61,* 188–190.

Cassidy, S. B. (1984). Prader–Willi syndrome. *Current Problems in Pediatrics, 14,* 1–55.

Cassidy, S. B. (1995, June). *Complexities of clinical diagnosis of Prader–Willi syndrome.* Paper presented at the 2nd Prader–Willi Syndrome International Conference, Oslo, Norway.

Cassidy, S. B., Devi, A., & Mukaida, C. (1994). Aging in Prader–Willi syndrome: 22 patients over age 30 years. *Proceedings of the Greenwood Genetics Center, 13,* 102–103.

Cassidy, S. B., Forsythe, M., Heeger, S., Nicholls, R. D., Schork, N., Benn, P., & Schwartz, S. (1997). Comparison of phenotype between patients with Prader–Willi syndrome due to deletion 15q and uniparental disomy 15. *American Journal of Medical Genetics, 68,* 433–440.

Cassidy, S. B., Geer, J. S., Holm, V. A., & Hudgins, L. (1996). African-Americans with Prader–Willi syndrome are phenotypically different. *American Journal of Human Genetics, 59,* A21.

Christian, S. L., Smith, A. C. M., Macha, M., Black, S. H., Elder, F. F. B., Johnson, J. M. P., Resta, R. G., Surti, U., Suslak, L., Verp, M. S., & Ledbetter, D. H. (1996). Prenatal diagnosis of uniparental disomy 15 following trisomy 15 mosaicism. *Prenatal Diagnosis, 16,* 323–332.

Clarke, D. J. (1993). Prader–Willi syndrome and psychoses. *British Journal of Psychiatry, 163,* 680–684.

Clarke, D. J., Webb, T., & Bachmann-Clarke, J. P. (1995). Prader–Willi syndrome and psychotic symptoms: Report of a further case. *Irish Journal of Psychological Medicine, 12,* 27–29.

Crnic, K. A., Sulzbacher, S., Snow, J., & Holm, V. A. (1980). Preventing mental retardation associated with gross obesity in the Prader–Willi syndrome. *Pediatrics, 66,* 787–789.

Curfs, L. G. (1992). Psychological profile and behavioral characteristics in Prader–Willi syndrome. In S. B. Cassidy (Ed.), *Prader–Willi syndrome and other 15q deletion disorders* (pp. 211–222). Berlin: Springer-Verlag.

Curfs, L. G., Wiegers, A. M., Sommers, J. R., Borghgraef, M., & Fryns, J. P. (1991). Strengths and weaknesses in the cognitive profile of youngsters with Prader–Willi syndrome. *Clinical Genetics, 40,* 430–434.

Dech, B., & Budow, L. (1991). The use of fluoxetine in an adolescent with Prader–Willi syndrome. *Journal of the American Academy of Child and Adolescent Psychiatry, 30,* 298–302.

Delach, J. A., Rosengren, S. S., Kaplan, L., Greenstein, R. M., Cassidy, S. B., & Benn, P. A. (1994). Comparison of high resolution chromosome banding and fluorescence *in situ* hybridization (FISH) for the laboratory evaluation of Prader–Willi syndrome and Angelman syndrome. *American Journal of Medical Genetics, 52,* 85–91.

Dunn, H. G. (1968). The Prader-Labhart-Willi syndrome: Review of the literature and report of nine cases. *Acta Paediatrica Scandanavica, 186,* 1–38.

Dykens, E. M. (1995). Measuring behavioral phenotypes: Provocations from the "new genetics." *American Journal of Mental Retardation, 99,* 522–532.

Dykens, E. M. (1996). DNA meets DSM: Genetic syndromes' growing importance in dual diagnosis. *Mental Retardation, 34,* 125–127.

Dykens, E. M., & Cassidy, S. B. (1995). Correlates of maladaptive behavior in children and adults with Prader–Willi syndrome. *American Journal of Medical Genetics, 60,* 546–549.

Dykens, E. M., & Clarke, D. J. (1997). Correlates of maladaptive behavior in individuals with 5p- (Cri-du-chart) syndrome. *Developmental Medicine and Child Neurology, 39,* 752–756.

Dykens, E. M., Finucane, B. M., & Gayley, C. (1997). Cognitive and behavioral profiles in persons with Smith–Magenis syndrome. *Journal of Autism and Developmental Disorders*, 27, 203–211.

Dykens, E. M., Goff, B. J., Hodapp, R. M., Davis, L., Devanzo, P., Moss, F., Halliday, J., Shah, B., State, M. W., & King, B. H. (1997). Eating themselves to death: Have "personal rights" gone too far in treating people with Prader–Willi Syndrome? *Mental Retardation*, 35, 312–314.

Dykens, E. M., & Hodapp, R. M. (1997). Treatment issues in genetic mental retardation syndromes. *Professional Psychology: Research and Practice*, 28, 263–270.

Dykens, E. M., Hodapp, R. M., & Evans, P. W. (1994). Profiles and development of adaptive behavior in children with Down syndrome. *American Journal of Mental Retardation*, 98, 580–587.

Dykens, E. M., Hodapp, R. M., & Leckman, J. F. (1994). *Behavior and development in fragile X syndrome*. Newbury Park, CA: Sage.

Dykens, E. M., Hodapp, R. M., Walsh, K., & Nash, L. J. (1992a). Profiles, correlates and trajectories of intelligence in individuals with Prader–Willi syndrome. *Journal of the American Academy of Child and Adolescent Psychiatry*, 31, 1125–1130.

Dykens, E. M., Hodapp, R. M., Walsh, K., & Nash, L. J. (1992b). Adaptive and maladaptive behavior in Prader–Willi syndrome. *Journal of the American Academy of Child and Adolescent Psychiatry*, 31, 1131–1136.

Dykens, E. M., & Kasari, C. (1997). Maladaptive behavior in children with Prader–Willi syndrome, Down syndrome and non-specific mental retardation. *American Journal of Mental Retardation*, 102, 228–237.

Dykens, E. M., Leckman, J. F., & Cassidy, S. B. (1996). Obsessions and compulsions in Prader–Willi syndrome. *Journal of Child Psychology and Psychiatry*, 37, 995–1002.

Freund, L. S., Reiss, A. L., & Abrams, M. T. (1993). Psychiatric disorders associated with fragile X in the young female. *Pediatrics*, 91, 321–329.

Gabel, S., Tarter, R. E., Gavaler, J., Golden, W., Hegedus, A. M., & Mair, B. (1986). Neuropsychological capacity of Prader–Willi children: General and specific aspects of impairment. *Applied Research in Mental Retardation*, 7, 459–466.

Garmezy, N., Masten, A. S., & Tellegen, A. (1984). The study of stress and competence in children: A building block for developmental psychopathology. *Child Development*, 55, 97–111.

Gillessen-Kaesbach, G., Robinson, W., Lohmann, D., Kaya-Westerloh, S., Passarge, E., & Horsthemke, B. (1995). Genotype–phenotype correlation in a series of 167 deletion and non-deletion patients with Prader–Willi syndrome. *Human Genetics*, 96, 638–643.

Glenn, C. C., Saitoh, S., Jong, M. T., Filbrandt, M. M., Surti, U., Driscoll, D. J., & Nicholls, R. D. (1996). Gene structure, DNA methylation and imprinted expression of the human *SNRPN* gene. *American Journal of Human Genetics*, 58, 335–346.

Goodman, W. K., Price, L. H., Rasmussen, S. A., Mazure, C., Fleischmann, R. L., Hill, C. L., Heninger, G. R., & Charney, D. S. (1989). The Yale–Brown Obsessive–Compulsive Scale: Development, use and reliability, *Archives of General Psychiatry*, 46, 1006–1011.

Greenswag, L. R. (1987). Adults with Prader–Willi syndrome: A survey of 232 cases. *Developmental Medicine and Child Neurology*, 29, 145–152.

Greenswag, L. R., & Alexander, R. A. (Eds.). (1995). *Management of Prader–Willi syndrome* (2nd ed.). New York: Springer-Verlag.

Gunay-Aygun, M., & Cassidy, S. B. (1997). Delayed diagnosis in Prader–Willi syndrome due to uniparental disomy. *American Journal of Medical Genetics*, 71, 106–110.

Gunay-Aygun, M., Cassidy, S. B., & Nicholls, R. D. (1997). Prader–Willi and other syndromes associated with obesity and mental retardation. *Behavior Genetics*, 27, 307–324.

Hellings, J. A., & Warnock, J. K. (1994). Self-injurious behavior and serotonin in Prader–Willi syndrome. *Psychopharmacology Bulletin*, 30, 245–250.

Hertz, G., Cataletto, M., Feinsilver, S. H., & Angulo, M. (1995). Developmental trends of sleep-disordered breathing in Prader–Willi syndrome: The role of obesity. *American Journal of Medical Genetics*, 56, 188–190.

Hodapp, R. M. (1996). Cross-domain relations in Down syndrome. In J. A. Rondal, J. Perera, L. Nadel, & A. Comblain (Eds.), *Down syndrome: Psychological, biopsychological and socio-educational perspectives* (pp. 65–79). London: Whurr.

Hodapp, R. M., & Dykens, E. M. (1994). Mental retardation's two cultures of behavioral research. *American Journal of Mental Retardation, 98,* 675–687.

Hodapp, R. M., Dykens, E. M., & Masino, L. (1997). Stress and support in families of persons with Prader–Willi syndrome. *Journal of Autism and Developmental Disorders, 27,* 11–23.

Hodapp, R. M., Freeman, S. F., & Kasari, C. (in press). Parental educational preferences for students with mental retardation: Effects of etiology and current placement. *Education and Training in Mental Retardation and Developmental Disabilities.*

Hodapp, R. M., & Zigler. E. (1990). Applying the developmental perspective to individuals with Down syndrome. In D. Cicchetti & M. Beeghly (Eds.), *Children with Down syndrome: A developmental perspective* (pp. 1–28). New York: Cambridge University Press.

Holland, A. J., Treasure, J., Coskeran, P., Dallow, J., Milton, N., & Hillhouse, E. (1993). Measurement of excessive appetite and metabolic changes in Prader–Willi syndrome. *International Journal of Obesity, 17,* 526–532.

Holm, V. A. (1981). The diagnosis of Prader–Willi syndrome. In V. A. Holm, S. Sulzbacher & P. L. Pipes (Eds.), *The Prader–Willi syndrome* (pp. 27–44). Baltimore: University Park Press.

Holm, V. A., Cassidy, S. B., Butler, M. G., Hanchett, J. M., Greenswag, L. R., Whitman, B. Y., & Greenberg, F. (1993). Prader–Willi syndrome: Consensus diagnostic criteria. *Pediatrics, 91,* 398–402.

Holm, V. A., & Pipes, P. L. (1976). Food and children with Prader–Willi syndrome. *American Journal of Diseases of Children, 130,* 1063–1067.

Hudgins, L. H., McKillop, J. A., & Cassidy, S. B. (1991). Hand and foot lengths in Prader–Willi syndrome. *American Journal of Medical Genetics, 41,* 5–9.

Kaufman, A. S., & Kaufman, N. L. (1984). *Kaufman Assessment Battery for Children.* Circle Pines, MN: American Guidance Service.

Kleppe, S. A., Katayama, K. M., Shipley, K. G., & Foushee, D. R. (1990). The speech and language characteristics of children with Prader–Willi syndrome. *Journal of Speech and Hearing Disorders, 55,* 300–309.

Kubota, T., Sutcliffe, J. S., Aradhya, S., Gillessen-Kaesbach, G., Christian, S. L., Horsthemke, B., Beaudet, A. L., & Ledbetter, D. H. (1996). Validation studies of *SNRPN* methylation as a diagnostic test for Prader–Willi syndrome. *American Journal of Medical Genetics, 66,* 77–80.

Ledbetter, D. H., Riccardi, V. M., Airhart, S. D., Strobel, R. J., Keenen, S. B., & Crawford, J. D. (1981). Deletion of chromosome 15 as a cause of Prader-Willi syndrome. *New England Journal of Medicine, 304,* 325–329.

Lee, P. D. (1995). Endocrine and metabolic aspects of Prader–Willi syndrome. In L. Greenswag & R. Alexander (Eds.), *Management of Prader–Willi syndrome* (pp. 32–57). New York: Springer-Verlag.

Levine, K., & Whenton, R. K. (1993). *Children with Prader–Willi syndrome: Information for school staff.* Rosyln Heights, NY: Visible Ink.

Luthar, S. S. (1991). Vulnerability and resilience: A study of at risk adolescents. *Child Development, 62,* 600–616.

Mascari, M. J., Gottlieb, W., Rogan, P. K., Butler, M. G., Waller, D. A., Armour, J. A. L., Jeffreys, A. J., Ladda, R. L., & Nicholls, R. D. (1992). The frequency of uniparental disomy in Prader–Willi syndrome. *New England Journal of Medicine, 326,* 599–607.

Meyers, B. A. (1987). Psychiatric problems in adolescents with developmental disabilities. *Journal of the American Academy of Child and Adolescent Psychiatry, 26,* 74–79.

Mitchell, J., Schinzel, A., Langlois, S., Gillessen-Kaesbach, G., Michaelis, R. C., Abeliovich, D., Lerer, I., Schuffenhauer, S., Christian, S., Guitart, M., McFadden, D. E., & Robinson, W. P. (1996). Comparison of phenotype in uniparental disomy and deletion Prader–Willi syndrome: Sex specific differences. *American Journal of Medical Genetics, 65,* 133–136.

Nicholls, R. D. (1993). Genomic imprinting and uniparental disomy in Angelman and Prader–Willi syndrome: A review. *American Journal of Medical Genetics, 46,* 16–25.

Nicholls, R. D., Knoll, J. H., Butler, M. G., Karam, S., & Lalande, M. (1989). Genetic imprinting suggested by maternal heterodisomy in nondeletion Prader–Willi syndrome. *Nature, 342,* 281–285.

Ozcelik, T., Leff, S., Robinson, W., Donlon, T., Lalande, M., Sanjines, E., Schinzel, A., & Francke, U. (1992). Small nuclear ribonucleoprotein polypeptide N (*SNRPN*), an expressed gene in the Prader–Willi syndrome critical region. *Nature Genetics, 2,* 265–269.

Prader, A., Labhart, A., & Willi, A. (1956). Ein syndrom von aidositas, kleinwuchs, kryptorchismus und oligophrenie nach myotonieartigem zustand im neugeborenenalter. *Schweizerische Medizinische Wochenschrift, 86,* 1260–1261.

Prasher, V. P. (1995). Overweight and obesity amongst Down syndrome adults. *Journal of Intellectual Disability Research, 39,* 437–441.

Robinson, W. P., Bottani, A., Yagang, X., Balakrishman, J., Binkert, F., Machler, M., Prader, A., & Schinzel, A. (1991). Molecular, cytogenetic and clinical investigations of Prader–Willi syndrome patients. *American Journal of Human Genetics, 49,* 1219–1234.

Rogan, P. K., Mascari, J., Ladda, R. L., Woodage, T., Trent, R. J., Smith, A., Lai, W., Erickson, R. P., Cassidy, S. B., Peterson, M. B., Mikkesen, M., Driscoll, D. J., Nicholls, R. D., & Butler, M. G. (1994, July). *Coinheritance of other chromosome 15 abnormalities with Prader–Willi syndrome: Genetic risk estimation and mapping.* Paper presented at the 16th Annual PWS(USA) National Scientific Day, Atlanta, GA.

Saitoh, S., Buiting, K., Cassidy, S. B., Conroy, J. M., Driscoll, D.J., Gabriel, J. M., Gillessen-Kaesbach, G., Clenn, C. C., Greenswag, L. R., Horsthemke, B., Kondo, I., Kuwajima, K., Niikawa, N., Rogan, P. K., Schwartz, S., Seip, J., Williams, C. A., Wiznitzer, M., & Nicholls, R. D. (1997). Clinical spectrum and molecular diagnosis of Angelman and Prader–Willi syndrome imprinting mutation patients. *American Journal of Medical Genetics, 68,* 195–206.

Silverstein, A. B. (1982). A note on the constancy of IQ. *American Journal of Mental Deficiency, 87,* 227–229.

Sparrow, S. S., Balla, D., & Cicchetti, D. V. (1984). *The Vineland Adaptive Behavior Scales.* Circle Pines, MN: American Guidance Service.

Spritz, R. A., Bailin, T., Nicholls, R. D., Lee, S. T., Park, S. K., Mascari, M. J., & Butler, M. G. (1997). Hypopigmentation in the Prader–Willi syndrome correlates with *P* gene deletion but not with haplotype of the hemizygous *P* allele. *American Journal of Medical Genetics, 71,* 57–62.

Stein, D. J., Keating, K., Zar, H. J., & Hollander, E. (1994). A survey of the phenomenology and pharmacotherapy of compulsive and impulsive–aggressive symptoms in Prader–Willi syndrome. *Journal of Neuropsychiatry and Clinical Neuroscience, 6,* 23–29.

Sulzbacher, S., Crnic, K., & Snow, J. (1981). Behavioral and cognitive disabilities in Prader–Willi syndrome. In V. Holm, S. Sulzbacher, & P. Pipes (Eds.), *The Prader–Willi syndrome* (pp. 147–169). Baltimore: University Park Press.

Swaab, D. F., Purba, J. S., & Hofman, M. A. (1995). Alterations in the hypothalamic paraventricular nucleus and its oxytocin neurons (putative satiety cells) in Prader–Willi syndrome: A study of 5 cases. *Journal of Clinical Endocrinology and Metabolism, 80,* 573–579.

Taylor, R. L. (1988). Cognitive and behavioral features. In M. L. Caldwell & R. L. Taylor (Eds.), *Prader–Willi syndrome: Selected research and management issues* (pp. 29–42). New York: Springer-Verlag.

Vitiello, B., Spreat, S., & Behar, D. (1989). Obsessive–compulsive disorder in mentally retarded patients. *Journal of Nervous and Mental Disease, 177,* 232–236.

Warnock, J. K., & Kestenbaum, T. (1992). Pharmacologic treatment of severe skin picking behaviors in Prader–Willi syndrome. *Archives of Dermatology, 128,* 1623–1625.

Warren, J., & Hunt, E. (1981). Cognitive processing in children with Prader–Willi syndrome. In V. Holm, S. Sulzbacher, & P. Pipes (Eds.), *The Prader–Willi syndrome* (pp. 161–177). Baltimore: University Park Press.

Waters, J. (1990). Prader–Willi syndrome. In J. Hogg, J. Sebba, & L. Lambe (Eds.), *Profound mental retardation and multiple impairment: Vol. 3. Medical and physical care and management* (pp. 54–67). London: Chapman & Hall.

Whitman, B. Y., & Accardo, P. (1987). Emotional problems in Prader–Willi adolescents. *American Journal of Medical Genetics, 28,* 897–905.

Williams, C. A., Angelman, H,, Clayton-Smith, J., Driscoll, D. J., Hendrickson, J. E., Knoll, J. H., Magenis, R. E., Schinzel, A., Wagstaff, J., Whidden, E. M., & Zori, R. T. (1995). Angelman syndrome: Consensus for diagnostic criteria. *American Journal of Medical Genetics, 56,* 237–238.

Zipf, W. B., & Bernston, G. G. (1987). Characteristics of abnormal food-intake patterns in children with Prader–Willi syndrome and study of effects of naloxone. *American Journal of Clinical Nutrition, 46,* 277–281.

24

WILLIAMS SYNDROME

COLLEEN A. MORRIS
CAROLYN B. MERVIS

Williams syndrome (WS) is characterized by a recognizable pattern of dysmorphic facial features, connective tissue abnormalities, cardiovascular disease, delayed development, a specific cognitive profile, and a unique personality. It usually occurs sporadically, with an incidence of 1 in 20,000 live births in all ethnic groups. The genetic etiology of WS, discovered in 1993, is a submicroscopic deletion of a portion of the long arm of chromosome 7 that contains the *elastin* gene (*ELN*) (Ewart et al., 1993a). The deletion of genes in the 7q11.23 region is responsible for the WS phenotype. The combination of a specific cognitive profile and unique personality make WS an important subject of research regarding the interrelationships of genes, neurodevelopment, cognition, and behavior. In this chapter, we discuss the genetic etiology, medical complications, pattern of cognitive strengths and weaknesses, and behavioral characteristics that constitute the WS phenotype.

GENETICS

WS is caused by a submicroscopic deletion of chromosome 7 at band q11.23 (Figure 24.1). The deletion is too small to be detected cytogenetically with standard banding techniques, but can be identified readily with fluorescent *in situ* hybridization (FISH). The FISH technique utilizes a DNA probe containing the *ELN* gene that is labeled with a fluorescent dye. The probe is applied to metaphase chromosomes of the subject. Normally, both chromosome 7s will show hybridization with the probe. In WS, only one of the chromosome pair (the normal one) will have the fluorescent marker. Several laboratories have demonstrated the *ELN* deletion in series of patients with WS, reporting an incidence of deletion of 97–100% (Ewart et al., 1993a; Lowery et al., 1995; Mari et al., 1995; Nickerson, Greenberg, Keating, McCaskill, & Shaffer, 1995).

WS usually occurs sporadically in families. The deletion of chromosome 7 can be either maternal or paternal in origin (Ewart et al., 1993a; Dutly & Schinzel, 1996; Urban et al., 1996). The occurrence of a deletion is probably related to the high number of repeti-

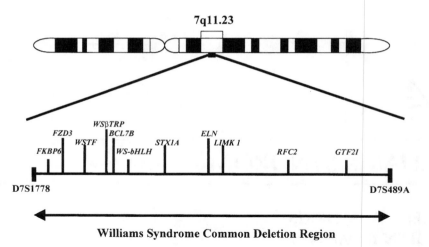

FIGURE 24.1. Physical map of the submicroscopic deletion of chromosome 7q11.23 that causes WS. The classic deletion is flanked by two polymorphic markers, D7S1778 and D7S489A. Relative positions of the genes within the region are shown, but the distances between the genes are not to scale.

tive DNA sequences in this region, since repetitive sequences are often associated with chromosome rearrangements. During meiosis, crossover occurs between regions of homologous chromosomes. The presence of a repetitive sequence increases the chance for a mismatch to occur, resulting in loss of chromosomal material. An individual with a deletion has a 50% chance with each pregnancy of passing on the deleted copy of chromosome 7 to offspring. Such cases of parent-to-child transmission of WS have been reported; both males and females have reproduced (Morris, Greenberg, & Thomas, 1993a; Sadler, Robinson, Verdaasdonk, & Gingell, 1993).

Chromosomes are paired, with one copy coming from the mother and one copy from the father. An individual with a deletion of a portion of a chromosome will have only one copy of each of the genes in the affected region, and therefore is hemizygous for those contiguous genes. The effect (phenotype) of the gene depends on its function. For some gene pairs, one copy of the gene is sufficient for normal outcome; for other gene pairs, *both* copies must be present for normal function or development. The abnormal phenotype in contiguous-gene deletion syndromes, then, results from the absence of some of the genes within the critical region. The object of genotype–phenotype correlation is to determine which genes contribute to the specific and individual phenotypic characteristics of the condition.

The size of the deletion in classic WS is approximately 1.5 megabases (a megabase equals 1 million base pairs of DNA) (Meng et al., 1998a). This region is large enough to contain several genes; 13 have been mapped within the region thus far (Ewart et al., 1993a; Frangiskakis et al., 1996; Jurado, Peoples, Kaplan, Hamel, & Francke, 1996; Osborne et al., 1996; Wang et al., 1997). Two of these contiguous genes, *ELN* and *LIM kinase 1* (*LIMK1*), have been associated with specific aspects of the WS phenotype (Ewart et al., 1993b; Frangiskakis et al., 1996). The function of the other genes relative to WS is unknown. They are *RFC2* (Peoples, Perez-Jurado, Wang, Kaplan, & Francke, 1996), *STX1A* (Osborne et al., 1997), *FZD3* (Wang et al., 1997), *FKBP6* (Meng, Lu, Morris, & Keating, 1998b), *GTF2I* (Jurado et al., 1998), *WSTF, WS-βTRP, WS-bHLH, BCL7B* (Meng et al., 1998a), *CPE-R*, and *RVP1* (Paperna, Peoples, Wang, & Francke, 1998).

ELN was the first known gene found to be deleted in WS (Ewart et al., 1993a). *ELN* codes for elastin, an important connective tissue protein found in skin, ligaments, organ walls, and (significantly) in the walls of arteries. Hemizygosity for *ELN* accounts for many of the connective tissue abnormalities of WS: generalized arteriopathy, including supravalvar aortic stenosis (SVAS); hernias; bowel and bladder diverticulae; premature aging of the skin; joint hypermobility in young children, followed by joint contractures in adults; hoarse voice quality; and some aspects of the dysmorphic face, such as periorbital fullness and full, jowly cheeks in infants and toddlers. Mutation of *ELN* has been shown to cause familial SVAS (Ewart et al., 1993b; Ensing et al., 1989; Olson et al., 1993). SVAS is inherited in an autosomal dominant fashion (Eisenberg, Young, Jacobson, & Boito, 1964; Grimm & Wesselhoeft, 1980). Families with SVAS typically have cardiovascular disease, hernias, and hoarse voice, but lack other WS features, such as developmental delay, growth retardation, and the WS personality. The second gene implicated in the WS phenotype was *LIMK1* (Frangiskakis et al., 1996). Hemizygosity of *LIMK1* is associated with the severe weakness in visual–spatial constructive cognition manifested by individuals with WS.

Variability is present in all disease, including genetic syndromes. The variability of expression of a gene has many etiologies. Some of the variability is the result of environmental factors. For instance, a lower socioeconomic status may account for decreased achievement scores on standardized tests. Another component of variability is the age of the individual, which always affects the phenotype. Certain characteristics change over time, such as the WS facial features (Morris, Leonard, Dilts, & Demsey, 1990). Some symptoms are more likely to be present at specific ages, such as hypercalcemia (which typically is symptomatic only in infancy) and joint limitations which are more common in older children and adults with WS). Some variability is due to a genetic cause. Examples of genetic variability include (1) different size of deletions, resulting in different numbers of deleted genes; (2) actions of other inherited genes on the phenotype, resulting in either an additive negative effect or an ameliorating positive effect; and (3) parent-of-origin effect, resulting from deletion of imprinted genes. Of these three possibilities for genetic variability, only the first, different deletion size, has been conclusively proven to occur in WS (Botta et al., 1998; Hirota et al., 1998). Regarding the third possibility, parent-of-origin effect, maternal origin of deletion had been implicated in more severe growth retardation in one series of individuals with WS (Jurado et al., 1996), but this finding was not replicated in subsequent series (Wu et al., 1998; Wang et al., 1998).

Prior to the molecular genetic discoveries, the relationship between WS and familial SVAS was unclear (Beuren, 1972; Grimm & Wesselhoeft, 1980; Merritt, Palmar, Lurie, & Petry, 1963). Most families with SVAS have a mutation in *ELN*. However, some rare families with SVAS have been found that have additional features of WS, showing a partial overlap with the WS phenotype (Frangiskakis et al., 1996; Sommer, Wheeller, Wagner, & Wegner, 1996). In two of these families, deletions of chromosome 7 have been characterized. Importantly, the size of the deletions is much less than in classic WS; the deletion was 83 kilobases in one family and approximately 300 kilobases in the other (Frangiskakis et al., 1996). Genotype–phenotype analysis has shown that these families have the cognitive profile and the connective tissue abnormalities of WS, associated with the deletion of *LIMK1* and *ELN*, respectively. Study of other families and individuals with partial or intermediate phenotypes may yield clues about the genes responsible for other aspects of the WS phenotype. Individuals with larger, microscopically visible deletions, including 7q11.23, have features of the WS phenotype such as cardiovascular disease. However, these patients also have additional birth defects or disability, and therefore would not be classified as having WS (Morris, Loker, Ensing, & Stock, 1993b).

CLINICAL/MEDICAL MANIFESTATIONS

WS is a multisystem disorder, and any of the medical complications detailed in this section may lead the clinician to consider the WS diagnosis. The diagnosis is considered earliest in infants with the most severe congenital heart disease. In young children, the diagnosis is typically suggested by the combination of developmental delay, idiopathic hypercalcemia, dysmorphic facies, and/or cardiovascular disease, especially SVAS. In older children, adolescents, and adults, the presence of the specific WS cognitive profile and the unique WS personality may contribute to a suspicion of the WS diagnosis. Prior to the availability of the FISH test for WS, mean age at diagnosis was 6.4 years and median age was 4 years (Morris, Dilts, Demsey, Leonard, & Blackburn, 1988). With the advent of an objective test, it is likely that the diagnosis will be made at a younger age in the future (Lowery et al., 1995). If WS is suspected in an individual, then FISH should be performed to establish the diagnosis.

The facial gestalt of the individual with WS is distinctive. Infants and young children with WS have a broad brow with bitemporal narrowing, periorbital fullness, a flat facial profile, a short upturned nose, a long philtrum, a wide mouth with full lips, full cheeks, and prominent earlobes (Figure 24.2). As children age, the face typically becomes more narrow, the neck has a long appearance, the nasal tip is bulbous, dental malocclusion is present, and facial asymmetry is common (Morris et al., 1988, 1990). In the remainder of this section, the WS medical complications and their treatment are discussed by organ system.

Ocular/Visual

Ocular and visual abnormalities are quite common in WS (Braddick & Atkinson, 1995; Greenberg & Lewis, 1988; Jones & Smith, 1975; Kapp, von Noorden, & Jenkins, 1995;

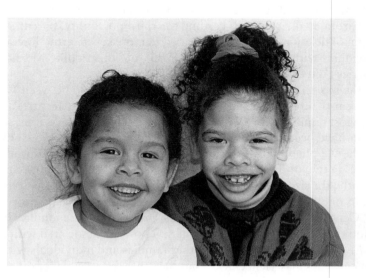

FIGURE 24.2. The distinctive facial gestalt of an individual with WS is seen in this 7-year-old girl with WS (right) as compared to her normally developing 4-year-old sister (left). Photograph used by permission of children's parents.

Morris et al., 1988). The stellate or lacy iris pattern observed in children with WS who have blue or hazel irides is secondary to hypoplasia of the anterior iris stroma and has no clinical consequence, though it is a helpful diagnostic sign (Greenberg & Lewis, 1988).

Refractive errors, most commonly hyperopia (farsightedness), are found in 25–50% of individuals with WS and are treated with corrective lenses. Strabismus, usually infantile esotropia, has its onset before age 6 months and is reported in 30–70% of children with WS, in contrast to an incidence of .1% in the general population. Because strabismus is seen at higher frequencies in children with other syndromes with impaired neurodevelopment, the strabismus in WS may be related to abnormalities of central visual pathways. One less likely possibility is that the elastin abnormality adversely affects the extraocular muscles (Kapp et al., 1995). The strabismus is usually treated with corrective lenses, patching, or surgery (medial rectus muscle recession).

Individuals with WS have problems with visual–motor integration. Examples include impaired visual–spatial construction and problems with depth perception, manifested in difficulty in negotiating curbs, stairs, and uneven surfaces. Many individuals with WS compensate by using handrails or by touching the heel to the back of the step for additional sensory input when descending stairs. With the high prevalence of vision problems in WS, Braddick and Atkinson (1995) looked for correlation between visual impairment and performance on spatial tasks, but did not find significant differences between the children with and without stereovision deficit. Sadler, Olitsky, and Reynolds (1996) also found significant reduction in stereoacuity resulting in abnormal binocular vision, and suggested that this sensory abnormality may be due to errors in brain morphogenesis. Since visual recognition skills (processed by the occipito*temporal* visual pathway called the "ventral stream") are preserved in WS, and visual–motor skills (processed by the occipito*parietal* visual pathway called the "dorsal stream") are weak in WS, it may be that the latter pathway is adversely affected by a gene deleted in WS. Atkinson et al. (1997) found deficits in performance on tasks requiring dorsal stream processing, but normal performance on tasks requiring ventral stream processing.

Children with WS should have ophthalmological evaluation and treatment when the diagnosis of WS is made, and will require periodic evaluations thereafter.

Ear/Auditory

Chronic otitis media is a significant problem in 40–60% of children with WS (Klein, Armstrong, Greer, & Brown, 1990; Morris et al., 1988). Hypotonia and connective tissue abnormalities affecting the pharynx and eustachian tube contribute to this problem. Tympanostomy tubes are often helpful to treat chronic disease. Like chronic otitis media in the general pediatric population, it tends to improve as a child gets older.

A more common auditory problem in WS is hypersensitivity to sound, reported in 85–95% (Klein et al., 1990; Martin, Snodgrass, & Cohen, 1984; Morris et al., 1988; Van Borsel, Curfs, & Fryns, 1997). Young children exhibit an exaggerated startle response to noise, cover their ears, or become upset in anticipation of some noises (e.g., seeing a vacuum cleaner). Older children and adults seem to become aware of environmental noises before others do, and complain that certain noises cause them to have a "nervous feeling." Though this symptom has been termed "hyperacusis" in the literature, Marriage and Barnes (1995) suggest that "phonophobia" may be a more correct designation. The auditory hypersensitivity is not associated with either hearing impairment or chronic otitis media in WS.

Possible explanations for this hypersensitivity include a connective tissue abnormality affecting the conduction of sound, or a difference in central processing pathways for auditory information, complicated by distractibility. Van Borsel et al. (1997) did not find a relationship between hyperactivity and hyperacusis in WS. Abnormality of serotonin function in sensory pathways has been proposed as one possible central nervous system mechanism (Marriage & Barnes, 1995). Loud and sudden noises should be avoided when possible, or earplugs may be used. Warning a child about an upcoming noise and explaining the origin of the sound is also helpful.

Respiratory

The voice in WS is distinctive. It has been variously described as hoarse, low-pitched, gravelly, or flat. Its pathogenesis is unknown, but it is probably related to the elastin abnormality, since it is also present in SVAS families. Other conditions that affect connective tissue, such as the myxedema of hypothyroidism, also alter voice quality.

Because elastin is an important component of the lung (i.e., damage to elastic fibers is seen in patients with emphysema), one might expect abnormalities of the pulmonary system in WS. However, there is no increase in the incidence of pulmonary disease in WS, suggesting that a single *ELN* allele is sufficient for production of elastic fibers in lung tissue.

Cardiovascular

The incidence of SVAS is 65–75% in WS. The detection of SVAS depends upon the sensitivity of the examination. The use of both two-dimensional and Doppler flow analysis is the preferable method (Ensing et al., 1989). The aortic narrowing may worsen over time, and monitoring of the cardiovascular system is warranted. On the other hand, the supravalvar pulmonic stenosis and peripheral pulmonic stenosis associated with the disease may improve clinically over time. One possible explanation for this difference between the pulmonic and the systemic systems in that the pulmonic vascular tree is subject to lower hemodynamic stress (pressure) than the systemic vasculature.

The effect of SVAS depends upon the degree of narrowing. It may be present as an hourglass narrowing of the aorta, or longer segments of the aorta may be involved, resulting in a generalized hypoplasia of the aorta. The aortic narrowing causes increased resistance, resulting in elevated left heart pressures and cardiac hypertrophy, which can lead to cardiac failure and death if untreated. Although the clinical findings are most significant in the aorta, it is important to realize that a generalized arteriopathy exists. Coronary artery stenosis has been implicated in some cases of sudden death in WS (Bird et al., 1996). Other localized arterial stenoses may account for additional symptoms in some patients with WS. For instance, renal artery stenosis is associated with hypertension (Deal, Snell, Marratt, & Dillon, 1992), and stenoses of mesenteric arteries may contribute to abdominal pain on the basis of bowel ischemia in some patients.

Involvement of the neurovasculature has been reported in rare patients (Ardinger, Goertz, & Mattioli, 1994; Soper et al., 1995). In isolated cases, a cerebrovascular accident has complicated the course of WS by causing additional neurological symptoms. However, it is unlikely that the arterial narrowing results in cerebral ischemia that in turn accounts for the neurodevelopmental abnormalities of WS. The pathological appearance of the arteries is identical in both familial SVAS, caused by a *mutation* in the *ELN* gene, and in WS, caused by *deletion* of the *ELN* gene (O'Connor et al., 1985). The degree of variability in the severity of the cardiovascular disease in both WS populations and in SVAS kindred is the same. Since there is no increased incidence of developmental delay or learning disability in *ELN*-mutation SVAS families, it is unlikely that the arteriopathy contributes significantly to either problem in patients with WS (Ewart et al., 1993b; Frangiskakis et al., 1996).

Hypertension is problematic for adult patients with WS and may be difficult to treat. A recent study indicates that blood pressures may be falsely elevated in WS, due to rigidity of arterial walls (Broder, Reinhardt, Lifton, Tamborlane, & Pober, 1995). Complicating measurement of blood pressure in WS is anxiety in medical situations, which alone results in temporary elevation of the blood pressure.

The incidence of structural congenital heart disease in WS, *excluding* abnormalities of the great vessels, is 17%.

Since the cardiovascular abnormalities contribute most to the mortality and morbidity of WS, early and ongoing monitoring and treatment of this system are warranted in order to optimize outcome.

Gastrointestinal

Feeding difficulties are reported in 70% of infants with WS (Morris et al., 1988). The majority (80%) have failure to thrive, which is probably the combined result of poor feeding, vomiting, constipation, and colic. Hypercalcemia, which occurs in 15% of infants with WS, has symptoms of abdominal pain, polyuria, and constipation that may also contribute to feeding difficulties. Both umbilical and inguinal hernias are common, occur in equal frequency in males and females, and require inguinal herniorrhaphy in 38%. Chronic constipation is reported by 40% of patients. The constipation may be the result of disturbed bowel motility or, in some cases, the result of hypothyroidism. Rectal prolapse has been reported in infants and children with WS, and is probably a result of the elastin deficit.

Chronic abdominal pain is a common complaint of adults. Possible causes of pain in this population include peptic ulcer disease, cholelethiasis, diverticulitis, ischemic bowel disease, constipation, and somatization of anxiety. The elastic fiber abnormality results in a high incidence of diverticulosis of the colon in WS (Morris et al., 1990; Pleatman & Dunbar, 1980). It is possible that this connective tissue abnormality also contributes to abdominal pain, primarily by resulting in painful overdistention of the bowel. Alternatively, a secondary hypersensitivity to normal bowel distention could result from dysfunction of sensory or autonomic nervous pathways caused by a deleted gene. It is likely that the abdominal pain is related to some combination of these factors. Because this pain can be debilitating, evaluation for a specific etiology is recommended in order to provide appropriate treatment.

Renal

Although kidney and urinary tract anomalies in the general population occur at a rate of 1.5%, patients with WS have an 18% incidence of renal anomalies (Pankau, Partsch, Winter, Gosch, & Wessel, 1996; Pober, Lacro, Rice, Mandell, & Teele, 1993). For this reason, a screening renal ultrasound is recommended for patients with WS. Structural anomalies reported include renal aplasia/hypoplasia, renal duplication, renal cysts, and hydroneph-rosis. Bladder diverticulae, vesicoureteral reflux, and urinary tract infections have been noted in series of patients with WS. Nephrocalcinosis has been observed, but the prevalence is low (<5%). Renal artery stenosis has been reported in 45–55% of patients who had had renal artery angiography (Ingelfinger & Newburger, 1991; Pankau et al., 1996; Pober et al., 1993).

Urinary frequency is common in children with WS; it is unknown whether this is the result of impulsivity, of diminished bladder capacity, or perhaps of hypercalciuria result-ing in increased production of urine. Enuresis is a common problem in WS, found in 50%. Recurrent urinary tract infections are a problem in one-third of adults with WS.

Puberty occurs early in WS, though the cause is unknown. Both males and females with WS have reproduced, but no systematic study of fertility has been done.

Musculoskeletal

The infant or young child with WS has hyperextensible joints (Morris et al., 1988). This joint instability contributes to delayed walking. The joint hypermobility may also be re-lated to a common childhood complaint in WS: nocturnal leg pains or cramps. These typi-cally occur after a day of high physical activity. Provision of joint support with elastic bandages and high-top shoes may ameliorate this problem. Physical therapy to strengthen knee muscles may also help. In many cases, the joint laxity leads to the development of abnormal compensatory postures to achieve stability. Gradual tightening of the heel cords and hamstrings occurs, resulting in a stiff and awkward gait by adolescence. Adults with WS frequently have kyphosis and lordosis. Limitation of supination of the forearm is seen in 10% of patients with WS and is sometimes due to radioulnar synostosis (Morris et al., 1988).

Kaplan, Kirschner, Watters, and Costa (1989) found joint contractures in 50% of individuals with WS, affecting hips, knees, ankles, wrists, elbows, and fingers. The con-tractures led to both gross motor and fine motor disability. The onset of contractures oc-curred in infancy in half of the patients. Voit et al. (1991) reported muscle weakness in four of six patients, a secondary carnitine deficiency in muscle in three of six patients, and nonspecific myopathic changes on muscle biopsy. Physical therapy and low-impact exer-cise with concentration on correct posture are recommended.

Metabolism/Growth

One of the first reports of a child with WS detailed the symptoms of hypercalcemia (Light-wood, 1952). This aspect of WS led to its early designation as "idiopathic hypercalcemia of childhood." Despite this appellation, however, hypercalcemia is documented in only 15% of children with WS (Morris et al., 1988). Multiple theories have been advanced re-garding the etiology of the hypercalcemia, but none has been proven (Culler, Jones, & Deftos, 1985; Forbes, Bryson, Manning, Amirhakmi, & Reina, 1972; Friedman & Mills, 1969). When hypercalcemia is diagnosed in WS, it is usually symptomatic, causing constipation, abdominal pain, and failure to thrive. In most instances, treatment with a low-calcium diet is adequate, but refractory cases are treated with oral steroids (Martin et al., 1984). Indi-viduals with WS are short compared to their families, and growth curves for WS are avail-able (Morris et al., 1988; Saul et al., 1988).

Neurological

The most prevalent neurological problem in the infant or young child with WS is hypotonia, whereas most older children and adults have hypertonia (Chapman, du Plessis, & Pober, 1996; Morris et al., 1988). Therefore a young child will have delayed attainment of gross motor milestones, because the combination of hypotonia and lax joints compromises stability in weight bearing. By adulthood, most patients have hyperactive deep tendon reflexes and an awkward gait. Fine motor difficulties are common at all ages.

Neuroimaging studies have shown few gross anatomical malformations. Jernigan, Bellugi, Sowell, Doherty, and Hesselink (1993) compared cerebral volume of WS and Down syndrome (DS) patients; they reported that individuals with both syndromes had reduced cerebral volume compared to controls, but that individuals with WS had preservation of cerebellar size. Rare patients with WS have had a Chiari I malformation of the brain, which is the displacement of the cerebellum through foramen magnum. Symptoms may include headache, dysphagia, dizziness, and weakness (Kaplan et al., 1989; Pober & Filiano, 1995; Wang, Hesselink, Jernigan, Doherty, & Bellugi, 1992). Pober and Filiano (1995) suggest that this finding is due to a mismatch between a normal-sized cerebellum and a small posterior fossa.

Rare cases of ischemic stroke have been reported in children with WS and are secondary to arterial stenoses of the cerebral vasculature (Ardinger et al., 1994; Soper et al., 1995).

COGNITIVE STRENGTHS AND WEAKNESSES

In addition to the characteristic multisystem medical manifestations, WS is associated with a particular pattern of cognitive strengths and weaknesses. Studies of cognition in children with WS have concentrated on three types of abilities: language, auditory rote memory, and visual–spatial construction (e.g., block design, drawing). The results of these studies have converged on a characteristic cognitive profile. At the same time, researchers have shown that there is a great deal of variability in the overall level of intellectual ability among children with WS. Below, we first review the results of studies focused on specific types of cognitive abilities. We then summarize the findings regarding overall level of intellectual ability. Finally, we consider a quantitative measure that we and our colleagues (Mervis et al., 1998b; Mervis, Morris, Bertrand, & Robinson, 1999) have developed for assessing the WS cognitive profile (WSCP).

Language

Studies of the language abilities of children and adolescents with WS have investigated both grammatical development and lexical (vocabulary) development. Most recently, a few studies of the language abilities of toddlers and preschoolers with WS have been reported. Each of these topics is considered separately below.

Grammar

The initial studies of the grammatical abilities of individuals with WS were conducted by Bellugi and her colleagues (e.g., Bellugi, Bihrle, Jernigan, Trauner, & Doherty, 1990; Bellugi, Marks, Bihrle, & Sabo, 1988; Bellugi, Wang, & Jernigan, 1994). Results of these studies, which involved adolescents, indicated excellent syntactic abilities. The participants were reliably able to comprehend reversible passives (e.g., "The dog is chased by the man"), conditionals, and negation. Their spoken language was grammatically correct and included complex grammatical constructions such as embedded clauses. When adolescents with WS heard sentences containing grammatical errors, they were able to detect these errors and in most cases to correct them. Moreover, they were able to form tag questions, which requires mastery of question formation rules, the verb auxiliary system, pronouns, and negation. In all these studies, the performance of adolescents with WS was compared to that of adolescents with DS matched for both chronological age (CA) and IQ. The adolescents with WS greatly outperformed those with DS. Klein and Mervis (in press) have compared the performance of 9- and 10-year-old children with WS to that of CA- and IQ-matched children with DS. Examination of the spontaneous expressive language produced by the two groups of children confirmed Bellugi et al.'s finding that the grammatical abilities of individuals with WS were more advanced than those of individuals with DS. Rice, Mervis, Klein, and Rice (1998) compared the morphological abilities of children with WS to those of younger children with specific language impairment (SLI) matched for mean length of utterance (MLU). The utterances of the children with WS were more complex than those of the children with SLI. In particular, the children with WS were much more likely to use morphemes encoding tense and aspect than were the children with SLI.

Individuals with DS and individuals with SLI are well known to have inordinate difficulty with morphosyntax (e.g., Chapman, 1997; Leonard, 1998; Rice & Wexler, 1997). When the grammatical abilities of children with WS are compared to those of other groups, a somewhat different pattern of findings emerges. In these studies, the grammatical abilities of children with WS generally have been found to be consistent with those of the individuals in the matched comparison group (e.g., Gosch, Stading, & Pankau, 1994; Udwin & Yule, 1990; Volterra, Capirci, Pezzini, Sabbadini, & Vicari, 1996). Klein (1995; Mervis et al., 1999) found that the grammatical abilities of English-speaking children with WS were considerably delayed. Although the mean CA of these children was 7 years, their mean MLU was lower than that reported by Scarborough (1990) for normally developing 3½-year-olds. Encouragingly, however, the relation between MLU and Index of Productive Syntax (IPSyn, a measure of emerging grammatical abilities; Scarborough, 1990) was the same for the children with WS as for the normally developing children. That is, the grammatical complexity of the children with WS was at the level expected for the length of their utterances. Rice et al. (1998) found that the morphological abilities (e.g., use of verb tense and aspect, noun plurals, and determiners) of these children with WS were similar to those of younger normally developing children matched for MLU.

The English language has relatively little morphology. For example, only pronouns are assigned grammatical gender or grammatical case (e.g., subject, object). Morphology in many languages is more complex. Recently, the use of grammatical gender has been considered for individuals with WS whose native language is either French or Italian— two languages with more complex grammatical gender systems. Karmiloff-Smith et al. (1997) considered the ability of French individuals with WS (mean age = 15 years, 9 months) to correctly produce determiner–noun–adjective phrases. In French, all three words must agree in grammatical gender. The individuals with WS made significantly more errors than did a contrast group of normally developing 5-year-olds. Volterra et al. (1996) reported that Italian children with WS also made more errors on grammatical gender than did the contrast group of younger normally developing children.

In summary, the syntactic abilities of children with WS are delayed relative to CA-matched normally developing children, advanced relative to matched children with DS or

SLI, consistent with those of matched children with mixed etiologies of mental retardation, and at the level expected for MLU. The morphological abilities of children with WS who are learning English are at the expected level for MLU. However, children with WS who are learning languages with more complex morphology have weaker morphological abilities than would be expected from MLU.

Lexicon

Most studies of the lexical ability of children and adolescents with WS have focused on performance on the Peabody Picture Vocabulary Test—Revised (PPVT-R; Dunn & Dunn, 1981). This measure requires a participant to choose, from a set of four pictures, the one that best matches the word that the researcher says. Words tested include names for objects, actions, descriptors, and abstractions. In a study of 85 children with WS between the ages of 4 and 17 years, we (Mervis et al., 1999) found a wide range of performance: Standard scores ranged from 19 (bottom of the 1st percentile) to 109 (73rd percentile), with a mean of 67.65 (SD = 18.88). The distribution of raw scores on the PPVT-R as a function of CA is presented in Figure 24.3. As is clear from the figure, vocabulary increases as children get older. The correlation between raw score and CA was .78 (p < .001). Standard scores were consistent across the age range sampled, indicating that the children with WS maintained their position relative to their normally developing peers across this age range. Although most of the children tested had Full Scale IQs in the mentally retarded range, 48% scored in the normal range on the PPVT-R, indicating that vocabulary is a strength for children with WS.

Other researchers have also considered the performance of children and adolescents with WS on the PPVT-R. Bellugi and her colleagues (e.g., Bellugi, Bihrle, Neville, & Doherty, 1992; Bellugi et al., 1988, 1990, 1994; Rossen, Klima, Bellugi, Bihrle, & Jones, 1996) have compared the performance of adolescents with WS on the PPVT-R to that of CA- and IQ-

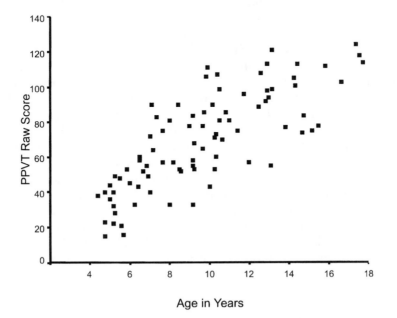

FIGURE 24.3. Distribution of raw scores on the PPVT-R as a function of CA.

matched adolescents with DS. The individuals with WS consistently scored higher than those with DS, and almost all of the individuals with WS earned higher age-equivalent scores on the PPVT-R than on a Full Scale IQ test (the Wechsler Intelligence Scale for Children—Revised [WISC-R]; Wechsler, 1974). In contrast, the results of studies of younger children with WS have indicated that these children's PPVT-R scores are consistent with those of the children in the matched contrast group, regardless of whether these children are normally developing (Volterra et al., 1996) or have DS (Klein & Mervis, in press).

Studies of the lexicon of individuals with WS have also been concerned with semantic organization (how a person cognitively relates the members of a particular category, such as "animals"). Semantic organization is typically measured by performance on semantic fluency tasks. These tasks require participants to name as many members of a given semantic category (e.g., "animals," "food," "clothing") as possible. Bellugi and her colleagues (Bellugi et al., 1992, 1994; Rossen et al., 1996) have compared the performance of adolescents with WS to that of either CA- and IQ-matched adolescents with DS or normally developing second-graders. Participants were asked to name as many animals as they could within 1 minute. Based on the findings of this study, Bellugi et al. concluded that the semantic organization of adolescents with WS was deviant. In particular, Bellugi and her colleagues found that adolescents with WS were much more likely than either of the contrast groups to list unusual animals (unusualness was defined as low word frequency), such as "yak" or "weasel."

More recently, the semantic organization of younger children with WS has been studied. Volterra et al. (1996) found no differences between the children with WS and the contrast group of younger normally developing children whose CA matched the mental age (MA) of the WS group. Most of the animals listed by the children in both groups were common (commonness was defined as high word frequency). Scott, Mervis, Klein, Armstrong, and Ford (1995; see Mervis et al., 1999) compared the performance of 12 children aged 9 and 10 years with WS to that of three other groups: CA- and IQ-matched children with DS, CA-matched children who were developing normally, and younger normally developing children matched for MA. Findings for word frequency matched those of Volterra et al. (1996). There were no differences among the three groups matched for MA. The CA-matched controls were more likely to produce infrequent animal names than any of the MA-matched groups. Scott et al. (1995) also considered the representativeness of the animals named (i.e., how well each animal named fit college students' idea or image of "animal"). This representativeness measure (also called "goodness of example" [GOE] or "typicality") is the most commonly used measure in studies of semantic organization of individuals who are developing normally (see, e.g., Rosch, 1973, 1975). The findings for mean representativeness value were the same as for word frequency: no differences among the three MA-matched groups, with a significantly higher (less representative) mean value for the normally developing CA-matched group. If only the GOE of the least representative animal named is considered, the performance of the WS and DS groups was equivalent to that of the CA matches. The least good exemplars named by the members of these groups were significantly less representative than the least good exemplars named by the younger normally developing MA matches. This latter finding probably reflects the increased life experience of the three CA-matched groups relative to the younger normally developing MA controls. These findings suggest that semantic organization in WS is appropriate, rather than deviant.

Early Language Development

Young children with WS do not begin to acquire language at the same CA as normally developing children. Singer Harris, Bellugi, Bates, Jones, and Rossen (1997) have stated that the acquisition of words is delayed by an average of 2 years. Furthermore, they have argued that in the earliest stages of language acquisition, children with DS have an advantage over children with WS. This is the polar opposite of their findings for adolescents: Adolescents with WS showed a strong advantage over adolescents with DS regarding all aspects of language ability. Over the entire age range considered (12 to 76 months), there was no difference between the two syndrome groups in vocabulary size. However, once grammatical development began, children with WS showed an advantage over children with DS. The findings from this study are problematic for several reasons. The two most important are that the diagnosis of WS was based on parental report rather than genetic test results,* and that comparisons between the two syndromes did not take CA into account.

Mervis, Robinson, Phelps, and Bertrand (1998c) have considered the early language development of 24 children with WS and 28 children with DS between the ages of 24 and 36 months. All diagnoses were verified by genetic testing. The findings of this study have confirmed that language onset is delayed for children with WS. On the MacArthur Communicative Development Inventories (Fenson et al., 1993)—the measure used in both the Singer Harris et al. (1997) and the Mervis et al. (1998c) studies—only about 30% of the 24- to 27-month-old children with WS in the Mervis et al. sample were at or above the 5th percentile (the lowest percentile included in the norms). However, in most cases, the delay was substantially less than that reported by Singer Harris et al. (1997). Furthermore, Mervis et al. (1998c) found that the language advantage for older individuals with WS relative to individuals with DS was present from the beginning of language acquisition. Even when only the age range from 24 to 27 months was considered, children with WS had much larger productive vocabularies (mean = 55 words) than children with DS (mean = 20 words). The discrepancy increased rapidly; for the age range from 32 to 36 months, mean vocabulary size was 191 for the children with WS and 83 for the children with DS.

Mervis and her colleagues (Mervis et al., 1995; Mervis & Robinson, 1998) have considered the early language development of 7 children with WS in more detail. These children were followed longitudinally from about the time they began to talk to at least age 5 years. The onset of language was delayed for all of these children. However, once they began to talk, the relation between the size of their receptive vocabulary and their productive vocabulary was consistently within normal limits (as defined by Bates, Dale, & Thal, 1995). The onset of novel (non-rote) two-word combinations was quite delayed, ranging from age 26 months to age 50 months. The onset of the spontaneous use of grammatical morphemes (e.g., plural, progressive) in two-word utterances (which occurs at about age 20 months for children who are developing normally) was further delayed. However, once this landmark was attained, grammatical development over the next year proceeded at about the same pace as for children who were developing normally. Until productive vocabulary size reached about 400 words, the relation between grammatical development and vocabulary size was within the normal range. Beginning at about 400 words, however, the grammatical development of the children with WS began to proceed more rapidly than expected from the rate of increase in vocabulary size.

---

*Approximately 20% of the "Williams syndrome" members of the Williams Syndrome Association do not actually have WS (T. Monkaba, personal communication, June 1998). Some of these individuals were clinically diagnosed with WS, but were later found not to have an *ELN* deletion. Other individuals received genetics reports indicating that they shared a few features with WS; this finding is often erroneously interpreted by parents as meaning that their children have WS. Given the manner in which participants were recruited for the Singer Harris et al. (1997) study, it is likely that about 20% of the WS group did not in fact have WS.

The relation between the onset of the ability to comprehend and produce referential pointing gestures and the onset of production of referential words has been considered for both normally developing children and children with a wide variety of developmental disabilities (see summary in Mervis & Bertrand, 1997). In almost all cases, comprehension and production of pointing gestures were found to precede the onset of referential production. Because of the consistency of this pattern, many early intervention programs use the onset of pointing gestures as a cue to begin working with children on vocabulary acquisition. This approach does not work for children with WS, however. Almost all children with WS begin to produce referential language well before they begin to comprehend or produce referential pointing gestures (Mervis & Bertrand, 1997). Given this pattern, a different cue for beginning intervention related to vocabulary acquisition is needed for children with WS. A possibility is to begin intervention related to vocabulary acquisition as soon as children begin to be able to maintain attention to both an object and a person at the same time (joint attention; Adamson, 1995).

Auditory Rote Memory

The results of several studies converge on the finding that auditory rote memory is a definite strength for children and adolescents with WS. Wang and Bellugi (1994) compared the auditory and visual rote memory abilities of 9 adolescents and young adults with WS to those of CA- and IQ-matched individuals with DS. Auditory rote memory was assessed with a forward digit span task. In this task, the researcher spoke a string of digits at a rate of one per second. Initial strings were two digits in length. If a participant was able to repeat a string of this length correctly, the researcher presented a string of three digits. The number of digits presented continued to increase until the participant was unable to repeat them correctly. Visual rote memory was measured with the Corsi blocks task (Milner, 1971). In this task, the researcher tapped a series of randomly placed blocks at a rate of one block per second, and the participant was then asked to tap the same sequence. As for the digit span task, initial strings involved tapping two blocks. If the participant was successful in repeating the sequence, the researcher increased the tapping sequence by one block at a time until the participant was unable to repeat the sequence correctly. Results indicated that the individuals with WS had significantly longer forward digit spans than the individuals with DS. In contrast, the individuals with DS had significantly longer Corsi spans than did the individuals with WS. Similarly, Klein and Mervis (in press) found that 9- and 10-year-olds with WS had significantly longer forward digit spans and word spans than CA- and MA-matched children with DS.

The results of studies including other types of comparison groups also have indicated that auditory rote memory is a strength for children with WS. Udwin and Yule (1991) found that children with WS recalled significantly more verbal items on the Rivermead Behavioural Memory Test (Wilson, Cockburn, & Baddeley, 1985) than did children of mixed etiologies of mental retardation matched for CA and WISC-R Verbal IQ. Finegan, Smith, Meschino, Vallance, and Sitarenios (1995) studied a sample of children, adolescents, and young adults with WS, and found that forward digit span, backward digit span, and word span were all greater than expected from MA.

We (Mervis et al., 1999) tested 65 children between the ages of 4 and 17 years on the Digit Recall subtest of the Differential Ability Scales (DAS; Elliott, 1990). In this measure, digits are presented at a rate of two per second, rather than the one-per-second rate used in the studies described previously. Because the DAS Digit Recall rate is more rapid, it more closely resembles the rate at which speech naturally occurs. A scatterplot of ability scores (similar to raw scores) on the DAS Digit Recall subtest as a function of CA is presented in Figure 24.4. As is clear from the figure, Digit Recall scores increased significantly as children got older ($r = .58$, $p < .001$). The mean T-score (standard score) was 34.83 ($SD = 8.87$), which is at the 7th percentile, definitely in the normal range. There was a great deal of variability among the children, however, with some obtaining the lowest possible T-score (bottom of the 1st percentile) while others earned T-scores as high as 55 (69th percentile). Although most of the children had Full Scale IQs within the mentally retarded range, 65% scored in the normal range (>2nd percentile) on DAS Digit Recall. These auditory rote memory abilities provide a solid foundation for both vocabulary acquisition and grammatical development (Mervis et al., 1999).

Visual–Spatial Construction

The most robust finding regarding the intellectual abilities of individuals with WS is the extreme difficulty they have with tasks involving visual–spatial construction. Two types of visual–spatial construction tasks have been studied: drawing and block design (pattern construction).

Drawing Measures

Studies of the drawing skills of individuals with WS have considered both the ability to copy geometric figures and the ability to draw and/or copy objects such as people or houses. Copying of geometric forms is usually assessed by performance on the Developmental Test

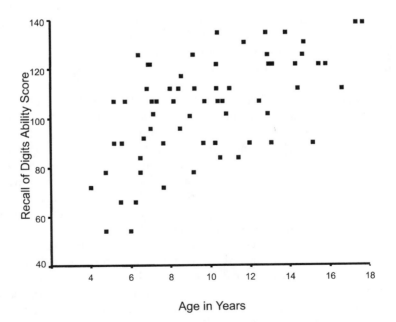

FIGURE 24.4. Distribution of ability scores (similar to raw scores) on DAS Digit Recall as a function of CA.

of Visual–Motor Integration (VMI; Beery, 1989). Completion of the VMI requires the participant to copy a series of line drawings, ranging from single lines and simple shapes to intersecting lines and shapes. Wang, Doherty, Rourke, and Bellugi (1995) compared the VMI performance of 10 adolescents and young adults with WS to that of CA- and IQ-matched individuals with DS. Although both groups performed poorly, the individuals with WS scored significantly lower than those with DS.

This discrepancy between individuals with WS and DS on ability to copy geometric figures is present by age 10 years. Klein and Mervis (in press) compared the performance of 13 children aged 9 and 10 years with WS on the Draw-a-Design subtest of the McCarthy Scales of Children's Abilities (McCarthy, 1972) to that of children with DS individually matched for CA and MA (based on total raw score on the McCarthy). The McCarthy Draw-a-Design subtest assesses the same types of drawings as the VMI. Once again, the children with WS earned significantly fewer points than the children with DS. Bertrand, Mervis, and Eisenberg (1997) compared the performance of 18 children aged 9 and 10 years with WS on the VMI to that of two groups of typically developing children: a group individually matched for CA, and a second group individually matched for MA (based on total raw score on the McCarthy). Both groups of typically developing children performed significantly better than the children with WS.

Research on the ability to draw and/or copy pictures of objects has yielded the same findings. These studies have typically used the flower, house, and elephant items from the Boston Diagnostic Aphasia Evaluation (BDAE; Goodglass & Kaplan, 1983). Participants are asked to first draw, and then copy a standard drawing of, a flower, a house, and an elephant. This task is often supplemented by asking participants to draw a person and a bicycle. Bellugi and her colleagues (e.g., Bellugi et al., 1988, 1994; Bellugi, Lai, & Wang, 1997) compared the performance of adolescents with WS to that of CA- and IQ-matched adolescents with DS on the BDAE drawing items. Findings from this comparison were reported qualitatively: Drawings by individuals with WS lacked both cohesion and overall global organization. Although many parts of each object were drawn, they were not connected to each other and were often scattered over the page. The drawings were typically unrecognizable. In contrast, drawings by matched adolescents with DS were simplified, but showed closure and maintained the correct overall global configuration among the parts. These drawings were typically recognizable.

The participants in Bertrand et al.'s (1997) study also completed the drawing component of the BDAE (as well as the person and bicycle drawing tasks). Results indicated that the drawings of the children with WS were significantly less likely to be recognizable as the intended object (e.g., a house) than the drawings of either group of typically developing children. Klein and Mervis (in press) also compared the performance of the matched pairs of 9- and 10-year-olds with WS and DS on the Draw-a-Child subtest of the McCarthy. The children with DS performed significantly better than the children with WS. It is important to note, however, that there was a wide range of performance across the children with WS; some drew primarily scribbles, whereas others were able to draw recognizable objects.

Thus children and adolescents with WS perform significantly worse than expected, even from their overall level of mental abilities, on measures of drawing skill. This discrepancy with MA has been shown in comparison to both children with DS and younger typically developing children. From these findings, it has often been concluded that the development of drawing by individuals with WS is deviant. In particular, individuals with WS have been argued to demonstrate a selective impairment for integration of parts—an impairment of global processing, with local processing relatively intact (e.g., Bellugi et al., 1988, 1994, 1997).

Bertrand and Mervis (1996), however, have argued that the problems evidenced by individuals with WS are probably developmental. Several types of evidence support this conclusion. First, in an accompanying study of the development of drawing ability of typically developing children between the ages of 4 and 8 years, Bertrand et al. (1997) found that some of the 4- and 5-year-olds produced drawings composed of parts scattered over the page. This production of disorganized drawings by typically developing preschoolers has also been reported by other researchers (see summary in Bertrand & Mervis, 1996). Second, in keeping with this result, Bertrand et al. (1997) did not find a significant difference between the 9- and 10-year-olds with WS and the MA-matched typically developing children with regard to the proportion of disorganized drawings produced. Analyses of the performance of the children with WS and the two groups of typically developing children confirmed the ordinality of the items on the VMI for each group of children. This finding offers further evidence that children with WS are following the same developmental sequence as typically developing children in learning to draw. Third, and most importantly, a longitudinal retest of the children with WS in the Bertrand et al. (1997) study when they were between 12 and 14 years of age showed considerable improvement in their drawing ability, in the direction that would be expected if their difficulty with drawing was developmental. At retest, almost all of the children improved their performance on the VMI. A Guttman scalogram again confirmed the ordinality of the items on the VMI for the children with WS. Significantly more of the drawings the children produced at ages 12–14 years were recognizable as the intended objects (or related objects) than were the drawings at ages 9–10 years, and significantly fewer of the drawings evidenced disorganization. An example of the change in one child's drawings of a house is presented in Figure 24.5.

Block Design Measures

The Klein and Mervis (in press) study also included a comparison of the performance on a third visual–spatial construction measure: the Block Building subtest of the McCarthy. On this subtest, the researcher constructs a design out of 1-inch wooden cubes, and the child is asked to construct the same design, while the model remains in view. Designs range from

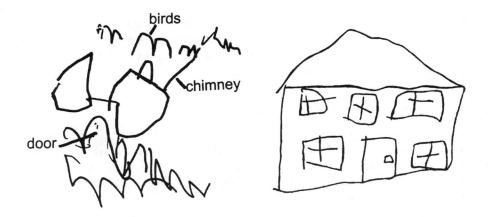

FIGURE 24.5. Two drawings of a house by a girl with WS. The child was 9 years, 2 months old when she drew the picture on the left and 12 years, 11 months old when she drew the picture on the right. (The words added to the picture on the left were provided spontaneously by the child after she finished her picture.)

simple towers to more complex houses. Once again, the children with DS performed significantly better than the children with WS.

The remaining studies of block design used either the Wechsler (WISC-R or Wechsler Adult Intelligence Scale—Revised [WAIS-R]) Block Design subtests or the Pattern Construction subtest from the DAS. On these measures, a participant is shown a colored picture of a block pattern and is asked to construct the same pattern out of colored cubes. On the Wechsler tests, the blocks have two solid red sides, two solid white sides, and two sides divided diagonally, forming red and white triangles. On the DAS, the blocks have one solid yellow side, one solid black side, two sides divided diagonally to form yellow and black triangles, and two sides divided horizontally (or vertically, depending on how the block is oriented) into yellow and black rectangles. The Wechsler patterns are composed of four or nine cubes. Bellugi and her colleagues (e.g., Bellugi et al., 1988, 1994, 1997) reported that most adolescents and adults with WS were unable to construct even the simplest four-block pattern (a checkerboard). Furthermore, the individuals with WS did not even maintain the appropriate 2×2 arrangement of the blocks. In contrast, although the participants with DS had trouble constructing the patterns, they consistently maintained the 2×2 arrangement. Udwin and Yule (1991) found that 6- to 15-year-old children with WS performed significantly worse on the WISC-R Block Design subtest than did control children with other etiologies of mental retardation, matched for CA and Verbal IQ. Pezzini, Vicari, Volterra, Milani, & Ossella (in press) replicated this finding, using a control group of typically developing children whose CA matched the MA obtained by the children with WS on the Leiter International Performance Scale (Leiter, 1980).

We (Mervis et al., 1999) considered the performance of 47 children with WS between the ages of 4 and 17 years on the Pattern Construction subtest of the DAS. The simplest cube patterns on this subtest are composed of two blocks, and thus are easier than the Wechsler patterns. Once again, the children with WS had great difficulty constructing the patterns. The modal standard score (*T*-score) was 20 (the lowest score possible). However, as illustrated in Figure 24.6, there was definite improvement as a function of age: The correlation between ability score and CA was .59 ($p < .001$). Most of the children were able to construct at least one of the patterns correctly. A few children were able to construct most patterns correctly, but took a very long time to do so. Many of the younger children had difficulty maintaining the overall configuration of the blocks for some of the patterns (Fonaryova Key, Pani, & Mervis, 1998). However, it is important to note that young typically developing children also sometimes have this problem. Older children and adults with WS usually conformed to this configuration, even when the pattern details were not reproduced correctly (Fonaryova Key et al., 1998).

Tasks Related to Visual–Spatial Construction

To consider the possibility that the difficulty individuals with WS have with visual–spatial construction tasks is related to problems in dorsal stream function, Atkinson et al. (1997) compared the performance of children with WS aged 4 to 14 years (mean = 9.7 years) on two postbox (mailbox) tasks. In the first task (dorsal stream), a child had to pick up a card from a table and then put it through the slot in a mailbox. The angle of the slot in the mailbox varied across trials. In the second task (ventral stream), the researcher placed the card in the rotatable hand of a mannequin, with the card 50 millimeters in front of the slot, and the child was asked to get the card ready to be mailed (i.e., to match the orientation of the letter to the orientation of the slot). Results indicated that in the matching task,

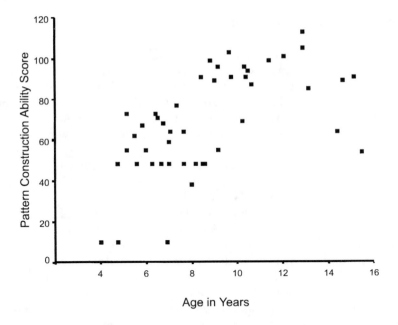

FIGURE 24.6. Distribution of ability scores on DAS Pattern Construction as a function of CA.

the children with WS performed almost as well as CA-matched controls. In contrast, performance in the first task, where the child actually had to put the letter through the slot, was considerably less accurate for the children with WS than for the controls. This pattern of findings suggests that children with WS have difficulty with tasks that involve extensive dorsal stream processing, but are more successful with tasks that depend on the same (or analogous) visual information but require primarily ventral stream processing. Mervis (1999) has compared the performance of children with WS on the DAS Pattern Construction task with their performance on a task in which they are shown each of the DAS patterns and asked to choose, from a set of three designs, the one that matches the target pattern. Even though the distractors on the matching task were very similar to the correct pattern, children performed much better on that task than on the construction task. Thus the difficulty for children with WS appears to involve visual–spatial construction per se, rather than visual perception in general.

Summary

In summary, children and adolescents with WS have a great deal of difficulty with tasks involving visual–spatial construction. Their abilities are substantially more limited than those of MA-matched typically developing children, MA-matched children with DS, or MA-matched children with mental retardation of mixed etiology. Nevertheless, there is a considerable variability across individuals with WS. There is substantial improvement as a function of increased CA. The developmental course of both drawing and pattern construction is similar to that for individuals who are developing normally, although for individuals with WS, this course is protracted and the endpoint is seldom as advanced as that for individuals of normal intelligence.

Williams Syndrome Cognitive Profile

As our review above has indicated, children and adults with WS evidence a characteristic cognitive profile, which we call the WSCP. Auditory rote memory ability is better than would be expected from overall level of cognitive ability. Language abilities are slightly better than would be expected from overall cognitive ability. Visual–spatial construction ability is substantially worse than overall level of cognitive ability. An examination of the literature regarding cognitive strengths and weaknesses associated with other syndromes involving mental retardation or borderline normal intelligence suggests that the pattern associated with WS may be relatively unique. However, the heterogeneity of methods and measures used in previous research has hampered the precise specification and testing of the cognitive profile associated with WS. To address this problem, we and our colleagues (Mervis et al., 1998b, 1999) have proposed an operationalization of the WSCP as a particular pattern of subtest scores on the DAS (Elliott, 1990). The DAS offers three important advantages over other standardized tests (e.g., the WISC-III; Wechsler, 1991) for the operationalization of the WSCP. First, the DAS was designed to provide specific information about an individual's strengths and weaknesses across a wide range of intellectual abilities. The core subtests of the DAS include assessments of verbal and visual–spatial constructive abilities, and a diagnostic subtest measures auditory rote memory. For each of these measures, the DAS covers the range of performance expected from very low-functioning 3-year-olds to very high-functioning 17-year-olds (equivalent to adult levels). Second, the very large range of possible standard scores (T-scores) for each subtest (from 20 to 80, with a mean of 50 and a standard deviation of 10) provides increased sensitivity to relative performance on the different subtests. Third, the Pattern Construction subtest includes much simpler patterns than those on the Block Design subtests of the Wechsler IQ tests, making it more likely that individuals with WS will pass at least some items assessing visual–spatial construction. The WSCP criteria are described in detail in Mervis et al. (1998b) and Frangiskakis et al. (1996).

To determine the sensitivity and specificity of the WSCP for individuals with WS, we considered the performance of 84 individuals with WS (mean age = 12 years, 9 months) and 56 individuals in a mixed-etiology comparison group (mean age = 12 years, 8 months). About two-thirds of the individuals in the WS group had been tested for a possible hemizygous deletion of the *ELN* gene; all were positive. Diagnosis for the remaining individuals was confirmed by Morris, based on the clinical criteria of Lowery et al. (1995). Of the 84 individuals with WS, 74 fit all four criteria for the WSCP, yielding a sensitivity (Se) of .88. Conversely, 52 of the 56 individuals in the mixed-etiology group did not fit all of the criteria, yielding a specificity (Sp) of .93. Eighteen individuals in the mixed etiology group had previously been clinically diagnosed with WS but had tested negative for an *ELN* deletion. Only 2 of these individuals fit the WSCP. Thus the WSCP evidenced excellent sensitivity and specificity: Most individuals with WS fit the WSCP, whereas most individuals who did not have WS (including people who had received a clinical diagnosis of WS, but did not meet the molecular genetic criterion) did not fit the WSCP.

Overall Level of Intellectual Ability

Overall cognitive ability is typically measured by Full Scale IQ tests. Studies of children with WS have used a variety of these tests, with similar results. Udwin, Yule, and Martin (1987) studied 44 children between the ages of 6 and 15 years, and found that Full Scale

IQs on the WISC-R (Wechsler, 1974) ranged from <40 (the lowest possible score) to 89. Ten of the children (23%) obtained Full Scale IQs below 40. These children were excluded from the authors' calculation of mean IQ. Mean IQ for the remaining children was 55. We (Mervis et al., 1998b) tested 67 children between the ages of 4 and 17 years on the DAS (Elliott, 1990). Mean General Conceptual Ability (GCA) (similar to IQ) was 59, with a range from 32 to 84. Greer, Brown, Pai, Choudry, and Klein (1997) administered the Stanford–Binet Intelligence Scale, fourth edition (Thorndike, Hagen, & Sattler, 1986) to 15 children aged 4 to 18 years. The mean IQ earned was 62; IQs ranged from 43 to 80. In all these studies, mean CA was between 9 and 11 years. In summary, the intelligence levels of children with WS (as measured by Full Scale IQ tests) vary from severe mental retardation to low average; IQs are typically in the mild mental retardation range.

The youngest participants in the Full Scale IQ studies were 4 years old. There have been almost no studies of overall level of cognitive ability in younger children with WS. Recently Mervis (1999) has assessed a group of 10 3-year-olds (mean age = 38 months) with WS, using the Bayley Scales of Infant Development, second edition (BSID II; Bayley, 1993). Mean developmental quotient (DQ) was 61, with a range from <30 (the lowest possible)* to 100.

Mean Full Scale scores IQs or DQs are misleading, however. Children with WS almost always score much better on subtests measuring verbal abilities than on subtests measuring visual–spatial construction. Performance on subtests measuring nonverbal reasoning is usually slightly lower than on verbal subtests, but considerably higher than on subtests measuring visual–spatial construction. These differences are well illustrated by a comparison of standard scores for the Verbal, Nonverbal Reasoning, and Spatial (measuring visual–spatial construction) clusters on the School Age form of the DAS. For a sample of 37 children between the ages of 7 and 17 years (mean CA = 10.6 years) who completed the School Age DAS, Mervis found a mean GCA of 58. The mean standard score for the Verbal cluster was 70, with a range from 51 (the lowest possible) to 96. For the Nonverbal Reasoning cluster, the mean standard score was 67, with a range from 52 (the lowest possible) to 89. In contrast, the mean standard score for the Spatial cluster was 55, with a range from 50 (the lowest possible) to 70.

This pattern of substantially better performance on verbal measures than on visual–spatial construction measures also is evidenced by younger children with WS. Mervis and Bertrand (1997) followed six toddlers longitudinally, from about age 1½ years to about age 3 years, administering the original BSID (Bayley, 1969) at intervals of approximately 6 months. The BSID does not include subscales; however, items may be divided into verbal or nonverbal. Across the entire age interval tested, the children with WS passed a significantly greater proportion of the verbal items than the nonverbal items. Most of the nonverbal items on the BSID assess visual–spatial construction. Thus toddlers with WS are already showing a pattern of cognitive strengths and weaknesses similar to that of older children.

Cognitive Assessment

As part of an intellectual assessment for children with WS, as for children with any type of developmental disability, it is important that a Full Scale IQ test be administered. How-

---

*The lowest standard score included in the BSID II manual (Bayley, 1993) is 50. Extrapolated standard scores for the range 30–49 are provided by Robinson and Mervis (1996).

ever, because of the unusual pattern of cognitive strengths and weaknesses associated with WS, it is inappropriate to assume that the composite IQ score obtained from that test provides an accurate measure of a child's abilities or intellectual potential. As we have just described, children with WS typically score much higher on verbal subtests than on tests measuring visual–spatial construction. Thus the focus should be on the standard scores obtained on the subscales, or even on the subtests within each subscale.

The school age DAS differs from the other Full Scale intellectual assessment measures described above, in that the Spatial cluster is devoted entirely to visual–spatial construction. Thus the cluster standard scores for the DAS best reflect the pattern of cognitive strengths and weaknesses associated with WS. For this reason, we consider the DAS to be the most appropriate Full Scale measure for assessing the intellectual abilities of children with WS. Norms are available for ages 5 years to 18 years. Typically, children with WS will score best on the Verbal cluster, not quite as well on the Nonverbal Reasoning cluster, and extremely poorly on the Spatial cluster. In addition to administering the six core subtests that contribute to the GCA (equivalent to a Full Scale IQ), it is helpful to administer the supplementary test measuring auditory short-term memory (Digit Recall). Children with WS characteristically perform well on this subtest. (Norms for Digit Recall are available for ages 2½ years to 18 years.)

The Preschool DAS includes just two clusters, Verbal and Nonverbal. Norms are available for ages 2½ years to 7 years. The Nonverbal cluster is composed of three subtests, two measuring visual–spatial construction, and one measuring reasoning (Picture Similarities). Children with WS perform relatively well on the Picture Similarities subtest, but extremely poorly on the visual–spatial construction subtests. Thus, the Nonverbal cluster score on the Preschool DAS typically is not useful for children with WS. Instead, it is important to consider the subtest scores individually.

The Kaufman Brief Intelligence Test (K-BIT; Kaufman & Kaufman, 1990) is composed of two subscales, one measuring verbal ability and one measuring nonverbal reasoning ability. (As on all "nonverbal" measures, it is possible, even likely, that the person being tested will use verbal mediation to solve the problems. People with WS almost always solve these problems verbally.) No measures of visual–spatial construction are included. Norms are available for ages 4 years through 90 years. As might be expected, the composite IQ obtained by children with WS on the K-BIT is almost always considerably higher than on the DAS (or any of the Wechsler IQ tests). The K-BIT IQ score provides a good indication of a child's potential intellectual ability, assuming that the child is able to develop strategies to circumvent his or her severe difficulty with visual–spatial construction. Helping the child to develop such strategies, at the same time as modifying the school, home, or work environment to diminish the need for the use of visual–spatial construction, is an important goal for intervention programs.

The BSID II (Bayley, 1993) is the most frequently used developmental assessment for infants, toddlers, and young preschoolers with WS; norms are available for ages 2 months through 3½ years. This measure provides only an overall DQ; subscales are not available. Thus, when one is considering the performance of a child with WS on this measure, it is important to keep in mind that the overall DQ is probably masking a pattern of relative strength on verbal items and serious weakness on items requiring visual–spatial construction. This pattern can be confirmed by examining the child's item-by-item performance. It is also important to remember that intelligence scores (whether DQs or IQs) obtained by toddlers or young children are not necessarily predictive of IQs or achievement levels during the school years or adulthood.

In addition to full-scale measures of cognitive abilities, there is a wide range of more narrowly focused assessments. For example, the third edition of the PPVT (Dunn & Dunn, 1997) provides a measure of receptive vocabulary for individuals aged 2½ to 90 years; the Expressive Vocabulary Test (Williams, 1997) measures productive vocabulary across the same age range for the same norming sample. The Clinical Evaluation of Language Fundamentals III (Semel, Wiig, & Secord, 1995) is used to assess both vocabulary and grammar; norms are available for ages 6 years through 21 years. There is also a preschool version of this measure (Wiig, Secord, & Semel, 1992). Specialized assessments are also available for memory, neuropsychology, reasoning, and visual–spatial construction.

BEHAVIORAL CHARACTERISTICS

Studies of the behavioral characteristics of children who have WS have focused on three areas: problem behaviors, personality characteristics, and adaptive behavior. Although additional research is definitely needed, the results of these studies are beginning to suggest a characteristic behavioral profile. Below, we review the findings of the available studies of behavioral characteristics.

Problem Behaviors

Studies of problem behaviors manifested by children with WS have typically used measures such as the Child Behavior Checklist (CBCL; Achenbach, 1991). The CBCL provides summary T-scores for Internalizing Problems (derived from the Withdrawn, Somatic Complaints, and Anxious/Depressed scales), Externalizing Problems (derived from the Delinquent Behavior and Aggressive Behavior scales), and Total Problems (composed of the Social Problems, Thought Problems, and Attention Problems scales, as well as those included in Internalizing and Externalizing Problems). This measure was used in the earliest studies of problem behaviors of children with WS (Dilts, Morris, & Leonard, 1990; Pagon, Bennett, LaVeck, Stewart, & Johnson, 1987). However, the published reports did not include overall findings for the CBCL. Both sets of authors concluded that children with WS have attention problems (probably due to distractibility). Dilts et al. (1990) reported that 67% of the 48 children in their study had significantly elevated clinical scores ($T > 70$) on the Attention Problems scale. Pagon et al. (1987) reported that the parents of most of the children endorsed the item "Can't concentrate or pay attention." Treatment of attention problems with methylphenidate has been helpful in some children with WS (Bawden, MacDonald, & Shea, 1997; Power, Blum, Jones, & Kaplan, 1997).

More recently, Greer et al. (1997) considered the behavior of 15 children with WS between the ages of 4 and 18 years, based on parental responses to the CBCL. Results again confirmed the presence of attention difficulties. Of the 15 children, 11 (73%) had significantly elevated clinical scores on the Attention Problems scale. Two additional children had borderline significant scores (T-scores from 67 through 70). The authors also reported that 9 of the children (60%) had borderline significant scores on the Social Problems scale (e.g., "Acts too young for age"), and 8 (53%) had borderline significant scores on the Thought Problems scale (e.g., "Mind wanders").

The results of these studies indicate that the majority of children with WS have attention problems, and that many also have social problems or thought problems. However, because the behavior of the children with WS was not compared to that of children with other syndromes (or with mental retardation of unknown etiology), it is impossible to know the extent to which this pattern of elevated scores is unique to WS, or is generally characteristic of children with mental retardation or borderline normal intelligence. This question has been addressed in one study in which the CBCL was used. Sarimski (1997) compared the CBCL (German version) results for 14 school-age children with WS to those of school-age children with Prader–Willi syndrome (PWS) and school-age boys with the fragile X mental retardation gene (FMR1). The mean T-scores for Total Problems were in the clinically elevated range for all three syndromes. Ten of the 14 children with WS (71%) had significantly elevated Total Problems scores, according to both parents and teachers. Sarimski also conducted an item analysis, and found several items that differentiated the children with WS from one or both of the other syndrome groups. Three characteristics were significantly more likely to be reported for children with WS than for children with either PWS or FMR1: worrying, talking too much, and not eating well. Three additional characteristics were significantly less likely to be reported for children with WS than for children with the other two syndromes: being self-conscious, overeating, and being overweight. The children with WS were significantly more likely than the children with PWS (but not the children with FMR1) to have difficulty concentrating, to be restless, and to be afraid of animals or situations. The children with WS were significantly more likely than the children with FMR1 (but not the children with PWS) to bite their fingernails and evidence nervous movements, and significantly less likely to prefer to be alone, to be shy, have speech problems, or to be unusually loud.

In addition, Sarimski administered a questionnaire designed to assess the social competence and behavioral problems of preschoolers (Döpfner, Berner, Fleischmann, & Schmidt, 1993) to the parents and teachers of 16 preschool-age children with WS, 20 preschool-age children with PWS, and 13 preschool-age boys with FMR1. Both parent and teacher results indicated that children with WS were significantly more hyperactive than children with PWS, but not than children with FMR1. Parent results also indicated that children with WS were significantly less aggressive and less emotionally labile than boys with FMR1, but not than children with PWS.

Sarimski (1997) also asked the parents of both the preschool-age and school-age children to complete the Society for the Study of Behavioral Phenotypes Postal Questionnaire (O'Brien, 1992). This measure assesses both developmental attainments and behavioral problems common among children with genetically based developmental disorders. Significantly more of the children with WS than of the children with PWS or FMR1 were overfriendly to strangers (97% of children with WS), had oversensitivity to certain sounds (hyperacusis; 82%), and/or had selective eating habits (63%). Significantly more of the children with PWS or FMR1 frequently made self-directed utterances than did children with WS (0%).

Udwin and Yule (1991) administered the Rutter (1967) questionnaire (similar to the CBCL) to the parents and teachers of 20 children aged 6 to 14 years with WS and 20 children of a variety of etiologies, matched for age, gender, and WISC-R Verbal IQ. The children with WS obtained higher scores from both parents and teachers on overall behavior disturbance and on hyperactivity. On the Teacher scale, significantly more children with WS (80%) than control children (35%) scored above the cutoff for deviant behavior. At the item level, parents reported that significantly more children with WS than children in the comparison group had poor concentration, had twitches or mannerisms, and/or were solitary. Teachers reported that significantly more children with WS than children in the comparison group were fearful, were fussy, and/or had twitches or mannerisms.

Gosch and Pankau (1994) asked parents to complete a 20-item questionnaire composed primarily of items from the CBCL, with the addition of a few items that previously had been described as characteristic of children with WS. The 19 children with WS ranged in age from 4 to 10 years; a comparison group of 19 children with nonspecific mental retardation was matched for CA, sex, and IQ. Only a few differences emerged between the children in the two groups. Significantly more of the children with WS were reported to evidence overreaction to sounds, and more of the children with WS evidenced extreme overfriendliness to strangers, including being willing to follow them without hesitation or fear. Gosch and Pankau also compared the behavior of the children with WS to normally developing children matched for CA. Relative to this group, significantly more children with WS were considered to be hyperactive, to be unable to engage themselves independently, to have sleep disturbances, and to lack a sense of shame. Significantly fewer children with WS than CA-matched children were considered obstinate or likely to tell lies.

Einfeld, Tonge, and Florio (1997) considered the responses of the parents of 70 children and adolescents with WS to the Developmental Behaviour Checklist (DBC; Einfeld & Tonge, 1994, 1995), a measure designed to assess behavioral and emotional problems of children with mental retardation. The parents' responses were compared to the norms for the DBC, which were derived from a sample of 454 children and adolescents with mental retardation. Results indicated that significantly more of the children with WS (61%) exceeded the cutoff score for behavior problems than children in the norming sample (41%). The scores for the children with WS were significantly higher than for the norming sample for Total Behavior Problems and for the Communication Disturbance and Anxiety subscales. With regard to individual items, significantly more of the children with WS evidenced anxiety, were overaffectionate, overreacted to sounds, were overactive, had a short attention span, had selective eating habits, were obsessed or preoccupied with a particular idea or activity, were overly attention-seeking, were inappropriately happy, and wandered aimlessly. The children with WS were significantly less likely to repeat words or phrases over and over. Although the authors had expected the children with WS to be more likely to evidence disturbed sleep (or too little sleep), to have tantrums, or to prefer to be alone, no differences were found between the children with WS and the norming sample on these items.

Personality Characteristics

"Personality" (or "temperament") is defined as a rubric of enduring behavioral characteristics, both positive and negative. As such, behavioral problems that occur consistently over time may be considered part of a child's temperament or personality. The four studies focusing on personality or temperamental characteristics of children with WS have considered both problem behaviors and more positive characteristics.

Tomc, Williamson, and Pauli (1990) examined the temperament of 204 children who had been diagnosed with WS. Children ranged in age from 1 through 12 years. Parents completed one of three temperament questionnaires, depending on the child's age. Each of the questionnaires yielded scores for nine temperamental characteristics, based on Thomas and Chess's (1977) approach to temperament. Relative to CA norms, the children with WS were rated as significantly more approaching; significantly higher in intensity, distractibility, and negative mood; and significantly lower in persistence and threshold of excitability. The researchers also estimated the MAs of the children with

WS and then compared the children to the norms for those ages. The same pattern of findings held.

Gosch and Pankau (1996, cited in Gosch & Pankau, 1997) compared the personality characteristics of children with WS to those of children with DS or Brachmann–de Lange syndrome. Results indicated that relative to the comparison groups, the children with WS were less reserved toward strangers and more curious. In addition, the children with WS were more restless, more anxious, and more tearful.

Van Lieshout, De Meyer, Curfs, and Fryns (1998) compared the personality characteristics of 28 children with WS ranging in age from 2½ to 19 years (mean = 9 years) to those of children with PWS or FMR1 and to CA-matched children who were developing normally. Parents completed the Dutch translation of the California Child Q-Set (CCQ; Block & Block, 1980). The CCQ yields scores for seven personality scales. There were no differences among the four groups on Extraversion. All three syndrome groups showed less Emotional Stability and less Openness than the normal controls. There were no differences between the syndrome groups on these two scales, however. The WS group scored as high on Agreeableness as the normal controls and higher than the PWS group. The WS group evidenced less Conscientiousness than either the normal controls or the PWS group, and scored lower on Motor Activity than either the normal or the FMR1 groups. Finally, the children in all three syndrome groups evidenced more Irritability than the normally developing children; there were no significant differences among the syndrome groups.

Van Lieshout et al. (1998) also considered the relation between these personality characteristics and CA. Results of correlational analyses indicated that as CA increased, children with WS became less extraverted, less open to new experiences, and less irritable. All of these findings also held for the other three groups. As CA increased, children with WS, as well as children with PWS or FMR1, showed a decrease in emotional stability. For the WS and FMR1 groups, motor activity also decreased.

Gosch and Pankau (1997) compared the personality characteristics of 48 children (age range = 2 to 10 years; mean = 6 years) and adolescents (age range = 10 to 20 years, mean = 15 years) with WS. Parents were given a series of 26 personality characteristics and asked to rate how typical each characteristic was of their child. The means for both age groups were above the scale mean for a number of characteristics: overfriendly, lively, cheerful, active, restless, eager to learn, happy, and hypersensitive to sound. For all characteristics except the last two, children were rated significantly higher than adolescents. The means for both groups were below the scale mean for three characteristics: calm, withdrawn, and inhibited. For these three characteristics, the adolescents were rated significantly higher than the children. The authors conclude that with increasing age, changes in personality characteristics toward more socially accepted values take place. Despite these changes, however, the authors argue that there is a typical WS personality profile, as evidenced by the consistently high (or low) ratings received for many of the characteristics, regardless of age.

Adaptive Behavior

"Adaptive behavior" refers to the functioning of a child in his or her environment. Assessments of adaptive behavior usually focus on such domains as communication, self-care, and interpersonal relationships. There have been only three studies of the adaptive behavior of children with WS. Gosch and Pankau (1994) used the Vineland Social Maturity Scale (an older version of the Vineland Scales of Adaptive Behavior; see below) to compare the adaptive behavior of 19 children with WS between the ages of 4 and 10 years and 19 children with nonspecific mental retardation matched for CA, IQ, and gender. The children with WS evidenced lower adaptive behavior abilities than the children in the contrast group, suggesting that the adaptive behavior abilities of children with WS are lower than would be expected from IQ. Gosch and Pankau pointed out that the Vineland Social Maturity Scale includes a large number of items that address independence and self-care, which are dependent on motor skills. Thus, the lower performance of the children with WS was likely due to their problems with visual–motor integration. The authors also concluded that despite their characteristic overfriendliness, the children with WS were less socially mature than the children in the contrast group.

The two other studies of adaptive behavior development by children with WS used the Vineland Scales of Adaptive Behavior (Sparrow, Balla, & Cicchetti, 1984) as the assessment measure. The Vineland involves a semistructured interview with a child's primary caregiver. For children less than 6 years old, four domains are assessed: Communication, Daily Living Skills, Socialization, and Motor Skills. For children aged 6 years or older, only the first three domains are assessed. Greer et al. (1997) measured the adaptive behavior of 15 children with WS between the ages of 4 and 18 years (mean = 9.5 years). Results indicated that overall adaptive skill was commensurate with intellectual abilities as assessed by the fourth edition of the Stanford–Binet. Performance on the Communication and Socialization domains was significantly better than performance on Daily Living Skills.

Mervis, Klein, and Rothstein (1998a) used the Vineland to examine the adaptive behavior of 41 children with WS ranging in age from 4 through 8 years (mean = 6.36 years). The mean Vineland Composite (standard score) was 62.98 (SD = 9.33). This score was similar to the children's mean DAS GCA of 59.32 (SD = 11.84). Thus, within this age range, the adaptive behavior abilities of the children with WS were consistent with their overall intellectual abilities. Performance on the Vineland differed as a function of domain: Standard scores were best for the Socialization domain; performance in this domain was significantly better than performance on Communication; and performance on Daily Living Skills was significantly lower than on either of the other domains. For the children aged 4 or 5 years, performance on Motor Skills was significantly lower than performance on any of the other domains. Within the Socialization domain, Interpersonal skills were found to be significantly more advanced than either Play/Leisure skills or Coping skills. Within the Daily Living Skills domain, Community skills and Domestic skills were significantly more advanced than Personal Care skills.

This pattern of adaptive behavior strengths and weaknesses for children with WS fits well with the findings we have described for patterns of cognitive abilities and personality and behavioral characteristics. The children had the most difficulty with the Daily Living Skills and Motor Skills domains. Both of these domains rely heavily on visual–spatial construction (visual–motor) skills—the area of greatest cognitive weakness. Within the Daily Living Skills domain, Personal Care skills, which are heavily dependent on visual–spatial constructive abilities, were considerably weaker than either Community or Domestic skills. Within the Socialization domain, children with WS evidenced a relative strength in the Interpersonal subdomain, where items involve the initiation of interactions and attunement to others' emotional states—two areas of strength in terms of personality and behavioral characteristics. The children performed less well on the Play/Leisure and Coping subdomains. Both of these depend on ability to continue or maintain an interaction and to control anxiety—definite behavioral weaknesses for children with WS.

ADULTS

In the few reports of adults with WS, a wide range of outcomes has been reported in all aspects of the phenotype. The possible medical complications of WS in adults include hyperopia, dental malocclusion, hypertension, progressive arterial stenoses, mitral valve prolapse, aortic insufficiency, hypercalcemia, chronic constipation, obesity, cholelithiasis, diabetes mellitus, progressive joint limitation, spasticity, bladder and bowel diverticuli, and chronic urinary tract infection (Kececioglu, Kotthoff, & Vogt, 1993; Lopez-Rangel, Maurice, McGillivray, & Friedman, 1992; Morris et al., 1990). Academically, individuals with WS typically perform best on reading; reading grade levels range from first-grade to college, with a mean of grade 5. Decoding grade level is often higher than comprehension grade level. However, individuals with WS have considerably more difficulty in writing, particularly with legibility and speed. Arithmetic is also a problem, with many individuals with WS not progressing beyond simple addition; however, some individuals have learned how to use a calculator. The level of independence achieved by adults with WS until now has been lower than expected for cognitive ability. Most adults live with their parents or in group homes and work in sheltered environments (Davies, Howlin, & Udwin, 1997). In the past few years, however, more adults have been moving into apartments with roommates; and with the help of job coaches, many adults with WS are now working in regular employment. The behavioral problems associated with WS (including attention problems, overfriendliness, and anxiety) contribute to level of functioning in the community; treatment of these problems should improve adaptive behavioral outcomes.

TREATMENT

Optimal management of the problems associated with WS requires a multidisciplinary approach. At the time of diagnosis, a medical evaluation should include a careful physical and neurological examination by the pediatrician; an evaluation for visual acuity, depth perception, strabismus, and amblyopia by the ophthalmologist; a clinical examination, echocardiogram with Doppler, and four-limb blood pressure determination by the cardiologist; and a dysmorphology examination and genetic counseling by the geneticist. Recommended laboratory and radiological investigations include an audiogram, thyroid function test, calcium studies (total serum calcium and spot urine calcium/creatinine), urinalysis, renal function tests (BUN/creatinine), and ultrasound of the bladder and kidneys. Additional studies may be indicated, depending on specific signs and symptoms (e.g., evaluation for gastroesophogeal reflux in the infant with feeding problems). Attentional problems and/or anxiety may require evaluation and treatment by a pediatric psychiatrist and/or neurobehavioral psychologist.

A comprehensive developmental evaluation is important to determine individualized therapy for the child with WS. A detailed psychological assessment is required to identify the individual's cognitive strengths and weaknesses and to suggest specific intervention strategies. A physical therapist should evaluate and treat joint contractures, postural abnormalities, and spasticity. The occupational therapist must address the greatest weakness seen in WS, visual–spatial construction (visual–motor integration). In addition to standard therapeutic methods, children with WS benefit from being taught to talk their way through fine motor tasks and to use verbal cues to help remember spatial information. Some children with WS will require speech therapy focused on all aspects of language and even the highest functioning children will benefit from therapy focused on pragmatics, including staying on topic in conversation. For most children with WS, phonics is the best teaching method for reading because it takes advantage of their strength in language and in verbal memory. It is important that children with WS have access to a computer for "written" work. Due to the extreme difficulty with handwriting, this task should be separated from the academic content in classroom assignments. The use of manipulatives and touch math is helpful in teaching numbers and number operations; eventually, children should be taught to use a calculator.

Adults with WS will require continued medical monitoring of neurologic, psychiatric, ophthalmologic, cardiovascular, gastrointestinal, genitourinary, and musculoskeletal systems. Adaptive behavior should be addressed by vocational training; physical, occupational, and/or speech therapy; and counseling and/or medication for anxiety.

Finally, the Williams Syndrome Association (WSA) is a support and advocacy group for individuals with WS and their families. The WSA is a good source for updated medical and educational information and recommendations for both families and professionals. Their website is www.williams-syndrome.org.

CONCLUSION

Syndromes have traditionally been defined by their medical signs and symptoms. More recently, the neurobehavioral components of genetic syndromes also have been recognized as characteristic and unique signs that not only may aid in diagnosis, but are important to recognize and treat for optimal outcome. In this chapter, we have discussed the complex phenotype of WS. The medically significant phenotype includes dysmorphic facial features; cardiovascular disease (elastin arteriopathy); infantile hypercalcemia; feeding difficulty resulting in failure to thrive; and connective tissue abnormalities affecting joints, bowel, bladder, and skin. Individuals with WS typically have mild mental retardation. However, there is wide variability, with some individuals having intelligence in the normal range, and others having moderate to severe mental retardation. The cognitive profile associated with WS (the WSCP) involves relative strengths in verbal rote memory and in language, but extreme weakness in visual–spatial construction. From a behavioral perspective, children with WS typically are overly friendly and quite sensitive to other people's feelings. At the same time, they are likely to manifest attention problems and anticipatory anxiety. Because WS is caused by a deletion of a finite number of genes on chromosome 7, it is likely that haplo-insufficiency of some of these gene products accounts for various components of the syndrome. Discovery of the roles of these genes in the phenotype will add to our understanding of the genetic bases of behavior. This knowledge, combined with continued study of the adaptations of individuals with WS to their disability, should lead to development of more effective multidisciplinary treatment strategies in the future.

ACKNOWLEDGMENTS

Preparation of this chapter was supported by Grant No. NS35102 from the National Institute of Neurological Disorders and Stroke and by Grant No. HD29957 from the National Institute of Child Health and Human Development. We thank the Williams Syndrome Association for helping us to identify potential participants and for permitting us to conduct research at national and regional meetings. The individuals who have participated in this research have been generous with their time and their commitment to the research; we are very grateful. We thank Stephanie Nelson for assistance in the preparation of this manuscript, and Cindy Mervis for taking the photograph for Figure 24.2.

REFERENCES

Achenbach, T. M. (1991). *Manual for the Child Behavior Checklist/4–18 and 1991 profile*. Burlington: University of Vermont, Department of Psychiatry.

Adamson, L. B. (1995). *Communication development during infancy*. Madison, WI: Brown & Benchmark.

Ardinger, R. H., Goertz, K. K., & Mattioli, L. F. (1994). Cerebrovascular stenosis with cerebral infarction in a child with Williams syndrome. *American Journal of Medical Genetics, 51,* 200–202.

Atkinson, J., King, J., Braddick, O., Nokes, L., Anker, S., & Braddick, F. (1997). A specific deficit of dorsal function in Williams' syndrome. *NeuroReport, 8,* 1919–1922.

Bates, E., Dale, P. S., & Thal, D. (1995). Individual differences and their implications for theories of language development. In P. Fletcher & B. MacWhinney (Eds.), *The handbook of child language* (pp. 96–151). Oxford: Blackwell Press.

Bawden, H. N., MacDonald, W., & Shea, S. (1997). Treatment of children with Williams syndrome with methylphenidate. *Journal of Child Neurology, 12,* 248–252.

Bayley, N. (1969). *Bayley Scales of Infant Development*. New York: Psychological Corporation.

Bayley, N. (1993). *Bayley Scales of Infant Development* (2nd ed.). San Antonio, TX: Psychological Corporation.

Beery, K. E. (1989). *Developmental Test of Visual–Motor Integration* (3rd rev.). Cleveland: Modern Curriculum Press.

Bellugi, U., Bihrle, A., Jernigan, T., Trauner, D., & Doherty, S. (1990). Neuropsychological, neurological, and neuroanatomical profile of Williams syndrome. *American Journal of Medical Genetics,* (Suppl. 6), 115–125.

Bellugi, U., Bihrle, A., Neville, H., & Doherty, S. (1992). Language, cognition, and brain organization in a neurodevelopmental disorder. In M. Gunnar & C. Nelson (Eds.), *Developmental behavioral neuroscience: The Minnesota symposium* (pp. 201–232). Hillsdale, NJ: Erlbaum.

Bellugi, U., Lai, Z., & Wang, P. (1997). Language, communication, and neural systems in Williams syndrome. *Mental Retardation and Developmental Disabilities Research Reviews, 3,* 334–342.

Bellugi, U., Marks, S., Bihrle, A., & Sabo, H. (1988). Dissociation between language and cognitive functions in Williams syndrome. In D. Bishop & K. Mogford (Eds.), *Language development in exceptional circumstances* (pp. 177–189). Edinburgh: Churchill Livingstone.

Bellugi, U., Wang, P. P., & Jernigan, T. L. (1994). Williams syndrome: An unusual neuropsychological profile. In S. H. Broman & J. Grafman (Eds.), *Atypical cognitive deficits in developmental disorders: Implications for brain function* (pp. 23–56). Hillsdale, NJ: Erlbaum.

Bertrand, J., & Mervis, C. B. (1996). Longitudinal analysis of drawings by children with Williams syndrome: Preliminary results. *Visual Arts Research, 22,* 19–34.

Bertrand, J., Mervis, C. B., & Eisenberg, J. D. (1997). Drawing by children with Williams syndrome: A developmental perspective. *Developmental Neuropsychology, 13,* 41–67.

Beuren, A. J. (1972). Supravalvular aortic stenosis: A complex syndrome with and without mental retardation. *Birth Defects Original Article Series, 8*(5), 45–56.

Bird, L. M., Billman, G. F., Lacro, R. V., Spicer, R. L., Jariwala, L. K., Hoyme, H. E., Zamora-Salinas, R., Morris, C. A., Viskochil, D., Frikke, M. J., & Jones, M. C. (1996). Sudden death in Williams syndrome: Report of ten cases. *Journal of Pediatrics, 129,* 926–931.

Block, J. H., & Block, J. (1980). The role of ego-control and ego-resiliency in the organization of behavior. In W. A. Collins (Ed.), *Minnesota Symposia on Child Psychology: Vol. 13. Development of cognition, affect, and social relations* (pp. 39–101). Hillsdale, NJ: Erlbaum.

Botta, A., Novelli, G., Mari, A., Novelli, A., Sabani, M., Korenberg, J., Osborne, L., Digilio, M. C., & Dallapiccola, B. (1998). Detection of an atypical 7q11.23 deletion in Williams syndrome patients which does not include STX1A and FZD3 genes [Abstract]. *American Journal of Human Genetics, 63*(4), A98.

Braddick, O., & Atkinson, J. (1995). Visual and visuo-spatial development in young Williams syndrome children. *Investigative Ophthalmology and Visual Science* (Suppl. 36), S954.

Broder, K., Reinhardt, E., Lifton, R., Tamborlane, W., & Pober, B. R. (1995). Ambulatory blood pressure monitoring in Williams syndrome. *Genetic Counseling, 6,* 150–151.

Chapman, C. A., du Plessis, A., & Pober, B. R. (1996). Neurologic findings in children and adults with Williams syndrome. *Journal of Child Neurology, 11,* 63–65.

Chapman, R. S. (1997). Language development in children and adolescents with Down syndrome. *Mental Retardation and Developmental Disabilities Research Reviews, 3,* 307–312.

Culler, F. L., Jones, K. L., & Deftos, L. J. (1985). Impaired calcitonin secretion in patients with Williams syndrome. *Journal of Pediatrics, 107,* 720–723.

Davies, M., Howlin, P., & Udwin, O. (1997). Independence and adaptive behavior in adults with Williams syndrome. *American Journal of Medical Genetics, 70,* 188–195.

Deal, J. E., Snell, M. F., Marratt, T. M., & Dillon, M. J. (1992). Renovascular disease in childhood. *Journal of Pediatrics, 131,* 378–384.

Dilts, C., Morris, C. A., & Leonard, C. O. (1990). Hypothesis for development of a behavioral phenotype in Williams syndrome. *American Journal of Medical Genetics,* (Suppl. 6), 126–131.

Döpfner, M., Berner, W., Fleischmann, T., & Schmidt, M. (1993). *Verhaltensbeurteilungsbogen für Vorschulkinder (VBV 3–6).* Weinheim, Germany: Beltz Test.

Dunn, L. E., & Dunn, L. E. (1981). *Peabody Picture Vocabulary Test—Revised.* Circle Pines, MN: American Guidance Service.

Dunn, L. E., & Dunn, L. E. (1997). *Peabody Picture Vocabulary Test* (3rd ed.). Circle Pines, MN: American Guidance Service.

Dutly, F., & Schinzel, A. (1996). Unequal interchromosomal rearrangements may result in elastin gene deletions causing the Williams–Beuren syndrome. *Human Molecular Genetics, 5,* 1893–1898.

Einfeld, S. L., & Tonge, B. J. (1994). *Manual for the Developmental Behaviour Checklist.* Sydney/Melbourne: University of New South Wales/Monash University.

Einfeld, S. L., & Tonge, B. J. (1995). The Developmental Behaviour Checklist: The development and validation of an instrument to assess behavioral and emotional disturbance in children and adolescents with mental retardation. *Journal of Autism and Developmental Disorders, 25,* 81–104.

Einfeld, S. L., Tonge, B. J., & Florio, T. (1997). Behavioral and emotional disturbance in individuals with Williams syndrome. *American Journal of Mental Retardation, 102,* 45–53.

Eisenberg, R., Young, D., Jacobson, B., & Boito, A. (1964). Familial supravalvular aortic stenosis. *American Journal of Diseases of Children, 108,* 341–347.

Elliott, C. D. (1990). *Differential Ability Scales.* San Diego, CA: Harcourt Brace Jovanovich.

Ensing, G. J., Schmidt, M. A., Hagler, D. J., Michels, V. V., Carter, G. A., & Feldt, R. H. (1989). Spectrum of findings in a family with nonsyndromic autosomal dominant supravalvular aortic stenosis: A Doppler echocardiographic study. *Journal of the American Academy of Cardiology, 13,* 413–419.

Ewart, A. K., Morris, C. A., Atkinson, D., Jin, W., Sternes, K., Spallone, P., Stock, A. D., Leppert, M., & Keating, M. T. (1993a). Hemizygosity at the elastin locus in a developmental disorder, Williams syndrome. *Nature Genetics, 5,* 11–16.

Ewart, A. K., Morris, C. A., Ensing, G. J., Loker, J., Moore, C., Leppert, M., & Keating, M. T. (1993b). A human vascular disorder, supravalvular aortic stenosis, maps to chromosome 7. *Proceedings of the National Academy of Sciences USA, 90,* 3226–3230.

Fenson, L., Dale, P. S., Reznick, J. S., Thal, D., Bates, E., Hartung, J. P., Pethick, S., & Reilly, J. S. (1993). *MacArthur Communicative Development Inventories: User's guide and technical manual.* San Diego, CA: Singular.

Finegan, J.-A., Smith, M. L., Meschino, W. S., Vallance, P. L., & Sitarenios, G. (1995, March). *Verbal memory in children with Williams syndrome.* Poster presented at the biennial meeting of the Society for Research in Child Development, Indianapolis, IN.

Fonaryova Key, A., Pani, J. R., & Mervis, C. B. (1998, November). *Visual–spatial constructive ability of people with Williams syndrome.* Kentucky Psychological Association, Louisville, KY.

Forbes, G. B., Bryson, M. F., Manning, J., Amirhakmi, G. H., & Reina, J. C. (1972). Impaired calcium homeostasis in the infantile hypercalcemic syndrome. *Acta Paediatrica Scandinavica, 61,* 305–309.

Frangiskakis, J. M., Ewart, A. K., Morris, C. A., Mervis, C. B., Bertrand, J., Robinson, B. F., Klein, B. P., Ensing, G. J., Everett, L. A., Green, E. D., Pröschel, C., Gutowski, N. J., Noble, M., Atkinson, D. L., Odelberg, S. J., & Keating, M. T. (1996). LIM–kinase1 hemizygosity implicated in impaired visuospatial constructive cognition. *Cell, 86,* 59–69.

Friedman, W. F., & Mills, L. F. (1969). The relationship between vitamin D and the craniofacial and dental anomalies of the supravalvular aortic stenosis syndrome. *Pediatrics, 43,* 12–18.

Goodglass, H., & Kaplan, E. (1983). *Assessment of Aphasia and Related Disorders—Revised.* Philadelphia: Lea & Febiger.

Gosch, A., & Pankau, R. (1994). Social–emotional and behavioral adjustment in children with Williams-Beuren syndrome. *American Journal of Medical Genetics, 53,* 335–339.

Gosch, A., & Pankau, R. (1997). Personality characteristics and behaviour problems in individuals of different ages with Williams syndrome. *Developmental Medicine and Child Neurology, 39,* 327–533.

Gosch, A., Stading, G., & Pankau, R. (1994). Linguistic abilities in children with Williams–Beuren syndrome. *American Journal of Medical Genetics, 52,* 291–296.

Greenberg, F., & Lewis, R. A. (1988). The Williams syndrome: Spectrum and significance of ocular features. *Ophthalmology, 95,* 1608–1612.

Greer, M. K., Brown, F. R., Pai, G. S., Choudry, S. H., & Klein, A. J. (1997). Cognitive, adaptive, and behavioral characteristics of Williams syndrome. *American Journal of Medical Genetics, 74,* 521–525.

Grimm, T., & Wesselhoeft, H. (1980). Zur Genetik des Williams–Beuren Syndroms und der Isolierten Form der Supravalvularen Aortenstenose: Untersuchungen von 128 Familien. *Zeitschrift für Kardiologie, 69,* 168–172.

Hirota, H., Chen, X. N., Shi, Z. Y., Matsuoka, R., Kimura, M., Bellugi, U., Lincoln, A., & Korenberg, J. R. (1998). Williams syndrome (WMS): From cognition to genes [Abstract]. *American Journal of Human Genetics, 63*(4), A138.

Ingelfinger, J. R., & Newburger, J. W. (1991). Spectrum of renal anomalies in patients with Williams syndrome. *Journal of Pediatrics, 119,* 771–773.

Jernigan, T. L., Bellugi, U., Sowell, E., Doherty, S., & Hesselink, J. R. (1993). Cerebral morphological distinctions between Williams and Down syndromes. *Archives of Neurology, 50,* 186–191.

Jones, K. L., & Smith, D. W. (1975). The Williams elfin facies syndrome. *Journal of Pediatrics, 86,* 718–723.

Jurado, L. A. P., Peoples, R., Kaplan, P., Hamel, B. C. J., & Francke, U. (1996). Molecular definition of the chromosome 7 deletions in Williams syndrome and parent-of-origin effects on growth. *American Journal of Human Genetics, 59,* 781–792.

Jurado, L. A. P., Wang, Y. K., Peoples, R., Coloma, A., Cruces, J., & Francke, U. (1998). A duplicated gene in the breakpoint regions of the 7q11.23 Williams–Beuren syndrome deletion encodes the initiator binding protein TFII-I and BAP-135, a phosphorylation target of BTK. *Human Molecular Genetics, 7,* 325–334.

Kaplan, P., Kirschner, M., Watters, G., & Costa, T. (1989). Contractures in patients with Williams syndrome. *Pediatrics, 84,* 895–899.

Kapp, M. E., von Noorden, G. K., & Jenkins, R. (1995). Strabismus in the Williams syndrome. *American Journal of Ophthalmology, 119,* 355–360.

Karmiloff-Smith, A., Grant, J., Berthoud, I., Davies, M., Howlin, P., & Udwin, O. (1997). Language and Williams syndrome: How intact is "intact"? *Child Development, 68,* 246–262.

Kaufman, A. S., & Kaufman, N. L. (1990). *Kaufman Brief Intelligence Test*. Circle Pines, MN: American Guidance Service.

Kececioglu, D., Kotthoff, S., & Vogt, J. (1993). Williams–Beuren syndrome: A 30-year follow-up of natural and postoperative course. *European Health Journal, 14*, 1458–1464.

Klein, A. J., Armstrong, B. L., Greer, M. K., & Brown, F. R. (1990). Hyperacusis and otitis media in individuals with Williams syndrome. *Journal of Speech and Hearing Disorders, 55*, 339–344.

Klein, B. P. (1995). *Grammatical abilities of children with Williams syndrome*. Unpublished master's thesis, Emory University.

Klein, B. P., & Mervis, C. B. (in press). Cognitive strengths and weaknesses of 9- and 10-year-olds with Williams syndrome or Down syndrome. *Developmental Neuropsychology*.

Leiter, R. G. (1980). *Leiter International Performance Scale*. Wood Dale, IL: Stoelting.

Leonard, L. B. (1998). *Children with specific language impairment*. Cambridge, MA: MIT Press.

Lightwood, R. (1952). Idiopathic hypercalcaemia with failure to thrive: Nephrocalcinosis. *Proceedings of the Royal Society of Medicine, 45*, 401.

Lopez-Rangel, E., Maurice, M., McGillivray, B., & Friedman, J. M. (1992). Williams syndrome in adults. *American Journal of Medical Genetics, 44*, 720–729.

Lowery, M. C., Morris, C. A., Ewart, A., Brothman, L., Zhu, X. L., Leonard, C. O., Carey, J. C., Keating, M., & Brothman, A. R. (1995). Strong correlation of elastin deletions, detected by FISH, with Williams syndrome: Evaluation of 235 patients. *American Journal of Human Genetics, 57*, 49–53.

Mari, A., Amati, F., Mingarelli, R. Giannotti, A., Sebastio, G., Colloridi, V., Novelli, G., & Dallapiccola, B. (1995). Analysis of the elastin gene in 60 patients with clinical diagnosis of Williams syndrome. *Human Genetics, 96*, 444–448.

Marriage, J., & Barnes, N. M. (1995). Is central hyperacusis a symptom of 5-hydroxytryptamine (5-HT) dysfunction? *Journal of Laryngology and Otology, 109*, 915–921.

Martin, N. D., Snodgrass, G., & Cohen, R. D. (1984). Idiopathic infantile hypercalcemia: A continuing enigma. *Archives of Diseases in Childhood, 59*, 605–613.

McCarthy, D. (1972). *McCarthy Scales of Children's Abilities*. New York: Psychological Corporation.

Meng, X., Lu, X. J., Li, Z. H., Green, E. D., Massa, H., Trask, B. J., Morris, C. A., Keating, M. T. (1998a). Molecular characterization of Williams syndrome deletion: An integrated physical, deletion and transcript map [Abstract]. *American Journal of Human Genetics, 63*(4), A335.

Meng, X., Lu, X., Morris, C. A., & Keating, M. T. (1998b). A novel human gene *FKBP6* is deleted in Williams syndrome. *Genomics, 52*, 130–137.

Merritt, D. A., Palmar, C. G., Lurie, P. R., & Petry, E. L. (1963). Supravalvular aortic stenosis: Genetic and clinical studies [Abstract]. *Journal of Laboratory and Clinical Medicine, 62*, 995.

Mervis, C. B. (1999). [Unpublished data.]

Mervis, C. B., & Bertrand, J. (1997). Developmental relations between cognition and language: Evidence from Williams syndrome. In L. B. Adamson & M. A. Romski (Eds.), *Communication and language acquisition: Discoveries from atypical development* (pp. 75–106). Baltimore: Paul H. Brookes.

Mervis, C. B., Bertrand, J., Robinson, B. F., Klein, B. P., Armstrong, S. C., Baker, D. E., Turner, N. D., & Reinberg, J. (1995, March). *Early language development of children with Williams syndrome*. Society for Research in Child Development, Indianapolis, IN.

Mervis, C. B., Klein, B. P., & Rothstein, M. (1998a). *Adaptive behavior of 4- to 9-year-olds with Williams syndrome*. Manuscript submitted for publication.

Mervis, C. B., Morris, C. A., Bertrand, J., & Robinson, B. F. (1999). Williams syndrome: Findings from an integrated program of research. In H. Tager-Flusberg (Ed.), *Neurodevelopmental disorders* (pp. 65–110). Cambridge, MA: MIT Press.

Mervis, C. B., & Robinson, B. F. (1998). *Language development of children with Williams syndrome*. Manuscript in preparation.

Mervis, C. B., Robinson, B. F., Bertrand, J., Morris, C. A., Klein, B. P., & Armstrong, S. C. (1998b). *The Williams syndrome cognitive profile*. Manuscript submitted for publication.

Mervis, C. B., Robinson, B. F., Phelps, E., & Bertrand, J. (1998c, November). *Early vocabulary acquisition by children who have Williams syndrome or Down syndrome.* Paper presented at the meeting of the Kentucky Psychological Association, Louisville.

Milner, B. (1971). Interhemispheric differences in the localization of psychological processes in man. *British Medical Bulletin, 27,* 272–277.

Morris, C. A., Dilts, C., Dempsey, S. A., Leonard, C. O., & Blackburn, B. (1988). The natural history of Williams syndrome: Physical characteristics. *Journal of Pediatrics, 113,* 318–326.

Morris, C. A., Greenberg, F., & Thomas, I. T. (1993a). Williams syndrome: Autosomal dominant inheritance. *American Journal of Medical Genetics, 47,* 478–481.

Morris, C. A., Leonard, C. O., Dilts, C., & Demsey, S. A. (1990). Adults with Williams syndrome. *American Journal of Medical Genetics,* (Suppl. 6), 102–107.

Morris, C. A., Loker, J., Ensing, G., & Stock, A. D. (1993b). Supravalvular aortic stenosis cosegregates with a familial 6;7 translocation which disrupts the elastin gene. *American Journal of Medical Genetics, 46,* 737–744.

Nickerson, E., Greenberg, F., Keating, M. T., McCaskill, C., & Shaffer, L. G. (1995). Deletions of the elastin gene at 7q11.23 occur in ~90% of patients with Williams syndrome. *American Journal of Human Genetics, 56,* 1156–1161.

O'Brien, G. (1992). Behavioural phenotypes and their measurement. *Developmental Medicine and Child Neurology, 34,* 365–367.

O'Connor, W., Davis, J., Geissler, R., Cottrill, C., Noonan, J., & Todd, E. (1985). Supravalvular aortic stenosis: Clinical and pathologic observations in six patients. *Archives of Pathology and Laboratory Medicine, 109,* 179–185.

Olson, T. M., Michels, V. V., Lindor, N. M., Pastores, G. M., Weber, J. L., Schaid, D. J., Driscoll, D. J., Feldt, R. H., & Thibodeau, S. N. (1993). Autosomal dominant supravalvular aortic stenosis: Localization to chromosome 7. *Human Molecular Genetics, 2,* 869–873.

Osborne, L. R., Martindale, D., Scherer, S. W., Shi, X.-M., Huizenga, J., Heng, H. H. Q., Costa, T., Pober, B., Lew, L., Brinkman, J., Rommens, J., Koop, B., & Tsui, L.-C. (1996). Identification of genes from a 500-kb region at 7q11.23 that is commonly deleted in Williams syndrome patients. *Genomics, 36,* 328–336.

Osborne, L. R., Soder, S., Shi, X.-M., Pober, B., Costa, T., Scherer, S. W., & Tsui, L. C. (1997). Hemizygous deletion of the syntaxin 1A gene in individuals with Williams syndrome. *American Journal of Human Genetics, 61,* 449–452.

Pagon, R., Bennett, F., LaVeck, B., Stewart, K., & Johnson, J. (1987). Williams syndrome: Features in late childhood and adolescence. *Pediatrics, 80,* 85–91.

Pankau, R., Partsch, C.-J., Winter, M., Gosch, A., & Wessel, A. (1996). Incidence and spectrum of renal abnormalities in Williams–Beuren syndrome. *American Journal of Medical Genetics, 63,* 301–304.

Paperna, T., Peoples, R., Wang, U.-K., & Francke, U. (1998). CPE-R and the human homolog of RVP1 are within the Williams–Beuren syndrome deletion [Abstract]. *American Journal of Human Genetics, 63*(4), A170.

Peoples, R., Perez-Jurado, L., Wang, Y. K., Kaplan, P., & Francke, U. (1996). The gene for replication factor C subunit 2 (RFC2) is within the 7q11.23 Williams syndrome deletion. *American Journal of Human Genetics, 58,* 1370–1373.

Pezzini, G., Vicari, S., Volterra, V., Milani, L., & Ossella, M. T. (in press). Children with Williams syndrome: Is there a single neuropsychological profile? *Developmental Neuropsychology.*

Pleatman, S. I., & Dunbar, J. S. (1980). Colon diverticulae in Williams elfin facies syndrome. *Radiology, 137,* 869–870.

Pober, B. R., & Filiano, J. J. (1995). Association of Chiari I malformations and Williams syndrome. *Pediatric Neurology, 12,* 84–88.

Pober, B. R., Lacro, R. V., Rice, C., Mandell, V., & Teele, R. L. (1993). Renal findings in 40 individuals with Williams syndrome. *American Journal of Medical Genetics, 46,* 271–274.

Power, T. J., Blum, N. J., Jones, S. M., & Kaplan, P. E. (1997). Response to methylphenidate in two children with Williams syndrome. *Journal of Autism and Developmental Disorders, 27,* 79–87.

Rice, M. L., Mervis, C. B., Klein, B. P., & Rice, K. (1998). *Morphological abilities of children with specific language impairment or Williams syndrome.* Manuscript in preparation.

Rice, M. L., & Wexler, K. (1996). A phenotype of specific language impairment: Extended optional infinitives. In M. L. Rice (Ed.), *Toward a genetics of language* (pp. 215–237). Mahwah, NJ: Erlbaum.

Robinson, B. F., & Mervis, C. B. (1996). Extrapolated raw scores for the second edition of the Bayley Scales of Infant Development. *American Journal of Mental Retardation, 100,* 666–671.

Rosch, E. (1973). On the internal structure of perceptual and semantic categories. In T. E. Moore (Ed.), *Cognitive development and the acquisition of language* (pp. 111–144). New York: Academic Press.

Rosch, E. (1975). Cognitive representations of semantic categories. *Journal of Experimental Psychology: General, 104,* 192–233.

Rossen, M., Klima, E. S., Bellugi, U., Bihrle, A., & Jones, W. (1996). Interaction between language and cognition: Evidence from Williams syndrome. In J. H. Beitchman, N. J. Cohen, M. M. Konstantares, & R. Tannock (Eds.), *Language, learning, and behavior disorders: Developmental, biological, and clinical perspectives* (pp. 367–392). Cambridge, England: Cambridge University Press.

Rutter, M. (1967). A children's behaviour questionnaire for completion by teachers: Preliminary findings. *Journal of Child Psychology and Psychiatry, 8,* 1–11.

Sadler, L. S., Olitsky, S. E., & Reynolds, J. D. (1996). Reduced stereoacuity in Williams syndrome. *American Journal of Medical Genetics, 66,* 287–288.

Sadler, L. S., Robinson, L. K., Verdaasdonk, K. R., & Gingell, R. (1993). The Williams syndrome: Evidence for possible autosomal dominant inheritance. *American Journal of Medical Genetics, 47,* 468–470.

Sarimski, K. (1997). Behavioral phenotypes and family stress in three mental retardation syndromes. *European Journal of Child and Adolescent Psychiatry, 6,* 26–31.

Saul, R. A., Stevenson, R. E., Rogers, R. C., Skinner, S. A., Prouty, L. A., & Flannery, D. B. (1988). Growth references from conception to adulthood. *Proceedings of the Greenwood Genetic Center* (Suppl. 1), 204–209.

Scarborough, H. S. (1990). Index of productive syntax. *Applied Psycholinguistics, 11,* 1–22.

Scott, P. Mervis, C. B., Bertrand, J., Klein, B. P., Armstrong, S. C., & Ford, A. L. (1995). Semantic organization and word fluency in 9- and 10-year-old children with Williams syndrome. *Genetic Counseling, 6,* 172–173.

Semel, E., Wiig, E. H., & Secord, W. A. (1995). *Clinical evaluation of language fundamentals* (3rd ed.). San Antonio, TX: Psychological Corporation.

Singer Harris, N. G., Bellugi, U., Bates, E., Jones, W., & Rossen, M. (1997). Contrasting profiles of language development in children with Williams and Down syndromes. *Developmental Neuropsychology, 13,* 345–370.

Sommer, A., Wheeller, J., Wagner, N., & Wenger, G. (1996). Large scale deletion of the elastin gene, but not "classical" Williams syndrome. *Proceedings of the Greenwood Genetic Center, 15,* 156–158.

Soper, R., Chaloupka, J. C., Fayad, P. B., Greally, J. M., Shaywitz, B. A., Awad, I. A., & Pober, B. R. (1995). Ischemic stroke and intracranial multifocal cerebral arteriopathy in Williams syndrome. *Journal of Pediatrics, 126,* 945–948.

Sparrow, S. S., Balla, D. A., & Cicchetti, D. V. (1984). *Vineland Adaptive Behavior Scales—Interview Edition.* Circle Pines, MN: American Guidance Service.

Thomas, S. A., & Chess, S. (1977). *Temperament and development.* New York: Brunner/Mazel.

Thorndike, R. L., Hagen, E. P., & Sattler, J. M. (1986). *Stanford–Binet Intelligence Scale* (4th ed.) Chicago: Riverside.

Tomc, S. A., Williamson, N. K., & Pauli, R. M. (1990). Temperament in Williams syndrome. *American Journal of Medical Genetics, 36,* 345–352.

Udwin, O., & Yule, W. (1990). Expressive language of children with Williams syndrome. *American Journal of Medical Genetics Supplment, 6,* 108–114.

Udwin, O., & Yule, W. (1991). A cognitive and behavioral phenotype in Williams syndrome. *Journal of Clinical and Experimental Neuropsychology, 13*, 232–244.

Udwin, O., Yule, W., & Martin, N. (1987). Cognitive abilities and behavioral characteristics of children with idiopathic infantile hypercalcemia. *Journal of Child Psychology and Psychiatry, 28*, 297–309.

Urban, Z., Helms, C., Fekete, G., Csiszar, K., Bonnet, D., Munich, A., Donis-Keller, H., & Boyd, C. (1996). 7q11.23 deletions in Williams syndrome arise as a consequence of unequal meiotic crossover. *American Journal of Human Genetics, 59*, 958–962.

Van Borsel, J., Curfs, L. M. G., & Fryns, J. P. (1997). Hyperacusis in Williams syndrome: A sample survey study. *Genetic Counseling, 8*, 121–126.

Van Lieshout, C. F. M., De Meyer, R. E., Curfs, L. M. G., & Fryns, J.-P. (1998). Family contexts, parental behavior, and personality profiles of children and adolescents with Prader–Willi, fragile-X, or Williams syndrome. *Journal of Child Psychology and Psychiatry, 39*, 699–710.

Voit, T., Kramer, H., Thomas, C., Wechsler, W., Reichmann, H., & Lenard, H. G. (1991). Myopathy in Williams–Beuren syndrome. *European Journal of Pediatrics, 150*, 521–526.

Volterra, V., Capirci, O., Pezzini, G., Sabbadini, L., & Vicari, S. (1996). Linguistic abilities in Italian children with Williams syndrome. *Cortex, 32*, 663–677.

Wang, M. S., Schinzel, A., Kotzot, D., Casey, R., Chodirker, B. N., Petersen, M. B., Gyftodimou, J., & Robinson, W. A. (1998). Clinical correlations in Williams–Beuren syndrome (WBS): No evidence of a parent of origin effect or influence of elastin (ELN) polymorphism [Abstract]. *American Journal of Human Genetics, 63*(4), A123.

Wang, P. P., & Bellugi, U. (1994). Evidence from two genetic syndromes for a dissociation between verbal and visual–spatial short-term memory. *Journal of Clinical and Experimental Neuropsychology, 16*, 317–322.

Wang, P. P., Doherty, S., Rourke, S. B., & Bellugi, U. (1995). Unique profile of visuo-perceptual skills in a genetic syndrome. *Brain and Cognition, 29*, 54–65.

Wang, P. P., Hesselink, J. R., Jernigan, T. L., Doherty, S., & Bellugi, U. (1992). Specific neurobehavioral profile of Williams syndrome is associated with neocerebellar hemispheric preservation. *Neurology, 42*, 1999–2002.

Wang, Y. K., Samos, C. H., Peoples, R., Perez-Jurado, L. A., Nusse, R., & Francke, U. (1997). A novel human homologue of the *Drosophila* frizzled wnt receptor gene binds wingless protein and is in the Williams syndrome deletion at 7q11.23. *Human Molecular Genetics, 6*, 465–472.

Wechsler, D. (1974). *Wechsler Intelligence Scale for Children—Revised*. New York: Psychological Corporation.

Wechsler, D. (1991). *Wechsler Intelligence Scale for Children* (3rd ed.). New York: Psychological Corporation.

Wiig, E. H., Secord, W., & Semel, E. (1992). *Clinical evaluation of language fundamentals—preschool*. San Antonio, TX: Psychological Corporation.

Williams, K. T. (1997). *Expressive Vocabulary Test*. Circle Pines, MN: American Guidance Service.

Wilson, B., Cockburn, J., & Baddeley, A. (1985). *Rivermead Behavioural Memory Test*. Reading, England: Thames Valley Test.

Wu, Y.-Q., Reid Sutton, V., Nickerson, E., Lupski, J. R., Potocki, L., Korenberg, J. R., Greenberg, F., Tassabehji, M., & Shaffer, L. G. (1998). Delineation of the common critical region in Williams syndrome and clinical correlation of growth, heart defects, ethnicity, and parental origin. *American Journal of Medical Genetics, 78*, 82–89.

INDEX